The Care Homes Guide

THE INDEPENDENT GUIDE TO CHOOSING A CARE HOME IN THE SOUTH-EAST OF ENGLAND

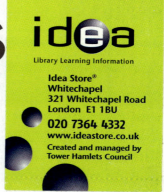

crimson

This edition first published in Great Britain 2008 by
Crimson Publishing, a division of Crimson Business Ltd
Westminster House
Kew Road
Richmond
Surrey
TW9 2ND

A catalogue record for this book is available from

ISBN 978-1-85458-405-2

Printed and bound in Turkey by Mega Printing.

Contents

Finding the right care

Today, almost half a million people in the UK live in care homes. Finding the right care home can often be a daunting task. With almost 1,600 in the south-east of England and 1,300 in the south-west, how do you go about finding the right one? How will you know that you or your loved ones will be well cared for? If you are searching for care for a relative, you will also feel a responsibility to meet their personal preferences, and ensure they are happy.

ASSESSING YOUR OPTIONS

Beginning the process

It is never easy to make the decision to move into a care home. Many are reluctant to leave their own homes and familiar surroundings and fear they will lose their privacy and independence by moving into residential care. Although the situation is undeniably difficult, more often than not, the decision to move can have a positive effect. Many elderly or disabled people struggle with household tasks such as doing the laundry, cooking, shopping or paying the bills. It can be a relief not to have to worry about coping with the difficulties of daily living.

Depending on the situation, it is sometimes best to plan for the future by looking for an appropriate care facility, so that you will be more prepared when the time comes to making a decision. The introduction to this book aims to guide you through each step of finding care for an elderly relative.It is always useful to make some enquiries and chat to friends and relatives about the different options available. Your GP and local council will also provide you with information about the different types of care available.

Care assessments

Care assessments are an evaluation of a person's individual needs, usually carried out by an occupational therapist, and organised by the local council. From this meeting, you will glean a better idea of the type of care your relative's needs, and therefore, where to begin looking. The assessment will also determine whether your relative is eligible for council funding. Based on their income, a Financial Assessment Officer will decide whether they are entitled to funds to assist with nursing or residential care.

Everyone is entitled to a free care assessment irrespective of their financial situation. The therapist will assess the difficulties your relative may be experiencing at home and try and find a way to help and support them. For example, if they are having difficulty with carrying the shopping or cleaning the home, then they may be entitled to home care help. Other services in the home might include the provision of disability equipment and adaptations to the home or the therapist may help your relative consider the option of day care and care homes. The main aim of the assessment is to provide your relative with the best support possible and to ensure that they are not putting themselves at risk by living on their own.

If your local council agrees that your relative is eligible to move into a care home, then they may receive some financial help, which would go towards the cost of the care home fees. (Please see *How to fund care* for more details on funding.)

If you or your relative is unhappy with the result of the assessment, you are fully entitled to make a complaint to your local council. The Citizens Advice Bureau also provides guidance about how to make a complaint of this nature.

Once a person's needs are assessed, then the necessary steps are put in place to ensure that their personal wishes have been taken into account. This is put into a document known as a 'care plan'. As people's health needs are likely to change over time, it is important that the care plan is reassessed and reviewed on a regular basis. If at any time you or your relative feel like you would like a reassessment, contact your local council.

To make an appointment to have a care assessment, contact your local council.

Types of care homes

There are many different types of care homes. Some simply cater for elderly residents, while others specialise in looking after those who need specific nursing care, such as those with disabilities or mental illnesses.

Terminology:
Care homes (previously known as residential homes)
Care homes with nursing (previously known as nursing homes)

Care homes

A care home is designed to provide care and security within a comfortable setting. It can be a relief not to have to worry about bills or running your own home and most residents enjoy the safety of being in a secure environment. Residents are not expected to cook, make their own beds, clean, do their laundry or do any housework – these tasks are carried out by the care assistants in the home.

Each resident has their own bedroom and bathroom which they are usually allowed to decorate themselves. Some homes offer shared accommodation. This is a less expensive option for an individual, and ideal for married couples wanting to remain together.

Most residents in care homes are quite active and mobile and need minimal assistance in carrying out day-to-day tasks. This means that there is no in-house nursing staff to provide medical assistance. However, there are care assistants on hand to help with personal care and many homes have a district nurse who visits when necessary.

In instances where residents fall ill, they have to be moved to a care home with nursing where they can receive the best medical care. Sometimes this move is upsetting for residents until they adjust to their new surrounings. It is worth considering the long-term when initially deciding on a care home – it is often a good idea to find a home that has both a residential wing and a nursing wing, so that if care needs increase, your relative will not have to change homes entirely.

Care homes with nursing

A care home with nursing is for people who are less mobile and need a higher level of care than those in a care home. Although the residents may be infirm, for the most part, they do not require hospitalisation but would be unable to care for themselves if they were to stay on their own homes.

These homes provide full-time highly qualified medical staff consisting of doctors and duty nurses who are on hand to assist with medical and other health needs.

Dual registered homes

Some homes offer both nursing and residential care. This means that in the event of illness, your relative would not have to endure the upheaval of being moved to a medical facility. This type of home is ideal for those who think that their level of care may change in the future, or for couples who have different health care needs.

Temporary stay/respite care

Many care homes reserve space for those who would only like to stay a short period of time. This option might appeal to those who have been ill and need some extra help in order to recover. If there is a carer involved, this is also a good way to give the carer a break if they both have been through a particularly difficult time.

This sort of home does not usually provide nursing care but everyone admitted is fully supervised. Respite care also allows you to assess what it is like to be in a care home without committing to it long-term.

Specialist care

Some care homes offer different levels of care and specialise in catering for specific illnesses including: dementia, Alzheimer's, Parkinson's, Huntington's, schizophrenia and depression. These homes have medical staff who are especially trained to deal with patients with these disabilities.

Caring for those with Alzheimer's and dementia

Discovering that loved ones are ill is always devastating and, depending on the stages of the disease, it can be difficult to care for them at home. Your doctor may recommend a clinic that specialises in the care of those with Alzheimer's or dementia. It can become increasingly difficult and distressing for the carer to cope with the more advanced stages of forgetfulness and odd behaviour. If you are a carer in this position and are finding it difficult to manage, the social services department within your local council will be able to advise you about different types of care. They should also provide you with a list of appropriate homes that would best suit your relative's needs.

Elderly Mentally Infirm (EMI) home

An Elderly Mentally Infirm (EMI) home typically cares for residents with dementia and Alzheimer's disease. Registered Mental Nurses (RMNs) are on duty at all times and are fully qualified to ensure that the residents are cared for and treated with respect and dignity. Doctors are also on hand to monitor the progress of the patients and prescribe medication where necessary.

Many of these homes run activities such bingo, cards or chess, and bring the residents out on day trips. Some even provide memory boxes and sensory gardens, which help to stimulate the senses. Usually, friends and relatives are allowed to visit at any time of the day.

Care homes for mental disorders

These are homes that specialise in caring for elderly residents with illnesses such as depression or schizophrenia. As with EMIs, the staff are fully trained to handle people with this sort of illness and provide them with a high level of care. Usually, a Community Psychiatric Nurse (CPN) pays frequent visits to the care home to examine the residents and monitor their progress.

Palliative care

If it is not appropriate for the patient to return home or go into a hospice, some care homes offer places for terminal or palliative care. Palliative care focuses on reducing the symptoms of the patient to relieve any pain and suffering and improving the quality of life.

Staff that care for the terminally ill provide physical, psychological, practical and spiritual support for the patient. They are also trained in dealing with bereavement and will help to support family members through this sad time.

This is a particularly difficult time for friends and family and you might feel you could benefit from some extra emotional support. The British Association for Counselling and Psychotherapy (0870 443 5252; www.bacp.co.uk) is the professional body for counsellors who should be able to provide you with comfort and advice.

Alternatives to care homes

The decision to move into a care home is not an easy one. It is best to consider all alternative options before making a final decision. There are many options available to those who would prefer not to move into a care home:

Staying in your own home

Many people choose to stay in their own homes rather than moving into a care home. Remaining in your own home is ideal for those who are still relatively healthy and active and feel that they would like to retain their independence.

If your relative does not want to move into a care home, your local council has a duty of care to ensure that they are comfortable, provide them with support and make their life as easy as possible. This might involve organising home help to assist them with personal care such as bathing, as well as helping with the shopping. Your relative can also choose to have meals delivered to their homes via a 'meals on wheels' service, which saves them the effort of preparing their own meals.

Often, the elderly are also given an option of a community alarm which is activated by pressing a button; this alerts a response centre which answers alarm calls any time of the day or night. Sometimes referred to as a 'lifeline', this button can be added to their phone or worn around their neck; whatever is more convenient for them. Once the response centre are alerted, they will contact your relative's next of kin to let them know there is a problem.

Sheltered housing/retirement housing

This option may appeal if your relative wishes to lead a more independent life and does not require the level of care provided by care homes. If they are over the age of 60 (single or in a couple) they are eligible to apply to most sheltered housing schemes. Typically, the scheme includes the provision of self-contained flats or bungalows, especially equipped to service the needs of the residents. There are also communal areas and some schemes even offer group activities.

There is a scheme manager (sometimes called a warden) who usually lives on the premises or nearby and can usually be contacted through an alarm system. The manager's responsibility is to keep in regular contact with the residents, check that they are comfortable, liaise with relatives or doctors where necessary and be there in case of an emergency. The manager is not there to carry out duties like shopping or cleaning, but it is worth remembering that residents can still apply for other services such as meals on wheels and home help.

Whether buying or renting their flat, residents are still obliged to pay a service charge that covers maintenance (garden, building repairs etc) and the cost of the onsite scheme manager. It is essential to verify what is and isn't included in the service charge as this can vary from scheme to scheme, for example, costs for electricity, phone etc may not be covered by the service charge. You might find it helpful to ask for a record of previous service charges and check if there have been any sudden increases in the past.

Extra care (assisted living) housing

In the last few years, new schemes have been set up to assist the needs of frailer, older people. This can be an ideal option for those who are unable to live on their own but, again, do not require the high level of care available in a care home. Like sheltered housing, the accommodation offered consists of mostly flats and bungalows and has the same communal areas, living rooms, dining rooms etc. However, with extra sheltered housing, there are usually a greater variety of communal facilities, for example, hobby rooms and health and fitness areas. There is also a number of onsite staff that provide domestic support such as preparing meals and helping with personal care.

The Commission for Social Care Inspection (CSCI)

The Commission for Social Care Inspection (CSCI) was created by the Health and Social Care (Community Health and Standards Act) 2003, as a means of promoting best practice, regulating, inspecting and reviewing all aspects of adult social care in England. Launched in 2004, the commission annually reports these findings to the government in a document called *The State of Social Care in England*, which is also available to the public.

Prior to the CSCI, the regulation of social care had been carried out by several different organisations including the Social Services Inspectorate (SSI) and the National Care Standards Commission (NCSC). The CSCI incorporated all these organisations and now acts as a single, independent body for the inspection of all the social care services in England, bringing with it a much-needed organised approach.

The CSCI works with local councils to ensure they are providing the highest quality services to members of the community and meeting the needs of different groups of people. The commission gives each council a rating and if they fall short of the expected standards, they are penalised.

The commission also inspects adult social care services and vets those who apply to run these services. They are also responsible for the treatment of the residents in care homes to ensure they are not at risk of abuse; a policy which is called 'protection of vulnerable adults' (POVA).

In 2008, the CSCI will also begin the process of rating care homes, awarding stars (from 0–3) to those that meet the right standards. This will make it a lot easier to choose a care home and assess the quality of care services in different areas. The introduction of the star system will be a gradual process, and this book pre-empts the government's selection (see *How to use this book* for more detail).

The commission assesses the care homes on a number of areas including the facilities, accommodation, communal space, overall care and services, and generally ensures that the needs of the residents are fully met. If the adult social care services fail to meet the national minimum standards, the CSCI has, by law, the right to impose the appropriate conditions. In the event that the care homes fail to improve and meet these conditions, then the CSCI has the legal right to shut them down.

Care home inspections

Care home inspectors from the CSCI carry out thorough inspections of all registered care homes periodically. The number of inspections made depends on the quality of care measured in the last report. If a home exceeds standards, the next inspection will be more infrequent than for a home that does not reach the required standards or where the inspectors are not happy with certain aspects of the running of the home.

During the inspection, the inspectors will spend time with the care home managers to go through their records and files relating to the daily operations of the home. Residents' care plans will be checked and medication records examined. They will also tour the home, chat to residents and observe them to assess their well-being. The inspector also monitors the staff while they are on duty to ensure they are treating the residents with the highest quality of care. When they have collated this information, they feed it back to the care home manager for further discussion.

CSCI reports

The CSCI create full reports based on these inspections that can be accessed online at www.csci.org.uk. We have used these reports, and interviewed each home, to provide you with a summarised, easily accessible list of the main information about each home. This includes contact details for the home, and information on the home's building, location and outdoor areas. See *How to use this book* for more details of what is included in this guide. Once you have cross-referenced the homes you are interested in, it is a good idea to then look at their reports and read some additional information about the home.

In addition to the information in this guide, you may want to read about:

- What kind of care the home offers residents. It is a good idea to check the number of beds the home has available for dementia, for example.
- The admissions process. The inspectors make sure this process it is as smooth as possible. The report will also specify how thorough care plans are and the efficiency of staff.
- How the staff interact with the residents and if the inspector believes the residents are treated with respect.
- Staffing levels and if there is a need to increase the level of staff.
- How the staff maintain residents' accounts and that files are organised and up to date If there should be additional staff training
- How the meals are presented and if they are based on a healthy balanced diet
- Whether the inspector has notes any improvements that the care home needs to make in time for the next inspection. At the following inspection, the care home will be assessed on how well they made these improvements.
- Information on the cleanliness of the care homes.
- Health and safety standards of the home.

HOW TO USE THIS BOOK

How we chose the homes included in our listings

Our choice of care homes has been based on the findings of the CSCI reports. Our team of researchers have only selected the care homes that have been considered by the CSCI to have met or exceeded government standards. Those who fell short of these standards at the time of the report have not been included in this book.

Understanding the information

Aabletone

Manager: Mary Nayakandi
Owner: Cedar Care Homes Ltd
Contact: Waltham House,
Stoke Park Road, Stoke Bishop,
Bristol BS9 1JF
) 0117 9682097
@ mimal@cedarcarehomes.com
⌐ www.cedarcarehomes.com

Aabletone is a period Cotswold-stone house near the Durdham Downs. It is next door to botanical gardens, and the home's grounds contain a cedar tree which is more than 100 years old. The home arranges a residents meeting every three months to allow residents to voice their opinions on any issues they may have. The home also has an activities coordinator who arranges daily activities such as armchair aerobics. Outings are offered to the residents and the home has its own minibus for transport.

1 Registered places: 42
2 Guide weekly rate: £472–£650
3 Specialist care: Nursing, respite
4 Medical services: Podiatry, dentist, optician, physiotherapy
5 Qualified staff: Undisclosed

Home details
Location: Rural area, 3.2 mile from Bristol
Communal areas: Lounge, dining room, conservatory, garden
6 Accessibility: *Floors:* 2 • *Access:* Lift • *Wheelchair access:* Good
7 Smoking: ✗
8 Pets: At manager's discretion
9 Routines: Flexible

Room details
Single: 31
10 Shared: 9
11 En suite: 33
12 Facilities: TV point, telephone point
13 Door lock: ✗
14 Lockable place: ✗

Services provided
Beauty services: Hairdressing
15 Mobile library: ✗
16 Religious services: ✗
17 Transport: Minibus
Activities: *Coordinator:* ✓ • *Examples:* Armchair aerobics, games
Outings: ✓
18 Meetings: ✓

Key

 nursing care

 wheelchair access

 no smoking

 pets allowed

 transport facility

General information

1. **Registered places:** Number of beds registered with CSCI. If the registered places does not equal the number of rooms, some shared rooms may have become single occupancy.
2. **Guide weekly rate:** The home's approximate weekly rate. These change annually in April/March and vary depending on the amount of care needed. Please contact the homes for their most up-to-date rates.
3. **Specialist care:** All of the homes care for 'old age'. Other care denotes any specialist care the home is registered to offer. These include: nursing care, dementia care, respite beds, palliative care, terminal care, physical disability, sensory impairment and learning disability. Each home will have a certain number of beds dedicated to the specialist care. Please contact the homes for details of this. If there is no specialist care, the home is purely a residential home. Some homes provide additional care to their registered categories: whether the home can provide the care you need is at the discretion of the home manager.
4. **Medical services:** Services that residents can access in the home; in-house visits organised. Most homes organise transport to local facilities, but this is not usually included in the weekly fee.
5. **Qualified staff:** The CSCI requirement is that 50% of staff must be qualified to NVQ level 2. The percentage of staff trained is included if this information was available.

Home details

6. **Accessibility:**Access: If 'None', there is no assisted access upstairs. This may not be appropriate for those in wheelchairs or the frail.
   Wheelchair access:
   Good: All rooms and communal areas are accessible in a wheelchair. The home has a lift.
   Limited: Wheelchair access may only be on the ground floor as there is no lift, or some areas may be accessed by steps.
   None: Cannot accommodate wheelchairs.
7. **Smoking:** Smoking is allowed inside care homes in designated areas. The areas must be clearly signposted and separate from the main lounge. Many homes are non-smoking or have a designated area outside.
8. **Pets:** Indicates whether residents' pets can live permanently in the home. Many managers will allow smaller pets such as budgies but not larger pets (this is signalled by 'At manager's discretion').
9. **Routines:** This indicates the home's daily routine. Most homes offer a flexible routine with some structure built in, eg set mealtimes. For homes that care for a large number of high-dependency residents, the routine may be more structured.

Room details

10. **Shared:** Either two single beds or one double bed (for couples).
11. **En suite:** The CSCI definition of en suite includes a basin and toilet, not necessarily a shower or bath.
12. **Facilities:** Indicates if rooms have a TV or telephone installed, or a TV point or telephone point for residents to bring their own appliances.
13. **Door lock:** All residents should have the choice of having a lock on their door, unless their risk assessment suggests otherwise.
14. **Lockable place:** All rooms should have a lockable facility to store valuables. 'Yes' indicates that there is a lockable place in residents' rooms. Some homes have a communal safe instead.

Services provided

15. **Mobile library:** Indicates whether a mobile library visits regularly. 'Library facilities' is used if the home has other facilities, such as its own library.
16. **Religious services:** Details any religious services that occur at the home – specifically, organised services or visits. All homes must make arrangements to meet residents' spiritual needs, so homes that do not offer religious services at the moment will organise this on an individual basis.
17. **Transport:** Some homes have their own transport, in which they take residents on outings or to appointments. Some will share transport with a nearby home, others order taxis or use dial-a-ride.
18. **Meetings:** In some homes, residents meet regularly to discuss the daily life of the home and raise any issues with the staff. These are sometimes called Residents Tenants' Associations, but many are more informal. Topics covered often include their likes and dislikes on the menu and activities they would like to repeat or new activities they would like to try. Where there are a large number of residents with dementia, or where residents are too frail, homes often organise regular relatives' meetings instead, as a forum to raise any issues and keep them informed about events at the home.

Frequently used terms

Residents: Those who live in care homes are often called 'service users'. Throughout the guide we have called them 'residents'.

Undisclosed: This information was either not available as it was subject to change or the homes would not divulge this information.

Pets As Therapy: www.petsastherapy.org. Pets As Therapy is a national charity now in its 25th year. It organises visits of assessed/vaccinated PAT Dogs and PAT Cats with registered volunteers to care homes, often providing comfort, companionship and therapy.

We have also only included homes that offer 'old age' care. Many offer other types of care as well, such as specialist dementia care, but all are equipped for elderly care.

Our researchers have spoken with each care home listed in this book to make sure the information we have provided is up-to-date and relevant to you.

The book is designed to help you quickly find essential information about a home, and be able to cross-reference this with other homes in the region. When you come to think about your priorities when looking for a home (discussed more in *How to choose a home*) you will be able to check if the home meets all your criteria. Read more about how to use the information in this book on in *Understanding the information*.

Regional concerns

This book is split into counties. In many cases, people prefer to move to a home near to the area they live in or where they already know some of the residents. For many, being located near to their relatives is an important consideration. Some even take this opportunity to move to the coast or to somewhere they have always wanted to live.

HOW TO FUND YOUR CARE

Most of us think financially as far as retirement and don't consider that we may need extra funds to pay for our care or the care of others. It is during a difficult time that your relative is faced with having to pay for care and the information provided can appear confusing.

Funding statistics
- More than 60% of residents in care homes have some or all of their fees paid by their local authority.
- 95,000 people in residential and nursing homes fund their own care.
- 32% of people in care homes are paying for their own care fees with little or no support from the state.

(source: Laing & Buisson UK Market Survey 2006)

Due to the nation's rising life expectancy, the government no longer pays for the increasing cost of caring for the elderly. There is a cost, whether you receive care at home or move into a care home. As the average care home costs between £20,000 and £30,000 a year, finding the funds can be a daunting prospect and a major cause for concern.

The cost of a home can depend on:
- The level of care you need
- The size of the home
- The facilities of the home

Usually, the basic fees cover:
- Accommodation
- Care
- Bed linen, towels etc
- Meals
- Laundry
- Heating

Government funding

The National Health Service and Community Care Act 1990, enforced in 1993, shifted the funding responsibility from the Department of Health to the social services department within local councils. In England, under this act, you are eligible to receive help with your care and accommodation if you have savings and assets of less than £21,000.

Although the government no longer pays wholly for care, there are still a number of benefits that your relative could be entitled to. You can find out more about their rights by contacting your local council. They will arrange a member of social services to meet with your relative to assess their situation and establish the type of care they need. See the *Care assessment* section on page vii.

Financial assessment

Based on the findings of your relative's care assessment carried out by your social services representative, a financial assessor will visit them to carry out a means test to evaluate their income. This will include:

- State pension
- Allowances (including disability allowance)
- Investments
- Savings
- Stocks and shares
- Other properties (if you own more than one)

Do they qualify?

Depending on this financial assessment, the local council will either contribute towards the costs of your relative's care or they may have to pay for it themselves. If their assets exceed £21,000, then they will have to fund the entire amount of fees themselves. If they are in a position to fund their own care for a certain amount of time, but know they will struggle to finance it at a later date, then their local council is obliged to assist them, but only up to a certain amount. Thus, it is worth reviewing their finances to establish if they can afford longer-term care.

They are entitled to some financial assistance from the State if the value of their total amount of assets falls below £21,000. However, they will still have to provide a large amount of their income towards their care. You may also find that the allowance provided by the State does not cover the fees required by your relative's chosen care home. In this case, a relative is permitted to contribute to the fees provided they can prove that they will be able to continue with the ongoing payments.

Property

There may be a number of reasons where the financial assessor would exclude your relative's property from their evaluation, for example, if their house is occupied by:

- A family member or spouse
- A relative over 60 years of age
- A child under the age of 16

Similarly, if they choose to receive care in their own home, their house will not be taken into consideration when it comes to evaluating their assets.

Joint savings and investments

The assessment does not include a spouse's sole assets but if they have joint savings and investments, it will be assumed that they each own half of the assets and this will be included when it comes to making a financial assessment.

Gifted assets

If they decide to 'gift' some of their assets, make sure they get the proper financial advice. If they have gifted assets and then attempt to claim state benefit, they may be accused of 'deprivation of assets' and their local council may still include the value of these assets as part of the financial assessment.

If you are seeking independent advice, always make sure the firm you use is a member of the FSA. Check their website www.fsa.gov.uk

---

Care in your own home

If your relative qualifies for care at home, their local council will provide them with a set amount of money through direct payments to contribute towards their care. Receiving care at home used to be free but some local councils do charge for the service so it is best to check the rates first. The payments also may not cover the cost of the care and your relative may be required to contribute some of their own income towards home help.

State benefits

Regardless of whether your relative does or doesn't qualify for funding, everyone is entitled to some welfare benefits:

Attendance allowance

This allowance is a tax-free benefit for those over 65 who are physically or mentally disabled and need help with personal care such as bathing, dressing, eating or assistance getting around their home. This benefit is rarely subject to a financial assessment and, therefore, usually applies to all those that qualify, irrespective of their financial circumstances.

The rate provided very much depends on the level of care required. For example, lower rates are paid if your relative only needs supervision and assistance either during the day or night. However, if your relative needs help throughout the day and night, they are paid a higher amount.

Disability living allowance (DLA)

This is a tax-free benefit for people under 65 who are physically and mentally disabled and need help with personal care or assistance with mobility. Again, the rates vary depending on the required level of care.

Registered nursing care contribution

The NHS now pays for nursing care if a resident is covering the entire cost of staying in a care home. This means that self-funded residents no longer have to pay the extra cost of receiving nursing care while they are living in a care home.

Self-funding your care

If your relative is paying for their own care, then you will need work out their own personal finances. There is no doubt that self-funding is expensive and requires a detailed overview of what they can afford.
You can start the process by:

- Evaluating their assets, including savings and investments
- Finding out how much money is annually generated by their assets
- Assessing how their assets can generate extra income and for how long.

It can be confusing to work out how to pay for long-term care over a number of years without running out of money and it is best to get some financial advice so you can assess the options.

Care Fee Annuity

If your relative doesn't wish to sell off all their assets to cover their long-term care, they may wish to consider purchasing a Care Fee Annuity. This involves paying a lump sum to an annuity provider who will guarantee a tax-free set amount towards care fees provided it is paid directly to the care home. The exact amount is determined by the provider and can vary widely depending on the annuity provider and circumstances.
When assessing the annuity, they will take into account:

- Age
- State of health
- Expected longevity of life.

Based on the above, they will make a decision on how much income to provide during your relative's stay in a care home. This option can be ideal for those who want to invest some of their capital but don't want to sell off all their assets. However, bear in mind that the annuity stops at the point of death and there is no compensation in the event of remaining monies. One way of ensuring against this loss is by purchasing a life assurance option, which guarantees a return of an agreed percentage of the lump sum. However, be aware that adding life assurance will increase the cost of the annuity.

Investing capital

Your relative may have a large amount of capital that they would like to invest in order to generate more income. However, no matter how financially experienced you may be, this can be a risky business as you are subject to the volatility of the financial markets. It can also take a long period of time before investments pay off so it is important to cater for that time when your relative will need to access to your funds. If your relative would like to invest some capital, then a financial adviser can help you to structure a portfolio and perhaps spread the capital across a range of low-risk investments.

Equity release scheme

There are different types of schemes available, but they are all based on loaning you money based on the value of your house. With house prices rising in many areas in the UK, many have found that the value of their home has doubled in price. Releasing cash from property is a popular option for retired people who still want to live in their home and have an income for it.

Generally, a company will assess the value of the house and then pay a set amount per month or sometimes even a lump sum. Many people use the lump sum to make alterations or improvements to their home to enable them to live comfortably in the long term.

The company will then reclaim the money by selling the house after death or if your relative decide to sell it. Generally, to be eligible for an equity release scheme you need:

- To be between 55 and 70 years of age
- To have a property worth at least £30,000 to £40,000
- To be a freeholder (although this can differ from scheme to scheme).

However, it is important to do your homework before entering into a scheme like this, as there can be some major pitfalls. For example, if your relative does enter into an equity release scheme, the company will eventually reclaim their money by selling their house. This means that they will not be able to leave their house as inheritance.

Depending on the value of their home, it might also mean that they do not qualify for State benefits. Therefore, it is essential that you or your relative seeks proper legal and financial advice before making the decision to enter into a scheme like this.

Deferred payment scheme

This is an option for those who are moving into residential care and do not wish to sell their homes. Alternatively, this scheme may also appeal to those who are moving into residential care but are unable to sell their homes quickly enough to pay for their care fees.

Under a deferred payment scheme, the local council may be able to give your relative an interest-free loan by taking a legal charge on their property; for example, they might take over the mortgage. The idea is that the loan would help to pay for care home fees. It is also based on the condition that the council reclaims the money after death by selling the home. They can also reclaim the loan if you decide to terminate the agreement or your relative sells the house. You can qualify for the scheme if:

- Your situation has been assessed by your local council and they agree that you require residential or nursing care
- Your home is of enough value to cover the fees of your stay in the care home
- You are able to pay a weekly contribution.

Again, there can be advantages and disadvantages to this option. While the loan is interest-free, it may affect the value of your relative's property. This means that when the property is sold, there may not be a large amount of inheritance left for family. Additionally, some councils do not offer this scheme or they only agree to pay a low amount which might not meet your relative's needs. Your relative may also be required to contribute a weekly amount based on their assets and income. It is best to check out the options with your local authority to find out how they operate the scheme, if available.

Other funding options

Renting out property

If your relative is not living in their own home and receiving care in a care home, then you may wish to consider letting out their property. You would have to ensure that the amount is enough to cover the mortgage (if applicable) and the care home fees. This option is appealing for those who would like to keep a property that may increase in value over time. It also means the family would be able to inherit the property after your relative's death.

However, there is no guarantee that the property will always be tenanted so it is important to have funds set aside for this potential situation. Be aware that you will still have to pay maintenance charges and buildings insurance and the rental income will be subject to income tax.

Charities

Many charities also provide useful information and some run care homes and offer full-time support for those with disabilities.

Financial assistance from friends and family

There are many ways for family to contribute towards care: they could either pay directly into your relative's account or help pay money towards other funding options such as a Care Fee Annuity.

Practicalities of paying

Self-funding

If residents are self-funding (ie paying for the care home themselves) then paying by direct debit is probably one of the most convenient ways of paying the fees. Many homes prefer fees to be paid on a monthly basis so it is worth checking with the home what date the money will be coming out of your relative's account. Make sure the date is convenient and works with the availability of finances.

Power of attorney

Your relative may wish to appoint a power of attorney to handle their financial affairs in the event that their health declines. Relatives are able to pay for care on their behalf if their power of attorney to do so.

You should ensure your relative appoints someone that they trust completely. Since 2007, you are now able to appoint someone to also make decisions about your health and general welfare, as well as looking after your legal and financial affairs.

It is relatively inexpensive to set up a power of attorney and it gives your relative reassurance that their affairs are being handled by someone that they trust. Without a power of attorney, the decisions about their finances and other matters rest with the Court of Protection which can involve higher costs and other added complications.

Contributions from social services

If care is being paid for partly by yourself or you relative and partly by social services, then social services will make their financial contributions directly to the care home. It is up to you to arrange with the care home how you or your relative will pay the remainder of the fees.

HOW TO CHOOSE A HOME

If, after your relative's care assessment, you both make the decision to move them into a care home, then it is important to know how to go about finding a home and organising the move.

The first step is to contact the social services department within your local council. Social services will send you all types of information about care homes, including a list of all the care homes in your area. However, be aware that it is entirely up to you what kind of home you choose as your local council is not permitted to recommend a particular home.

Choosing care for a relative

Choosing a care home for a relative is never an easy task. There is so much to consider and it is important to ensure your relative is given the best care possible. The first thing to do is to sit down with your relative and write down the following essential facts:

- Full name
- Date of birth
- Address
- Past profession
- Your relation to them

- Medications
- Medical history
- Mobility/wheelchair-dependent
- Doctor's name

A great concern of most people is that they will choose a home that their relative does not like or becomes unhappy with your decision. To ensure you meet your relative's needs and preferences, you might find it helpful to discuss the following areas with your relative and ask them some questions to help determine the type of care they are looking for:

Food and drink

- Does your relative have any food or drink intolerances or allergies?
- Do they need a special diet? For example, if your relative has diabetes or suffers from obesity, they will need to be on a very strict diet.
- What sort of food preferences do they have?
- Are they able to eat on their own?

Mobility

- Are they able to walk without assistance?
- Are they able to use the toilet on their own?
- Would they benefit from handrails on the walls of the bedroom and bathroom?
- Is there enough space for them to move around?

Speech

- What is their speech like? Is it clear enough to understand?

Hearing

- What is the extent of your relative's hearing problems?
- Do they use sign language? If so, it is important to ensure that the staff are also skilled in this area.
- Do they use a hearing aid? If so, note down the type of hearing aid and the sort of batteries it uses.

Sight

- Do they have difficulties with their sight?
- Do they use glasses? How many pairs do they have?
- What kind of prescription do they use?
- If your relative has a guide dog, does the home cater for pets?
- Is there any reading material available for the sight-impaired such as documents and literature printed in Braille?

Personality

Personality is very important in deciding which sort of care home is most suitable for your relative. If they are outgoing, then they may enjoy a wide range of social activities. Similarly, if they are a more private person who values peace and quiet, they may prefer a library or a garden on the premises.

The following questions are useful to keep in mind when assessing your relative's personality:

- What sort of person is your relative?
- Does he/she still have an active mind?
- What kind of hobbies would they enjoy?
- What kind of people do they get on best with?

Spiritual needs

- Does your relative have any religious preferences or spiritual needs?

Hobbies

- What kind of hobbies or activities does your relative enjoy?
- What kinds of facilities should the care homes offer that would fit their needs?

Be sure to make notes from talking with your relative, and take these with you when visiting homes as they will be useful when talking to the managers or matrons of them. The answers to these questions will give you a guide to make sure a home covers all your relative's needs.

Know your priorities

It really important to take time to think about what your relative would like and expect from a care home. They
might prefer to move to a care home that is near friends and family, or choose one that allows pets. Their personal
preferences are very important and having a clear idea of what these are before you begin your search will help to
ensure that their needs are fully met.

Everybody will have different priorities when choosing a care home. Some will want to be near the centre of
town; others will want a quiet lounge; others, a large garden where they can help in. For many, the deciding
factors come down to cost and location. It is a good idea to write down these priorities and number them. Keep
referring to this list throughout the process.

Remember, you are not just choosing a place to live – you are choosing a home.
The people are just as important as the place.

The categories below are a few examples of points you may want think about – everyone will have different
preferences, you need to work out what your relative's are. The considerations are numerous, so take time to think
about all aspects of daily life.

Size of the home
Larger homes often have better facilities, and a choice of communal areas; while smaller homes will often have
a homely feel. It is not always as black and white as this: many large homes have a great atmosphere, and small
homes can have ample communal space. Often it is better to consider the type of home your relative would like,
without considering its size.

Single or shared rooms
Is it very important for you to have your own room, or would you consider sharing if other aspects of the home
were suitable?

Purpose-built/conversions
Many care homes have been converted from older, grander buildings such as manor houses. These buildings
can look beautiful and are usually set in large grounds. The cost of staying in one of these homes is higher as
it takes a lot of money to run such a large estate. Also, the accommodation might not be as modern as it would
be in newer builds. If the care home is situated far outside a city, public transport may be a problem. As these
homes are larger, they can hold a greater number of residents. These buildings usually have many floors and can
be quite spread out. If you have difficulty with mobility, do take these points into consideration if you are thinking
about moving into a large, country estate. Care homes that have been purpose-built for elderly residents are more
modern and usually lower in cost. Many have fully functioning lifts and modern facilities.

Location
There are some very picturesque homes in wonderful rural settings; there are also care homes in the centre of
towns. Think about the location your relative would like. Do they love the countryside and fresh air or do they value

being able to pop to the shops or meet friends independently for a coffee? A large consideration is the availability of public transport around the home, and if the home has its own transport.

Do your homework

There are probably a number of nursing homes in your area – some that you have heard have good reputations, some that you don't know anything about. This is when this book becomes invaluable, as, when researched, the homes included all met CSCI standards. The information in this guide will give you a good grounding for your research.

Once you have established your budget, care needs and priorities, you can begin your search. Begin by going through the listings in this book and choosing the homes that meet your list of priorities. Don't restrict yourself to only looking at care homes in your local area; also check out the ones a little farther afield. Consider homes in the surrounding counties, or ones with good transport links.

This is when your numbered priorities list will come in useful: the reality is you may have to compromise on some of your choices. If you have decided that your home must have a garden, you may not be able to be as near to town as you would like. Keep your priorities in mind when looking through the homes.

Short-listing the homes

Jot down your top 10 or 20 homes. With this list, you can conduct some further research into the homes that you and your relative like the sound of.

Gathering a few brochures together always helps to narrow down the number of suitable choices. Begin by acquiring all 10–20 brochures and then decide on a shortlist. Be aware that the information in these brochures can sometimes be limited or out of date or the photos may not be an accurate representation of the size of the bedrooms or dining rooms etc, so it is best to visit the homes to get a feel for them first-hand.

Visiting care homes

Preparation

Before you pay a visit to the care homes of your choice, call first and speak to the care manager or matron. Ask if there is room currently available at the care home or if there is a waiting list and double-check if they can cater for your relative's needs. If you don't already have the brochure of that particular care home, then ask them to send you one.

If you are satisfied that the care home may be a suitable option, then make an appointment with the care manager to further discuss your relative's needs.

Visiting the home

Try not to visit too many care homes in one day. It can be an exhausting and an emotionally draining experience and with so many details to remember, it is easy to become confused and forget what each of them has to offer.

On your first visit, take your relative's list of priorities with you and ensure that you are armed with as much information about your relative as possible, including the answers to the questions in *Choosing care for a relative*.

Typically, you will be given a tour of the premises so try to note down as much detail as possible about each home. Notice whether each home meets your priorities, and make notes of distinguishing features. This will really help when you are looking back at your visit, trying to remember which home had the lovely water feature in the garden! Things to keep in mind are as follows:

First impressions

First impressions do count. Think about the presentation of the home from the exterior.
Are the gardens well maintained?
Is the driveway swept?
Assess how you are greeted as you walk in. *Are you given a warm welcome or are you ignored?*

Staff

Are the staff friendly and polite?

Observe how the staff treat the residents. Have a chat with some members of the staff and see if you can find out what they think of their own working environment. Discontented staff can have a negative impact on the residents. Staff should be warm, respectful, good humoured, calm and sensitive towards the residents. Residents should always feel comfortable in approaching staff with any problems and staff should support the residents to the best of their ability.

Are the staff fully qualified?

The CSCI requires that 50% of staff working in care homes are fully qualified to National Vocational Qualification (NVQ) level 2 status. Ask for this information when you are visiting care homes. We have indicated whether a home meets the standard in this guide, but bear in mind that the percentage of qualified staff can change dramatically if staff leave, or if unqualified staff pass their NVQ. Many care homes also conduct in-house training on 'Abuse in the Care Home' to learn about how to protect vulnerable residents from abuse. Find out what kind of staff training each care home offers.

Other training

If your relative suffers from a mental illness such as dementia or Alzheimer's, ask the care manager if the staff keep up-to-date about any medical progress in these areas and if they undergo any further training on how to handle residents with these type of illnesses.

What are the staffing levels like?

Ask to see a copy of the staff rota and check how many staff are on duty at night and during the day. If the care home is in the process of hiring new staff, ask about their recruitment policy and procedures. Usually all new staff are subject to mandatory induction training which includes fire drills, manual handling and health and safety.

Fees

Find out exactly what the fees cover. Are there extra fees for:

- Single room
- En suite
- Refreshments for visitors
- Services like hairdresser, chiropodist
- Outings
- Laundry
- Prescriptions
- Visits from the GP

The residents

Do the residents seem healthy and happy?

What is the general atmosphere like?

Note how the staff and residents interact with each other. Depending on what you see, you might want to consider making a surprise visit on another occasion to make sure that you get a realistic view of the care home.

Try and have a chat with a few of the residents to gauge their opinions on the care home and their general environment. Ask the residents to describe an average day in the home.

Accommodation

Are the rooms clean?

Make sure you thoroughly inspect the bedrooms, bathrooms and all communal areas to ensure that they have been cleaned to a high standard and that they smell nice and fresh.

Are the bedrooms big enough?

The size of the rooms vary from home to home. Check the size of the room and ensure that it is a comfortable size for your relative. The CSCI have a minimum size a single and shared room must be: you will see in the report if there are any rooms that are too small. Bear in mind, a room may meet government standards but still feel too small if you have a lot of furniture!

Can your relative bring in their own furniture?

Most homes will allow you to bring in your furniture from home provided it is in good shape (no woodworm etc). However, some bedrooms can be quite small and there may not be enough space for larger items of furniture.

Do residents have to bring their own appliances?

Some care homes will have already furnished the bedrooms with a telephone and television. However, if they don't provide these appliances, check that there are the right electrical points in the rooms so you can connect your own electrical equipment.

Can the rooms be personalised and decorated according to the resident's wishes?

Moving to an entirely different setting can be a traumatic affair. Being surrounded by familiar items from home can help with the adjustment period. Check with the care home to ascertain exactly what kinds of items you can bring. Some care homes do permit the bedroom to be repainted; at task which is usually carried out by their own maintenance man. Some homes even make a point of redecorating before a new resident arrives.

Are there en suites available?

Again, the provision of en suite bathrooms can vary from home to home. Remember that 'en suite' might not mean a fully equipped bathroom, but simply a basin and a toilet. In some care homes, the bedrooms do not have an adjoining bathroom as there is not enough space. Some residents prefer communal bathrooms as they are usually very large and they are easier to manoeuvre through.

Accessibility and space

What is accessibility like?

Are there enough handrails to make it easier to get around?

Many homes have excellent access, due to the high percentage of wheelchair-users. Check that there is assisted access on the ground floor as well as the upper floors. If you are quite frail and has difficulty with stairs, then ensure the home has a lift. If there is no lift on the premises, check if the staff help to assist the residents when they wish to get to the upper floors.

Is there proper wheelchair access?

If you use a wheelchair, check and see if the care home can accommodate it. Again, some care homes may not have a lift and may only allow for ground floor wheelchair access. Check that the route to the bedroom you are looking at is also accessible – even if a home has a lift, there may be a few steps up to a room.

Is there enough inside and outside space?

If you use a wheelchair, ensure that there is enough room to move around comfortably. The amount of space also depends on your personality. If you value your privacy, you will appreciate as much space as possible and may like a care home with a large garden or well-stocked library.

Meals

What's the menu like?

Ask to see a copy of the menu. Usually, this will change on a daily basis so request the week's menu to get a comprehensive idea of what kind of food is being served. Ask about the ingredients and produce they use. If you are used to organic food and home cooking, check with the care home manager or matron if this is available.

If possible, have a chat with the chef and ensure that he can prepare meals to suit special dietary requirements and personal preferences. In some care homes, the chef regularly meets with the residents to get their feedback on the meals provided and some even attend the residents meetings.

Does the food/drink look, taste and smell good?

Most homes are happy to let you try the food. Make sure it is presented nicely, tastes fresh and smells appealing. Ensure your cup of tea or coffee is hot (rather than lukewarm) and the milk is fresh.

Rules

What are the rules of the home?

Many care homes are very flexible but they will still have a number of rules, mostly concerning the personal safety of their residents.

Rules on pets

The decision to allow pets is usually at the manager's discretion. Many homes allow small pets such as budgies but it is more difficult to find a care home that permits larger pets to live in with the resident. If you having difficulty finding a care home that allows larger pets, then check with the care manager if a relative is able to bring the pet when they visit.

Access to GP and other services

Will you still have access to a GP?

This very much depends on where the care home is located. If it is near your relative's home, then it is likely that the local GP will make visits to the care home. However, if the care home is situated elsewhere, the likelihood is your relative will have to change to a local practice. The care manager should be able to advise you on this matter.

Will there be visits from a hairdresser, chiropodist, physiotherapist and dentist?

Many care homes organise weekly appointments with people from the above professions and a list of these services is included in the information in the book. You need to find out how often these services occur and if there is an extra cost. These services usually benefit residents and need to be taken into account when choosing a care home.

Entertainment and activities

What kind of entertainment is available in the care home?

We have included some example activities that homes partake in. While visiting the home, ensure you ask for a complete list of activities and entertainment that is organised.

Many care homes consult with the residents about their preferences in entertainment and activities. Depending on the feedback, the staff will draw up a monthly timetable and post it in communal areas so residents and their visitors are aware of any upcoming planned activities and events. Check with the care home if they draw up a schedule of events and ask if you can see their most recent one.

Ask the care manager if they have any photos of past events that you can take a look at.

Exercise activities are usually held daily in most care homes. It is essential that the residents keep mobile (where possible) and do a certain amount of gentle physical exercise. However, do check with your relative's GP to ensure that these exercises are suitable.

If gardening is a preference, are residents allowed to get involved in gardening?

Some homes have lovely gardens, and many let residents help with gardening. An increasing number of homes, especially purpose-built homes, have raised flowerbeds so that wheelchair-users can also participate in gardening.

Are church services organised at the home or do the residents have to travel to where the service is taking place?

This is often a very important consideration. Many homes offer an in-house service, but these are sometimes only once a month. If your relative would like to attend a service more regularly, or if it is important to attend a specific denomination, make sure there is a service nearby and that there is transport available.

Facilities

What are the facilities like?

Most care homes will have communal rooms where the residents can gather together and watch television or play games. Check the chairs are comfortable and whether the communal rooms are pleasant places to sit. Some homes have spectacular views from their lounges, which is much appreciated by residents.

Cleaning services

Do the care homes have laundry services?

The majority of care homes have an in-house laundry where they wash and dry clothes and return them to the residents' rooms. They do not usually have dry cleaning facilities and may ask for an extra charge for this service.

How often are the bedrooms cleaned and linen changed?

Transport

Does the home have its own transport?

Many care homes have a minibus or people carrier to bring the residents to local places of interest or on shopping trips. Most residents enjoy the change from their own environment and like to experience new things. The information in this guide will tell you whether transport is available. It is a good idea to ask how frequently the transport is used, to go on outings etc.

If not, what is the public transport like?

Ask about local bus services, dial-a-ride and any council-run transport services for older people. This is especially important if your relative wants to retain some independence.

Is there a trolley shop?

Some residents in care homes may be physically unable to partake in shopping excursions. If this is the case, then many care homes offer a weekly shopping trolley which contains useful items that the residents can purchase. Check with the care home if they have a trolley like this available and ask for a list of the items and prices offered.

The daily routine

What is the daily routine?

Try and get a sense of what takes place during a typical day at the home. Depending on the type of home, the routine will either be flexible or structured. Generally, mealtimes are usually set, but it is useful to find out how the residents fill their days. Check what happens if residents miss their meals or 'stray' from the routine.

Resident's charter

Most homes have a resident's charter which sets out the rights of the resident during their stay in the care home. Usually, this charter is on display in the home; if you can't see it, ask for a copy to review. Sometimes the charter is on the care home website. The charter includes information on the rights and privileges that residents are entitled to and outlines the standards and quality of services provided by the care home.

Typically, the charter would include the following with regards to the rights of the residents:

- To observe the residents' right to privacy
- To encourage and maintain independence of the residents
- To be treated with courtesy, dignity and respect
- To be provided with appetising food according to their diet and personal wishes
- To be given the opportunity to pursue new hobbies and activities
- The right to complain about any aspect of the home and its services without fear of reprisal
- To have full information about his/her health
- To have individual preferences and personal wishes taken into account
- To always have access to own room whenever they want
- To rise and go to bed any time they wish
- To manage their own finances
- To freely choose how to spend their day
- To be free to worship and attend religious services

Registration and insurance certificates

The CSCI are responsible for registering all facilities that provide personal and nursing care. If the care home meets the required standards, they will be granted a certificate of registration which should be displayed on the wall of the care home. Insurance certificates should also be exhibited prominently. Look out for both while you are touring the home.

Options for visitors

As relatives (and others) will most likely be regularly visiting, you and your relative will need to know some information about the following:

Car parking

Assess the car-parking situation and ensure that there is either space within the grounds of the care home or nearby. Some care homes are situated on busy roads and sometimes there can be very little room to park.

Public transport

If the care home is in the middle of the countryside, the public transport may not be too frequent. Check and see if there are regular buses or trains to the care home.

Visiting hours

Make sure you find out what times of the day people are able to visit. Some homes have an open-door policy, in that they allow visitors any time of the day. However, depending on the home, there might be restrictions around visiting hours so it is best to check this out.

The second visit

Once you have visited a few care homes and created a short list of those that you think might appeal, ask your relative to come with you on a second round of visits so you can gauge their opinion. This is important as it includes your relative in the decision-making process and will help them adjust to the idea once they become familiar with the types of homes available. It is also important to get a second opinion as they may notice things you may not have.

Make sure you have all your questions prepared for the care managers you are seeing so you can address any concerns you both may have.

After your second visit

If you and your relative cannot decide between homes and like one or more, check if your relative can stay for a day or two so they can get a feel for the environment. If there is a waiting list on the care home of your choice, check with social services and see if they can assist you. The care manager or matron of the care home can also visit your relative at home to ensure that they are a suitable candidate for the home and will also check if they can afford the fees. They will also advise you on the fees involved when reserving a room. If everything goes well, then your relative might decide to move into one of the care homes.

MOVING HOME AND SETTLING IN

Preparing for the move

Moving into a care home can be a very stressful experience. In the months prior to the move, it is important that you keep informed about everything to do with the home and include your relative in every decision you make. You can also take your relative on several visits to the care home so they become a bit more familiar with their surroundings. It is also helpful for you and your relative to have frequent chats with the manager of the care home and the staff to ensure that all your questions are answered.

Packing

If you are helping a relative pack for the move, be aware that this can be quite a big job and needs careful organisation before transporting belongings to their new home. Assess how much space there is in your relative's new bedroom for furnishings, equipment and clothes.

Clothing

There may only be a small single wardrobe available in the bedroom so do not pack too many items of clothing. It is important to choose a combination of warm and light clothes, even in the summer. Many elderly people feel cold even when it's warm outside and need appropriate clothing on hand to make them feel comfortable. At the beginning of each season, do check that your relative has the appropriate clothes for the weather ahead. Make sure that all the clothes are suitable for a commercial washing machine and tumble dryer.

Labelling

It is essential that you mark every item your relative is bringing to the care home as they can get lost or go missing very easily. You can mark clothes by sewing on name labels or using a marking pen. Do check these labels regularly as sometimes they can come off or become faded after the clothes are washed repeatedly. Some care homes order labels for the residents' clothing so check with the care manager if they offer that facility.

Apart from marking clothes, it is very important to label all other belongings. If your relative is bringing in their own electrical appliances such as a television, radio or portable/mobile phone, make sure they are labelled appropriately.

You will also need to mark any medical equipment your relative may be bringing with them. For example, if they have dentures, there are dentists that can label them. However, this can incur a charge that varies from dentist to dentist. Do shop around to find the most reasonable fee for carrying out this work.

If your relative has a hearing aid, there should be enough space to mark their name. If not, then store it in a container that is marked clearly. Similarly, make sure spectacles are also labelled appropriately.

Your relative might also be bringing in walking aids such as a Zimmer frame, walking stick or wheelchair. Their name can be painted on to the back of the wheelchair but it is trickier to mark smaller items such as walking sticks etc. In this case, you should either carefully paint their name on or use sticky labels. Marking all their belongings will make it significantly easier for the staff to return any missing items to your relative.

Toiletries

Remember to also pack some toiletries. The care home will provide some of these, so check with them first before packing. There is no need to pack six months' worth of toiletries. There will be facilities to buy toiletries, such as a trolley shop or trips into town.

Moving day

Ensure your relative has a friend or relative on hand to help on moving day. Bear in mind they will need all the support they can get on the day of the move. Make sure you or someone else is available to bring your relative to the care home or at least be there when they arrive. It can be a traumatic experience and it will help your relative to have a familiar face around. Staff will help to answer any questions you both may have and then assist your relative by unpacking their belongings and settling them into their new bedroom. They may also be introduced to some of the other residents.

Admissions process

This can be a difficult time and it is important that the admissions process is as smooth as possible and that the staff are kind, comforting and supportive of their new residents.

The care home should provide you with a contract of terms and conditions on admission which your relative will have to sign. They will also explain how the residents' care is assessed and evaluated.

Care plans

On the day of admission, the care manager will discuss your relative's needs, create a care plan to include their requirements and make sure they are carried out. Care plans are personalised for each resident and include a list of their social care, cultural, personal and health needs. Each plan should also contain a medication profile that details prescriptions and include details of any medicinal side effects.

The care home manager will also ask about your relative's daily routine and likes and dislikes. Friends and family should also be consulted during the creation of the care plan to give their input. Photographs may also be taken to include in their file. Care plans should be checked regularly to ensure that the needs of the residents are being met and updated to include any changes in their requirements.

End of life care plans

After a period in the care home, your relative may wish to establish their wishes relating to palliative care and the provisions they would like to be made. This is a very difficult subject to discuss but the care home staff are trained in this area and should advise you and your family appropriately and treat the matter with the sensitivity it deserves.

Preparing for your arrival

The staff should have prepared your relative's bedroom in anticipation of their arrival to the care home. The room should be clean with fresh sheets on the bed and towels in the bathroom, if it is an en suite room. Each room should have a fully functioning call bell, which the staff will ensure is in working order before your relative arrives. They should also ensure that a jug of fresh water is placed within reach of the bed.

Make sure that this preparation has been done before your arrival and also ensure that any of your relative's belongings, such as furniture etc have been arranged appropriately in the room.

Staff in the care home

It can be confusing and emotional to be surrounded by so many new faces, especially if your relative has been used to living alone. Try to visit as many times as you can prior to the move so your relative gets to know some of the staff. This will help them adjust more quickly to the environment if they are greeted by a familiar face on moving day.

In most care homes, the staff will wear a uniform which is traditionally navy blue.

Once you have moved

Culture shock

Adjusting to a new environment can be difficult to begin with. Your relative may not be used to being surrounded by so many other people and might also find it hard to adapt to the routine of the care home. They may also miss the familiarity of home and well-known surroundings.

The adjustment period can be difficult for all involved, especially family that visit. Your relative might be withdrawn and upset for the first while and might feel self-conscious about needing help with bathing or dressing. During your visits with your relative, it is important to encourage them to adopt a more positive attitude and try and lift their spirits as much as possible. You can help with the settling in period by:

- Visiting your relative as often as you can
- Encouraging other friends and family to also visit frequently
- Giving them all the contact details for their closest friends and family
- Hanging a calendar on their bedroom wall marked with significant occasions
- Putting photos and messages on their wall
- Bringing in meaningful gifts to cheer them up
- Taking them out for walks or short trips
- Bringing in their pet if the care home permits it
- Chatting to them about how they are feeling and offering comfort and advice.

It will take time for your relative to settle in but after a period, you may notice that they are more contented and may even be enjoying the experience of meeting new people and taking part in the different activities.

Changing routine

Depending on your relative's situation, they will most likely have settled into their own routine according to their lifestyle. They might have risen at a certain time every morning and prepared meals at the time of day that suited them best. Care homes do have a routine but it is a flexible one. The residents can to go to bed whenever they wish and rise at their preferred time in the morning. Mealtimes are generally at set times but some care homes also serve the meals in the residents' bedrooms if they prefer.

For the most part, residents have the freedom to do as much or as little as they wish on every given day. Some care homes impose a set time for bathing and washing etc. As many of the residents need help with their personal care, it can be helpful to know what day this will be taking place. Most care homes have specialist baths which are designed to make the experience as easy and comfortable as possible. A member of staff will always be on hand to help with getting in and out of the bath.

Resolving problems

There might be instances where your relative may feel uncomfortable about certain aspects of the care home and wish to air their grievances. This could be anything from noise volume to complaints about the staff or the meals. Some care homes hold weekly meetings to discuss any issues that the residents may have. Minutes might also be taken and circulated to the families of the residents to keep them up to date on any new decisions.

If your relative would prefer to talk privately about their problem, the best thing would be for you or your relative to have a chat with the care manager about the problem. If the problem persists then you can also write a letter to the proprietor explaining the nature of your complaint and why you feel it needs to be addressed. Most care home managers are willing to listen when you do have a grievance and it is always best to air your complaint as early as possible so it can be resolved quickly.

Quality assurance

Care homes are required to enforce a formal quality assurance system to accurately assess the needs of the residents, gather feedback and act on it if necessary. This might come in the form of surveys and comment cards which the residents and their relatives will be asked to complete. It is not compulsory to fill out these forms but it is an excellent way for the care home to assess the level of satisfaction with regards to the services they offer.

Visiting protocol

Taking your relative out

You may wish to take your relative out for lunch, bring them shopping or even take them back to your home for the day. Make sure you notify the care manager of your intentions and ask about any medication you might need for your relative while they are away from the home.

If you choose to take your relative and others from the care home on an outing, make sure your car is insured to cover all your passengers. If it is a special occasion, such as your relative's birthday, Christmas etc, inform the care home and let them know of your plans to take them out. It is always best to check with the care home about the most suitable times of day to pick up your relative and to let them know what time you will return.

Holiday

You may wish to bring your relative away on holiday. In this case, you must inform the care manager at least one month prior to the trip. Let them know how long you will be away, your contact details at your destination and the dates of your absence.

Meals

You may wish to have a meal with your relative during your visit. It is best to call ahead and let the home know that you are planning to stay for the meal. Some homes do not impose a charge for the meals, but there are homes that put the cost of the meal onto the resident's account. When you are looking around for suitable care homes, confirm what their policy is on accompanying your relative for meals.

Other visitors

There may be a number of people who would like to pay a visit to the home to see your relative. Some might be friends and may be elderly themselves. Therefore, it is important that their visit is made as comfortable as possible. Most care homes will provide visitors with free cups of tea and biscuits, but do confirm what sort of refreshments they offer and if there is a cost involved.

Other information

Telephone calls

Most care homes will have pay phones available to make calls to friends and family. These phones may be fixed to the wall or will be brought around on a trolley to cater for residents with mobility problems. The bedrooms will generally not have telephones already installed and it might be expensive for to set this up. They also may not need a telephone in their room if they only make calls a couple of times a week.

Some homes offer a facility whereby the resident can make calls from their own room through the care home's switchboard and the price of the calls charged to their account. If this is a facility that may appeal to your relative, make enquiries during your visits to the care home.

If you do decide to install a telephone for your relative, it is best to take into account the following:

- Does your relative have a hearing problem? If so, telephone providers can supply a phones that amplify the sound to make it easier for your relative to receive the call.
- Does your relative have failing sight? There are telephones available for the visually impaired that are equipped with large buttons, extra-bright ring flashers and Braille keypads.
- Payment for the calls will be made from a private account between your relative and a telecommunications company, so the care home will not be involved in the payment of the bills.

Mobile phones

If you are considering purchasing a mobile phone for your relative, then check with the care home first. Depending on the type of care home, some may forbid the use of mobiles in case they interfere with sensitive medical equipment.

TV licence

If your relative wishes to take their own TV into the care home, then they will have to purchase a TV licence. However, if they are over 75 years of age, then they no longer have to pay this fee.

Useful contacts

Please see page 465 for a list of useful contacts for financial and medical advice and further information about care homes.

Action plan

When faced with the prospect of going into a care home, the process can be daunting and rather confusing. We have broken it down into 10 steps which will help you on the way to finding the right care for you or your relative. Details of how to go about each step are found in the relevant sections of this introduction.

- [ ] Care assessment
- [ ] Care home or other care options?
- [ ] What are your care needs? (nursing/dementia etc)
- [ ] Are you eligible for council funding?
- [ ] With or without funding, what is your budget?
- [ ] What are your priorities?
- [ ] Shortlist 10–20 homes
- [ ] Request their brochures/look up reports
- [ ] Visit a few homes; visit top 2 or 3 again
- [ ] Make a decision and reserve a place

Abbeycrest Nursing Home

Manager: Lesley Wright
Owner: Abbeycrest Ltd
Contact: Essex Way, Sonning Common, Reading, Berkshire RG4 9RG
☏ 0118 9724414

Originally a school, Abbeycrest is at the edge of Sonning Common village, near Reading. There is a bus stop a quarter of a mile away, and a shop, post office and library one and a half miles away. Reading town centre which is a large shopping centre is 15 minutes' drive by car. There is a lawned garden and a patio area with views across fields. Residents are welcome to help maintain the garden. Activities coordinators organise activities for the residents on a daily basis to keep them stimulated which includes bingo, scrabble and coffee mornings.

Registered places: 24
Guide weekly rate: £518–£720
Specialist care: Nursing, learning disability, respite
Medical services: Podiatry
Qualified staff: Meets standard

Home details
Location: Rural area, 5 miles from Reading centre
Communal areas: Lounge, lounge/dining room, dining room, patio and garden
Accessibility: *Floors:* 2 • *Access:* Lift • *Wheelchair access:* Good
Smoking: In designated area
Pets: ✓
Routines: Flexible

Room details
Single: 14
Shared: 5
En suite: Undisclosed
Facilities: TV point, telephone point

Door lock: ✗
Lockable place: ✓

Services provided
Beauty services: Hairdressing
Mobile library: ✓
Religious services: Monthly church service
Transport: ✗
Activities: *Coordinator:* ✓ • *Examples:* Bingo, gardening, scrabble *Outings:* ✗
Meetings: ✓

Abbeyfield Home

Manager: Bernadette Yanquoi
Owner: Abbeyfield Society Ltd
Contact: 11 Maitland Road, Reading, Berkshire RG1 6NL
☏ 0118 957 2826

Abbeyfield Home is situated in a quiet conservation area one mile from Reading town centre. The home is run by Abbeyfield Society, a voluntary group with a Christian ethos. There is a small public park at the rear of the landscape garden. Public transport links into town include Readibus, a service that collects residents from the home. There are two lounges, one equipped with an organ and the other designated a quiet area, as well as a conservatory overlooking the garden and hairdressing salon. The home also has a resident cat.

Registered places: 28
Guide weekly rate: £540–£610
Specialist care: Respite
Medical services: Podiatry
Qualified staff: Meets standard

Home details
Location: Residential area, 1 mile from Reading centre
Communal areas: 2 lounges, dining room, hairdressing salon, conservatory, garden
Accessibility: *Floors:* 3 • *Access:* Lift • *Wheelchair access:* Good
Smoking: ✗
Pets: ✗
Routines: Flexible

Room details
Single: 28
Shared: 0
En suite: 28
Facilities: TV point, telephone point

Door lock: ✓
Lockable place: ✓

Services provided
Beauty services: Hairdressing
Mobile library: ✓
Religious services: Weekly Anglican Communion service
Transport: ✗
Activities: *Coordinator:* ✓ • *Examples:* Cruise afternoon, songs of praise • *Outings:* ✓
Meetings: ✓

Applegarth Care Home

Manager: Jennifer Poole
Owner: Harbhajan Surdhar
Contact: 24 Huntercombe Lane North, Maidenhead, Berkshire SL6 0LG
☏ 01628 663287

Applegate is a privately owned care home in an urban location. It is approximately five miles from Slough and a few miles from Maidenhead. There is a local shop, post office, chemist, GP surgery, bank, bus stop, social centre, shopping centre, train station and pub within a quarter of a mile. There is a garden with seating area for the residents to enjoy. The home organises monthly visiting entertainment such as pottery, live music and darts competitions. It is a small home, and as a result the residents have a lot of input in daily activities and planning.

Registered places: 14
Guide weekly rate: £385–£450
Specialist care: None
Medical services: Podiatry, physiotherapy
Qualified staff: Exceeds standard: 71% at NVQ Level 2

Home details
Location: Urban area, 5 miles from Slough
Communal areas: Lounge, dining room, conservatory, garden
Accessibility: *Floors:* 2 • *Access:* Lift • *Wheelchair access:* Good
Smoking: In designated area
Pets: At manager's discretion
Routines: Flexible

Room details
Single: 14
Shared: 1
En suite: 15
Facilities: TV point, telephone point

Door lock: ✗
Lockable place: ✓

Services provided
Beauty services: Hairdressing
Mobile library: ✓
Religious services: Weekly prayer services
Transport: ✗
Activities: *Coordinator:* ✗ • *Examples:* Quizzes, bowls, darts, visiting entertainers • *Outings:* ✓
Meetings: ✓

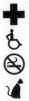

Argyles Nursing Home

Manager: Sue Smith
Owner: BUPA Care Homes Ltd
Contact: Pound Street, Newbury, Berkshire RG14 6AE
☏ 01635 551166
@ Abbotsleighmewsall@BUPA.com
🖰 www.bupacarehomes.co.uk

A purpose-designed Tudor-style home, the Argyles is situated within a residential area of Newbury, convenient for local shops and public transport. Furnished to a high standard throughout, and with lift access, it offers a choice of four lounge areas and a conservatory. The dining room overlooks the garden and patio. Daily activities include flower arranging, crafts, coffee mornings and reminiscence sessions, as well as trips to local attractions and church services and concerts.

Registered places: 57
Guide weekly rate: Undisclosed
Specialist care: Nursing, respite
Medical services: Podiatry, physiotherapy
Qualified staff: Undisclosed

Home details
Location: Residential area, in Newbury centre
Communal areas: 4 lounges, dining room, conservatory, hairdressing salon, patio and garden
Accessibility: *Floors:* 2 • *Access:* Lift • *Wheelchair access:* Good
Smoking: ✗
Pets: ✓
Routines: Flexible

Room details
Single: 43
Shared: 7
En suite: 12
Facilities: TV, telephone point

Door lock: ✓
Lockable place: ✗

Services provided
Beauty services: Hairdressing, aromatherapy
Mobile library: ✓
Religious services: ✓
Transport: ✓
Activities: *Coordinator:* ✓ • *Examples:* Flower arranging, crafts, coffee mornings, reminiscence sessions • *Outings:* ✓
Meetings: ✓

Registered places: 79
Guide weekly rate: From £1,000
Specialist care: Nursing, dementia, physical disability, respite
Medical services: Podiatry, optician, physiotherapy
Qualified staff: Meets standard

Home details
Location: Residential area, 5 miles from Reading
Communal areas: 4 lounges, 4 dining rooms, library, garden
Accessibility: *Floors:* 2 • *Access:* Lift
    Wheelchair access: Good
Smoking: ✗
Pets: At manager's discretion
Routines: Flexible

Room details
Single: 79
Shared: 0
En suite: 72
Facilities: TV point, telephone point

Door lock: ✗
Lockable place: ✓

Services provided
Beauty services: Hairdressing
Mobile library: Library facilities
Religious services: Monthly church service
Transport: Minibus
Activities: *Coordinator:* ✓ • *Examples:* Crafts, gardening club
    Outings: ✓
Meetings: ✓

Austen House
Manager: Lynne Geeves
Owner: Barchester Healthcare Ltd
Contact: Kilnsea Drive, Lower Earley, Reading, Berkshire RG6 3UJ
☏ 01189 266100
🖥 www.barchester.com

Austen House is situated in a residential area, close the local amenities and five miles from Reading town centre. The home has a sensory garden with raised beds and organises a gardening club for residents. There is a church service once a month and the home has its own bus for outings. There are regular residents meetings and the home has its own library as well as themed areas such as a shoeshine area, a music area and a war museum.

Registered places: 17
Guide weekly rate: £520
Specialist care: None
Medical services: Podiatry
Qualified staff: Undisclosed

Home details
Location: Residential area, 0.5 miles from Reading centre
Communal areas: Lounge, dining room, patio and garden
Accessibility: *Floors:* 2 • *Access:* Stair lift
    Wheelchair access: Limited
Smoking: In designated area
Pets: ✓
Routines: Flexible

Room details
Single: 9
Shared: 4
En suite: 0
Facilities: TV point, telephone point

Door lock: ✓
Lockable place: ✓

Services provided
Beauty services: Hairdressing
Mobile library: ✓
Religious services: ✗
Transport: ✗
Activities: *Coordinator:* ✗ • *Examples:* Bingo, board games, gentle exercise • *Outings:* ✓
Meetings: ✓

Bath Lodge

Manager: Jacqueline Foster
Owner: Michael Bissell
Contact: 8 Bath Road, Reading, Berkshire RG1 6NB
☏ 0118 9589726
@ relax@beechhousehotel.com

Bath Lodge is close to the M4 and all local amenities. The home is on the main A4 road into Reading and is only half a mile from the town centre. There are extensive and well-kept gardens for residents to enjoy in the summer. The home organises its own activities for the residents with active and more restful choices. These include bingo, board games and gentle exercises. The staff aim for a homely and friendly atmosphere and pets are welcome. Routines are flexible with structured meal times.

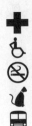

Bayford House

Manager: Jenny Dawkins
Owner: BUPA Care Homes Ltd
Contact: Rookwood, Stockcross,
Newbury, Berkshire RG20 8LB
☎ 01488 608632
@ bayfordhouseeveryone@bupa.com
🖰 www.bupacarehomes.co.uk

Bayford House is located in the rural village of Stockcross – four miles from Newbury. The home lies within six acres of grounds which offer countryside walks with extensive wildlife such as squirrels, rabbits and pheasants. Originally a private residence built at the turn of the century, Bayford House has been extended and modernised. In the summer residents can use the patio area to relax and take in the fresh air and watch the various bird life. The home links with two local care homes in the area for activity sessions which include trips, afternoon tea and live entertainment.

Registered places: 53
Guide weekly rate: Undisclosed
Specialist care: Nursing, respite
Medical services: Podiatry, optician, physiotherapy
Qualified staff: Undisclosed

Home details
Location: Rural area, 4 miles from Newbury
Communal areas: 2 lounges, 2 dining rooms, patio and garden
Accessibility: *Floors:* 3 • *Access:* Lift and stair lift
  Wheelchair access: Good
Smoking: ✗
Pets: ✓
Routines: Flexible

Room details
Single: 45
Shared: 0
En suite: 41
Facilities: TV

Door lock: ✓
Lockable place: ✓

Services provided
Beauty services: Hairdressing, aromatherapy
Mobile library: ✓
Religious services: ✓
Transport: ✓
Activities: *Coordinator:* ✓ • *Examples:* Crafts, gardening
  Outings: ✓
Meetings: ✓

Beacher Hall

Manager: Chrissie Whitmore
Owner: BUPA Care Homes Ltd
Contact: 42 Bath Road, Reading,
Berkshire RG1 6PG
☎ 01189 530600
@ BeacherHallEveryone@BUPA.com
🖰 www.bupacarehomes.co.uk

On the outskirts of Reading, Beacher Hall is a listed building that has been converted to provide long-term nursing, respite and convalescence care for elderly residents and young physically disabled people. All bedrooms at Beacher Hall are single occupancy and have en suite facilities; some have direct access to the garden. The home has seven lounges including a TV lounge, quiet lounge and place to receive visitors. Beacher Hall boasts attractive grounds and has a patio area, a solar-powered water feature and a wild-flower walk. Activities include gardening, bowls, walks, themed parties, discussions and reminiscent times.

Registered places: 70
Guide weekly rate: Undisclosed
Specialist care: Nursing, respite, physically disabled
Medical services: Podiatry, physiotherapy, occupational therapy
Qualified staff: Undisclosed

Home details
Location: Residential area, 1.5 miles from Reading centre
Communal areas: 7 lounges, 3 dining rooms, hairdressing salon,
  computer room, patio and garden
Accessibility: *Floors:* 3 • *Access:* Lift • *Wheelchair access:* Good
Smoking: In designated area
Pets: ✗
Routines: Flexible

Room details
Single: 68
Shared: 1
En suite: 69
Facilities: TV, telephone point

Door lock: ✓
Lockable place: ✗

Services provided
Beauty services: Hairdressing, aromatherapy
Mobile library: ✓
Religious services: ✓
Transport: ✓
Activities: *Coordinator:* ✓ • *Examples:* Art class, music therapy,
  visiting entertainers • *Outings:* ✓
Meetings: ✓

Registered places: 87
Guide weekly rate: £561–£770
Specialist care: Nursing, dementia, respite
Medical services: Podiatry, hygienist, physiotherapy
Qualified staff: Exceeds standard: 70% at NVQ Level 2

Home details

Location: Residential area, 0.3 miles from Bracknell centre
Communal areas: Lounge, dining room, activities room, garden
Accessibility: *Floors:* 2 • *Access:* Lift • *Wheelchair access:* Good
Smoking: In designated area
Pets: ✗
Routines: Flexible

Room details

Single: 77
Shared: 11
En suite: 9
Facilities: TV, telephone point

Door lock: ✗
Lockable place: ✓

Services provided

Beauty services: Hairdressing, aromatherapy, manicures
Mobile library: ✓
Religious services: ✗
Transport: ✗
Activities: *Coordinator:* ✗ • *Examples:* Bingo, exercise sessions,
    dancing, crafts • *Outings:* ✗
Meetings: ✓

Birdsgrove Nursing Home

Manager: Mary Slater
Owner: Southern Counties Care Ltd
Contact: Warfield Road, Bracknell,
Berkshire RG12 2JA
☎ 01344 422261
@ jslater@asterhealthcare.co.uk
🖱 www.asterhealthcare.co.uk

Birdsgrove Nursing Home is situated in a residential area on the borders of Bracknell. The home is within walking distance from a bus stop and station. Split into three units, one specialises in dementia care. Staff ensure a variety of activities for residents such as games of bingo, dancing and craft. They also have regular soloists or groups coming to perform. The home also makes use of the Pets As Therapy scheme.

Registered places: 18
Guide weekly rate: £315–£500
Specialist care: Mental disorder, respite
Medical services: Podiatry
Qualified staff: Meets standard

Home details

Location: Residential area, 2 miles from Reading centre
Communal areas: Lounge, dining room, patio and garden
Accessibility: *Floors:* 2 • *Access:* Lift • *Wheelchair access:* Limited
Smoking: ✓
Pets: ✗
Routines: Flexible

Room details

Single: 17
Shared: 1
En suite: 4
Facilities: TV point

Door lock: ✓
Lockable place: ✓

Services provided

Beauty services: Hairdressing
Mobile library: ✓
Religious services: Weekly Anglican service, Catholic visits
Transport: Car
Activities: *Coordinator:* ✗ • *Examples:* Card games, bingo, jigsaw,
    music sessions • *Outings:* ✓
Meetings: ✓

The Boltons

Manager: Vijaye Juggurnauth
Owner: Vijaye and Premila Juggurnauth
Contact: 4 College Road, Reading,
Berkshire RG6 1QB
☎ 0118 9261712
@ djuggurnauth@hotmail.com

The Boltons is situated in a residential area of Reading. It is a Victorian house, and therefore has limited wheelchair access. There is a large garden with seating areas.

Residents have the opportunity of using mobile handsets so that staff are always accessible anywhere in the home. Weekly exercise sessions and frequent outings are organised, although the home does not have an activities coordinator. The home aims to cater for any culture, and assures residents have the opportunity to attend their chosen religious service, and even eat their preferred cuisine.

Boulters Lock Residential Home

Manager: Amanda Gardiner
Owner: Amanda Gardiner
Contact: 56 Sheephouse Road, Maidenhead, Berkshire SL6 8HP
) 01628 634985

Boulters Lock is a large detached house in a private residential road, close to the River Thames. To the rear of the property there is a small, mature garden with a patio area that can be accessed from the lounges and dining room. The home offers a variety of activities including manicures and a Pets As Therapy scheme is in place. There are also monthly outings with trips to the cinema and afternoon teas. The residents meet monthly to discuss aspects of their daily routine and activities that they enjoy, or would like altered.

Registered places: 27
Guide weekly rate: £650–£795
Specialist care: Dementia
Medical services: Podiatry
Qualified staff: Meets standard

Home details
Location: Residential area, 2.5 miles from Maidenhead
Communal areas: 2 lounges, dining room, patio and garden
Accessibility: *Floors:* 2 • *Access:* Lift • *Wheelchair access:* Good
Smoking: ✗
Pets: At manager's discretion
Routines: Flexible

Room details
Single: 27
Shared: 0
En suite: 27
Facilities: TV point, telephone point

Door lock: ✓
Lockable place: ✓

Services provided
Beauty services: Hairdressing
Mobile library: ✓
Religious services: Fortnightly Catholic visits, monthly Anglican Communion service
Transport: ✗
Activities: *Coordinator:* ✓ • *Examples:* Arts and crafts, games
Outings: ✓
Meetings: ✓

Broadmead Rest Home

Manager: Jan Bunton
Owner: Broadmead Rest Home Ltd
Contact: Broad Layings, Woolton Hill, Newbury, Berkshire RG20 9TS
) 01635 253517
@ broadmead@dsl.pipex.com

Broadmead is a privately run nursing home consisting of a large old house and a new single storey extension. It is set in large gardens and is in a rural area of Berkshire, three miles from Newbury. There is a small post office in walking distance, but other facilities are further away. There is a bus service available and the home has its own transport. There is a communal phone for residents' use. Pets are allowed to visit the home. There is a fortnightly Communion service and a vicar makes visits every fortnight.

Registered places: 38
Guide weekly rate: £527
Specialist care: Dementia, mental disorder
Medical services: Podiatry, dentist, optician
Qualified staff: Exceeds standard: 100% at NVQ Level 2

Home details
Location: Rural area, 3 miles from Newbury
Communal areas: 2 lounges, dining room, garden
Accessibility: *Floors:* 2 • *Access:* Stair lift
Wheelchair access: Limited
Smoking: In designated area
Pets: ✗
Routines: Flexible

Room details
Single: 20
Shared: 10
En suite: 0
Facilities: TV point

Door lock: ✓
Lockable place: ✓

Services provided
Beauty services: Hairdressing
Mobile library: ✓
Religious services: Fortnightly Communion service
Transport: ✓
Activities: *Coordinator:* ✗ • *Examples:* Quizzes, singalongs, visits from accordion player • *Outings:* ✗
Meetings: Undisclosed

Registered places: 35
Guide weekly rate: £825–£1,150
Specialist care: Nursing, respite, emergency care
Medical services: Podiatry, physiotherapy
Qualified staff: Exceeds standard: 75% at NVQ level 2

Home details

Location: Rural area, 2.5 miles from Maidenhead
Communal areas: Lounge, dining room, conservatory,
    patio and garden
Accessibility: *Floors:*2 • *Access:* Lift • *Wheelchair access:* Good
Smoking: ✗
Pets: ✗
Routines: Flexible

Room details

Single: 35
Shared: 0
En suite: 0
Facilities: TV point, Telephone point

Door lock: ✗
Lockable place: ✓

Services provided

Beauty services: Hairdressing
Mobile library: ✓
Religious services: ✓
Transport: ✓
Activities: *Coordinator:* ✓ • *Examples:* River walks, gardening,
    quiz nights • *Outings:* ✓
Meetings: ✓

Cookham Riverside Nursing Home

Manager: Mary Clay
Owner: Hamilton House Medical Ltd
Contact: Berries Road, Cookham,
Berkshire SL6 9SD
☎ 01628 521249
🖰 www.hamiltoncare.com

The Cookham Riverside was founded and for many years operated by the Civil Service Benevolent Fund. The Home continues to attract retired civil servants. Most bedrooms have glorious views over the gardens and of the Cookham Reach. It is this stretch of the Thames that inspired Kenneth Graham's *Wind in the Willows*. The Home is 100 yards level walk from the Cookham village centre and the church is a very similar distance down the river. The home enjoys the benefits of a dedicated activity organiser and its own transport service.

Registered places: 24
Guide weekly rate: £520–£580
Specialist care: Day care, respite
Medical services: Podiatry, hygienist, physiotherapy
Qualified staff: Meets standard

Home details

Location: Village location, 1 mile fro Goring centre
Communal areas: Lounge, dining room, conservatory,
    patio and garden
Accessibility: *Floors:* 2 • *Access:* Lift
    Wheelchair access: Limited
Smoking: ✗
Pets: At manager's discretion
Routines: Flexible

Room details

Single: 22
Shared: 2
En suite: 21
Facilities: TV point, telephone point

Door lock: ✓
Lockable place: ✓

Services provided

Beauty services: Hairdressing, aromatherapy
Mobile library: ✓
Religious services: Monthly Anglican Communion service
Transport: Car
Activities: *Coordinator:* ✓ • *Examples:* Music, quiz, reminiscence,
    mobility classes • *Outings:* ✓
Meetings: ✓

The Coombe House

Manager: Susan Hutchinson
Owner: Marianne Windibank
Contact: Streatley-on-Thames,
Berkshire RG8 9QL
☎ 01491 872174

The Coombe House is set in a rural village, in walking distance to local amenities.
  Residents are encouraged to lead independent lives in a safe and accommodating environment. If any Catholic residents ask for a service, one will be provided along with the monthly Anglican service. Visitors are welcome any time and have a meal at no extra charge. The home has an annexe separate from the main building with five bedrooms. Activities are arranged in consultation with residents and the home maintains strong links with the local community.

Crossways Residential Care Home

Manager: Tom Neehaul

Owner: Mr and Mrs Neehaul

Contact: 306 Yorktown Road, Sandhurst, Berkshire GU47 0PZ

☎ 01276 34691

Situated in Sandhurst, Crossways is an extended domestic dwelling, with good local amenities within a quarter of a mile. It is also close to main transport routes (M3 and M4) and a train station is within one and a half miles of the home. The home has an activities organiser who arranges weekly activities including exercise and gentle dancing. Residents hold meetings two or three times a year.

Registered places: 10
Guide weekly rate: £420–£670
Specialist care: None
Medical services: Podiatry, physiotherapy
Qualified staff: Exceeds standard: 80% at NVQ Level 2

Home details
Location: Residential area, in Sandhurst
Communal areas: Dining room, lounge, conservatory, patio and garden
Accessibility: *Floors:* 2 • *Access:* lift • *Wheelchair access:* Good
Smoking: In designated area
Pets: ✓
Routines: Flexible

Room details
Single: 10
Shared: 0
En suite: 0
Facilities: TV point, telephone point

Door lock: ✓
Lockable place: ✓

Services provided
Beauty services: Hairdressing
Mobile library: ✓
Religious services: Monthly Catholic and Anglican service
Transport: ✗
Activities: *Coordinator:* ✓ • *Examples:* Board games, exercise, dancing • *Outings:* ✗
Meetings: ✓

Donnington Nursing Home

Manager: Jo Taylor

Owner: BUPA Care Homes Ltd

Contact: Wantage Road, Newbury, Berkshire RG14 3BE

☎ 01635 521272

@ TheDonningtonALL@BUPA.com

🖰 www.bupacarehomes.co.uk

This red brick Victorian private house has been extended and converted into a care home with nursing. Situated in the Berkshire countryside, in the suburb of Donnington near Newbury, the home stands in landscaped gardens, with seating areas to enjoy a sunny afternoon. There are four lounges, so residents may meet and chat with other residents, or find a peaceful room. Personal interests are encouraged, and among the daily activities offered are art classes, gardening and musical recitals.

Registered places: 45
Guide weekly rate: Undisclosed
Specialist care: Nursing, palliative care, respite, terminal care
Medical services: Podiatry, physiotherapy
Qualified staff: Exceeds standard: 75% at NVQ Level 2

Home details
Location: Rural area, 1.5 miles from Newbury
Communal areas: 4 lounges, dining room, hairdressing salon, computer room, patio and garden
Accessibility: *Floors:* 2 • *Access:* Lift and stair lift *Wheelchair access:* Good
Smoking: In designated area
Pets: ✗
Routines: Flexible

Room details
Single: 37
Shared: 1
En suite: 27
Facilities: TV

Door lock: ✓
Lockable place: ✗

Services provided
Beauty services: Hairdressing, aromatherapy
Mobile library: ✓
Religious services: ✓
Transport: ✓
Activities: *Coordinator:* ✓ • *Examples:* Arts and crafts, exercise, visiting entertainers • *Outings:* ✓
Meetings: ✓

Registered places: 16
Guide weekly rate: £450–£525
Specialist care: Day care, respite
Medical services: Podiatry, dentist, physiotherapy, optician
Qualified staff: Exceeds standard: 95% at NVQ Level 2

Home details
Location: Residential area, 150 yards from Wokingham centre
Communal areas: Lounge, dining room, conservatory, garden
Accessibility: *Floors:* 2 • *Access:* Lift • *Wheelchair access:* Good
Smoking: ✗
Pets: ✗
Routines: Structured

Room details
Single: 14
Shared: 1
En suite: 7
Facilities: TV

Door lock: ✓
Lockable place: ✓

Services provided
Beauty services: Hairdressing, manicures
Mobile library: ✓
Religious services: Monthly Catholic service
Transport: ✗
Activities: *Coordinator:* ✓ • *Examples:* Board games, aerobics, games • *Outings:* ✓
Meetings: ✓

Down Lodge

Manager: Graham Casselden
Owner: Graham Casselden
Contact: 11 Sturges Road, Wokingham, Berkshire RG40 2HG
☏ 0118 978 6484

Down Lodge is a care home set 150 yards from Wokingham town centre. The home has ample communal living space, with a large, south-facing conservatory. Recently refurbished, the home has 14 single rooms and one double room. There are two residents meetings a year and the home also offers respite and day care. There is a pleasant garden, where parties and barbecues are held in the summer months. An activities coordinator organises daily activities including board games and exercise sessions. There are also occasional outings for residents. There is a Catholic service once a month in the home.

Registered places: 26
Guide weekly rate: £390–£450
Specialist care: Dementia
Medical services: Podiatry, dentist, occupational therapy, optician
Qualified staff: Exceeds standard: 100% at NVQ Level 2

Home details
Location: Rural area, 1 mile from Slough
Communal areas: Lounge, dining room, patio and garden
Accessibility: *Floors:* 3 • *Access:* Lift • *Wheelchair access:* Good
Smoking: ✓
Pets: At manager's discretion
Routines: Flexible

Room details
Single: 26
Shared: 0
En suite: 26
Facilities: TV point, telephone point

Door lock: ✓
Lockable place: ✓

Services provided
Beauty services: Hairdressing
Mobile library: ✓
Religious services: Weekly Anglican church service
Transport: ✓
Activities: *Coordinator:* ✗ • *Examples:* Bingo, games, visiting entertainers • *Outings:* ✓
Meetings: ✗

Eton House Residential Home

Manager: Keith Stenning
Owner: Akberali Abdeali
Contact: 68 Eton Road, Datchet, Berkshire SL3 9AY
☏ 01753 547251
@ Etonhouse2@aol.com
🖰 www.eton-house.co.uk

A converted church school building situated in a semi-rural location next door to a Catholic church, Eton House is half a mile from the local village. Much of the garden is paved and its features include raised flowerbeds. The home has its own transport which it uses to take two or three outings a year, for example on a boat trip. There are also daily activities and visits from entertainers. Pets are allowed if the residents can care for the animal themselves. Smoking is permitted in the resident's own room.

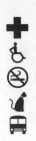

Foxleigh Grove

Manager: Mark Aram
Owner: The Aram family
Contact: Forest Green Road, Holyport,
Maidenhead, Berkshire SL6 3LQ
) 01628 673332
@ info@foxleighgrove.co.uk
⌂ www.foxleighgrove.co.uk

Foxleigh Grove was a private home originally built in the 18th century. An extension, complementing earlier brickwork, has been added and the house has been redesigned to accommodate residents' needs. Situated on the Green Belt, the home is set in six acres of grounds with formal lawns, wooded areas, a walled garden and a pond. Foxleigh Grove is a family-run home, following a multidisciplinary approach with a large team of staff to make this possible. The home also has good public transport links. As well as in-house entertainment, trips are organised to Buckingham Palace, and to the cinema and theatre.

Registered places: 39
Guide weekly rate: £750–£1,000
Specialist care: Nursing, emergency admission, physical disability, respite
Medical services: Podiatry, physiotherapy
Qualified staff: Undisclosed

Home details
Location: Rural area, 3 miles from Maidenhead
Communal areas: Lounge, quiet room, 2 conservatories, dining room, garden
Accessibility: *Floors:* 2 • *Access:* Lift • *Wheelchair access:* Good
Smoking: ✗
Pets: ✓
Routines: Flexible

Room details
Single: 35
Shared: 4
En suite: 31
Facilities: TV point, telephone point

Door lock: ✓
Lockable place: ✓

Services provided
Beauty services: Hairdressing
Mobile Library: ✓
Religious services: Local clergy visit
Transport: Minibus
Activities: *Coordinator:* ✓ • *Examples:* Games and music, outside activities • *Outings:* ✓
Meetings: ✓

Gurney House

Manager: Sheila Gallo
Owner: BUPA Care Homes Ltd
Contact: Upton Road, Slough,
Berkshire SL1 2AE
) 01753 521060
@ GurneyHouseALL@BUPA.com
⌂ www.bupacarehomes.co.uk

Gurney House is managed on behalf of Slough Borough Council, and is only able to accept residents referred by social services. It is set in a residential area of Slough, close to the eastern end of the high street and its shops. This purpose-built home has been designed to meet the needs of elderly residents. There is a conservatory and large landscaped garden. Most bedrooms are for single occupancy. Daily activities are arranged, as well as entertainers and trips to local places of interest. For further information on referrals to Gurney House please contact Slough social services.

Registered places: 35
Guide weekly rate: Undisclosed
Specialist care: Nursing, respite
Medical services: Podiatry, occupational therapy, physiotherapy
Qualified staff: Undisclosed

Home details
Location: Urban area, 0.5 miles from Slough centre
Communal areas: 3 lounges, dining room, conservatory, hairdressing salon, garden
Accessibility: *Floors:* 2 • *Access:* Lift • *Wheelchair access:* Good
Smoking: In designated area
Pets: ✗
Routines: Flexible

Room details
Single: 33
Shared: 1
En suite: 0
Facilities: TV point, telephone point

Door lock: ✓
Lockable place: ✗

Services provided
Beauty services: Hairdressing, aromatherapy
Mobile library: ✓
Religious services: ✓
Transport: ✓
Activities: *Coordinator:* ✓ • *Examples:* Quizzes, games, crafts
Outings: ✓
Meetings: ✓

Registered places: 30
Guide weekly rate: £995–£1,030
Specialist care: Nursing, day care, physical disability, respite
Medical services: Podiatry, optician, physiotherapy
Qualified staff: Meets standard

Home details

Location: Rural area, 3 miles from Maidenhead
Communal areas: 2 lounges, dining room, conservatory, patio and garden
Accessibility: *Floors:* 3 • *Access:* Lift • *Wheelchair access:* Good
Smoking: ✗
Pets: ✓
Routines: Flexible

Room details

Single: 18
Shared: 6
En suite: 14
Facilities: TV, telephone

Door lock: ✗
Lockable place: ✓

Services provided

Beauty services: Hairdressing, manicures, aromatherapy
Mobile library: ✓
Religious services: Weekly church service
Transport: ✗
Activities: *Coordinator:* ✓ • *Examples:* Sherry and card afternoons *Outings:* ✓
Meetings: ✓

Harwood House Nursing Home

Manager: Morag Forsyth
Owner: Harwood House Ltd
Contact: Spring Lane, Cookham Dean, Berkshire SL6 6PW
☏ 01628 478000
@ harwoodhouse@btconnect.com
🖰 www.harwoodhouse.co.uk

Harwood House is approximately three miles from Maidenhead in a rural setting with views over trees and fields with Windsor and the Thames Valley beyond. The home has well-maintained gardens with a conservatory and a patio area. There are two lounges in the home as well as a dining room. Hairdressing, aromatherapy and manicures are organised at the home, as well as sociable activities such as sherry and card afternoons. The home also organises reading to individuals. There are monthly residents meetings. The home also organises visits from a mobile library and a weekly church service.

Registered places: 79
Guide weekly rate: £527–£880
Specialist care: Nursing, physical disability, respite, terminal care
Medical services: Podiatry, dentist, optician
Qualified staff: Exceeds standard: 80% at NVQ Level 2

Home details

Location: Residential area, in Reading
Communal areas: 2 lounges, 2 dining rooms, patio and garden
Accessibility: *Floors:* 3 • *Access:* 2 lifts • *Wheelchair access:* Good
Smoking: ✗
Pets: At manager's discretion
Routines: Flexible

Room details

Single: Undisclosed
Shared: Undisclosed
En suite: 40
Facilities: TV, telephone point

Door lock: ✓
Lockable place: ✓

Services provided

Beauty services: Hairdressing, manicures
Mobile library: ✓
Religious services: Monthly church services
Transport: ✗
Activities: *Coordinator:* ✓ • *Examples:* Painting, reminiscence, bingo • *Outings:* ✗
Meetings: ✓

Jasmine House

Manager: Helena Hawkins
Owner: Jasmine Care Ltd
Contact: 22 Westcote Road, Reading, Berkshire RG30 2DE
☏ 0118 9590684
@ Jasminecare@btconnect.com

Jasmine House comprises of two Edwardian semi-detached properties that have been converted into a care home. A care worker spends time organising social activities for the residents and two young people volunteer an evening a week to provide companionship. There are two lounges and two dining rooms, providing choice for the residents. Three denominations visit the home every month to minister to residents. There are no organised outings but Reading town centre is only 10 minutes' walk away. The home has an activities coordinator who arranges painting, reminiscence sessions and bingo.

Lady Astor Court Nursing Home

Manager: Jeanette Chell
Owner: Southern Cross Healthcare Ltd
Contact: Burlington Avenue, Slough,
Berkshire SL1 2LD
📞 01753 517789
@ ladyastor@schealthcare.co.uk
🖥 www.schealthcare.co.uk

Lady Astor Court Nursing Home is a modern, purpose-built building in the centre of Slough. There is easy access to the shops and local resources, 10 minutes' walk away. The home has a garden surrounding it, part of which is accessible by the residents on the first floor. An activities coordinator posts a regular programme of activities and one-to-one sessions with residents which includes a bingo night, quiz night and arts and craft afternoon.

Registered places: 72
Guide weekly rate: £556–£880
Specialist care: Nursing, dementia, physical disability
Medical services: Podiatry
Qualified staff: Fails standard: 45% at NVQ Level 2

Home details
Location: Residential area, in Slough
Communal areas: 3 lounges, dining rooms, garden
Accessibility: *Floors:* 2 • *Access:* Lift • *Wheelchair access:* Good
Smoking: ✗
Pets: ✗
Routines: Flexible

Room details
Single: 72
Shared: 0
En suite: 72
Facilities: TV point, telephone point

Door lock: ✓
Lockable place: ✗

Services provided
Beauty services: Hairdressing
Mobile library: ✗
Religious services: ✓
Transport: ✗
Activities: *Coordinator:* ✓ • *Examples:* Bingo, arts and crafts
   Outings: ✓
Meetings: ✓

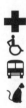

Langley Nursing Home

Manager: Veeda Gill
Owner: Langley Nursing Home Ltd
Contact: 44 Langley Road, Slough,
Berkshire SL3 7AD
📞 01753 676500

Langley Nursing Home is situated on a main road in Langley, close to its shops and local amenities. It is a 15-minute drive into Slough town centre. There is a large landscaped garden to the rear of the property, which boasts many flowers and shrubs. Activities are organised on a daily basis and include darts, music sessions, light exercise and gardening. There is live music for the residents enjoy every month. The staff hold weekly coffee mornings to discuss how residents are feeling and what activities they would like to plan for the next week.

Registered places: 11
Guide weekly rate: £565–£800
Specialist care: Nursing, dementia
Medical services: Podiatry, physiotherapy
Qualified staff: Meets standard

Home details
Location: Residential area, 1.5 miles from Slough centre
Communal areas: Lounge/dining room, conservatory, garden
Accessibility: *Floors:* 2 • *Access:* Lift • *Wheelchair access:* Good
Smoking: In designated area
Pets: At manager's discretion
Routines: Flexible

Room details
Single: 3
Shared: 4
En suite: 0
Facilities: TV point, telephone point

Door lock: ✗
Lockable place: ✗

Services provided
Beauty services: Hairdressing
Mobile library: ✓
Religious services: Monthly visit from local priest
Transport: ✗
Activities: *Coordinator:* ✓ • *Examples:* Games, music, gentle
   exercise, live music • *Outings:* ✗
Meetings: ✗

Registered places: 22
Guide weekly rate: £800–£850
Specialist care: Nursing
Medical services: Podiatry, hygienist, physiotherapy
Qualified staff: Meets standard

Home details

Location: Rural area, 4 miles from Windsor centre
Communal areas: Lounge, dining room, conservatory,
    patio and garden
Accessibility: *Floors:* 2 • *Access:* Lift • *Wheelchair access:* Good
Smoking: In designated area
Pets: ✗
Routines: Flexible

Room details

Single: 18
Shared: 2
En suite: 22
Facilities: Telephone point

Door lock: ✓
Lockable place: ✓

Services provided

Beauty services: Hairdressing
Mobile library: ✓
Religious services: ✓
Transport: ✓
Activities: *Coordinator:* ✓ • *Examples:* Quizzes, themed events,
    visiting entertainers • *Outings:* ✓
Meetings: ✓

Longlea Nursing Home

Manager: Mary Stone
Owner: Rowen Atkinson
Contact: Fifield Road, Fifield,
Maidenhead, Berkshire SL6 2PG
☎ 01628 634201
🖰 www.atkinsonshomes.co.uk

Situated on the outskirts of Fifield, Longlea Nursing Home is near both Windsor and Slough town centres. All bedrooms are en suite and most are single rooms.

The home has a large garden that is often visited by wildlife and birds, and can be accessed through the lounge and conservatory. Activities such as painting, bingo and quizzes are all organised by an activities coordinator. Residents are regularly visited by musicians and entertainers. A monthly church service is held at the home.

Registered places: 26
Guide weekly rate: £375–£585
Specialist care: Day care, respite
Medical services: Podiatry, physiotherapy
Qualified staff: Meets standard

Home details

Location: Residential area, in Wokingham
Communal areas: Dining room, lounge, garden
Accessibility: *Floors:* 3 • *Access:* Lift • *Wheelchair access:* Good
Smoking: ✗
Pets: At manager's discretion
Routines: Flexible

Room details

Single: 22
Shared: 2
En suite: 18
Facilities: TV point, telephone point

Door lock: ✓
Lockable place: ✓

Services provided

Beauty services: Hairdressing
Mobile library: ✓
Religious services: Monthly Anglican Communion service,
    weekly Catholic Communion service
Transport: ✗
Activities: *Coordinator:* ✓ • *Examples:* Exercise, board games,
    singalongs • *Outings:* ✓
Meetings: ✗

Lovat House

Manager: Fiona Honeyman
Owner: Mr and Mrs Tappin
Contact: 6 Crescent Road, Wokingham,
Berkshire RG40 2DB
☎ 0118 978 6750

Lovat House is a converted Edwardian property, with later extensions, in a residential area of Wokingham. There is a large rear garden, with raised flowerbeds, level paths, sunny and shady areas and plenty of seating. The home employs an activities coordinator to organise activities and take residents on outings to places such as garden centres and riverside towns. Events such as barbecues, birthday parties and a visiting farm have taken place.

Lynwood Nursing Home

Manager: Julie Way
Owner: BEN – Motor & Allied Trades Benevolent Fund
Contact: Rise Road, Sunninghill, Berkshire SL5 0AJ
☎ 01344 620191

Lynwood's accommodation is arranged in five units. The home has 20 acres of ground for residents to enjoy walking or admiring the wildlife. There is a bar that is open for residents to enjoy from Friday to Sunday. The home has a variety of activities and outings include trips to the London Eye and pubs. There are also musical entertainers who come in to entertain the residents. The League of Friends organises a calendar of social events – up to six per month.

Registered places: 87
Guide weekly rate: £500–£850
Specialist care: Nursing, dementia, respite
Medical services: Podiatry, physiotherapy
Qualified staff: Meets standard

Home details
Location: Residential area, in Sunninghill
Communal areas: Dining room, lounge, bar, chapel, garden
Accessibility: *Floors:* 3 • *Access:* Lift • *Wheelchair access:* Good
Smoking: In designated area
Pets: ✗
Routines: Flexible

Room details
Single: 87
Shared: 0
En suite: Undisclosed
Facilities: TV point, telephone point

Door lock: ✓
Lockable place: ✓

Services provided
Beauty services: Hairdressing
Mobile library: ✓
Religious services: Nondenominational service
Transport: 3 minibuses
Activities: *Coordinator:* ✓ • *Examples:* Bingo, exercises to music, quizzes • *Outings:* ✓
Meetings: ✓

The Manor House

Manager: Shanaaz Mohamad
Owner: Southern Cross OCPO Ltd
Contact: Church Road, Windsor SL4 2JW
☎ 01753 832920
@ manorhouse@ southerncrosshealthcare.co.uk
🖰 www.schealthcare.co.uk

The Manor House is located in a residential area of Old Windsor. The home's gardens have views of the Thames and there is ample communal space within the home itself with four lounges and three dining rooms. There are also three quiet rooms with library facilities. There is an activities coordinator who arranges a variety of activities and there are regular residents meetings.

Registered places: 62
Guide weekly rate: £800–£1,200
Specialist care: Nursing, dementia, respite
Medical services: Podiatry, dentist, optician
Qualified staff: Fails standard

Home details
Location: Residential area, 2.5 miles from Windsor
Communal areas: 4 lounges, 3 dining rooms, 3 quiet rooms, hairdressing salon
Accessibility: *Floors:* 3 *Access:* Lift • *Wheelchair access:* Good
Smoking: ✗
Pets: ✓
Routines: Flexible

Room details
Single: 60
Shared: 1
En suite: 60
Facilities: TV, telephone

Door lock: ✓
Lockable place: ✓

Services provided
Beauty services: Hairdressing, reflexology, reiki
Mobile library: Library facilities
Religious services: Religious visits
Transport: ✗
Activities: *Coordinator:* ✓ • *Examples:* Games *Outings:* ✓
Meetings: ✓

Registered places: 15
Guide weekly rate: £600–£750
Specialist care: Day care, respite
Medical services: Podiatry, physiotherapy
Qualified staff: Exceeds standard: 65% at NVQ level 2

Home details

Location: Residential area, in Maidenhead centre
Communal areas: 4 lounges, dining room, conservatory,
   patio and garden
Accessibility: *Floors:* 2 • *Access:* Lift • *Wheelchair access:* Good
Smoking: ✗
Pets: At manager's discretion
Routines: Flexible

Room details

Single: 15
Shared: 0
En suite: 5
Facilities: TV point, telephone point

Door lock: ✓
Lockable place: ✓

Services provided

Beauty services: Hairdressing
Mobile library: ✓
Religious services: Monthly Anglican service
Transport: ✗
Activities: *Coordinator:* ✗ • *Examples:* Baking, exercise,
   gardening, sewing • *Outings:* ✓
Meetings: ✓

Meadowbank Care

Manager: Caroline Li
Owner: Meadowbank Care Home Ltd
Contact: 44 Braywick Road,
Maidenhead, Berkshire SL6 1DA
☎ 01628 781186
@ meadowbank.uk@btinternet.com
🖰 www.meadowbankcare.com

Meadowbank is a residential care home with views overlooking the local park. It is situated close to train station; local amenities and only a five-minute walk to the town centre. The home has four communal areas for residents' use and a large garden and patio area. A short drive from River Thames, Henley and Marlow, the home organises outings and expeditions on a regular basis. Every resident has a personal radio paging and call system. An emphasis is put on creating a homely atmosphere, and residents have as much independence as they wish.

Registered places: 17
Guide weekly rate: £500–£750
Specialist care: None
Medical services: Podiatry, dentist, optician, physiotherapy
Qualified staff: Exceeds standard: 90% at NVQ Level 2

Home details

Location: Village location, 2 miles from Maidenhead
Communal areas: Lounge, dining room, conservatory, garden
Accessibility: *Floors:* 2 • *Access:* Lift • *Wheelchair access:* Good
Smoking: ✗
Pets: ✓
Routines: Flexible

Room details

Single: 14
Shared: 3
En suite: 6
Facilities: TV, telephone point

Door lock: ✗
Lockable place: ✗

Services provided

Beauty services: Hairdressing, manicures
Mobile library: ✗
Religious services: ✓
Transport: ✗
Activities: *Coordinator:* ✗ • *Examples:* One-to-ones, reading
   Outings: ✓
Meetings: ✓

Moor Cottage Residential Home

Manager: Helen King
Owner: Rana Rezajooi
Contact: High Street, Cookham,
Berkshire SL6 9SF
☎ 01628 526036
@ info@moorcottagecare.co.uk
🖰 www.moorcottagecare.co.uk

Moor Cottage is situated in a small village, two miles from Maidenhead with good train and bus services. The home is also close to the river Thames where residents are taken on outings. The home has a dining room, a lounge, a new conservatory and a large garden. The activity coordinator spends time with each resident and there are visitors who read to the residents. The home arranges for a vicar to visit once a month and pets are allowed in the home. The home is run as a family home and residents are not restricted in the personal items they can bring.

Moorlands Rest Home

Manager: Koomari Ramdany
Owner: Sundith and Koomari Ramdany
Contact: 987 Oxford Road, Tilehurst, Reading, Berkshire RG31 6TN
☎ 0118 942 7522

Moorlands Rest Home is situated two miles from Reading town centre and is close to the local railway station. The home provides care for those with middle to low dependency needs. Activities offered include exercise classes, beauty classes with foot spas and manicures, quizzes and music. Outings are also organised and church services are held in the home. Home-cooked food is prepared and residents have the option of eating in their room, conservatory or dining room. Staff aim to create a warm and friendly environment throughout the home.

Registered places: 12
Guide weekly rate: £300–£360
Specialist care: Physical disability, respite
Medical services: Podiatry, physiotherapy
Qualified staff: Meets standard

Home details
Location: Residential area, 2 miles from Reading centre
Communal areas: Lounge, dining room, conservatory, garden
Accessibility: *Floors:* 2 • *Access:* Lift • *Wheelchair access:* Good
Smoking: ✗
Pets: At manager's discretion
Routines: Flexible

Room details
Single: 8
Shared: 2
En suite: 0
Facilities: TV

Door lock: ✓
Lockable place: ✓

Services provided
Beauty services: Hairdressing, manicures
Mobile library: ✓
Religious services: Monthly Anglican service
Transport: ✗
Activities: *Coordinator:* ✓ • *Examples:* Exercise classes, quizzes, music • *Outings:* ✓
Meetings: ✓

The Mount

Manager: Sarah Ntshudu
Owner: Majestic Number One Ltd
Contact: School Hill, Wargrave, Berkshire RG10 8DY
☎ 01189402046

The Mount is a converted and extended Victorian home situated on the banks of a river. The home is located in a village with good access to the town of Wargrave. No religious services are organised in the home, but clergy visits when required. The home has a large garden with a seating area for residents to enjoy. There are residents meetings every quarter and there are also regular relatives meetings. The activities coordinator arranges a variety of activities, including arts and crafts, reminiscence sessions and quizzes. The home also has access to a minibus to take the residents on outings.

Registered places: 37
Guide weekly rate: £500–£675
Specialist care: Nursing
Medical services: Audiologist, podiatry, optician, psychologist, speech and language therapy
Qualified staff: Meets standard

Home details
Location: Village location, 7 miles from Reading
Communal areas: 2 lounges, dining room, garden
Accessibility: *Floors:* 2 • *Access:* Lift • *Wheelchair access:* Good
Smoking: ✗
Pets: Undisclosed
Routines: Structured

Room details
Single: 35
Shared: 2
En suite: 0
Facilities: TV

Door lock: ✗
Lockable place: ✗

Services provided
Beauty services: Hairdressing
Mobile library: ✗
Religious services: ✗
Transport: Shared minibus
Activities: *Coordinator:* ✓ • *Examples:* Arts and crafts, games, quizzes, reminiscence sessions • *Outings:* ✓
Meetings: ✓

Registered places: 27
Guide weekly rate: £475–£550
Specialist care: None
Medical services: Podiatry, dentist, optician, physiotherapy
Qualified staff: Exceeds standard: 60% at NVQ Level 2

Home details

Location: Residential area, in Wokingham
Communal areas: 3 lounges, dining room, garden, patio, conservatory
Accessibility: *Floors:* 3 • *Access:* Lift • *Wheelchair access:* Good
Routines: Flexible
Pets: ✓
Smoking: In designated area

Room details

Single: 25
Shared: 1
En suite: Undisclosed
Facilities: TV point, telephone point

Door lock: ✓
Lockable place: ✓

Services provided

Beauty services: Hairdressing, manicures
Mobile library: ✓
Religious services: ✓
Transport: ✗
Activities: *Coordinator:* ✓ • *Examples:* Bingo, flower arranging, visiting entertainers • *Outings:* ✓
Meetings: ✓

Murdoch House

Manager: Pamela O'Donnell
Owner: Southern Cross Healthcare Ltd
Contact: 1 Murdoch Road, Wokingham, Berkshire RG11 2DL
☎ 0118 978 5423
@ murdochhouseuk@
　　southerncrosshealthcare.com
🖰 www.southerncrosshealthcare.com

Situated in a residential area, Murdoch House lies close to a park and a three-minute walk from the town centre which has a wide variety of amenities including a train station. The home offers a weekly hairdressing service and manicures are available. The home has its own activities coordinator and there is a residents meeting every month to discuss what activities and outings the residents would enjoy. As part of a comprehensive weekly activities programme, seasonal events are also celebrated and a pantomime and carol singers perform at the home at Christmas.

Registered places: 18
Guide weekly rate: £335–£400
Specialist care: None
Medical services: Podiatry, dentist, optician, physiotherapy
Qualified staff: Meets standard

Home details

Location: Residential area, 1.5 miles from Reading centre
Communal areas: 2 lounges, dining room, patio and garden
Accessibility: *Floors:* 2 • *Access:* Lift • *Wheelchair access:* Good
Smoking: In designated area
Pets: ✗
Routines: Flexible

Room details

Single: 16
Shared: 1
En suite: 0
Facilities: TV, telephone point

Door lock: ✓
Lockable place: ✓

Services provided

Beauty services: Hairdressing
Mobile library: ✓
Religious services: ✓
Transport: ✓
Activities: *Coordinator:* ✓ • *Examples:* Bingo, mobility sessions *Outings:* ✓
Meetings: ✓

Navara Lodge

Manager: Poorun Bhugooa
Owner: Poorun and Malawutty Bhugooa
Contact: 1009 Oxford Road, Tilehurst, Reading, Berkshire RG31 6TL
☎ 0118 942 4692

Navara Lodge is a home for those with low to medium-dependency needs, therefore a strong emphasis is put on the residents' independence. Occasional outings are organised for individuals and the home has its own transport. There is a covered area in the garden so residents can still enjoy the garden when the sun is too strong. There is also a gazebo for smokers to use. The lodge provides a very homely atmosphere and keeps family members and friends very involved. The home has visits from a mobile library and there are also regular religious services.

Nightingales Care Home

Manager: Richelle Dix
Owner: Thames Carehome Ltd
Contact: Islet Road, Maidenhead,
Berkshire SL6 8LD
☎ 01628 621494

Situated close to the River Thames in Maidenhead, Nightingales is a converted house which set in its own grounds. Maidenhead is the nearest town centre and is approximately two miles from the home. The home offers a comprehensive activities programme. This includes visitors who provide Pets As Therapy and reminiscence therapy.

Registered places: 14
Guide weekly rate: £375–£600
Specialist care: Respite
Medical services: Podiatry, dentist, optician
Qualified staff: Undisclosed

Home details
Location: Residential area, 2.5 miles to Maidenhead
Communal areas: Lounge, dining room, conservatory, library facilities, garden
Accessibility: *Floors:* 2 • *Access:* Lift • *Wheelchair access:* Good
Smoking: ✗
Pets: ✗
Routines: Flexible

Room details
Single: 12
Shared: 1
En suite: 3
Facilities: TV point

Door lock: ✓
Lockable place: ✓

Services provided
Beauty services: Hairdressing, manicures
Mobile library: ✗
Religious services: Monthly Methodist church services
Transport: ✗
Activities: *Coordinator:* ✗ • *Examples:* Light exercise, reminiscence therapy, visiting entertainers • *Outings:* ✓
Meetings: ✓

Northcourt Lodge

Manager: Rozina Hashwani
Owner: Harbhajan Surdhar and Dr Ramnath Narayan
Contact: 65 Northcourt Avenue, Reading, Berkshire RG2 7HF
☎ 0118 987 5062

Northcourt Lodge is situated in the suburbs of Reading. The home aims for a friendly atmosphere for residents and encourages families to come visit. The activities coordinator helps with individual hobbies being retained such as gardening and singing. Board games and quizzes are also offered for residents to play. There is a garden and patio area for residents to sit out in during the warm weather. Anglican and Catholic ministers visit the home once a fortnight.

Registered places: 22
Guide weekly rate: £450–£650
Specialist care: Nursing, day care, respite
Medical services: Podiatry
Qualified staff: Exceeds standard: 58% at NVQ Level 2

Home details
Location: Residential area, 1.5 miles from Reading centre
Communal areas: Dining room, lounge, patio and garden
Accessibility: *Floors:* 2 • *Access:* Lift • *Wheelchair access:* Good
Smoking: In designated area
Pets: ✗
Routines: Flexible

Room details
Single: 21
Shared: 1
En suite: 9
Facilities: TV point, telephone point

Door lock: ✗
Lockable place: ✓

Services provided
Beauty services: Hairdressing
Mobile library: ✓
Religious services: ✓
Transport: ✗
Activities: *Coordinator:* ✓ • *Examples:* Gardening, singalongs, quizzes • *Outings:* ✓
Meetings: ✗

Registered places: 34
Guide weekly rate: £490–£600
Specialist care: Nursing, respite
Medical services: Podiatry
Qualified staff: Exceeds standard: 88% at NVQ Level 2

Home details

Location: Residential area, in Slough
Communal areas: Lounge, dining room, garden
Accessibility: *Floors:* 2 • *Access:* Lift • *Wheelchair access:* Good
Smoking: In designated area
Pets: ✗
Routines: Flexible

Room details

Single: 28
Shared: 3
En suite: 4
Facilities: TV point

Door lock: ✗
Lockable place: ✓

Services provided

Beauty services: Hairdressing
Mobile library: ✓
Religious services: Weekly nondenominational service
Transport: ✗
Activities: *Coordinator:* ✓ • *Examples:* Arts and crafts, bingo, music and movement • *Outings:* ✗
Meetings: ✗

Oxford House Nursing Home

Manager: Angela Cole
Owner: Edward and Abina Johnston
Contact: 204 Stoke Road, Slough, Berkshire SL2 5AY
☎ 01753 536842
@ info@oxfordhousenursinghome.co.uk
🖰 www.oxfordhousenursinghome.co.uk

Originally an Edwardian house, Oxford House opened in 1980. It is situated in a quiet residential area on the northern outskirts of Slough. The home offers views over an adjoining school playing field. The home organises many activities including bingo, arts and crafts and visiting entertainers. Visits to the library are regular occurrences as well as a mobile library that comes to change books often. There is a Pets As Therapy scheme in place. The staff endeavour to create a warm and caring environment for residents to enjoy and pick up or continue hobbies and activities.

Registered places: 75
Guide weekly rate: £495–£850
Specialist care: Nursing, physical disability, palliative care, respite, terminal care
Medical services: Podiatry, physiotherapy, dentist, optician
Qualified staff: Undisclosed

Home details

Location: Urban area, 1 mile from Reading centre
Communal areas: 3 lounges, dining room, kitchenette, hairdressing salon, garden
Accessibility: *Floors:* 3 • *Access:* Lift • *Wheelchair access:* Good
Smoking: ✗
Pets: ✓
Routines: Flexible

Room details

Single: 75
Shared: 0
En suite: 75
Facilities: TV point, telephone point

Door lock: ✓
Lockable place: ✓

Services provided

Beauty services: Hairdressing, aromatherapy
Mobile library: ✓
Religious services: ✓
Transport: ✗
Activities: *Coordinator:* ✓ • *Examples:* Games, reminiscence sessions • *Outings:* ✓
Meetings: ✗

Parkside House Nursing Home

Manager: Debbie Brewer
Owner: BUPA Care Homes Ltd
Contact: Parkside Road, Reading, Berkshire RG30 2DR
☎ 0118 381 6100
@ ParksidehouseEveryone@BUPA.com
🖰 www.bupacarehomes.co.uk

Parkside House is situated in a residential area of Reading, approximately one mile from the city centre. Opened in summer 2005, it is a purpose-built nursing home designed specifically to meet the needs of elderly residents. Some bedrooms have patio access or views onto the attractive gardens. The lounge and dining room on each floor offer a comfortable area for residents to relax and entertain guests. The home's activities programme features a varied and entertaining social calendar including trips to local places of interest and visits by local entertainers. Personal interests and hobbies, such as arts and crafts, are encouraged.

Pembroke Lodge

Manager: Charles D'Cruz
Owner: Charles D'Cruz
Contact: 32 Alexandra Road, Reading, Berkshire RG1 5PF

📞 0118 926 6255
@ enquires@pembrokelodge.net
🖱 www.pembrokelodge.net

Pembroke Lodge is a large adapted Edwardian house, situated near the town centre of Reading. Toilets and bathrooms are situated on each of its three floors, including a bath with integral hoist and shower on the first floor. Outings to local shops or areas of interest are often organised, and all birthdays are celebrated by the home. Families are welcome to use the facilities of the home for parties. The home has two pet Bichon Frises – a brother and sister, by the names of Benson and Peaches – to provide ad-hoc entertainment. They are very popular amongst the residents.

Registered places: 20
Guide weekly rate: £550–£750
Specialist care: None
Medical services: Podiatry, physiotherapy
Qualified staff: Exceeds standard: 60% at NVQ Level 2

Home details
Location: Residential area, 2.5 miles from Reading centre
Communal areas: Lounge, dining room, garden
Accessibility: *Floors:* 3 • *Access:* Lift • *Wheelchair access:* Good
Smoking: In designated area
Pets: ✓
Routines: Flexible

Room details
Single: 10
Shared: 5
En suite: 0
Facilities: TV point, telephone point

Door lock: ✗
Lockable place: ✓

Services provided
Beauty services: Hairdressing
Mobile library: ✓
Religious services: ✓
Transport: ✓
Activities: *Coordinator:* ✓ • *Examples:* Games, music, bingo
   Outings: ✓
Meetings: ✓

Pinehurst

Manager: Christine Hazlewood
Owner: Pinehurst Care Ltd
Contact: 38–44 Duke's Ride, Crowthorne, Berkshire RG45 6ND

📞 01344 774233
@ pinehurstcare@btconnect.com

Pinehurst is found in the town of Crowthorne, close to local amenities. Its activities programme includes themed events such as garden parties, barbecues, Christmas parties and the occasional outing to the theatre and garden centres. The home is split into three sections: Hurst, Cedar and Pine/Fern, and in these different wings different disabilities are cared for. Pinehurst boasts a Gold Award for their kitchen, offering a wide selection of menus for residents to enjoy. They see mealtimes as a central part of the residents' daily routine and therefore take pride in making sure residents enjoy their food.

Registered places: 50
Guide weekly rate: £499–£535
Specialist care: Respite
Medical services: Podiatry, hygienist, physiotherapy
Qualified staff: Exceeds standard: 97% at NVQ Level 2

Home details
Location: Residential area, 1 mile from Crowhurst centre
Communal areas: 4 lounges, 3 dining rooms, patio and 2 gardens
Accessibility: *Floors:* Undisclosed • *Access:* Undisclosed
   Wheelchair access: Good
Smoking: In designated area
Pets: ✗
Routines: Flexible

Room details
Single: 37
Shared: 13
En suite: 13
Facilities: TV point, telephone point

Door lock: ✓
Lockable place: ✓

Services provided
Beauty services: Hairdressing, manicures
Mobile library: ✗
Religious services: ✓
Transport: ✗
Activities: *Coordinator:* ✗ • *Examples:* Exercise, games, parrot feeding, reminiscence • *Outings:* ✓
Meetings: ✓

Registered places: 137
Guide weekly rate: From £761
Specialist care: Nursing, dementia, respite
Medical services: Podiatry, physiotherapy
Qualified staff: Undisclosed

Home details
Location: Residential area, 1 mile from Tilehurst centre
Communal areas: Dining room, multi-sensory room,
     hairdressing salon, activities rooms, patio and garden
Accessibility: *Floors:* 2 • *Access:* Lift • *Wheelchair access:* Good
Smoking: In designated area
Pets: At manager's discretion
Routines: Structured

Room details
Single: 137
Shared: 0
En suite: 137
Facilities: TV point, telephone point

Door lock: ✓
Lockable place: ✓

Services provided
Beauty services: Hairdressing
Mobile library: ✗
Religious services: ✓
Transport: ✗
Activities: *Coordinator:* ✓ • *Examples:* Reminiscence groups,
     knitting, puzzles • *Outings:* ✗
Meetings: ✓

Riverview Care Home

Manager: Maria Foster
Owner: Southern Cross Healthcare Ltd
Contact: Rodway Road, Tilehurst,
Reading, Berkshire RG30 6TP
☎ 0118 9728360
@ riverview@
     southerncrosshealthcare.co.uk
🖰 www.southerncrosshealthcare.co.uk

Riverview Care Home is well situated, in proximity to the River Thames and local shops. There are a wide range of activities for residents to participate in, run by three activities coordinators, including a multi-sensory room to aid individual or group relaxation. There are budgies in the home, and other pets are allowed, at the discretion of the manager. The Friends of Riverview group ensures good links between the home and community. Where possible, residents are encouraged to integrate into mainstream community resources. Although Riverview is a large home, every effort is taken to create a homely atmosphere for its residents.

Registered places: 25
Guide weekly rate: £500–£700
Specialist care: Respite
Medical services: Physiotherapy
Qualified staff: Meets standard

Home details
Location: Rural area, 1 mile from Ascot centre
Communal areas: Lounge, dining room, conservatory,
     chapel, garden
Accessibility: *Floors:* 2 • *Access:* Lift • *Wheelchair access:* Good
Smoking: In designated area
Pets: ✓
Routines: Flexible

Room details
Single: 17
Shared: 4
En suite: Undisclosed
Facilities: TV, telephone point

Door lock: ✓
Lockable place: ✓

Services provided
Beauty services: Hairdressing, acupuncture, aromatherapy,
     reflexology
Mobile library: ✓
Religious services: Weekly church service
Transport: ✗
Activities: *Coordinator:* ✓ • *Examples:* Bingo, quizzes, exercises
     Outings: ✓
Meetings: ✓

St Christopher's

Manager: Gill Gwyther
Owner: Ascot Residential Homes Ltd
Contact: Ascot Priory, Priory Road,
Ascot, Berkshire SL5 8RS
☎ 01344 891198
@ info@arhltd.com
🖰 www.arhltd.com

St Christopher's is set within 40 acres of grounds at Ascot Priory and offers residential care, while its sister home, St David's, offers a nursing facility. The homes are in close proximity to each other and share many events, creating a communal atmosphere. There is an activities coordinator who organises a range of activities for residents. Services offered at the home include aromatherapy and acupuncture. A mobile library and hairdresser also visit the home. Close links are kept with the local church and a weekly service is held in the home's chapel.

St David's Nursing Home

Manager: Gill Gwyther
Owner: Ascot Residential Homes Ltd
Contact: Ascot Priory, Priory Road, Ascot, Berkshire SL5 8RS

☎ 01344 884079
@ info@arhltd.com
🖰 www.arhltd.com

St David's is situated near its sister home, St Christopher's, in 35 acres of Ascot Priory. The building, which was once part of the priory itself, retains many original features and is adorned with ivy. The home encourages residents to maintain their independence and pursue personal hobbies, as well as arranging activities and outings. It has strong ties with the local church and holds regular services in the home. There is a library at the home that is supplemented by a visiting library, adding new titles regularly to the selection.

Registered places: 39
Guide weekly rate: £500–950
Specialist care: Nursing, respite, terminal care
Medical services: Physiotherapy
Qualified staff: Undisclosed

Home details
Location: Rural area, 1 mile from Ascot centre
Communal areas: Lounge, dining room, conservatory, recourse room, garden
Accessibility: *Floors:* 2 • *Access:* Lift • *Wheelchair access:* Good
Smoking: In designated area
Pets: ✓
Routines: Flexible

Room details
Single: 31
Shared: 5
En suite: Undisclosed
Facilities: TV, telephone point

Door lock: ✓
Lockable place: ✓

Services provided
Beauty services: Hairdressing, aromatherapy, acupuncture
Mobile library: ✓
Religious services: Weekly church service
Transport: ✗
Activities: *Coordinator:* ✓ • *Examples:* Craft, films, musical events
Outings: ✓
Meetings: ✓

St Luke's and The Oaks Residential Home

Manager: Kim Franks
Owner: B&M Care
Contact: Marshlands Square, Caversham, Reading, Berkshire RG4 8RP

☎ 0118 946 1424
@ st.lukesbm@btopenworld.com
🖰 www.bmcare.co.uk

St Luke's and The Oaks is situated in Caversham, just a short distance from the village of Emmer Green and close to Reading. The home is in close proximity to a small parade of shops, and Reading town centre is only a short car journey away. The home is purpose built, and there is a variety of large very well kept, landscaped gardens with different decking areas throughout with level access. Residents have a choice of single, superior single or companion rooms, all with en suite facilities, all of which may be personalised with their own possessions.

Registered places: 80
Guide weekly rate: £600–£700
Specialist care: Dementia, respite
Medical services: Podiatry, physiotherapy
Qualified staff: Exceeds standard: 70% at NVQ Level 2

Home details
Location: Village location, 3 miles from Reading
Communal areas: Lounge, dining room, hairdressing salon, computer access, garden
Accessibility: *Floors:* 1 • *Wheelchair access:* Good
Smoking: ✗
Pets: At manager's discretion
Routines: Flexible

Room details
Single: 74
Shared: 3
En suite: 77
Facilities: TV point, telephone point

Door lock: ✗
Lockable place: ✓

Services provided
Beauty services: Hairdressing
Mobile library: ✓
Religious services: ✓
Transport: ✓
Activities: *Coordinator:* ✓ • *Examples:* Cake-making, crafts, music and movement • *Outings:* ✗
Meetings: ✓

Registered places: 15
Guide weekly rate: £475–£525
Specialist care: None
Medical services: Podiatry
Qualified staff: Undisclosed

Home details

Location: Residential area, 1.5 miles from Reading centre
Communal areas: Lounge, dining room, patio and garden
Accessibility: *Floors:* 2 • *Access:* Lift • *Wheelchair access:* Good
Smoking: In designated area
Pets: ✗
Routines: Flexible

Room details

Single: 11
Shared: 2
En suite: 0
Facilities: TV point, telephone point

Door lock: ✗
Lockable place: ✓

Services provided

Beauty services: Hairdressing, manicures
Mobile library: ✗
Religious services: ✓
Transport: ✓
Activities: *Coordinator:* ✗ • *Examples:* Exercises, word games,
   themed events • *Outings:* ✗
Meetings: ✓

Summerfield

Manager: Tracy Jane Clark
Owner: Colin Robbins
Contact: 4 Kidmore Road,
Caversham Heights, Reading,
Berkshire RG4 7LU
☏ 0118 947 2164

Summerfield is a Victorian property in a quiet residential area on the outskirts of Reading. The home is accessible by public transport, and it is only a 10-minute drive into the centre of Reading town. Activities that the staff organise for residents include keep fit, games, birthday parties, teas and seasonal events such as bonfire night. Often there is a themed night with different foods or costumes. There is a garden with decking area and a gazebo is used for shade in the summer. If residents enjoy gardening they are encourage to help maintain the garden.

Registered places: 47
Guide weekly rate: £301–£500
Specialist care: Respite
Medical services: Podiatry
Qualified staff: Exceeds standard: 70% at NVQ Level 2

Home details

Location: Residential area
Communal areas: Lounge, dining room, patio and garden,
   roof garden
Accessibility: *Floors:* 2 • *Access:* Lift • *Wheelchair access:* Good
Smoking: ✗
Pets: At manager's discretion
Routines: Flexible

Room details

Single: 45
Shared: 1
En suite: 13
Facilities: TV point, telephone point

Door lock: ✓
Lockable place: ✓

Services provided

Beauty services: Hairdressing
Mobile library: ✓
Religious services: Monthly Communion service,
   Anglican and Catholic visits
Transport: ✗
Activities: *Coordinator:* ✗ • *Examples:* Arts and crafts, exercise,
   musical entertainment • *Outings:* ✗
Meetings: ✓

Trafalgar Court

Manager: Valerie Fearns
Owner: Sovereign Housing Association
Contact: Play Platt, Theale, Reading,
Berkshire RG7 5HW
☏ 0118 930 2029

Trafalgar Court is situated is a quiet residential area, close to local amenities. The home also has a sensory garden, snooker table, bar, and sky on a wide screen TV. The home also class this as the residents' home and aim to provide as much care as possible without infringing upon their dignity and independence. Although the home does not have an activities coordinator, care workers organise activities with residents such as art and musical entertainment.

The Whispers Care Home

Manager: Mohanjit Hyare
Owner: Mohanjit Hyare
Contact: 30 Rambler Lane, Langley, Slough, Berkshire SL3 7RR
☎ 01753 527300

A small home set in a quiet cul-de-sac, The Whispers is located one and a half miles from Slough town centre. The town offers an extensive variety of amenities including shops, restaurants, pubs and Upton Hospital. There are extensive local and national transport links surrounding the home. To the rear of the home is a large garden with seating area for residents' use.

Registered places: 19
Guide weekly rate: £430–£550
Specialist care: Respite
Medical services: Podiatry, dentist, optician, physiotherapy
Qualified staff: Exceeds standard: 75% at NVQ Level 2

Home details
Location: Residential area, 1.5 miles from Slough
Communal areas: Lounge, dining room, conservatory, garden
Accessibility: *Floors:* 1 • *Wheelchair access:* Good
Smoking: ✗
Pets: ✓
Routines: Flexible

Room details
Single: 17
Shared: 1
En suite: 19
Facilities: TV point, telephone point

Door lock: ✓
Lockable place: ✓

Services provided
Beauty services: Hairdressing, manicures
Mobile library: ✗
Religious services: Monthly Anglican services
Transport: ✗
Activities: *Coordinator:* ✗ • *Examples:* Games, passive exercise, singalongs • *Outings:* ✓
Meetings: ✓

Wild Acres Rest Home

Manager: Janet Elliott
Owner: Harbhajan Surdhar
Contact: 440 Finchampstead Road, Finchampstead, Wokingham, Berkshire RG40 3RB
☎ 0118 973 3670
@ wildacresresthome@tiscali.co.uk

Set back from the road, Wild Acres is situated a short walk from local amenities which can be easily accessed by public transport. Each en suite bedroom opens out onto the garden's raised terrace where there are views of the surrounding countryside. The home has a lounge with a TV, a dining room and three communal bathrooms, one of which is a wet room. Pets are allowed and the home has its own cat. There are outings to nearby garden centres and country parks. The home has its own transport and access to a mobile library.

Registered places: 20
Guide weekly rate: £500
Specialist care: None
Medical services: Podiatry, dentist, optician.
Qualified staff: Exceeds standard: 60% at NVQ Level 2

Home details
Location: Village location, 4 miles from Wokingham
Communal areas: Lounge, dining room, garden
Accessibility: *Floors:* 1 • *Wheelchair access:* Good
Smoking: ✗
Pets: ✓
Routines: Flexible

Room details
Single: 20
Shared: 0
En suite: 5
Facilities: TV point, telephone

Door lock: ✓
Lockable place: ✓

Services provided
Beauty services: Hairdressing, manicures
Mobile library: ✓
Religious services: Monthly Communion service
Transport: ✓
Activities: *Coordinator:* ✓ • *Examples:* Quizzes, chair exercises, reminiscence sessions • *Outings:* ✓
Meetings: ✓

Registered places: 45
Guide weekly rate: £550–£825
Specialist care: Nursing, dementia
Medical services: Podiatry
Qualified staff: Meets standard

Home details
Location: Rural area, on the outskirts of Farley Hill near Reading
Communal areas: Lounge, dining room, garden
Accessibility: *Floors:* Undisclosed • *Access:* Undisclosed
   Wheelchair access: Good
Smoking: In designated area
Pets: ✗
Routines: Flexible

Room details
Single: 43
Shared: 2
En suite: 45
Facilities: TV point, telephone point

Door lock: ✗
Lockable place: ✓

Services provided
Beauty services: Hairdressing
Mobile library: ✓
Religious services: ✓
Transport: ✓
Activities: *Coordinator:* ✓ • *Examples:* Painting/drawing,
   country walks, gardening • *Outings:* ✓
Meetings: ✓

Woodbury House

Manager: Sara Baker
Owner: Exceler Healthcare Services Ltd
Contact: Joulding Lane, Farley Hill,
Swallowfield, Berkshire RG7 1UR
  ☎ 0118 9733885

Woodbury House is a large converted country house that has views across the Berkshire countryside on the outskirts of Farley Hill near Reading. It is not close to any shops, however the home has it's own transport to there are regular shopping trips into Reading town centre. Daily activities include gardening, country walks and painting and drawing. If residents enjoy gardening, they are welcome to help maintain the garden as a hobby.

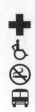

Ashby House

Manager: Karen Welch
Owner: Barchester Healthcare Ltd
Contact: 100 Chadwick Drive, Milton Keynes. Buckinghamshire MK6 5LS
) 01908 696676
@ ashby@barchester.net
www.barchester.com

Ashby House is a purpose-built home situated in a residential area three miles from the town of Milton Keynes. The home has a lounge and a quiet room, as well as large gardens. The home arranges for visiting entertainers to come to the home and there are also regular meetings with residents and their relatives. The home holds an Anglican service once a month and there is a Communion service held on a weekly basis. The home has its own minibus and takes residents on outings in the local area.

Registered places: 64
Guide weekly rate: £545–£1,094
Specialist care: Nursing, dementia, respite
Medical services: Podiatry, optician, physiotherapy
Qualified staff: Meets standard

Home details
Location: Residential area, 3 miles from Milton Keynes
Communal areas: 2 lounges, dining room, garden
Accessibility: *Floors:* 1 • *Wheelchair access:* Good
Smoking: ✗
Pets: ✗
Routines: Flexible

Room details
Single: 64
Shared: 0
En suite: 64
Facilities: None

Door lock: ✓
Lockable place: ✓

Services provided
Beauty services: Hairdressing
Mobile library: ✓
Religious services: Monthly Anglican service, weekly Communion service
Transport: Minibus
Activities: *Coordinator:* ✓ • *Examples:* Visiting entertainers *Outings:* ✓
Meetings: ✓

Becket House Nursing Home

Manager: Olusegun Adetunji
Owner: C Jeyaratnam
Contact: Pitcher Lane, Loughton Village, Milton Keynes, Buckinghamshire MK5 8AU
) 01908 231981

Becket House is situated in a quiet residential area, a short distance from central Milton Keynes. Milton Keynes has numerous shops and other local amenities and is served by local and national rail and bus links. The residents benefit from a flexible daily routine with set meal times. Pets are not allowed but the home provides services such as hairdressing and arranges for a vicar to visit every fortnight.

Registered places: 27
Guide weekly rate: £529–£550
Specialist care: Nursing, dementia
Medical services: Podiatry, dentist, hygienist, optician, physiotherapy
Qualified staff: Exceeds standard: 98% at NVQ Level 2

Home details
Location: Residential area, 5.5 miles from Milton Keynes
Communal areas: 3 lounges, dining room, garden
Accessibility: *Floors:* 2 • *Access:* Lift • *Wheelchair access:* Good
Smoking: ✗
Pets: ✗
Routines: Flexible

Room details
Single: 23
Double: 2
En suite: 11
Facilities: TV, telephone point

Door lock: ✗
Lockable place: ✗

Services provided
Beauty services: Hairdressing
Mobile library: ✗
Religious services: ✓
Transport: ✗
Activities: *Coordinator:* ✓ • *Examples:* Knitting, singing, visiting entertainers • *Outings:* ✓
Meetings: ✗

Registered places: 32
Guide weekly rate: £495–£510
Specialist care: Dementia, learning disability
Medical services: Podiatry, optician
Qualified staff: Exceeds standard: 60% at NVQ Level 2

Home details

Location: Residential area, 0.5 miles from Newport Pagnell
Communal areas: 3 lounges, dining room, garden
Accessibility: *Floors:* 2 • *Access:* Stair lift
Wheelchair access: Limited
Smoking: ✓
Pets: ✓
Routines: Structured

Room details

Single: 18
Shared:
En suite: 11
Facilities: TV point, telephone point

Door lock: ✗
Lockable place: ✓

Services provided

Beauty services: Hairdressing
Mobile library: ✓
Religious services: Monthly church service
Transport: ✗
Activities: *Coordinator:* ✗ • *Examples:* Bingo, newspaper night
Outings: ✗
Meetings: ✗

The Beeches

Manager: Annmarie Sweeney
Owner: Brancaster Care Homes Ltd
Contact: 16 Lakes Lane,
Newport Pagnell, Buckinghamshire
MK16 8HP
☏ 01908 210650
@ thebeeches@
brancastercarehomes.co.uk
🖥 www.brancastercarehomes.co.uk

The Beeches is a two-storey care home divided into three areas. It is in a residential area in Newport Pagnell, a five-minute walk to the high street where there is an abundance of shops and facilities. The home does not have an activities coordinator because they feel it is an equal responsibility for every staff member to make sure the residents stay active by organising activities such as bingo night and cooking night. The home is also animal friendly and has visit from Pets As Therapy once a week. Residents' animals are also welcome to come and visit at any time.

Registered places: 41
Guide weekly rate: £568–£653
Specialist care: None
Medical services: Podiatry, physiotherapy
Qualified staff: Exceeds standard: 87% at NVQ Level 2

Home details

Location: Residential area, 1 mile from Beaconsfield centre
Communal areas: 5 lounges, dining room, 4 kitchenettes,
patio and garden
Accessibility: *Floors:* 2 • *Access:* Lift • *Wheelchair access:* Good
Smoking: In designated area
Pets: At manager's discretion
Routines: Flexible

Room details

Single: 30
Shared: 1
En suite: 40
Facilities: TV point, telephone point

Door lock: ✓
Lockable place: ✓

Services provided

Beauty services: Hairdressing
Mobile library: ✓
Religious services: ✓
Transport: ✗
Activities: *Coordinator:* ✓ • *Examples:* Arts and crafts, cake making,
music and movement • *Outings:* ✓
Meetings: ✗

Bradbury House

Manager: Wendy Stallwood
Owner: Abbeyfield Society Ltd
Contact: Windsor End, Beaconsfield,
Buckinghamshire HP9 2JW
☏ 01494 671780
@ wendys@bradburyhouse.co.uk
🖥 www.bradburyhouse.co.uk

Bradbury House is a purpose-built care home with accessible, well-kept gardens. The home focuses on retaining residents' dignity and independence and aims to promote socialising. There are meetings organised for staff and residents to get together and discuss any items or issues residents might have. The staff acknowledge that the home is the home of the residents and aim to create a comfortable and caring environment. There is a weekly Anglican service in the home.

Byron House Nursing Home

Manager: Sheila James
Owner: Mr and Mrs Patel
Contact: 141–143 Wendover Road, Aylesbury, Buckinghamshire HP21 9LP
☎ 01296 424325

Byron House Nursing Home is situated two miles outside the town of Aylesbury, and a small distance from local shops. The home comprises of a large landscaped garden which has a seating area, level access and a sun umbrella. There is a multi-discipline team which sees to the needs of all residents and makes sure they are happy and comfortable at all times. A dietician also regularly visits to ensure the residents are receiving a healthy balanced diet, and are happy with the meals that are being provided.

Registered places: 33
Guide weekly rate: £472–£600
Specialist care: Nursing, respite
Medical services: Podiatry, dietician, physiotherapy
Qualified staff: Meets standard

Home details

Location: Residential area, 2 miles from Aylesbury
Communal areas: Lounge, dining room, quite room, garden
Accessibility: *Floors:* 3 • *Access:* Lift • *Wheelchair access:* Good
Smoking: ✗
Pets: ✗
Routines: Flexible

Room details

Single: 19
Shared: 7
En suite: 0
Facilities: TV point

Door lock: ✗
Lockable place: ✓

Services provided

Beauty services: Hairdressing
Mobile library: ✓
Religious services: ✓
Transport: ✗
Activities: *Coordinator:* ✓ • *Examples:* Quizzes, painting, knitting, drawing • *Outings:* ✓
Meetings: ✓

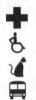

Castle Mead Court

Manager: Tracy Shepherd
Owner: Excelcare Holdings
Contact: Wolverton Road, Newport Pagnell, Buckinghamshire MK16 8HW
☎ 020 8313 5000
@ tracy.shepherd@ excelcareholdings.com

Castle Mead Court is a purpose-built home located in Newton Pagnell. The home has direct access the high street and its amenities. The home has ample communal space including a computer with internet access. The home has an enclosed garden with a patio and decking area. There is an activities coordinator who arranges seasonal parties for the residents, for example at Halloween and daily activities which include baking and quizzes. The home also arranges visits to other homes for tea parties.

Registered places: 79
Guide weekly rate: £575–£700
Specialist care: Nursing, dementia, respite
Medical services: Podiatry, dentist, optician
Qualified staff: Meets standard

Home details

Location: Residential area, 4.5 miles from Milton Keynes
Communal areas: 3 lounges, 2 quiet rooms, 3 dining rooms, prayer room, hairdressing salon, patio and garden
Accessibility: *Floors:* 3 • *Access:* Lift • *Wheelchair access:* Good
Smoking: In designated area
Pets: ✓
Routines: Flexible

Room details

Single: 79
Shared: 0
En suite: 79
Facilities: None

Door lock: ✓
Lockable place: ✓

Services provided

Beauty services: Hairdressing
Mobile library: ✓
Religious services: Monthly service
Transport: Minibus
Activities: *Coordinator:* ✓ • *Examples:* Baking, bingo, visiting entertainers • *Outings:* ✓
Meetings: Monthly

Registered places: 60
Guide weekly rate: £800
Specialist care: Nursing, day care, dementia, respite
Medical services: Podiatry
Qualified staff: Undisclosed

Home details
Location: Residential area, 3 miles from High Wycombe centre
Communal areas: 4 lounges, 2 dining rooms, garden
Accessibility: *Floors:* 2 • *Access:* Lift • *Wheelchair access:* Good
Smoking: x
Pets: x
Routines: Flexible

Room details
Single: 52
Shared: 4
En suite: 56
Facilities: TV point, telephone point

Door lock: ✓
Lockable place: ✓

Services provided
Beauty Services: Hairdressing
Mobile library: x
Religious services: ✓
Transport: x
Activities: *Coordinators:* 3 • *Examples:* Arts and crafts, games, quizzes • *Outings:* ✓
Meetings: x

Catherine Court Nursing Home

Manager: Ann Hill
Owner: Community Health Services Ltd
Contact: Cressex Road, Booker, High Wycombe, Buckinghamshire HP12 4QF
) 01494 524850
@ manager.catherinecourt@careuk.com
⌂ www.careuk.com

Situated approximately three miles from High Wycombe town centre, Catherine Court Nursing Home is a purpose-built home with a spacious rear garden. The home is set in a residential area and the town possesses a variety of shops and local amenities, and provides access to local and national transport networks. There is a keypad security system at entrance to the home. The home has weekly visits from an Anglican minister.

Registered places: 20
Guide weekly rate: £580–£600
Specialist care: Respite
Medical services: Podiatry
Qualified staff: Undisclosed

Home details
Location: Residential area, 300 yards from centre of Wendover
Communal areas: Lounge, conservatory/dining room
Accessibility: *Floors:* 1 • *Wheelchair access:* Good
Smoking: x
Pets: ✓
Routines: Flexible

Room details
Single: 20
Double: 0
En suite: 5
Facilities: TV point, telephone point

Door lock: x
Lockable place: ✓

Services provided
Beauty services: x
Mobile library: x
Religious services: x
Transport: x
Activities: *Coordinator:* x • *Examples:* Bingo, exercise, quizzes • *Outings:* ✓
Meetings: ✓

Cherry Tree House

Manager: Janet Parker
Owner: Peter Hall and Janet Parker
Contact: 49 Dobbins Lane, Wendover, Aylesbury, Buckinghamshire HP22 6DH
) 01296 623350

Cherry Tree House is a private care home in the village of Wendover, 300 yards from the centre of town. Residents enjoy outings to the local garden centre to choose plants and flowers for the garden. The conservatory, which doubles as a dining area, looks out onto the garden which has a fishpond. There is a seating area in the garden which residents enjoy to sit at when the weather is nice. In good weather coffee mornings are transferred into the garden for residents to enjoy the sun.

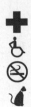

Cherry Tree Nursing Home

Manager: Maxine Bennell
Owner: A Dhot
Contact: Bledlow Road, Saunderton, Princes Risborough, Buckinhamshire HP27 9NG
) 01844 346259

Cherry Tree is situated in a rural location, close to the market town of Princes Risborough. The garden is well maintained with a millstream and large millpond, which attracts wildlife and birds. There is a patio area with wheelchair access and shaded seating throughout the garden. Seasonal social occasions are arranged, such as an annual Strawberry Tea day, to which relatives are also invited. The remote location of the home makes interaction with a community difficult, but is solved by bringing groups to the home.

Registered places: 42
Guide weekly rate: £670–690
Specialist care: Nursing
Medical services: Podiatry
Qualified staff: Fails standard: 18% at NVQ Level 2

Home details
Location: Residential area, 1 mile from Princes Risborough centre
Communal areas: Lounge, dining room, conservatory, garden
Accessibility: *Floors:* 2 • *Access:* Lift • *Wheelchair access:* Good
Smoking: ✗
Pets: At manager's discretion
Routines: Flexible

Room details
Single: 42
Shared: 0
En suite: 0
Facilities: None

Door lock: ✓
Lockable place: ✓

Services provided
Beauty services: Hairdressing
Mobile library: ✗
Religious service: Monthly
Transport: ✗
Activities: *Coordinator:* ✓ • *Examples:* Quizzes, bingo, charades
Outings: ✗
Meetings: ✗

Chiltern View Nursing Home

Manager: Susan Lovelace
Owner: The Brendoncare Foundation
Contact: St John's Drive, Stone, Aylesbury, Buckinghamshire HP17 8PP
) 01296 747463
@ slovelace@brendoncare.org.uk
www.brendoncare.org.uk

Divided into two distinct units and catering primarily for those suffering from dementia, Chiltern View is situated in the village of Stone and permits residents rural views of the countryside to the Chiltern Hills. Although it is a quiet village, there are still main bus routes to Oxford, Thame and Aylsebury. The well maintained landscaped gardens are easily accessible to residents and have been designed to promote interest in gardening.

Registered places: 31
Guide weekly rate: £847
Specialist care: Nursing, dementia, mental disorder
Medical services: Podiatry, physiotherapy
Qualified staff: Exceeds standard: 70% at NVQ level 2

Home details
Location: Residential area, 2 miles from Aylesbury
Communal areas: Undisclosed
Accessibility: *Floors:* Undisclosed • *Access:* Lift
Wheelchair access: Good
Smoking: ✗
Pets: ✗
Routines: Flexible

Room details
Single: 26
Shared: 2
En suite: 0
Facilities: TV point, telephone point

Door lock: ✗
Lockable place: ✗

Services provided
Beauty services: Hairdressing
Mobile library: ✗
Religious services: Weekly Catholic visits
Transport: ✗
Activities: *Coordinator:* ✓ • *Examples:* Visiting entertainer
Outings: ✗
Meetings: ✓

Registered places: 45
Guide weekly rate: From £900
Specialist care: Nursing, respite
Medical services: Podiatry, physiotherapy, reflexology
Qualified staff: Meets standard

Home details

Location: Residential area, 10 miles to Aylesbury
Communal areas: Lounge, dining room, exercise room, hairdressing salon, library, garden
Accessibility: *Floors:* 3 • *Access:* Lift • *Wheelchair access:* Good
Pets: At manager's discretion
Smoking: ✗
Routines: Flexible

Room details

Single: 45
Shared: 0
En suite: 45
Facilities: TV, telephone

Door lock: ✗
Lockable place: ✓

Services provided

Beauty Services: Hairdressing, beautician, massages, manicures, pedicures
Mobile library: ✗
Religious services: Monthly Anglican Communion service
Transport: Cars
Activities: *Coordinator:* ✗ • *Examples:* Book club, bridge games, pianist • *Outings:* ✓
Meetings: ✗

Chilton House

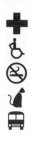

Manager: Lynne Breakell
Owner: Chilton House Ltd
Contact: Chilton, Aylesbury, Buckinghamshire HP18 9LR
☎ 01844 265200
@ enquiries@chiltonhouse.co.uk
🖰 www.chiltonhouse.co.uk

Chilton House is a Grade II listed manor house, situated in countryside 20 minutes from Oxford. The home aims to support residents' style of life and adapt to cater for individual needs. Residents are welcome to join in the varied weekly activities, or enjoy their surroundings in one of the quiet seating areas or terrace. Although the home is not served by public transport links, it possesses two cars which ensure residents can visit local attractions and amenities. Some ground floor rooms have French doors opening on to a terrace. A daily newspaper is included in the fees.

Registered places: 26
Guide weekly rate: From £530
Specialist care: Respite
Medical services: Podiatry, dentist, optician, physiotherapy
Qualified staff: Exceeds standard: 97% at NVQ Level 2

Home details

Location: Rural area, 5 miles to Milton Keynes
Communal areas: 2 lounges, conservatory/dining room, library, garden
Accessibility: *Floors:* 2 • *Access:* 2 lifts • *Wheelchair access:* Good
Smoking: ✗
Pets: ✗
Routines: Flexible

Room details

Single: 20
Shared: 3
En suite: 20
Facilities: TV, telephone point

Door lock: ✗
Lockable place: ✓

Services provided

Beauty services: Hairdressing, aromatherapy, manicures
Mobile library: Library facilities
Religious services: ✓
Transport: ✗
Activities: *Coordinator:* ✓ • *Examples:* Arts and crafts, bingo, singalongs, board games • *Outings:* ✓
Meetings: ✓

Devon Lodge Retirement Home

Manager: Elizabeth Fellows
Owner: Amberley Healthcare Ltd
Contact: 18 Theydon Avenue, Woburn Sands, Milton Keynes, Buckinghamshire MK17 8PL
☎ 01908 281470
@ Elizabeth@devonlodgecare.co.uk
🖰 www.devonlodgecare.co.uk

Devon Lodge is a two-storey retirement home located in the village of Woburn Sands, a five-minute drive to Milton Keynes. The home has three lounges which serve as a main TV lounge, a quiet room and a conservatory. The home also has a separate dining room and library facilities. The books in the library are changed regularly. The staff are insured to drive the residents and take the residents on outings to the garden centre. There are regular residents meetings. Although pets are not allowed the manager and staff regularly bring pets to visit the residents.

Fayreways

Manager: Carmen Burnham
Owner: Carmen Burnham
Contact: Main Street,
Grendon Underwood, Buckinghamshire
HP18 0SP
☎ 01296 770620

This home is situated in a rural area a conservatory for residents to enjoy in the summer. Menus are varied and reflective of the season. These meals can be taken into the residents' own bedroom if wished. Three cooked meals a day are offered with drinks made readily available. Transport to church services is arranged by the home.

Registered places: 12
Guide weekly rate: £500
Specialist care: Nursing, dementia
Medical services: Podiatry
Qualified staff: Undisclosed

Home details
Location: Rural area, 10.5 miles from Aylesbury
Communal areas: Lounge, dining room, conservatory, garden
Accessibility: *Floors:* 2 • *Access:* Stair lift
    Wheelchair access: Limited
Smoking: ✗
Pets: ✗
Routines: Flexible

Room details
Single: 8	**Door lock:** ✓
Shared: 2	**Lockable place:** ✓
En suite: 0	
Facilities: TV, telephone	

Services provided
Beauty Services: Hairdressing
Mobile library: ✗
Religious services: ✓
Transport: ✗
Activities: *Coordinator:* ✓ • *Examples:* Arts and crafts, bingo
    Outings: ✗
Meetings: ✗

Five Acres Nursing Home

Manager: Terri Walker
Owner: Five Acres Nursing Home Ltd
Contact: Simpson Village, Milton Keynes,
Buckinghamshire MK6 3AD
☎ 01908 690292

Five Acres is an older building set in private grounds in Simpson. The village of Simpson is situated on the outskirts of Milton Keynes, with public transport links into the city centre where there is an abundance of shops and facilities. The home offers Independent Living Training, as staff think it is important for residents to stay as proactive and independent as they possibly can.

Registered places: 32
Guide weekly rate: £540–£670
Specialist care: Nursing, dementia
Medical services: Podiatry, physiotherapy
Qualified staff: Meets standard

Home details
Location: Residential area, 3 miles to Milton Keynes
Communal areas: Lounge, dining room, garden
Accessibility: *Floors:* Undisclosed • *Access:* Undisclosed
    Wheelchair access: Good
Smoking: In designated area
Pets: ✓
Routines: Structured

Room details
Single: 20	**Door lock:** ✗
Shared: 6	**Lockable place:** ✓
En suite: 1	
Facilities: TV point	

Services provided
Beauty Services: Hairdressing
Mobile library: ✓
Religious services: Monthly church services
Transport: ✗
Activities: *Coordinator:* ✓ • *Examples:* Sewing, flower arranging,
    gardening • *Outings:* ✗
Meetings: ✓

Registered places: 8
Guide weekly rate: £493–£503
Specialist care: Respite
Medical services: Podiatry, hygienist, optician, physiotherapy
Qualified staff: Exceeds standard: 80% at NVQ Level 2

Home details

Location: Residential area, 3 miles from High Wycombe
Communal areas: Lounge, lounge/dining room, garden
Accessibility: *Floors:* 2 • *Access:* None
    Wheelchair access: Limited
Smoking: ✗
Pets: ✓
Routines: Flexible

Room details

Single: 8
Shared: 0
En suite: 1
Facilities: TV point, telephone point

Door lock: ✗
Lockable place: ✓

Services provided

Beauty services: Hairdressing, massages
Mobile library: ✓
Religious services: ✓
Transport: ✗
Activities: *Coordinator:* ✗ • *Examples:* Board games, gentle exercise, knitting • *Outings:* ✓
Meetings: ✗

The Havens

Manager: Wendy Harris
Owner: Wendy Harris
Contact: 13–20 Derehams Lane,
Loudwater, High Wycombe,
Buckinghamshire HP10 9RH
✆ 01494 532709
@ wendyharris@waitrose.com

The Havens care home consists of two small houses opposite each other on a small country lane in Loudwater near High Wycombe. One house is the residence of the manager and her husband and five residents. It is on two floors, and does not have a lift or stair lift. Over the road, a bungalow provides accommodation and has its own lounge/dining area. The Home also has a Cinnamon Trust certificate that enables residents to have pets as companions.

Registered places: 41
Guide weekly rate: Undisclosed
Specialist care: Nursing, dementia, palliative care, respite, terminal care
Medical services: Podiatry, physiotherapy
Qualified staff: Undisclosed

Home details

Location: Residential area, 2.5 miles from Milton Keynes centre
Communal areas: 5 lounges, dining room, activities room, hairdressing salon, kitchenette, garden
Accessibility: *Floors:* 2 • *Access:* Lift • *Wheelchair access:* Good
Smoking: In designated area
Pets: ✓
Routines: Flexible

Room details

Single: 37
Shared: 4
En suite: 26
Facilities: TV, telephone point

Door lock: ✓
Lockable place: ✗

Services provided

Beauty services: Hairdressing, aromatherapy
Mobile library: ✗
Transport: ✓
Religious services: Monthly church service
Activities: *Coordinator:* ✓ • *Examples:* Card games gardening, board games • *Outings:* ✓
Meetings: ✗

Highclere Nursing Home

Manager: Cheryl Edwards
Owner: BUPA Care Homes Ltd
Contact: Chapman Avenue,
Downs Barn, Milton Keynes,
Buckinghamshire MK14 7NH
✆ 01908 667568
@ HighclereALL@BUPA.com
🌐 www.bupacarehomes.com

Situated in a residential area and within walking distance of local amenities, Highclere is a purpose-built nursing home specially designed for the elderly. It is set in beautiful landscaped grounds with attractive shrubs and flowers. Highclere has been thoughtfully laid out with several lounges and has a light spacious dining room, which overlooks the attractive gardens. Most of the bedrooms offer en suite facilities and are light and airy. Daily activities include flower arranging, gardening and board games. Highclere offers nursing care, dementia care and palliative and terminal care.

Hillside Nursing Home

Manager: Elizabeth Nicholas
Owner: Trinity Care Ltd
Contact: Bicester Road, Aylesbury,
Buckinghamshire HP19 8AB
☎ 01296 710011

Divided into three distinct units, Hillside Nursing Home accommodates individuals with a range of needs. The home has 11 places allocated to younger adults with physical disabilities. The home is situated in the centre of Aylesbury town and is therefore very central and accessible to shops and amenities. The home also has its own minibus to take residents on outings which occur twice monthly. Pets are welcome to come and visit.

Registered places: 67
Guide weekly rate: £481–£1,143
Specialist care: Nursing, day care, dementia, physical disability, respite
Medical services: Podiatry, physiotherapy
Qualified staff: Undisclosed

Home details
Location: Urban area, in Aylesbury
Communal areas: Lounge, hairdressing salon, patio and garden
Accessibility: *Floors:* Undisclosed • *Access:* Undisclosed
  Wheelchair access: Undisclosed
Smoking: ✗
Pets: ✗
Routines: Flexible

Room details
Single: 67
Shared: 0
En suite: 67
Facilities: TV point, telephone point

Door lock: ✗
Lockable place: ✓

Services provided
Beauty Services: Undisclosed
Mobile library: ✗
Religious services: ✓
Transport: ✓
Activities: *Coordinator:* ✓ • *Examples:* Audio books • *Outings:* ✓
Meetings: ✓

Kents Hill Care Home

Manager: Karen Daw
Owner: James Halton and
Mr and Mrs Dhanani
Contact: Tunbridge Grove, Kents Hill,
Milton Keynes, Buckinghamshire
MK7 6JD
☎ 01908 355900
@ susan.gildner@carebase.org.uk
🖰 www.carebase.org.uk

Kents Hill Care Home is purpose-built facility in the centre of Milton Keynes. The home hosts 'sherry mornings' and arranges Pets As Therapy visits for the residents. There is an enclosed spacious garden with seating area for residents to enjoy. There is CCTV monitoring in the home and a keypad security system at the entrance.

Registered places: 62
Guide weekly rate: £550–£700
Specialist care: Nursing, dementia, respite
Medical services: Podiatry, physiotherapy
Qualified staff: Exceeds standard: 100% at NVQ Level 2

Home details
Location: Urban area, in Milton Keynes
Communal areas: 3 lounges, dining room, conservatory, garden
Accessibility: *Floors:* 3 • *Access:* 2 lifts • *Wheelchair access:* Good
Smoking: In designated area
Pets: At manager's discretion
Routines: Flexible

Room details
Single: 62
Shared: 0
En suite: 62
Facilities: TV point, telephone point

Door lock: ✓
Lockable place: ✓

Services provided
Beauty services: Hairdressing, manicures.
Mobile library: ✗
Religious services: Monthly multi-faith services
Transport: ✗
Activities: *Coordinator:* ✓ • *Examples:* Cooking, flower arranging, games • *Outings:* ✗
Meetings: ✗

Registered places: 46
Guide weekly rate: £650–£850
Specialist care: Nursing
Medical services: Podiatry, dentist, optician
Qualified staff: Exceeds standard: 75% at NVQ Level 2

Home details
Location: Village location, 4 miles from Marlow
Communal areas: 2 lounges, dining room, library,
    patio and garden
Accessibility: *Floors:* 2 • *Access:* Lift • *Wheelchair access:* Good
Smoking: ✗
Pets: At manager's discretion
Routines: Flexible

Room details
Single: 25
Shared: 9
En suite: 15
Facilities: TV point, telephone point

Door lock: ✓
Lockable place: ✓

Services provided
Beauty services: Hairdressing
Mobile library: ✗
Religious services: ✓
Transport: ✗
Activities: *Coordinator:* ✓ • *Examples:* Bingo, quizzes, music,
    school visits • *Outings:* ✓
Meetings: ✓

Kingfishers Nursing Home

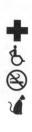

Manager: Shelley Ackland-Snow
Owner: Kingfisher Carehome Ltd
Contact: Fieldhead Gardens, Bourne End,
Buckinghamshire SL8 5RA
☎ 01628 520020
@ King.scare@aol.com

Kingfishers Nursing Home is a large three-storey Edwardian house situated in the village of Bourne End, close to the shops and amenities of a small town. Marlow and the River Thames are a short drive away. There is a train station 200 yards away.

The property has been sympathetically adapted and extended to meet the needs of its residents. Pets are allowed at the manager's discretion but there are visits from therapy dogs as part of the activities program. Communion is offered every month with weekly visits from other religious denominations.

Registered places: 59
Guide weekly rate: £550–£880
Specialist care: Nursing
Medical services: Podiatry, dentist, optician, physiotherapy
Qualified staff: Meets standard

Home details
Location: Residential area, 1 mile from Aylesbury
Communal areas: Lounge, dining room, patio and garden
Accessibility: *Floors:* 3 • *Access:* None
    Wheelchair access: Limited
Smoking: In designated area
Pets: ✓
Routines: Flexible

Room details
Single: 53
Shared: 6
En suite: Undisclosed
Facilities: TV point, telephone point

Door lock: ✓
Lockable place: ✓

Services provided
Beauty services: Hairdressing, aromatherapy
Mobile library: ✗
Religious services: Weekly church service
Transport: ✗
Activities: *Coordinator:* ✓ • *Examples:* Raffles, seasonal activities
    Outings: ✓
Meetings: ✓

Lakeside Nursing Home

Manager: Angela Jones
Owner: Ashbourne Homes Ltd
Contact: Brambling, Watermead,
Aylesbury, Buckinghamshire HP19 3WH
☎ 01296 393166

Lakeside is a purpose-built home in Watermead. The garden leads down to the lake and the home has views from bedrooms, the lounge and veranda leading off it. Residents are allowed to choose how to spend and what to do with their day. There is a good activities coordinator, who organises regular group programmes or activities for individuals. The standard of cleanliness is good, enabling residents to live in a comfortable place environment.

Lathbury Manor Residential Home for the Elderly

Manager: Gillian Broadway

Owner: Edward and Gillian Broadway

Contact: Lathbury, Nr Newport, Pagnell, Buckinghamshire MK16 8JX

☎ 01908 615245

Lathbury Manor specialises in dementia care and has recently received government funding to increase their facilities for dementia sufferers. There is one TV lounge and one activities lounge. Visiting entertainers often come in for activities such as art and music and movement sessions. There is also a garden for residents to enjoy. For more frail users, adjustable beds have been provided to offer more comfort.

Registered places: 23

Guide weekly rate: £475

Specialist care: Dementia, learning disability, physical disability

Medical services: Podiatry, hygienist, optician, physiotherapy

Qualified staff: Exceeds standard: 85% at NVQ Level 2

Home details

Location: Rural area, 13 miles from Bedford

Communal areas: 3 lounges, dining room garden

Accessibility: *Floors:* 2 • *Access:* Lift • *Wheelchair access:* Good

Smoking: In designated area

Pets: At manager's discretion

Routines: Flexible

Room details

Single: 20

Shared: 2

En suite: 0

Facilities: TV point, telephone point

Door lock: ✗

Lockable place: ✓

Services provided

Beauty services: Hairdressing

Mobile library: ✓

Religious services: Monthly visits from local vicar

Transport: ✓

Activities: *Coordinator:* ✗ • *Examples:* Arts and crafts, music and movement • *Outings:* ✗

Meetings: ✓

The Leonard Pulham

Manager: Kim Anwyl

Owner: Abbeyfield Society Ltd

Contact: Tring Road, Halton, Aylesbury, Buckinghamshire HP22 5PN

☎ 01296 625188

The Leonard Pulham nursing home is a purpose-built home, situated on the edge of the Chilterns, just outside Wendover. The home maintains close links with the Royal Air Force and is adjacent to the RAF at Halton. Out of the 33 beds, the home maintains five RAF beds and three Masonic beds. The home's dining room overlooks a large garden, which is well maintained and has seating outside for residents to socialise.

Registered places: 33

Guide weekly rate: £794

Specialist care: Nursing

Medical services: Podiatry, hygienist, optician

Qualified staff: Meets standard

Home details

Location: Residential area, 6 miles from Aylesbury

Communal areas: 3 lounges, dining room, garden

Accessibility: *Floors:* 2 • *Access:* Lift • *Wheelchair access:* Good

Smoking: ✗

Pets: ✗

Routines: Flexible

Room details

Single: 33

Shared: 0

En suite: 1

Facilities: TV point, telephone point

Door lock: ✗

Lockable place: ✓

Services provided

Beauty services: Hairdressing

Mobile library: ✓

Religious services: Monthly

Transport: ✗

Activities: *Coordinator:* ✗ • *Examples:* Bingo, dominoes, exercise *Outings:* ✓

Meetings: ✓

Registered places: 23
Guide weekly rate: From £500
Specialist care: Dementia
Medical services: Podiatry, dentist, optician, dietician,
    physiotherapy, occupational therapy
Qualified staff: Meets standard

Home details

Location: Village location, 8 miles from Bichester
Communal areas: 2 lounges, dining room, garden
Accessibility: *Floors:* 2 • *Access:* Lift • *Wheelchair access:* Good
Smoking: In designated area
Pets: At manager's discretion
Routines: Flexible

Room details

Single: 11
Shared: 5
En suite: 0
Facilities: TV point

Door lock: ✓
Lockable place: ✓

Services provided

Beauty services: Hairdressing
Mobile library: ✓
Religious services: ✓
Transport: ✗
Activities: *Coordinator:* ✓ • *Examples:* Cooking, quizzes, ball games
    Outings: ✗
Meetings: ✗

Lime Tree Court

Manager: Georgina Rixon
Owner: Georgina Rixon
Contact: Church Street, Twyford,
Buckinghamshire MK18 4EX
☎ 01296 730556
@ georgierixon@hotmail.com
🖥 www.limetreecourt.co.uk

Lime Tree Court is in a quiet cul-de-sac at the end of a country lane in the village of Twyford, north east of Bicester. The village shop is within easy walking distance. It is also near a pub, frequented by residents accompanied by staff. The garden is professionally maintained with a south-facing patio. The home is in close proximity to the local church and maintains strong ties with it. The home also has a resident cat. There is a dedicated TV lounge and independently controlled heating in the rooms. The activities coordinator comes to the home four days a week.

Registered places: 19
Guide weekly rate: £575
Specialist care: None
Medical services: Podiatry, dentist, optician, physiotherapy
Qualified staff: Meets standard

Home details

Location: Residential area, 1.5 miles from High Wycombe
Communal areas: 3 lounges, dining room, conservatory, garden
Accessibility: *Floors:* 2 • *Access:* Lift and stair lift
    Wheelchair access: Good
Smoking: ✗
Pets: ✗
Routines: Structured

Room details

Single: 15
Shared: 2
En suite: 1
Facilities: TV, telephone

Door lock: ✓
Lockable place: ✓

Services provided

Beauty services: Hairdressing, manicures, aromatherapy
Mobile library: ✓
Religious services: ✗
Transport: ✓
Activities: *Coordinator:* ✓ • *Examples:* Reminiscence sessions,
    card games, quizzes • *Outings:* ✓
Meetings: ✓

Little Oaks

Manager: Monica Tillotson
Owner: Mr and Mrs Tillotson
Contact: Daws Lea, High Wycombe,
Buckinghamshire HP11 1QG
☎ 01494 446878
@ andytillotson@msn.com

Little Oaks is a detached and spacious house situated near to the town centre of High Wycombe. There are two alcoves where the residents enjoy sitting in when they have visitors. The home has its own transport and arranges outings for boat trips and picnics as well as a visit to Ascot racecourse. The home aims to provide a welcoming and cosy atmosphere for its residents.

BUCKINGHAMSHIRE

Mandeville Grange

Manager: Minerva Patti
Owner: Mandeville Care Services Ltd
Contact: 201–203 Wendover Road,
Aylesbury, Buckinghamshire HP21 9PB
☎ 01296 435320
@ mcsmand@gmail.com

An extended Edwardian house, Mandeville Grange is a family-run nursing home. The home itself is situated on a bus route and is approximately two miles from the centre of Aylesbury. The manager of the home is a registered nurse. The home has an activities coordinator who organises daily and seasonal activities, including dances, singalongs and pantomimes. The daily routine of the home is flexible, yet a structured routine is gently encouraged.

Registered places: 31
Guide weekly rate: From £650
Specialist care: Nursing, day care, respite
Medical services: Podiatry, physiotherapy, dentist, optician
Qualified staff: Meets standard

Home details
Location: Residential area, 2 miles from Aylesbury centre
Communal areas: 3 lounges, dining room/conservatory, garden
Accessibility: *Floors:* 2 • *Access:* Lift • *Wheelchair access:* Good
Smoking: In designated area
Pets: At manager's discretion
Routines: Flexible

Room details
Single: 27
Shared: 2
En suite: 2
Facilities: TV

Door lock: ✓
Lockable place: ✓

Services provided
Beauty services: Hairdressing, aromatherapy, manicures
Mobile library: ✗
Religious services: Monthly church service
Transport: ✗
Activities: *Coordinator:* ✓ • *Examples:* Conversation group, games, reminiscence • *Outings:* ✗
Meetings: ✗

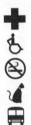

The Marguerite Centre

Manager: Janet Sillitoe
Owner: J Clarke
Contact: The Royal Bucks Hospital,
Buckingham Road, Aylesbury,
Buckinghamshire HP19 9AB
☎ 01296 678800
@ jan@royalbucks.co.uk
🖰 www.royalbucks.co.uk

Located on the first floor of the Royal Buckinghamshire Hospital, this one-level home offers excellent wheelchair accessibility for residents. The home is close to Aylesbury town centre which offers level access to restaurants, a library, a shopping centre, cinema and other local amenities. There is an adequate bus service. Outings are arranged to the theatre and the cinema.

Registered places: 25
Guide weekly rate: From £480
Specialist care: Nursing, physical disability
Medical services: Podiatry, dentist, optician, physiotherapy
Qualified staff: Exceeds standard: 70% at NVQ Level 2

Home details
Location: Urban area, 0.5 miles from Aylesbury
Communal areas: Lounge, dining room, patio and garden
Accessibility: *Floors:* 1st floor of hospital • *Access:* Lift
Wheelchair access: Good
Smoking: ✗
Pets: At manager's discretion
Routines: Flexible

Room details
Single: 21
Shared: 2
En suite: 0
Facilities: TV, telephone

Door lock: ✓
Lockable place: ✓

Services provided
Beauty services: Hairdressing
Mobile library: ✓
Religious services: ✓
Transport: ✓
Activities: *Coordinator:* ✓ • *Examples:* Bingo, exercises, entertainers • *Outings:* ✓
Meetings: ✗

Registered places: 8
Guide weekly rate: £450–£735
Specialist care: Dementia
Medical services: Podiatry
Qualified staff: Undisclosed

Home details

Location: Residential area, 1.5 miles from High Wycombe
Communal areas: Lounge, dining room, conservatory, kitchen, patio and garden
Accessibility: *Floors:* 2 • *Access:* None
   Wheelchair access: Limited
Smoking: ×
Pets: ×
Routines: Structured

Room details

Single: 8
Shared: 0
En suite: 0
Facilities: TV, telephone point

Door lock: ✓
Lockable place: ×

Services provided

Beauty services: Hairdressing
Mobile library: ✓
Religious services: ×
Transport: ×
Activities: *Coordinator:* ✓ • *Examples:* Games, puzzles
   Outings: ×
Meetings: ×

Maria Residential Home

Manager: Zulfiqar Ahmad
Owner: Maria Ahmad
Contact: Silver Birches, Kendalls Close, High Wycombe, Buckinghamshire HP13 7NJ
☏ 01494 530042

Given its small size and capacity, the manager and carers on duty have an excellent rapport with the residents. The manager allows visitors to enter the home most afternoons. The home itself is clean and tidy, which should have a positive impact and ensures the residents are living in a pleasant environment.

Registered places: 11
Guide weekly rate: £454–£499
Specialist care: Day care
Medical services: Podiatry, dentist, optician
Qualified staff: Undisclosed

Home details

Location: Urban area, 1 mile from Marlow centre
Communal areas: Lounge, dining room, patio and garden
Accessibility: *Floors:* 2 • *Access:* Lift • *Wheelchair access:* Good
Smoking: ×
Pets: ×
Routines: Flexible

Room details

Single: 9
Shared: 1
En suite: 9
Facilities: TV point, telephone point

Door lock: ✓
Lockable place: ✓

Services provided

Beauty services: Hairdressing
Mobile library: ×
Religious services: ✓
Transport: ×
Activities: *Coordinator:* ✓ • *Examples:* Arts and crafts, games, visiting entertainers • *Outings:* ✓
Meetings: ×

Meadowside Rest Home Ltd

Manager: Lorraine Hughes
Owner: Eileen Spiers
Contact: 202 Little Marlow Road, Marlow, Buckinghamshire SL7 1HX
☏ 01628 898068

Meadowside Rest Home is located approximately one mile from Marlow town centre. Accessible by car and the area is served by buses from Marlow, Bourne End and High Wycombe. The home was established in 1989 and is a large, detached Edwardian house which has been adapted to meet all the residents' needs. There is a monthly Communion service and weekly visits from a Catholic priest.

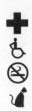

Paganell Grange Nursing Home

Manager: Linda Stubbs
Owner: The Extra Care Charitable Trust.
Contact: Westbury Lane,
Newport Pagnell, Buckinghamshire
MK16 8JA
☎ 01908 210322

Pagnell Grange is situated one mile from the town centre of Newport Pagnell, which includes a variety of shops and other local amenities. The home is five miles from the larger town of Milton Keynes. Residents are treated to several trips outside the home, which include a trip to Woburn Abbey, and Whipsnade Zoo, as well as a picnic by the stream and trips to the city centre for shopping.

Registered places: 30
Guide weekly rate: £377
Specialist care: Nursing, dementia
Medical services: Podiatry, dentist, optician
Qualified staff: Exceeds standard: 100% at NVQ Level 2

Home details
Location: Residential area, 5 miles from Milton Keynes
Communal areas: Lounge, dining room, conservatory, garden
Accessibility: *Floors:* 2 • *Access:* Lift • *Wheelchair access:* Good
Smoking: ✗
Pets: At manager's discretion
Routines: Flexible

Room details
Single: 30
Shared: 0
En suite: 30
Facilities: TV, telephone point

Door lock: ✗
Lockable place: ✓

Services provided
Beauty services: Hairdressing, massage therapy
Mobile library: ✗
Religious services: Monthly
Transport: ✗
Activities: *Coordinator:* ✓ • *Examples:* Glass painting, flower arranging, cooking • *Outings:* ✓
Meetings: ✗

Park House

Manager: Gillian Broadway
Owner: Edward and Gillian Broadway
Contact: Tyringham, Nr Newport Pagnell,
Buckinghamshire MK16 9ES
☎ 01908 613386

Park House is situated in the country estate of Tyringham, three miles from Newport Pagnell, with its shops and amenities. The home has ample grounds, including two courtyard gardens. There are a range of activities for residents to choose from including reminiscence and arts and crafts. The home also arranges for frequent trips out, such as shopping and going to the theatre. Entertainers also come to the home including one entertainer who organises quizzes for the residents.

Registered places: 24
Guide weekly rate: From £488
Specialist care: Dementia, respite
Medical services: Podiatry, dentist, optician, physiotherapy
Qualified staff: Exceeds standard: 70% at NVQ Level 2

Home details
Location: Residential area, 3 miles from Newport Pagnell
Communal areas: 2 lounges, dining room, patio and garden
Accessibility: *Floors:* 2 • *Access:* Lift • *Wheelchair access:* Good
Smoking: In designated area
Pets: At manager's discretion
Routines: Flexible

Room details
Single: 24
Shared: 0
En suite: 19
Facilities: TV point, telephone point

Door lock: ✓
Lockable place: ✓

Services provided
Beauty services: Hairdressing
Mobile library: ✓
Religious services: ✗
Transport: 7-seater vehicle
Activities: *Coordinator:* ✓ • *Examples:* Reminiscence, shopping, arts and crafts • *Outings:* ✓
Meetings: ✓

Registered places: 45
Guide weekly rate: £577–£677
Specialist care: Dementia, respite
Medical services: Podiatry, dentist, optician, physiotherapy
Qualified staff: Exceeds standard: 75% at NVQ Level 2

Home details

Location: Rural area, 3.5 miles from Amersham
Communal areas: Lounge, dining room, TV area, patio and garden
Accessibility: *Floors:* 2 • *Access:* Lift • *Wheelchair access:* Good
Smoking: In designated area
Pets: ✗
Routines: Flexible

Room details

Single: 45
Shared: 0
En suite: Undisclosed
Facilities: TV, telephone

Door lock: ✗
Lockable place: ✗

Services provided

Beauty services: Hairdressing, aromatherapy, manicures
Mobile library: ✓
Religious services: ✓
Transport: Minibus
Activities: *Coordinator:* ✓ • *Examples:* Bingo, flower arranging, visiting entertainers • *Outings:* ✓
Meetings: ✗

Rayners Residential Care Home

Manager: Christopher Matthews
Owner: Rayners Ltd
Contact: Weedon Hill, Hyde Heath, Amersham, Buckinghamshire HP6 5UH
☏ 01494 773606
@ chris@careatrayners.co.uk
🖱 www.careatrayners.co.uk

A purpose-built home situated in Hyde Heath close to the village green and amenities such as a village store and pub, Rayners is a family-run home offering dementia care. The home is three and a half miles from Amersham. The home has an activities coordinator who organises day trips as well as daily activities such as flower arranging and visiting entertainers. The home also offers respite care.

Registered places: 54
Guide weekly rate: £900–£950
Specialist care: Nursing
Medical services: Podiatry, optician
Qualified staff: Meets standard

Home details

Location: Residential area, 1 mile from High Wycombe
Communal areas: Reception area, seating area, garden
Accessibility: *Floors:* 2 • *Access:* Lift • *Wheelchair access:* Good
Smoking: ✗
Pets: At manager's discretion
Routines: Flexible

Room details

Single: 50
Shared: 2
En suite: 50
Facilities: TV, telephone point

Door lock: ✗
Lockable place: ✓

Services provided

Beauty services: Hairdressing
Mobile library: ✓
Religious services: Fortnightly service, visits by Catholic and Anglican clergy
Transport: Minibus
Activities: *Coordinator:* ✓ • *Examples:* Bingo, gardening, quizzes *Outings:* ✓
Meetings: ✓

Shelburne Lodge

Manager: Pam Camichel
Owner: Barchester Healthcare Ltd
Contact: Rutland Street, High Wycombe, Buckinghamshire HP11 2LJ
☏ 01494 440404
@ shelburne@barchester.com
🖱 www.barchester.com

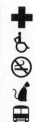

Shelburne Lodge is located in a residential area, approximately one mile from High Wycombe. The home has a garden for residents to enjoy and a minibus to take residents on outings. There is also a varied activities programme, which includes gardening, quizzes and bingo. The residents also have access to a mobile shop. There is a religious service every two weeks and Catholic and Anglican clergy visit the home on a regular basis.

Stone House Nursing Home

Manager: Philomena Heritage

Owner: Mr and Mrs Dhanani

Contact: Bishopstone Road, Stone, Aylesbury, Buckinghamshire HP17 8BX

☎ 01296 747122

@ stonehousehome@aol.com

Stone House Nursing Home is situated on a country road, six and a half miles from Aylesbury. The home is a large older house set in well-kept, gardens that residents can enjoy, particularly in the warmer months. Residents are encouraged to personalise their rooms with their own furniture and personal belongings to create a more homely environment. The daily activities are posted in the entrance hall of the home, with an activities coordinator providing residents with craft sessions, quizzes and outings to the local garden centre, and Bucks Goat Farm.

Registered places: 29

Guide weekly rate: £550–£900

Specialist care: Nursing, dementia

Medical services: None

Qualified staff: Undisclosed

Home details

Location: Village location, 6.5 miles from Aylesbury

Communal areas: 3 lounges, dining room, conservatory, garden

Accessibility: *Floors:* 3 • *Access:* Lift • *Wheelchair access:* Good

Smoking: ✗

Pets: ✗

Routines: Flexible

Room details

Single: 26

Shared: 3

En suite: Undisclosed

Facilities: TV point, telephone point

Door lock: ✗

Lockable place: ✗

Services provided

Beauty services: Hairdressing

Mobile library: ✗

Religious services: Monthly church service

Transport: ✗

Activities: *Coordinator:* ✓ • *Examples:* Craft sessions, quizzes, entertainers • *Outings:* ✓

Meetings: ✗

Tweed House Nursing Home

Manager: Mr Chirinuuta

Owner: ExtraCare Charitable Trust

Contact: 1 Witham Court, Tweed Drive, Bletchley, Milton Keynes, Buckinghamshire MK3 7QU

☎ 01908 366702

The home is situated on the outskirts of Bletchley, five miles from Milton Keynes. The property is a bungalow, which has wheelchair access throughout There are regular outings to Milton Keynes and the surrounding area to historical points of interest, a pub lunch, or simply a shopping trip. Residents' pets are welcome to visit.

Registered places: 30

Guide weekly rate: £388

Specialist care: Nursing, dementia

Medical services: Podiatry, dentist, optician, physiotherapy

Qualified staff: Exceeds standard: 100% at NVQ Level 2

Home details

Location: Residential area, 5 miles from Milton Keynes

Communal areas: Lounge, dining room, sensory relaxation area, garden

Accessibility: *Floors:* 1 • *Wheelchair access:* Good

Smoking: In designated area

Pets: ✗

Routines: Flexible

Room details

Single: 30

Shared: 0

En suite: 0

Facilities: TV point

Door lock: ✗

Lockable place: ✓

Services provided

Beauty services: Hairdressing

Mobile library: ✓

Religious services: Monthly church service

Transport: ✗

Activities: *Coordinator:* ✓ • *Examples:* Walks, darts, carpet bowls *Outings:* ✓

Meetings: ✓

Registered places: 23
Guide weekly rate: £695–£905
Specialist care: Respite
Medical services: Podiatry, dentist, occupational therapy, optician, physiotherapy
Qualified staff: Exceeds standard: 100% at NVQ Level 2

Home details

Location: Village location, 0.5 miles from Marlow
Communal areas: 3 lounges, dining room, garden
Accessibility: *Floors:* 3 • *Access:* 2 lifts • *Wheelchair access:* Good
Smoking: In designated area
Pets: At manager's discretion
Routines: Flexible

Room details

Single: 19
Shared: 2
En suite: 21
Facilities: TV, telephone point

Door lock: ✓
Lockable place: ✓

Services provided

Beauty services: Hairdressing, aromatherapy, beautician
Mobile library: ✗
Religious services: Fortnightly Communion service
Transport: ✗
Activities: *Coordinator:* ✓ • *Examples:* Bowling, exercise classes, visiting performers • *Outings:* ✓
Meetings: ✗

White Lodge

Manager: Roderick Ting
Owner: Roderick and Amy Ting and Ming and Annie Chiu
Contact: Marlow Road, Bisham, Marlow, Buckinghamshire SL7 1RP
) 01628 898281

This country house is only half a mile from Marlow town and the River Thames. White Lodge is surrounded by a large, well-maintained garden with a raised deck giving a view of the surrounding fields. All areas of the garden and house are accessible by wheelchair so can be enjoyed by all. An activities coordinator is available four days a week. Summer barbecues and trips to the theatre feature in a varied programme of events. Friends and relatives are also invited to various social occasions throughout the year including celebrating resident's birthdays.

Registered places: 38
Guide weekly rate: £625–£725
Specialist care: Dementia
Medical services: Podiatry, dentist, optician, physiotherapy
Qualified staff: Meets standard

Home details

Location: Village location, 4.2 miles from Uxbridge
Communal areas: Lounge, dining room, garden
Accessibility: *Floors:* 2 • *Access:* Lift • *Wheelchair access:* Good
Smoking: ✗
Pets: ✗
Routines: Flexible

Room details

Single: 38
Shared: 0
En suite: 14
Facilities: TV point, telephone point

Door lock: ✗
Lockable place: ✓

Services provided

Beauty services: Hairdressing
Mobile Library: ✓
Religious services: Monthly Communion service
Transport: ✓
Activities: *Coordinator:* ✓ • *Examples:* Visiting entertainers *Outings:* ✓
Meetings: ✓

White Plains

Manager: Yvonne O'Connor
Owner: B & M Investments Ltd
Contact: Tilehouse Lane, Denham, Nr Uxbridge, Buckinghamshire UB9 6AA
) 01895 832190

White Plains is located in Denham next to a small airfield and close to Denham village. Denham Green is opposite the home, and Collsels Wood, Nightingale Wood and Northmoor Nature Reserve are close to the home. As a result of its surroundings the home often organises walks around the local area. The home also has visiting entertainers, who come in on a monthly basis. This includes actors, magicians and live singing.

The Willow

Manager: Lynne Woodstock
Owner: Lynne Woodstock and
Mason Duke
Contact: 110 Chartridge Lane,
Chesham, Buckinghamshire HP5 2RG
) 01494 773451
@ woodstockconkers@aol.com

The Willow can be found in a residential area approximately one mile from local facilities and from Chesham town centre. The home does not have a lift and therefore residents moving into the home must be relatively mobile. The Willow issues a newsletter twice a year for residents and relatives. There is a garden to the rear of the home which includes a secluded seating area.

Registered places: 10
Guide weekly rate: £550
Specialist care: None
Medical services: Podiatry, dentist, optician.
Qualified staff: Fails standard: 30% at NVQ Level 2

Home details

Location: Residential area, 0.7 miles from Chesham
Communal areas: Lounge, dining room, conservatory, garden
Accessibility: *Floors:* 2 • *Access:* None
   Wheelchair access: Limited
Smoking: ✗
Pets: ✓
Routines: Flexible

Room details

Single: 10	**Door lock:** ✓
Shared: 0	**Lockable place:** ✓
En suite: 8	
Facilities: Telephone point	

Services provided

Beauty services: Hairdressing, beautician
Mobile library: ✗
Religious services: ✗
Transport: 7-seater vehicle
Activities: *Coordinator:* ✓ • *Examples:* games, quizzes
   Outings: ✓
Meetings: ✓

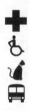

The Willows Care Centre

Manager: Kay Shephard
Owner: Willows Care Centre Ltd
Contact: Heathercroft,
Great Linford, Milton Keynes,
Buckinghamshire MK14 5EG
) 01908 679505

The Willows is a purpose-built care home, situated in the Great Linford area of Milton Keynes. It is situated in a residential area, close to local shops. The home specialises in care for dementia sufferers, and there is 24-hour nursing for these sufferers. The home provides a range of activities such as outings for the residents and there are activities coordinators on each floor as well as a garden for residents to enjoy.

Registered places: 116
Guide weekly rate: Undisclosed
Specialist care: Nursing, dementia
Medical services: Podiatry, hygienist, optician, physiotherapy
Qualified staff: Exceeds standard: 70% at NVQ Level 2

Home details

Location: Residential area, 3.8 miles from Milton Keynes
Communal areas: 6 lounges, dining room, conservatory, cinema room
Accessibility: *Floors:* 3 • *Access:* 3 lifts
   Wheelchair access: Good
Smoking: In designated area
Pets: At manager's discretion
Routines: Flexible

Room details

Single: 116	**Door lock:** ✓
Shared: 0	**Lockable place:** ✓
En suite: 116	
Facilities: TV point, telephone point	

Services provided

Beauty services: Hairdressing
Mobile library: ✓
Religious services: Monthly Catholic and Anglican visits
Transport: ✓
Activities: *Coordinator:* ✓ • *Examples:* Bowling, music nights
   Outings: ✓
Meetings: ✓

Registered places: 9
Guide weekly rate: £550–£700
Specialist care: Day care, respite
Medical services: Podiatry, hygienist, optician, physiotherapy
Qualified staff: Meets standard

Home details

Location: Rural area, 1.9 miles from Gerrards Cross
Communal areas: Lounge, dining room, garden
Accessibility: *Floors:* 1 • *Wheelchair access:* Good
Smoking: In designated area
Pets: ✗
Routines: Flexible

Room details

Single: 7
Shared: 1
En suite: 2
Facilities: TV point, telephone point

Door lock: ✗
Lockable place: ✓

Services provided

Beauty services: Hairdressing, manicures
Mobile library: ✗
Religious services: Monthly Catholic visits
Transport: ✗
Activities: *Coordinator:* ✗ • *Examples:* Crafts, musician
     Outings: ✓
Meetings: ✓

Windsor Lodge

Manager: Deborah Dry
Owner: Mr and Mrs Glynn
Contact: Windsor Road, Gerrards Cross,
Buckinghamshire SL9 8SS
☎ 01753 662342

Windsor Lodge is the family home of the proprietors and consists of a large bungalow set in its own grounds. Accommodation for the residents is on the ground floor. The home is accessed through electronically controlled gates. A homely environment has been created for residents, which is safe and clean, providing residents with adequate surroundings. An induction is in place for all new staff, to make sure that they have the necessary skills and knowledge to meet the care needs of the residents.

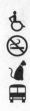

Abbey House

Manager: Leah Ramshaw
Owner: Angel Healthcare Ltd
Contact: 20–22 Albert Road,
Bexhill-on-Sea, East Sussex TN40 1DG
) 01424 222534
✆ www.angelhealthcare.co.uk

Abbey House is a detached Victorian property near the seafront in Bexhill-on-Sea. At the rear of the building there is a small, private rear garden. The shops and amenities are in easy reach of the home. The home is hoping to go on outings further a field than the seafront with the new purchase of a minibus. Residents meetings are also starting after an influx of new residents. There are two resident cats in the home at the moment and other pets may be approved. The home also offers interesting activities including t'ai chi and aromatherapy.

Registered places: 23
Guide weekly rate: £339–£425
Specialist care: Day care, respite
Medical services: Podiatry, dentist, optician, physiotherapy
Qualified staff: Fails standard: 40% at NVQ Level 2

Home details
Location: Residential area, in Bexhill
Communal areas: Lounge, dining room, garden
Accessibility: *Floors:* 3 • *Access:* Lift • *Wheelchair access:* Good
Smoking: ✗
Pets: At manager's discretion
Routines: Flexible

Room details
Single: 23
Shared: 0
En suite: 22
Facilities: TV point, telephone point

Door lock: ✓
Lockable place: ✓

Services provided
Beauty services: Hairdressing, aromatherapy
Mobile library: ✓
Religious services: Monthly Communion service
Transport: Minibus
Activities: *Coordinator:* ✓ • *Examples:* Quizzes, t'ai chi
 Outings: ✗
Meetings: ✗

Alma Lodge Residential Care

Manager: Dawn Owasil
Owner: Mr and Mrs Owasil
Contact: 5 Staveley Road, Eastbourne,
East Sussex BN20 7LH
) 01323 734208

Alma Lodge is a detached, two-storey property situated in a suburban area. It is very near the seafront and only one mile from the centre of Eastbourne. There are shops, a bank, chemist, post office and pub within one quarter of a mile. There is also a bus stop close by and a train station two miles away for the more mobile residents and families to visit. The home focuses on creating a homely atmosphere for the residents with a vast variety of activities.

Registered places: 14
Guide weekly rate: £352–£410
Specialist care: None
Medical services: Podiatry, dentist, optician, physiotherapy
Qualified staff: Exceeds standard: 90% at NVQ Level 2

Home details
Location: Residential area, 1 mile from Eastbourne centre
Communal areas: Lounge/dining room, conservatory,
 patio and garden
Accessibility: *Floors:* 2 • *Access:* Lift • *Wheelchair access:* Good
Smoking: In designated area
Pets: ✓
Routines: Flexible

Room details
Single: 9
Shared: 3
En suite: 1
Facilities: TV point, telephone point

Door lock: ✓
Lockable place: ✓

Services provided
Beauty services: Hairdressing
Mobile library: ✓
Religious services: Monthly Anglican service
Transport: Car
Activities: *Coordinator:* ✓ • *Examples:* Board games,
 reminiscence, quizzes • *Outings:* ✓
Meetings: ✓

Registered places: 36
Guide weekly rate: £417–£750
Specialist care: Nursing
Medical services: Podiatry, dentist, optician, physiotherapy
Qualified staff: Meets standard

Home details

Location: Residential area, 1 mile from Bexhill centre
Communal areas: Lounge, dining room, garden
Accessibility: *Floors:* 3 • *Access:* Lift • *Wheelchair access:* Good
Smoking: In designated area
Pets: ✓
Routines: Flexible

Room details

Single: 8
Shared: 14
En suite: 15
Facilities: TV point, telephone point

Door lock: ✗
Lockable place: ✓

Services provided

Beauty services: Hairdressing
Mobile library: ✓
Religious services: ✓
Transport: ✗
Activities: *Coordinator:* ✗ • *Examples:* Bingo, darts, walks
  Outings: ✓
Meetings: ✓

Amber Beach

Manager: Claire Avery
Owner: Mr Manji
Contact: 2–3 Middlesex Road,
Bexhill-on-Sea, East Sussex TN40 1LP
☎ 01424 210202

Amber Beach is a converted Victorian property that was formerly a guesthouse. It is situated in a quiet residential area of Bexhill close to the seafront, town centre and mainline railway station. The home has a pretty garden with seating for residents to enjoy, which is popular in the summer months when the weather is warm. The garden is used for barbecues and Pimm's evenings in the summer. Regular daily activities include bingo, quizzes, flower arranging, and on occasion there are beachfront walks for residents accompanied by carers.

Registered places: 14
Guide weekly rate: £395–£420
Specialist care: Day care
Medical services: Podiatry, optician
Qualified staff: Fails standard: 45% at NVQ Level 2

Home details

Location: Residential area, 1 mile from Hove centre
Communal areas: Lounge, dining room, garden
Accessibility: *Floors:* 2 • *Access:* Lift • *Wheelchair access:* Good
Smoking: ✗
Pets: ✓
Routines: Flexible

Room details

Single: 6
Shared: 4
En suite: 10
Facilities: TV point, telephone point

Door lock: ✗
Lockable place: ✓

Services provided

Beauty services: Hairdressing
Mobile library: ✓
Religious services: ✓
Transport: ✓
Activities: *Coordinator:* ✗ • *Examples:* Poetry reading, quizzes,
  reminiscence • *Outings:* ✓
Meetings: ✓

Amberley House Residential Home

Manager: Elizabeth Lamacraft
Owner: Elizabeth Lamacraft and Dr Rosalind Sinka
Contact: 19 Vallance Gardens, Hove,
East Sussex BN3 2DB
☎ 01273 779225
@ amberleyhouse@gicham.co.uk

Amberley is a large detached house on a residential road close to Hove seafront and the town centre. It is within walking distance from the library and Hove Museum is just round the corner. Activities are organised by an ex-employee of the home on a voluntary basis. They include poetry reading, walks into the village and music and movement. At the rear of the home is a large, peaceful walled garden where residents can sit and enjoy peace and quiet, and in good weather there are frequent barbecues and party evenings.

Ancaster Court

Manager: Alison Sowerby
Owner: BUPA Care Homes Ltd
Contact: 24 Hastings Road,
Bexhill-on-Sea, East Sussex TN40 2HH
) 01424 213532
@ AncasterCourtALL@BUPA.com
www.bupacarehomes.co.uk

Formerly two Victorian private houses, Ancaster Court has been converted into a care home. It is situated in a peaceful residential area on the outskirts of Bexhill-on-Sea with local shops within half a mile and a short bus journey into Bexhill centre. The home has three lounges and there are two spacious dining rooms. A conservatory, patio and large gardens can be enjoyed by residents. Many of the bedrooms have views over the gardens to the sea. Daily activities are offered including singing, Pets As Therapy and entertainers, as well as trips to local attractions and the seafront.

Registered places: 37
Guide weekly rate: Undisclosed
Specialist care: Respite, dementia
Medical services: Podiatry, physiotherapy
Qualified staff: Undisclosed

Home details

Location: Residential area, 0.5 miles from Bexhill centre
Communal areas: 4 lounges, 2 dining rooms, hairdressing salon, garden
Accessibility: *Floors:* 3 • *Access:* Lift • *Wheelchair access:* Good
Smoking: In designated area
Pets: ✓
Routines: Flexible

Room details

Single: 43
Shared: 3
En suite: 14
Facilities: TV point, telephone point

Door lock: ✓
Lockable place: ✗

Services provided

Beauty services: Hairdressing
Mobile library: ✓
Religious services: ✓
Transport: ✓
Activities: *Coordinator:* ✓ • *Examples:* Entertainers, exercise, singing • *Outings:* ✓
Meetings: ✓

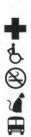

Arundel Park Lodge

Manager: Anita Redwood
Owner: Michael and Anita Redwood
Contact: 22–24 Arundel Drive East,
Saltdean, Brighton, East Sussex
BN2 8SL
) 01273 303449

Arundel Park Lodge is situated in a residential area of Saltdean, with views over the town and sea. It has ample communal space, with two lounge areas, two dining rooms and a large garden with wheelchair access. The home is on a bus route with access to the local town and connecting the residents to local amenities. The activities programme includes trips to the theatre, pub lunches, and musical entertainers. The home is also involved with the University of the Third Age, and welcomes visitors giving poetry readings and other activities of interest.

Registered places: 30
Guide weekly rate: £380–£660
Specialist care: Nursing, respite
Medical services: Podiatry, dentist, optician, occupational therapy, physiotherapy
Qualified staff: Exceeds standard: 70% at NVQ Level 2

Home details

Location: Residential area, 5 miles from Brighton centre
Communal areas: 2 lounges, lounge/dining room, dining room, garden
Accessibility: *Floors:* 2 • *Access:* Lift • *Wheelchair access:* Good
Smoking: ✗
Pets: At manager's discretion
Routines: Flexible

Room details

Single: 25
Shared: 3
En suite: 21
Facilities: TV point, telephone point

Door lock: ✓
Lockable place: ✓

Services provided

Beauty services: Hairdressing
Mobile library: ✓
Religious services: Monthly Anglican service
Transport: Car
Activities: *Coordinator:* ✓ • *Examples:* Arts and crafts, music *Outings:* ✓
Meetings: ✗

Registered places: 22
Guide weekly rate: £325–£500
Specialist care: Respite
Medical services: Podiatry, dentist, optician
Qualified staff: Meets standard

Home details
Location: Residential area, 1 mile from Eastbourne centre
Communal areas: 2 lounges, 2 dining rooms, garden
Accessibility: *Floors:* 4 • *Access:* Lift • *Wheelchair access:* Limited
Smoking: In designated area
Pets: x
Routines: Flexible

Room details
Single: 16
Shared: 3
En suite: 14
Facilities: TV point

Door lock: ✓
Lockable place: ✓

Services provided
Beauty services: Hairdressing
Mobile library: x
Religious services: Monthly visit from pastor
Transport: x
Activities: *Coordinator:* x • *Examples:* Musical entertainment, arts and crafts, games • *Outings:* x
Meetings: ✓

Ashberry Court

Manager: David Short
Owner: Ramachandran Jalatheepan and Varunatheepan Ramachandran
Contact: 39 Lewes Road, Eastbourne, East Sussex BN21 2BU
☎ 01323 722335
@ ashberry@broadgate-healthcare.co.uk

Ashberry Court is one mile from the centre of Eastbourne and there are bus routes into the centre. The home prides itself on being a relaxed and friendly atmosphere. There is a variety of activities for residents to take part in, including weekly musical entertainment and fortnightly exercise classes. The home has two dining rooms and two lounges for residents to choose from.

Registered places: 26
Guide weekly rate: £322–£450
Specialist care: None
Medical services: Podiatry, optician
Qualified staff: Exceeds standard: 80% at NVQ Level 2

Home details
Location: Residential area, in St Leonards-on-Sea
Communal areas: 2 lounges, 2 dining rooms, conservatory, garden
Accessibility: *Floors:* 4 • *Access:* Lift and stair lift
Wheelchair access: Good
Smoking: x
Pets: x
Routines: Flexible

Room details
Single: 26
Shared: 0
En suite: 26
Facilities: TV point, telephone

Door lock: ✓
Lockable place: ✓

Services provided
Beauty services: Hairdressing, manicures, pedicures
Mobile library: x
Religious services: x
Transport: x
Activities: *Coordinator:* ✓ • *Examples:* Bingo, exercise, singalongs
Outings: x
Meetings: ✓

Ashburnham Lodge

Manager: Malcolm Kay
Owner: Malcolm Kay
Contact: 62 London Road, St Leonards-on-Sea, East Sussex TN37 6AS
☎ 01424 438575
@ malcolmkay@supanet.com

Ashburnham Lodge is a large, detached property that boasts a well maintained garden, located in a residential area of St Leonards-on-Sea. Although all the rooms are singles, doubles are available and all rooms also have an en suite facility.

Ashburnham Lodge is located a short distance from the main shopping area of St Leonards-on-Sea, and a 10-minute walk to the seafront. The home sets up a caring and respectful relationship between carers and residents, thereby personal knowledge of an individual residents needs are tended to effectively.

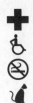

Ashridge Court Nursing Home

Manager: Ashridge Court Ltd
Owner: Elizabeth Van Eugen
Contact: 163 Barnhorn Road,
Bexhill-on-Sea, East Sussex TN39 4QL
☎ 01424 842357

Ashridge Court is located on the main road between Eastbourne and Bexhill, approximately half a mile from Little Common Village. Local amenities are accessible by public transport. The home is set in well-maintained gardens that have extensive views to the rear of the property overlooking a large fishpond which attracts a lot of local wildlife, such as birds, foxes and dragon flies.

Registered places: 53
Guide weekly rate: £450–£850
Specialist care: Nursing, physical disability
Medical services: Podiatry
Qualified staff: Meets standard

Home details
Location: Village location, 2.5 miles from Bexhill
Communal areas: Lounge, dining room, garden
Accessibility: *Floors:* 2 • *Access:* Lift • *Wheelchair access:* Good
Smoking: ✗
Pets: ✓
Routines: Flexible

Room details
Single: 44
Shared: 1
En suite: 27
Facilities: TV point, telephone point

Door lock: ✗
Lockable place: ✓

Services provided
Beauty services: Hairdressing
Mobile library: ✗
Religious services: ✗
Transport: ✗
Activities: *Coordinator:* ✓ • *Examples:* Country walks, knitting, films • *Outings:* ✗
Meetings: ✓

Bannow Retirement Home

Manager: Karen Tracey
Owner: Terence and Mary Tracey
Contact: Quarry Hill,
St Leonards-on-Sea,
East Sussex TN38 0HG
☎ 01424 433021
@ bannowretirement@hotmail.com

Bannows is a detached, listed building, set in its own grounds in the quiet residential area of West Hill in St Leonard's-on-Sea. There are many activities for residents to take part in, giving individual choice with a gardening club and board and card games. For those who enjoy outings there are afternoon tea trips and going to see local points of interest. Though pets are not allowed to stay at the home they can visit.

Registered places: 26
Guide weekly rate: £398–£530
Specialist care: Respite
Medical services: Podiatry, dentist, optician
Qualified staff: Fails standard: 44% at NVQ Level 2

Home details
Location: Residential area, 1 mile from Hastings
Communal areas: Lounge, dining room, library, garden
Accessibility: *Floors:* 3 • *Access:* Lift • *Wheelchair access:* Good
Smoking: In designated area
Pets: ✗
Routines: Flexible

Room details
Single: 17
Shared: 4
En suite: 21
Facilities: TV point, telephone point

Door lock: ✓
Lockable place: ✓

Services provided
Beauty services: Hairdressing
Mobile library: ✓
Religious services: Anglican Communion service every 3 months
Transport: Minibus
Activities: *Coordinator:* ✓ • *Examples:* Gardening club, whist, scrabble • *Outings:* ✓
Meetings: ✗

Registered places: 40
Guide weekly rate: £531–£755
Specialist care: Nursing
Medical services: Podiatry, optician, physiotherapy
Qualified staff: Meets standard

Home details

Location: Residential area, 0.25 miles from Hove centre
Communal areas: 4 lounges, 4 dining rooms, garden
Accessibility: *Floors:* 2 • *Access:* Lift • *Wheelchair access:* Good
Smoking: In designated area
Pets: At manager's discretion
Routines: Flexible

Room details

Single: 40
Shared: 0
En suite: 40
Facilities: TV point, telephone point

Door lock: ✓
Lockable place: ✗

Services provided

Beauty services: Hairdressing
Mobile library: Library facilities
Religious services: ✗
Transport: Minibus
Activities: *Coordinator:* ✓ • *Examples:* Keep fit, snooker, visiting entertainers • *Outings:* ✓
Meetings: ✓

Barford Court

Manager: Susan Hale
Owner: Royal Masonic Benevolent Institution
Contact: 157 Kingsway, Hove, East Sussex BN3 4GR
☎ 01273 777736
@ barford@rmbi.org.uk
🖰 www.rmbi.org.uk

On the seafront, a few minutes from the beautiful South Downs, this Art Deco-style house has been converted to include a purpose-built extension and conservatory overlooking elegant gardens. It is divided into four 'family-style' house group units, each with about 10 residents. Each house group has its own lounge, dining room and kitchen. There is a large landscaped garden with seating, a pond, and tropical foliage. The home is close to amenities, five minutes' walk into Hove and three miles from Brighton. The home also has a snooker table.

Registered places: 29
Guide weekly rate: £400–£495
Specialist care: Day care, respite
Medical services: Podiatry, dentist, optician
Qualified staff: Exceeds standard: 70% at NVQ Level 2

Home details

Location: Residential area, 0.5 miles from Seaford centre
Communal areas: 7 lounge/dining rooms, conservatory, patio and garden
Accessibility: *Floors:* 2 • *Access:* Lift • *Wheelchair access:* Good
Smoking: In designated area
Pets: At manager's discretion
Routines: Flexible

Room details

Single: 27
Shared: 1
En suite: 20
Facilities: TV point, telephone point

Door lock: ✓
Lockable place: ✓

Services provided

Beauty services: Hairdressing, aromatherapy
Mobile library: ✗
Religious services: Monthly multi-faith church service
Transport: Minibus
Activities: *Coordinator:* ✓ • *Examples:* Craft classes, music groups *Outings:* ✓
Meetings: ✓

Beachlands Care Ltd

Manager: Vacant
Owner: Beachlands Care Ltd
Contact: Marine Parade, Seaford, East Sussex BN25 2PY
☎ 01323 891004

A family-owned home, Beachlands is situated on the seafront giving residents views across the English Channel. The home is approximately 100 yards from local shops and half a mile from Seaford town centre and it's amenities. There is an attractive garden to the rear of the home with a fishpond and seating area. Local people of an older age are invited to the home for meals. It gives an opportunity for residents to socialise with people from outside the home.

Beachside Rest Home

Manager: Abdoollah Peersaib
Owner: Abdoollah and Maryam Peersaib
Contact: Cricketfield Road, Seaford,
East Sussex BN25 1BU
☎ 01323 893756

Beachside Rest Home is situated within walking distance from the seafront and from Seaford town centre. The town centre offers various shops and restaurants as well as having extensive bus routes and a train station. There are gardens to the rear and front of the home along with seating areas for the residents' use. The home offers a variety of therapies such as art and music therapy, particularly for residents with mental disorders.

Registered places: 11
Guide weekly rate: £363–£550
Specialist care: Mental disorder, respite
Medical services: Podiatry, dentist, optician, psychiatry
Qualified staff: Exceeds standard: 60% at NVQ Level 2

Home details
Location: Residential area, 0.5 miles from Seaford centre
Communal areas: Lounge, dining room, patio and garden
Accessibility: *Floors:* 3 • *Access:* None
    Wheelchair access: Limited
Smoking: ✗
Pets: ✗
Routines: Flexible

Room details
Single: 7	**Door lock:** ✓
Shared: 2	**Lockable place:** ✓
En suite: 1	
Facilities: TV point	

Services provided
Beauty services: Hairdressing
Mobile library: ✗
Religious services: ✗
Transport: 7-seater vehicle
Activities: *Coordinator:* ✗ • *Examples:* Arts and crafts, exercises, reminiscence • *Outings:* ✗
Meetings: ✓

Beeches Retirement Home

Manager: Darren Sinclair
Owner: Mr and Mrs Sinclair
Contact: 4 De Roos Road, Eastbourne,
East Sussex BN21 2QA
☎ 01323 731307

The Beeches is a detached, two-storey Victorian house set in its own grounds.
    Residents hold meetings to discuss daily life at the home every one or two months. The home arranges for a range of outings such as drives out. There are also a range of activities including music and motivation and quizzes. There are two resident cats, but residents' own pets are not allowed in the home.

Registered places: 20
Guide weekly rate: £322–£400
Specialist care: Respite
Medical services: Podiatry, optician
Qualified staff: Meets standard

Home details
Location: Residential area, 0.5 miles from Eastbourne centre
Communal areas: Lounge, dining room, conservatory, garden
Accessibility: *Floors:* 2 • *Access:* Lift • *Wheelchair access:* Good
Routines: Flexible
Pets: ✗
Smoking: ✗

Room details
Single: 14	**Door lock:** ✓
Shared: 3	**Lockable place:** ✓
En suite: 17	
Facilities: TV point, telephone point	

Services provided
Beauty services: Hairdressing
Mobile library: ✓
Religious services: Salvation Army service, Communion service
Transport: ✗
Activities: *Coordinator:* ✗ • *Examples:* Bingo, music and motivation, quizzes • *Outings:* ✓
Meetings: ✓

Registered places: 25
Guide weekly rate: £500–£800
Specialist care: Nursing, physical disability, respite
Medical services: Podiatry, dentist, optician
Qualified staff: Exceeds standard: 65% at NVQ Level 2

Home details

Location: Residential area, 1 mile from Eastbourne centre
Communal areas: Lounge, dining room, garden
Accessibility: *Floors:* 3 • *Access:* Lift and stair lift
　　Wheelchair access: Good
Smoking: In designated area
Pets: ✓
Routines: Flexible

Room details

Single: 19
Shared: 3
En suite: 0
Facilities: TV, telephone point

Door lock: ✗
Lockable place: ✓

Services provided

Beauty services: Hairdressing, manicures
Mobile library: ✗
Religious services: ✗
Transport: ✗
Activities: *Coordinator:* ✓ • *Examples:* Arts and crafts, bingo,
　　knitting • *Outings:* ✓
Meetings: ✗

Bendigo Nursing Home

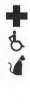

Manager: Mariana Philipova
Owner: Kindcare UK Ltd
Contact: 22 Arundel Road, Eastbourne,
East Sussex BN21 2EL
☏ 01323 642599
@ Marianamp9565@hotmail.co.uk
🖱 www.kindcare.co.uk

Bendigo Nursing Home is a converted detached property situated in a residential area of Eastbourne and is close to the town centre with its variety of shops, public transport facilities and other amenities. Residents have a menu in their room and although there are set meal times the residents can choose when they wish to have their meals. The home offers services such as hairdressing and manicures and has a range of activities and outings available to the residents. Smoking is not permitted in communal areas but is allowed in the resident's own room.

Registered places: 60
Guide weekly rate: £465–£850
Specialist care: Nursing, day care, dementia, physical disability,
　　terminal care
Medical services: None
Qualified staff: Meets standard

Home details

Location: Residential area, 1.5 miles from Brighton centre
Communal areas: Dining room, garden
Accessibility: *Floors:* 5 • *Access:* Lift and stair lift
　　Wheelchair access: Good
Routines: Flexible
Pets: At manager's discretion
Smoking: ✗

Room details

Single: 18
Shared: 42
En suite: 60
Facilities: TV point, telephone point

Door lock: ✓
Lockable place: ✗

Services provided

Beauty services: Hairdressing
Mobile library: ✗
Religious services: ✓
Transport: ✗
Activities: *Coordinator:* ✓ • *Examples:* Arts and crafts, shows,
　　pottery evenings • *Outings:* ✓
Meetings: ✓

Birch Grove Nursing Home

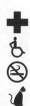

Manager: Christine Turnbull
Owner: Mr and Mrs Shookhye
Contact: 1 Stanford Avenue, Brighton,
East Sussex BN1 6AD
☏ 01273 566111
@ birchcarehome@aol.com

Birch Grove Nursing Home is situated in Brighton town centre very close to the pier and all central amenities. The home provides a large range of activities which are based around residents at the time. Activities such as belly dancing shows, pottery classes and poetry writing are arranged on a regular basis to suit the residents' desires. The home caters for a wide range of patients, such as those with dementia, those who are terminal care, the physically disabled and the frail.

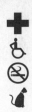

Blatchington House

Manager: Carol Breeds
Owner: AHLE Ltd
Contact: Firle Road, Seaford,
East Sussex BN25 2HH

) 01323 891702
@ info@ahle.co.uk
⌂ www.ahle.co.uk

Blatchington House is located in a quiet residential area approximately one mile from the seafront. The home has its own small shop where the less-mobile residents can access confectionary and toiletries. Seaford town centre is approximately a mile from the home, which provides shops, restaurants, a doctor's surgery and a library. There is an attractive garden to the rear of the property with a seating area for residents use during good weather.

Registered places: 34
Guide weekly rate: £450–£650
Specialist care: Nursing, physical disability, respite
Medical services: Podiatry, dentist
Qualified staff: Meets standard

Home details
Location: Residential area, 1 mile from Seaford centre
Communal areas: 3 lounges, dining room, garden
Accessibility: *Floors:* 3 • *Access:* Lift • *Wheelchair access:* Good
Smoking: ✗
Pets: ✓
Routines: Flexible

Room details
Single: 30   **Door lock:** ✓
Shared: 2   **Lockable place:** ✓
En suite: 3
Facilities: TV point, telephone point

Services provided
Beauty services: Hairdressing, manicures
Mobile library: ✗
Religious services: Fortnightly Anglican visits
Transport: ✗
Activities: *Coordinator:* ✓ • *Examples:* Exercises, visiting entertainers • *Outings:* ✗
Meetings: ✓

Bramble Cottage Retirement Home

Manager: Diana Shaw
Owner: Bramble Care Homes Ltd
Contact: 18 Carden Avenue, Brighton,
East Sussex BN1 8NA

) 01273 565821
⌂ www.bramblecottagebrighton.com

Bramble Cottage is located in Brighton, half a mile from Patcham and three miles from Brighton town centre. There is ample communal space, with a large lounge, separate dining room and large garden. There are weekly activities organised, which include outings. Summer barbecues are also provided on a yearly basis for residents, cooked by an in-house chef. The home encourages residents to keep active; one resident built a waterwheel for the waterfall in the garden, named 'The Bramble Eye'.

Registered places: 28
Guide weekly rate: £575–£825
Specialist care: Respite
Medical services: Podiatry, dentist, optician, physiotherapy
Qualified staff: Exceeds standard: 75% at NVQ Level 2

Home details
Location: Residential area, 3 miles from Brighton
Communal areas: 2 Lounges, dining room, garden
Accessibility: *Floors:* 3 • *Access:* Lift • *Wheelchair access:* Good
Smoking: ✗
Pets: At manager's discretion
Routines: Flexible

Room details
Single: 24   **Door lock:** ✓
Shared: 2   **Lockable place:** ✓
En suite: 26
Facilities: TV point, telephone point

Services provided
Beauty services: Hairdressing, massages, aromatherapy
Mobile library: ✗
Religious services: ✓
Transport: ✗
Activities: *Coordinator:* ✓ • *Examples:* Discussions, painting, poetry reading, quizzes • *Outings:* ✗
Meetings: ✓

Registered places: 15
Guide weekly rate: £371–£450
Specialist care: Respite
Medical services: Podiatry, dentist, optician
Qualified staff: Exceeds standard: 80% at NVQ Level 2

Home details

Location: Residential area, 1.5 miles from Hove
Communal areas: Lounge, dining room, patio and garden
Accessibility: *Floors:* 2 • *Access:* Stair lift
    Wheelchair access: Good
Smoking: In designated area
Pets: ×
Routines: Flexible

Room details

Single: 12	Door lock: ✓
Shared: 2	Lockable place: ✓
En suite: 10	
Facilities: TV point	

Services provided

Beauty services: Hairdressing
Mobile library: ✓
Religious services: Fortnightly Communion service
Transport: ×
Activities: *Coordinator:* ✓ • *Examples:* Arts and crafts, poetry,
    writing, reading • *Outings:* ✓
Meetings: ✓

Brittany Lodge

Manager: Anna Bromham
Owner: Deborah Dunne
Contact: 32 Brittany Road, Hove,
East Sussex BN3 4PB
☏ 01273 413413

Brittany Lodge is situated in a quiet residential area of Hove, near the seafront. The home is suitable for those who do not need a high level of care. The home's philosophy is that they do not use agency staff and there is not a high staff turnover which gives continuity for the residents. The carers also come in on set days and times without changing for increased consistency. The kitchen remains open all day for residents to make themselves a snack or tea and though pets are not allowed there is a goldfish.

Registered places: 29
Guide weekly rate: £750–£780
Specialist care: Nursing, day care, physical disability, respite
Medical services: Podiatry, dentist, optician, physiotherapy
Qualified staff: Meets standard

Home details

Location: Rural area, 3 miles from Forest Row
Communal areas: Dining room, lounge, garden
Accessibility: *Floors:* 2 • *Access:* Lift • *Wheelchair access:* Good
Smoking: In designated area
Pets: ×
Routines: Flexible

Room details

Single: 25	Door lock: ✓
Shared: 2	Lockable place: ✓
En suite: 25	
Facilities: TV point, telephone point	

Services provided

Beauty services: Hairdressing
Mobile library: ×
Religious services: Fortnightly Catholic service
Transport: Car
Activities: *Coordinator:* ✓ • *Examples:* Gentle exercise,
    reminiscence therapy • *Outings:* ✓
Meetings: ✓

Brooklands

Manager: Catherine Sheil
Owner: Hadi and Shehnaz Rajabali
Contact: Wych Cross, Forest Row,
East Sussex RH18 5JN
☏ 01825 712005

Brooklands is an old, converted building found three miles south of Forest Row village. The home's rural location means that shops and amenities are only available to residents by private transport as there is no bus route near the home. The home does have its own car, to facilitate *outings* for residents. The garden is extensive and accessible to residents.

Bybuckle Court

Manager: Sylvia Lord

Owner: James and Sylvia Lord

Contact: 5 Marine Parade, Seaford, East Sussex BN25 2PZ

) 01323 898094

@ Samantha_bickerstaff@yahoo.co.uk

Bybuckle Court is a large detached property, overlooking the seafront in Seaford. The home is within easy walking distance of the town centre's shops, amenities and railway station. There is also a bus stop located just outside the home with a service to the town centre. The residents have a flexible daily routine and the only set mealtime is for breakfast. A patio provides outside space. Pets are allowed in a cage and smoking is permitted outside. There is also a visiting book club. The activities programme includes games such as darts and bingo and quizzes.

Registered places: 17
Guide weekly rate: £310–£400
Specialist care: None
Medical services: Podiatry, dentist, optician, physiotherapy
Qualified staff: Meets standard

Home details

Location: Residential area, 1 mile from Seaford centre
Communal areas: Lounge, dining room, patio
Accessibility: *Floors:* 2 • *Access:* Lift • *Wheelchair access:* Good
Smoking: In designated area
Pets: At manager's discretion
Routines: Flexible

Room details

Single: 15
Shared: 1
En suite: Undisclosed
Facilities: TV, telephone point

Door lock: ✓
Lockable place: ✓

Services provided

Beauty services: Hairdressing, manicures
Mobile library: ✗
Religious services: ✗
Transport: ✗
Activities: *Coordinator:* ✗ • *Examples:* Bingo, exercises, games, darts, quizzes • *Outings:* ✗
Meetings: ✓

Camelot Retirement Home

Manager: Anthony White

Owner: Mr and Mrs White

Contact: 7 Darley Road, Eastbourne, East Sussex BN20 7PB

) 01323 735996

@ Camelot1@btconnect.com

Camelot is a semi-detached property on four floors in the Meads area of Eastbourne, near the seafront. The home has two resident cats and a residents meeting bi-monthly. There are a variety of activities to choose from including exercises, music and quizzes. The home also goes on outings in its minibus to local points of interest and afternoon tea trips. The staff aim to create a homely and caring environment for the residents and relatives' peace of mind.

Registered places: 17
Guide weekly rate: £350–£420
Specialist care: Respite
Medical services: Podiatry, dentist, optician
Qualified staff: Meets standard

Home details

Location: Residential area, 1.5 miles from Eastbourne centre
Communal areas: 2 lounges, dining room, garden
Accessibility: *Floors:* 4 • *Access:* Lift • *Wheelchair access:* Good
Smoking: ✗
Pets: At manager's discretion
Routines: Flexible

Room details

Single: 15
Shared: 1
En suite: 15
Facilities: TV point, telephone point

Door lock: ✓
Lockable place: ✓

Services provided

Beauty services: Hairdressing
Mobile library: ✓
Religious services: ✓
Transport: Minibus
Activities: *Coordinator:* ✓ • *Examples:* Exercises, music, quizzes *Outings:* ✓
Meetings: ✓

Registered places: 20
Guide weekly rate: £520–£725
Specialist care: None
Medical services: Podiatry, dentist, optician, physiotherapy
Qualified staff: Meets standard

Home details

Location: Residential area, 1 mile from Eastbourne centre
Communal areas: Lounge, dining room, conservatory, garden
Accessibility: *Floors:* Undisclosed • *Access:* Lift
    Wheelchair access: Good
Smoking: x
Pets: ✓
Routines: Flexible

Room details

Single: 18
Shared: 1
En suite: 19
Facilities: TV point, telephone point

Door lock: x
Lockable place: ✓

Services provided

Beauty services: Hairdressing
Mobile library: x
Religious services: x
Transport: Minibus
Activities: *Coordinator:* ✓ • *Examples:* Singalongs, musical
    evenings, cheese and wine parties • *Outings:* ✓
Meetings: ✓

Carlisle Lodge

Manager: Diane Lawson
Owner: The Croll Group
Contact: 103 Carlisle Road, Eastbourne,
East Sussex BN20 7TD
) 01323 646149
@ Diane@carlislelodge.plus.com
🖰 www.carlislelodge.co.uk

Carlisle Lodge is a detached property and a former family home converted for use as a care home. The home is situated one mile from the town centre and the seafront. Carlisle Lodge has extensive gardens to the rear of the building. The lounge, dining room and conservatory have recently been redecorated. The home has its own activities coordinator who organises a monthly activities programme for the residents. Each resident receives a copy of this program. There are special and seasonal events throughout the year and friends and relatives are included in social events.

Registered places: 24
Guide weekly rate: £385–£600
Specialist care: None
Medical services: Podiatry, dentist, hygienist, optician,
    physiotherapy
Qualified staff: Fails standard

Home details

Location: Residential area, 0.5 miles from Hailsham centre
Communal areas: 2 lounges, dining room, library,
    patio and garden
Accessibility: *Floors:* 2 • *Access:* Lift • *Wheelchair access:* Good
Smoking: x
Pets: At manager's discretion
Routines: Flexible

Room details

Single: 22
Shared: 1
En suite: 9
Facilities: TV point, telephone

Door lock: x
Lockable place: ✓

Services provided

Beauty services: Hairdressing
Mobile library: Library facilities
Religious services: Fortnightly church service
Transport: x
Activities: *Coordinator:* ✓ • *Examples:* Bingo, darts, musical
    entertainment • *Outings:* ✓
Meetings: ✓

Caroline House

Manager: Karen Mitchell
Owner: Mr and Mrs Ravichandran and
Mr and Mrs Suganthakumaran
Contact: 7–9 Ersham Road, Hailsham,
East Sussex BN27 3LG
) 01323 841073

Caroline House is a large, detached Victorian house situated in a quiet residential area of Hailsham, close to the town centre. There is an activities coordinator who arranges activities such as bingo, darts and musical entertainment. Outings are also arranged. The residents have both a flexible routine and meal times and pets are allowed at the manager's discretion. The home has a resident tenant's association which meets every two months. The home arranges a hairdressing service and a fortnightly church service.

Cedarwood House

Manager: Christine Butcher
Owner: Cedarwood House Ltd
Contact: Hastings Road, Battle,
East Sussex TN33 0TG
☎ 01424 772428

Cedarwood House is located in a rural area, approximately one mile from Battle. The home is surrounded by fields offering country views. The home has a garden with a patio area as well as a lounge and a dining room. The home has a daily activities programme, which includes quizzes and performances by visiting entertainers. There are also outings arranged for the residents in the local area.

Registered places: 20
Guide weekly rate: £350–£410
Specialist care: Dementia, respite
Medical services: Podiatry, dentist, optician
Qualified staff: Meets standard

Home details
Location: Rural area, 1 mile from Battle
Communal areas: Lounge, dining room, patio and garden
Accessibility: *Floors:* 2 • *Access:* Lift • *Wheelchair access:* Good
Smoking: ✗
Pets: ✗
Routines: Flexible

Room details
Single: 18
Shared: 1
En suite: 7
Facilities: TV, telephone point

Door lock: ✓
Lockable place: ✓

Services provided
Beauty services: Hairdressing
Mobile library: ✗
Religious services: ✓
Transport: ✗
Activities: *Coordinator:* ✗ • *Examples:* Quizzes, visiting entertainers *Outings:* ✓
Meetings: ✓

Chardwood Rest Home

Manager: Ashley Richardson
Owner: Mr and Mrs Richardson
Contact: 127 Eastbourne Road,
Pevensey Bay, East Sussex BN24 6BN
☎ 01323 766058
@ Ash35@freeserve.co.uk

Chardwood is half a mile from Pevensey village and four miles from Eastbourne. Exercises and outings with Age Concern are offered for residents to keep busy and active. There had been a residents' meeting but as residents didn't want such a formal approach the home now send out a newsletter every six weeks. Though no pets are allowed there is a Pets As Therapy scheme in place.

Registered places: 15
Guide weekly rate: £324–£400
Specialist care: Respite
Medical services: Podiatry, dentist, optician, physiotherapy
Qualified staff: Exceeds standard: 65% at NVQ Level 2

Home details
Location: Village location, 4 miles from Eastbourne
Communal areas: Lounge, dining room, conservatory, patio and garden
Accessibility: *Floors:* 2 • *Access:* Lift • *Wheelchair access:* Limited
Smoking: ✗
Pets: ✗
Routines: Flexible

Room details
Single: 13
Shared: 1
En suite: 11
Facilities: TV point, telephone point

Door lock: ✓
Lockable place: ✓

Services provided
Beauty services: Hairdressing
Mobile library: ✓
Religious services: Monthly Anglican service
Transport: Car
Activities: *Coordinator:* ✗ • *Examples:* Exercises, handicrafts, musical sessions • *Outings:* ✗
Meetings: ✗

Registered places: 18
Guide weekly rate: £361
Specialist care: None
Medical services: Podiatry
Qualified staff: Fails standard: 30% at NVQ Level 2

Home details

Location: Residential area, 2 miles from Brighton centre
Communal areas: Lounge, dining room, conservatory
Accessibility: *Floors:* 3 • *Access:* Lift • *Wheelchair access:* Limited
Smoking: In designated area
Pets: ✓
Routines: Flexible

Room details

Single: 14	Door lock: ✓
Shared: 2	Lockable place: ✓
En suite: 0	

Facilities: TV point, telephone point

Services provided

Beauty services: Hairdressing
Mobile library: Library facilities
Religious services: Weekly Communion service
Transport: ✗
Activities: *Coordinator:* ✓ • *Examples:* Morning newspaper debates, gardening, coffee mornings • *Outings:* ✗
Meetings: ✓

Charlesworth Rest Home

Manager: Eileen Horne
Owner: Eileen Horne
Contact: 37 Beaconsfield Villas, Brighton, East Sussex BN1 6HB
☎ 01273 565561

Charlesworth Rest Home is situated near to the Preston Park area of Brighton and is a large double fronted semi-detached Victorian house. The town centre is half a mile away as well as the seafront. The home has a very large garden, which has a family of foxes. There is seating and a veranda in the garden and in nice weather there are often barbecues. There is also a resident cat called Poppy who is lively and keeps the residents entertained. Morning newspaper discussions about world news are very popular in the home.

Registered places: 18
Guide weekly rate: £361–£500
Specialist care: None
Medical services: Podiatry
Qualified staff: Fails standard: 25% at NVQ Level 2

Home details

Location: Residential area, 1 mile from Hove centre
Communal areas: Lounge, dining room, garden
Accessibility: *Floors:* 3 • *Access:* Lift and stair lift
   Wheelchair access: Good
Smoking: ✗
Pets: ✗
Routines: Flexible

Room details

Single: 14	Door lock: ✗
Shared: 2	Lockable place: ✓
En suite: 7	

Facilities: TV point

Services provided

Beauty services: Hairdressing
Mobile library: ✓
Religious services: ✓
Transport: ✓
Activities: *Coordinator:* ✗ • *Examples:* Art classes, visiting entertainers • *Outings:* ✓
Meetings: ✓

The Churchley Rest Home

Manager: Karen Lewis
Owner: The Churchley Rest Home Ltd
Contact: 91 New Church Road, Hove, East Sussex BN3 4BB
☎ 01273 725185

The Churchley Rest Home is a large property set over three floors with lift and stair lift access. The home is situated on a main road which leads into Hove town centre. The home is close to the seafront, although sea views cannot be seen from the home itself. There is a varied activity programme including monthly art classes, and outside visiting entertainers who come in such as live music, singing and interesting talks about points of interest. In Hove, only a short distance way, there is the seafront, an abundance of shops. Brighton pier is 10 minutes' drive up the coast.

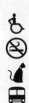

Claremont House

Manager: Karon Crouch
Owner: Claremont House Rest Home Ltd
Contact: 40–42 Claremont Road,
Seaford, East Sussex BN25 2BD
☎ 01323 893591
@ claremonthouse@f2s.com

Claremont House is located less than half a mile from the centre of Seaford where there is a library and is found in a residential area. The home has a conservatory and a recently landscaped garden and offers sea views. The home arranges a variety of activities including one to one sessions and film afternoons. There are also regular outings organised for the residents. There is a residents meeting held every month.

Registered places: 19
Guide weekly rate: From £386
Specialist care: Respite
Medical services: Podiatry, dentist, optician
Qualified staff: Exceeds standard: 100% at NVQ level 2

Home details
Location: Residential area, 0.2 miles from Seaford
Communal areas: Lounge, dining room, conservatory, garden
Accessibility: *Floors:* 4 • *Access:* Lift • *Wheelchair access:* Good
Smoking: ✗
Pets: At manager's discretion
Routines: Flexible

Room details
Single: 19
Shared: 0
En suite: 19
Facilities: TV, telephone point

Door lock: ✓
Lockable place: ✓

Services provided
Beauty services: Hairdressing
Mobile library: ✗
Religious services: ✗
Transport: ✓
Activities: *Coordinator:* ✗ • *Examples:* Film afternoons, one-to-one sessions • *Outings:* ✓
Meetings: ✓

Claydon House

Manager: Rachel Bekaert
Owner: Claydon House Ltd
Contact: 8 Wallands Crescent,
Lewes, East Sussex BN7 2QT
☎ 01273 474844

Claydon House is a detached Victorian property quietly situated in one of the most sought-after parts of Lewes. The home has strong links with the local churches, clubs and associations for many opportunities for residents to get involved. There is also a varied activity plan which is made after consultation with residents. Wallands Park is five minutes' walk away. The home has links with another local home, where residents visit for tea. The home also helps raise money for the local school. Residents also work with the activities coordinator to create the home's newsletter.

Registered places: 32
Guide weekly rate: £324–£700
Specialist care: Respite
Medical services: Podiatry, dentist, optician
Qualified staff: Undisclosed

Home details
Location: Residential area, 0.5 miles from Lewes centre
Communal areas: 2 lounges, 2 dining rooms, conservatory, garden
Accessibility: *Floors:* 4 • *Access:* Lift • *Wheelchair access:* Good
Smoking: ✗
Pets: ✗
Routines: Flexible

Room details
Single: 25
Shared: 3
En suite: 12
Facilities: TV point, Telephone point

Door lock: ✓
Lockable place: ✓

Services provided
Beauty services: Hairdressing
Mobile library: ✗
Religious services: Monthly Communion service
Transport: Minibus
Activities: *Coordinator:* ✓ • *Examples:* Armchair exercises, knitting, cooking, gardening • *Outings:* ✓
Meetings: ✓

Registered places: 48
Guide weekly rate: £500–£1,200
Specialist care: Nursing, dementia, physical disability, respite
Medical services: Podiatry, hygienist, optician, physiotherapy
Qualified staff: Meets standard

Home details

Location: Residential area, 2 miles from Hastings centre
Communal areas: Lounge, dining room, conservatory, garden
Accessibility: *Floors:* 3 • *Access:* Lift and stair lift
    Wheelchair access: Good
Smoking: ✗
Pets: At manager's discretion
Routines: Flexible

Room details

Single: 40
Shared: 4
En suite: 44
Facilities: TV point, telephone point

Door lock: ✗
Lockable place: ✗

Services provided

Beauty services: Hairdressing
Mobile library: ✓
Religious services: Weekly Catholic visits
Transport: Minibus
Activities: *Coordinator:* ✓ • *Examples:* Arts and craft, exercise,
    scrabble • *Outings:* ✓
Meetings: ✓

Clyde House

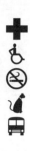

Manager: Linda Davidson
Owner: New Century Care Ltd
Contact: 258 Sedlescombe Road North,
St Leonards-on-Sea, East Sussex
TN37 7JN
☎ 01424 751002
@ clydehouse@new-meronden.co.uk
🖰 www.newcenturycare.co.uk

The owners of Clyde House, own a number of care home in East Sussex. Clyde House is in a residential area and is not very near any shops; however the homes minibus takes residents into town on weekly shopping trips. The home has a separate floor, the Tay Unit, for residents who have dementia. There are accommodation facilities for relatives of residents to stay over at the home. Pets are welcome at the home and there is a large garden at the rear of the property for residents to enjoy.

Registered places: 34
Guide weekly rate: £460–£650
Specialist care: Respite
Medical services: Podiatry, dentist, optician
Qualified staff: Undisclosed

Home details

Location: Residential area, 0.5 miles from Hove centre
Communal areas: Dining room, lounge, garden
Accessibility: *Floors:* 3 • *Access:* Stair lifts
    Wheelchair access: Limited
Smoking: In designated area
Pets: At manager's discretion
Routines: Flexible

Room details

Single: 24
Shared: 5
En suite: 29
Facilities: TV point, telephone point

Door lock: ✓
Lockable place: ✓

Services provided

Beauty services: Hairdressing, beautician, manicures
Mobile library: ✓
Religious services: ✗
Transport: ✗
Activities: *Coordinator:* ✗ • *Examples:* Entertainers, quizzes,
    board games • *Outings:* ✓
Meetings: ✓

Conifer Lodge

Manager: Josephine Lowe
Owner: Macleod Pinsent Care Conifer Ltd
Contact: Pembroke House,
91 Pembroke Crescent, Hove,
East Sussex BN3 5DE
☎ 01273 701888
@ mpc@ntlbusiness.com

Conifer Lodge is in a quiet residential area near Hove town centre. The home consists of three houses converted into a single care home. There are many activities available including classic board games, quizzes and visiting entertainers. The home also takes residents on outings to garden centres and for afternoon teas. Staff endeavour to create a friendly and comfortable environment for residents to relax in and enjoy such services as manicures and a beautician.

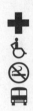

Copper Beech House Nursing Centre

Manager: Patricia High

Owner: BUPA Care Homes Ltd

Contact: Eastbourne Road, Ridgewood, Uckfield, East Sussex TN22 5ST

☏ 01825 769947

@ CopperBeechHouseEveryone@ BUPA.com

🖰 www.bupacarehomes.co.uk

Copper Beech House is situated in a quiet area one mile from the town of Uckfield. The centre has been purpose-built and caters for residents requiring long-term nursing care, short-term respite care, as well as convalescent, post-operative, palliative and rehabilitation care. All of the centre's bedrooms are single occupancy with en suite facilities. Many bedrooms have views out onto the gardens, which have patio areas and a gazebo. Residents can get involved in the home's stimulating and varied activities programme. The activities team arranges everything from games of bingo to arts and crafts sessions, and trips to the local cinema.

Registered places: 48

Guide weekly rate: Undisclosed

Specialist care: Nursing, palliative care, respite

Medical services: Podiatry, dentist, optician, physiotherapy, occupational therapy

Qualified staff: Undisclosed

Home details

Location: Rural area, 1 mile from Uckfield centre

Communal areas: 3 lounges, 2 dining rooms, kitchenette, hairdressing salon, patio and garden

Accessibility: *Floors:* 2 • *Access:* Lift • *Wheelchair access:* Good

Smoking: ✗

Pets: ✗

Routines: Flexible

Room details

Single: 48

Shared: 0

En suite: 48

Facilities: TV, telephone point

Door lock: ✓

Lockable place: ✓

Services provided

Beauty services: Hairdressing, aromatherapy

Mobile library: ✗

Religious services: Church services

Transport: ✓

Activities: *Coordinator:* ✓ • *Examples:* Arts and crafts, bingo *Outings:* ✓

Meetings: ✓

Cross Lane House

Manager: Amanda Newport

Owner: Amanda and Vincent Newport

Contact: Cross Lane, Ticehurst, Wadhurst, East Sussex TN5 7HQ

☏ 01580 200747

Cross Lane House is a converted country house set back from the road a few hundred yards from the high street. Here, more independent residents may enjoy taking advantage of the bus routes while Stonegate train station is approximately three miles away. There are daily activities such as bingo, keep fit and musical entertainment and regular outings. The home is set in two acres of land, which is very well kept, by a gardener who visits weekly. There are four lawns which have different seating and decking areas for residents to sit outside.

Registered places: 18

Guide weekly rate: £430–£650

Specialist care: None

Medical services: Podiatry, dentist, optician, physiotherapy

Qualified staff: Meets standard

Home details

Location: Village location, 100 yards from Ticehurst centre

Communal areas: Lounge, dining room, garden

Accessibility: *Floors:* 3 • *Access:* Lift • *Wheelchair access:* Good

Smoking: ✗

Pets: ✓

Routines: Flexible

Room details

Single: 14

Shared: 2

En suite: 12

Facilities: TV point, Telephone point

Door lock: ✗

Lockable place: ✓

Services provided

Beauty services: Hairdressing

Mobile library: ✓

Religious services: Monthly church service

Transport: ✗

Activities: *Coordinator:* ✗ • *Examples:* Bingo, keep fit, musical entertainment • *Outings:* ✓

Meetings: ✓

Registered places: 30
Guide weekly rate: Up to £465
Specialist care: None
Medical services: Podiatry, hygienist, optician, physiotherapy
Qualified staff: Undisclosed

Home details

Location: Residential area, in Saltdean
Communal areas: Lounge, dining room, patio and garden
Accessibility: *Floors:* 3 • *Access:* Lift • *Wheelchair access:* Good
Smoking: In designated area
Pets: ✓
Routines: Flexible

Room details

Single: 28
Shared: 2
En suite: 30
Facilities: TV point, telephone point

Door lock: ✓
Lockable place: ✓

Services provided

Beauty services: Hairdressing
Mobile library: ✗
Religious services: ✓
Transport: ✗
Activities: *Coordinator:* ✗ • *Examples:* Singing, quizzes, exercise sessions • *Outings:* ✓
Meetings: ✓

Crowborough Lodge

Manager: Bernadette Weller
Owner: Evans Care Ltd
Contact: 2 Crowborough Road, Saltdean, East Sussex BN2 8EA
☎ 01273 302614

A large detached residence situated off the A259 main road, Crowborough Lodge boats sea views that adds to the friendly and relaxed environment. Residents are given reasonably flexible daily routines, and are given the opportunity to participate in activities such as quizzes, short walks and visits to the local pub. Access to local transport, shops and other amenities are located close to the home. Crowborough Lodge has recently expanded to accommodate more residents in the adjoining property.

Registered places: 20
Guide weekly rate: £364–£408
Specialist care: Respite
Medical services: Podiatry, optician, physiotherapy
Qualified staff: Exceeds standard: 100% at NVQ Level 2

Home details

Location: Residential area, 1 mile from Hastings centre
Communal areas: Lounge, dining room, garden
Accessibility: *Floors:* 4 • *Access:* Lift
   Wheelchair access: Limited
Smoking: ✗
Pets: ✗
Routines: Flexible

Room details

Single: 16
Shared: 2
En suite: 11
Facilities: TV point, telephone point

Door lock: ✓
Lockable place: ✓

Services provided

Beauty services: Hairdressing, manicures
Mobile library: ✓
Religious services: Salvation Army and Anglican visits
Transport: ✗
Activities: *Coordinator:* ✗ • *Examples:* Art club, Bingo, exercise, bunny cuddling • *Outings:* ✓
Meetings: ✓

Cumberland Court

Manager: Elizabeth Crotty
Owner: PJP Care Ltd
Contact: 6 Cumberland Gardens, St Leonards-on-Sea, East Sussex TN38 0QL
☎ 01424 432949
@ office@cumberlandcourt.co.uk
🖰 www.cumberlandcourt.co.uk

Situated in a residential area of St Leonard-on-Sea, Cumberland Court is a Victorian property situated a short walk from a pleasant park, local shop, a mainline railway station and near the promenade and beach of St Leonards. The home organises a variety of outings, especially in the summer and Pantomime season. Visits from the Salvation Army and musicians provide residents with an enjoyable array of entertainment throughout the week.

Dalling House

Manager: Pamela Wickens
Owner: Aspenglade Ltd
Contact: Croft Road, Crowborough,
East Sussex TN6 1HA
) 01892 662917

Dalling House is located in the town of Crowborough, near Tunbridge Wells. Communication and consultation with residents' family members is effective and ongoing. Effective systems for consultation enable residents to make choices and decisions about their day-to-day living. Activities also take place such as video or DVD afternoons, musical movement, gentle exercise sessions and a weekly hand massage keep the residents enthused.

Registered places: 21
Guide weekly rate: £340–£450
Specialist care: None
Medical services: Podiatry
Qualified staff: Undisclosed

Home details
Location: Residential area, 0.5 miles from Crowborough centre
Communal areas: Dining room, lounge, garden
Accessibility: *Floors:* Undisclosed • *Access:* Lift
   Wheelchair access: Good
Smoking: ✗
Pets: At manager's discretion
Routines: Structured

Room details
Single: 17
Shared: 2
En suite: 0
Facilities: TV, telephone

Door lock: ✓
Lockable place: ✓

Services provided
Beauty services: Hairdressing, manicures
Mobile library: ✗
Religious services: ✗
Transport: ✗
Activities: *Coordinator:* ✗ • *Examples:* Music, arts and crafts
   Outings: ✗
Meetings: ✗

Derwent Residential Care Home

Manager: Denise King
Owner: The Derwent Residential Care Ltd
Contact: 38 Sedlescombe Road South,
St Leonards-on-Sea, East Sussex
TN38 0TB
) 01424 436044
@ derwent@cedarscaregroup.co.uk
🖰 www.cerdarscaregroup.co.uk

The Derwent Residential Care Home is a large detached house situated on the outskirts of St Leonards-on-Sea. There are good transport links with a bus stop located across the road from the home. The home is within walking distance of Silverhill and the local shops and cafés. The home arranges a variety of outings such as a 'bangers and mash' evening at another care home and trips to the theatre. The home is looking in to forming a Resident Tenants Association. The home has a landscaped garden with a handrail and a large entrance hall with a seating area.

Registered places: 35
Guide weekly rate: £425
Specialist care: Dementia, respite
Medical services: Podiatry, dentist, optician
Qualified staff: Meets standard

Home details
Location: Residential area, 1 mile from Hastings centre
Communal areas: Lounge, dining room, garden
Accessibility: *Floors:* 3 • *Access:* 2 stair lifts
   Wheelchair access: Limited
Smoking: In designated area
Pets: ✗
Routines: Flexible

Room details
Single: 25
Shared: 5
En suite: 35
Facilities: TV, telephone

Door lock: ✓
Lockable place: ✓

Services provided
Beauty services: Hairdressing, manicures
Mobile library: ✓
Religious services: Monthly visits from local vicar
Transport: ✗
Activities: *Coordinator:* ✗ • *Examples:* Motivation class, movement to music, visiting singers • *Outings:* ✓
Meetings: ✗

Registered places: 7
Guide weekly rate: £500
Specialist care: None
Medical services: Podiatry, dentist, optician
Qualified staff: Exceeds standard: 60% at NVQ Level 2

Home details

Location: Village location, 1.5 miles from Lewes
Communal areas: Dining room, patio lounge, garden
Accessibility: *Floors:* 2 • *Access:* Lift • *Wheelchair access:* Good
Smoking: ✗
Pets: At manager's discretion
Routines: Flexible

Room details

Single: 7   **Door lock:** ✓
Shared: 0   **Lockable place:** ✓
En suite: 7
Facilities: TV, telephone point

Services provided

Beauty services: Hairdressing
Mobile library: ✗
Religious services: Monthly visit from vicar
Transport: ✗
Activities: *Coordinator:* ✗ • *Examples:* Crafts, films, exercises, visiting speakers, flower arranging • *Outings:* ✓
Meetings: ✗

Dove Cottage

Manager: Jane Smythe
Owner: Mr and Mrs Smythe
Contact: Kingstonridge, Kingston, Lewes, East Sussex BN7 3JX
☏ 01273 486677

Dove Cottage is situated one and a half miles from the village of Lewes, nine miles from Eastbourne. There are train and bus links to the town centre. The home is a purpose-built, two-storey extension to the provider's own residence and is suitable for low-dependency residents. The home is set in beautiful surroundings with views over the downs and gardens for the residents to enjoy. Daily activities include flower arranging and visiting speakers and the residents are sometimes taken out for lunch and to watch ice skating. The daily routine is quite flexible with lunch being the only scheduled meal.

Registered places: 25
Guide weekly rate: £700
Specialist care: Nursing
Medical services: Podiatry
Qualified staff: Exceeds standard: 60% at NVQ Level 2

Home details

Location: Residential area, 2 miles from Hove centre
Communal areas: Lounge, lounge/dining room, garden
Accessibility: *Floors:* 3 • *Access:* Lift • *Wheelchair access:* Good
Smoking: In designated area
Pets: ✓
Routines: Flexible

Room details

Single: 25   **Door lock:** ✗
Shared: 0   **Lockable place:** ✓
En suite: 25
Facilities: TV point, telephone point

Services provided

Beauty services: Hairdressing
Mobile library: Library facilities
Religious services: Weekly church service
Transport: ✗
Activities: *Coordinator:* ✓ • *Examples:* Flower arranging, film afternoon, knitting • *Outings:* ✗
Meetings: ✓

The Downs Care Centre

Manager: G Whitmore
Owner: Trinity Care Ltd
Contact: Laburnum Avenue, Hove, East Sussex BN3 7JW
☏ 01273 746611

The Downs is situated in a residential area of Hove, a 10-minute drive from the seafront and town centre. The entrance is shared with the South Downs Health Trust, which provides an inpatient facility in a separate area of the building. Outings to the seafront are frequent: residents take a walk, followed by fish and chips looking on at the sea. Brighton is only a 15-minute drive away with it pier and amusement arcades. Daily activities include gardening, flower arranging, film afternoon, knitting or bingo. This keeps the residents stimulated and active.

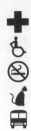

Dudwell St Mary New Building

Manager: Sue Glover
Owner: Barchester Healthcare Ltd
Contact: Etchingham Road, Burwash, East Sussex TN19 7BE

) 01435 883688
@ dudwell@barchester.com
🖰 www.barchester.com

An attractive purpose-built red-bricked building that is sited in the grounds of a former convent, Dudwell St Mary New Building provides panoramic view across the countryside. The home is a 10-minute drive from Etchingham and Heathfield where there good transport links. For those with dementia, corridors with textured walls feature interesting memorabilia such as clothes and shoes which act as sensory awareness tools. The home has a walled garden with fountain and for residents with an interest in gardening, there is a gardening club. The home has four lounges, four dining rooms and a garden with a patio area.

Registered places: 67
Guide weekly rate: From £850
Specialist care: Nursing, dementia, respite
Medical services: Podiatry, dietician, dentist, occupational therapy, optician, physiotherapy
Qualified staff: Meets standard

Home details
Location: Rural area, 1 mile from Etchingham
Communal areas: 4 lounges, 4 dining rooms, hairdressing salon, patio and garden
Accessibility: *Floors:* Undisclosed • *Access:* Lift *Wheelchair access:* Good
Smoking: ✗
Pets: At manager's discretion
Routines: Flexible

Room details
Single: 67
Shared: 0
En suite: 67
Facilities: TV, telephone

Door lock: ✓
Lockable place: ✓

Services provided
Beauty services: Hairdressing, aromatherapy, manicures
Mobile library: ✓
Religious services: ✓
Transport: Minibus
Activities: *Coordinator:* ✓ • *Examples:* Exercise classes, skittles *Outings:* ✓
Meetings: ✓

Dudwell St Mary Old Building

Manager: Alan Risk
Owner: Barchester Healthcare Ltd
Contact: Etchingham Road, Burwash, East Sussex TN19 7BE

) 01435 883688
@ dudwell@barchester.com
🖰 www.barchester.com

Dudwell St Mary Old Building is a Victorian country house located close to the village of Burwash. Its sister home, a new build is next to the home. Situated in the lovely setting of a former convent with its own extensive grounds, Dudwell St Mary exudes a calm and welcoming atmosphere. It boasts panoramic views of the local countryside. The building has been carefully adapted to meet the needs of its residents and in combination with our new, state-of-the-art purpose-built centre can happily accommodate you whether your requirement is for residential or nursing services, respite stay and holiday breaks or specialist dementia care.

Registered places: 31
Guide weekly rate: £500–£900
Specialist care: Nursing
Medical services: Podiatry, dentist, optician, physiotherapy
Qualified staff: Meets standard

Home details
Location: Rural area, 1 mile from Etchingham centre
Communal areas: Lounge, dining room, garden
Accessibility: *Floors:* 3 • *Access:* Lift • *Wheelchair access:* Good
Smoking: ✗
Pets: ✓
Routines: Flexible

Room details
Single: 23
Shared: 4
En suite: Undisclosed
Facilities: TV point, telephone point

Door lock: ✗
Lockable place: ✓

Services provided
Beauty services: Hairdressing
Mobile library: ✓
Religious services: Monthly church service
Transport: ✗
Activities: *Coordinator:* ✓ • *Examples:* Visiting entertainers *Outings:* ✗
Meetings: ✓

Registered places: 25
Guide weekly rate: £350–£425
Specialist care: None
Medical services: Podiatry, dentist, optician
Qualified staff: Exceeds standard: 75% at NVQ Level 2

Home details
Location: Residential area, in Eastbourne
Communal areas: 2 lounges, dining room, library
Accessibility: *Floors:* Undisclosed • *Access:* Lift
   Wheelchair access: Good
Smoking: ✗
Pets: At manager's discretion
Routines: Flexible

Room details
Single: 15
Shared: 5
En suite: 20
Facilities: TV point, telephone point

Door lock: ✗
Lockable place: ✗

Services provided
Beauty services: Hairdressing
Mobile library: Library facilities
Religious services: ✓
Transport: ✗
Activities: *Coordinator:* ✓ • *Examples:* Bingo, quizzes, arts and
   crafts, exercises • *Outings:* ✗
Meetings: ✗

Eastbourne Grange

Manager: Patricia Pearce
Owner: Trevor and Patricia Pearce
Contact: 2 Grange Gardens,
Blackwater Road, Eastbourne,
East Sussex BN20 7DE
☎ 01323 733466

Eastbourne Grange is located 10 minutes from the seafront, in a residential area of Eastbourne. Residents able to personalise their individual rooms and the daily life of the home is flexible. The home has its own library facilities and an activities coordinator organises a variety of activities for residents to join in if they wish. These include gentle exercise, quizzes and arts and crafts. All rooms are en suite.

Registered places: 40
Guide weekly rate: £374
Specialist care: Nursing, mental disorder
Medical services: Podiatry, dentist, optician
Qualified staff: Undisclosed

Home details
Location: Residential area, 1 mile from Eastbourne centre
Communal areas: 2 lounges, dining room, library, garden
Accessibility: *Floors:* 4 • *Access:* Lift • *Wheelchair access:* Good
Smoking: In designated area
Pets: At manager's discretion
Routines: Structured

Room details
Single: 40
Shared: 0
En suite: Undisclosed
Facilities: TV

Door lock: ✓
Lockable place: ✓

Services provided
Beauty services: Hairdressing
Mobile library: Library facilities
Religious services: ✗
Transport: ✗
Activities: *Coordinator:* ✓ • *Examples:* Bingo, cricket, skittles
   Outings: ✗
Meetings: ✗

Ennis House

Manager: Michael Baldry
Owner: Michael Baldry
Contact: 59–61 Enys Road,
Eastbourne, East Sussex BN21 2DN
☎ 01323 720719
@ ennishouse@baldry59freeserve.co.uk

Ennis House is a large property converted from three terrace houses. The home is located in a residential area close to Eastbourne town centre. There are good transport links the town centre and good wheelchair access. Smoking is permitted in the designated lounge and the home has its own library. There are two lounges in the home, one with a TV and the other a designated quiet room. Activities include bingo, cricket and skittles. The home has its own cats and other pets would be allowed to visit at the owner's discretion.

Eridge House Rest Home

Manager: Linda Stevens
Owner: Heidi Haddow
Contact: 12 Richmond Road,
Bexhill-on-Sea, East Sussex
TN39 3DN
☎ 01424 214500

Eridge House is situated in a residential area of Bexhill-on-Sea close to the seafront and near to Collington railway station. The town and shops are a 10-minute walk away. There are regular activities planned for residents including games, gardening and music exercises there are also regular outings to the seafront for a walk and fish and chips or a leisurely pub lunch. There is a patio garden with seating which then extends into a lawned garden. There is seating for residents to socialise and if they wish they can help maintain the garden as a hobby.

Registered places: 40
Guide weekly rate: £294–£500
Specialist care: None
Medical services: Podiatry, dentist, optician, physiotherapy
Qualified staff: Meets standard

Home details
Location: Residential area, 1 mile from Eastbourne centre
Communal areas: 2 lounges, conservatory, patio and garden
Accessibility: *Floors:* Undisclosed • *Access:* Lift
   Wheelchair access: Good
Smoking: ✗
Pets: ✓
Routines: Flexible

Room details
Single: 34
Shared: 3
En suite: 36
Facilities: TV point, telephone point

Door lock: ✗
Lockable place: ✓

Services provided
Beauty services: Hairdressing
Mobile library: ✓
Religious services: Monthly church visits
Transport: ✗
Activities: *Coordinator:* ✗ • *Examples:* Games, gardening, music
   Outings: ✓
Meetings: ✗

Ersham House Nursing Home

Manager: Sharon Sugars
Owner: Lakeglide Ltd
Contact: Ersham Road, Hailsham,
East Sussex BN27 3PN
☎ 01323–442727

Ersham House is set in grounds of approximately one acre, on the rural outskirts of Hailsham, with extensive views to the South Downs. It is a short 10-minute drive to local shops and amenities. The grounds have various decking and seating areas that have views over the surrounding countryside. If residents wish, they are welcome to help with gardening and maintenance of the grounds. Daily activities arranged for residents include walks, flower arranging and bingo.

Registered places: 41
Guide weekly rate: £490–£790
Specialist care: Nursing, physical disability, terminal care
Medical services: Podiatry, dentist, optician, physiotherapy
Qualified staff: Meets standard

Home details
Location: Rural area, 1 mile from Hailsham centre
Communal areas: 2 lounges, lounge/dining room, garden
Accessibility: *Floors:* 2 • *Access:* Lift • *Wheelchair access:* Good
Smoking: In designated area
Pets: ✗
Routines: Flexible

Room details
Single: 39
Shared: 1
En suite: 30
Facilities: TV point, telephone point

Door lock: ✗
Lockable place: ✓

Services provided
Beauty services: Hairdressing
Mobile library: ✓
Religious services: Monthly church services
Transport: ✓
Activities: *Coordinator:* ✓ • *Examples:* Bingo, flower arranging,
   walks • *Outings:* ✗
Meetings: ✓

Registered places: 17
Guide weekly rate: £482
Specialist care: Nursing, respite
Medical services: Podiatry, dentist, optician
Qualified staff: Meets standard

Home details

Location: Residential area, 1.3 miles from Hastings
Communal areas: Lounge, dining room, patio and garden
Accessibility: *Floors:* 1 • *Access:* Lift • *Wheelchair access:* Good
Smoking: ×
Pets: At manager's discretion
Routines: Flexible

Room details

Single: 11
Shared: 3
En suite: 2
Facilities: Telephone

Door lock: ✓
Lockable place: ✓

Services provided

Beauty services: Hairdressing, manicures
Mobile library: Library facilities
Religious services: Monthly Anglican Communion
Transport: ✓
Activities: *Coordinator:* × • *Examples:* Card games, visiting
   entertainers • *Outings:* ✓
Meetings: ✓

Fabee Nursing Home

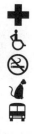

Manager: Rita Cripps
Owner: Reshad Nahoor
Contact: 35 Fearon Road, Hastings, East
Sussex TN34 2DL
☎ 01424 436485

Fabee Nursing Home is situated approximately two miles from Hastings in a residential area. The home has a patio area and a garden. However access to the garden is provided by steep steps and therefore is not accessible to all residents. There is an Anglican Communion service held once a month in the home and there are also regular outings organised. The home arranges a varied activities programme, which includes card games, ball games and performances by visiting entertainers.

Registered places: 20
Guide weekly rate: £325–£425
Specialist care: None
Medical services: Podiatry, optician
Qualified staff: Meets standard

Home details

Location: Residential area, 1 mile from Eastbourne centre
Communal areas: 2 lounges, dining room, garden
Accessibility: *Floors:* 2 • *Access:* Lift and stair lift
   Wheelchair access: Good
Smoking: ×
Pets: ×
Routines: Flexible

Room details

Single: 18
Shared: 2
En suite: 14
Facilities: TV point, telephone point

Door lock: ×
Lockable place: ✓

Services provided

Beauty services: Hairdressing
Mobile library: ✓
Religious services: Monthly church visit
Transport: ×
Activities: *Coordinator:* ✓ • *Examples:* Gardening, cooking, bingo
   Outings: ✓
Meetings: ✓

Felix Home

Manager: Karenne Karchinski
Owner: William and Elizabeth Keyworth
Contact: 15 Arundel Road, Eastbourne,
East Sussex BN21 2EL
☎ 01323 641848

Felix Home is a large detached care home set back from the road. It is in a quiet residential area of Eastbourne about quarter of a mile from Eastbourne train station making it very accessible. The home has a large, well-maintained garden that is accessible to wheelchair users. There are also two lounges – one with a TV, the other a quiet area – a separate dining room which boasts views of the homes large gardens. Visiting entertainers visit regularly, such as a monthly pianist, and the church and Salvation Army visit once a month.

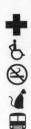

Filsham Lodge Residential Care Home

Manager: Olive Dunford
Owner: Mr and Mrs Ravichandran and Mr and Mrs Suganthakumaran
Contact: 137 South Road, Hailsham, East Sussex BN27 3NN
☎ 01323 844008
@ filsham.lodge@tiscali.co.uk

Filsham Lodge is a mile from Hailsham where the high street has a variety of shops and amenities. Staff at Filsham Lodge organise regular minibus Outings into Eastbourne and the surrounding area for coffees, lunches and local theatre trips. The home manager also organises monthly parties for residents and their families and puts on a buffet for friends and family. In the summer months it is held in the garden and often a barbecue is held. The activities coordinator organises weekly activities such as arts and crafts, exercises, games, music and quizzes to keep the residents stimulated in a variety of ways.

Registered places: 53
Guide weekly rate: £410–£700
Specialist care: Nursing, dementia
Medical services: Podiatry, dentist, optician, physiotherapy
Qualified staff: Meets standard

Home details
Location: Residential area, 1 mile from Hailsham
Communal areas: Lounge, 3 lounge/dining rooms, conservatory
Accessibility: *Floors:* 2 • *Access:* Lift • *Wheelchair access:* Good
Smoking: ✗
Pets: ✓
Routines: Flexible

Room details
Single: 53   **Door lock:** ✓
Shared: 0   **Lockable place:** ✓
En suite: 14
Facilities: TV point, telephone point

Services provided
Beauty services: Hairdressing
Mobile library: ✓
Religious services: Monthly church visits
Transport: Minibus
Activities: *Coordinator:* ✓ • *Examples:* Arts and craft, exercise, games, music, quizzes • *Outings:* ✓
Meetings: ✗

Fourways

Manager: Pamela Darch
Owner: Pamela and David Darch
Contact: 3 Bramber Avenue, Peacehaven, East Sussex BN10 8LR
☎ 01273 585670
@ 4-ways@tiscali.co.uk

Situated in Peacehaven, in a residential area on the coast, Fourways specialises in caring for those with Huntington's disease. The home also cares for the physically disabled, from 18 years old. Residents of the home are of a variety of ages, and therefore has an 'extended family' feel. Activities are designed to draw residents together and so special occasions such as birthday parties and Valentine's Day celebrations are organised.

Registered places: 21
Guide weekly rate: £420–£800
Specialist care: Nursing, respite, physical disability
Medical services: Podiatry, hygienist, optician, physiotherapy
Qualified staff: Meets standard

Home details
Location: Residential area, in Peachaven
Communal areas: Lounge, dining room, garden
Accessibility: *Floors:* 2 • *Access:* Stair lift • *Wheelchair access:* Good
Smoking: ✓
Pets: ✓
Routines: Flexible

Room details
Single: 21   **Door lock:** ✓
Shared: 0   **Lockable place:** ✓
En suite: Undisclosed
Facilities: TV point, telephone point

Services provided
Beauty services: Hairdressing, aromatherapy, massage
Mobile library: ✗
Religious services: Twice a week
Transport: ✗
Activities: *Coordinator:* ✗ • *Examples:* Parties, one-to-one sessions • *Outings:* ✓
Meetings: ✓

Registered places: 11
Guide weekly rate: £535–£625
Specialist care: None
Medical services: Podiatry, dentist, optician
Qualified staff: Exceeds standard: 80% at NVQ Level 2

Home details

Location: Residential area, in Rottingdean
Communal areas: Lounge/dining room, conservatory, garden
Accessibility: *Floors:* 2 • *Access:* Lift • *Wheelchair access:* Good
Smoking: x
Pets: x
Routines: Flexible

Room details

Single: 11
Shared: 0
En suite: 11
Facilities: TV point, telephone point

Door lock: x
Lockable place: ✓

Services provided

Beauty services: Hairdressing
Mobile library: x
Religious services: x
Transport: Minibus
Activities: *Coordinator:* x • *Examples:* Cards, black-jack, puzzles, scrabble • *Outings:* ✓
Meetings: ✓

Gate Cottage

Manager: Brenda Sodeau
Owner: Michael and Brenda Sodeau
Contact: Bazehill Road, Rottingdean, Brighton, East Sussex BN2 7DB
) 01273 301890

Gate Cottage is in the quiet residential area of Rottingdean, close to local amenities, transport links and the seafront, and is dour miles from Brighton seafront. Some activities organised include weekly drives along the coast and occasional outings in the home's own minibus. There is also a garden for residents to enjoy and caterers adapt for dietary requirements such as allergies and personal preferences.

Registered places: 33
Guide weekly rate: Up to £650
Specialist care: Nursing, physical disability
Medical services: Podiatry, optician, physiotherapy
Qualified staff: Undisclosed

Home details

Location: Residential area, 0.5 miles from Hove centre
Communal areas: Lounge, dining room, conservatory, quiet room, garden
Accessibility: *Floors:* 2 • *Access:* Lift • *Wheelchair access:* Good
Smoking: In designated area
Pets: ✓
Routines: Structured

Room details

Single: 21
Shared: 6
En suite: Undisclosed
Facilities: TV, telephone

Door lock: ✓
Lockable place: ✓

Services provided

Beauty services: Hairdressing, manicures
Mobile library: x
Religious services: ✓
Transport: x
Activities: *Coordinator:* ✓ • *Examples:* Bingo, arts and crafts, visiting entertainers • *Outings:* ✓
Meetings: Undisclosed

Glentworth House

Manager: Anita Redwood
Owner: Whytecliffe Ltd
Contact: 40–42 Pembroke Avenue, Hove, East Sussex BN3 5DB
) 01273 720044

Glentworth House is situated in a residential area of Hove, close to local shops and has good public transport links. The home has a well-maintained garden, which is easily accessed from the ground floor lounge. The home arranges daily activities for all the residents to enjoy and occasional outings, for example Christmas shopping. Pets are allowed and the home has its own cat. The residents have a structured daily routine due to their high dependency needs but residents do have the option to have their meals in their room.

The Grange Rest Home

Manager: Suzanne Leahy
Owner: The Grange Rest Home Ltd
Contact: 11 Sackville Gardens, Hove, East Sussex BN3 4GJ
☎ 01273 298746

The Grange Rest Home is a privately owned home in an extended Victorian property. There is a small garden at the rear with a patio and conservatory area. The home is close to the shopping areas of Hove, teashops, the local library and Sussex County Cricket Ground. Activities include listening to live music, group games and trips to the theatre or going for a walk. The home has its own organ in the dining room.

Registered places: 26
Guide weekly rate: £368–£450
Specialist care: None
Medical services: Podiatry, dentist, optician
Qualified staff: Fails standards

Home details

Location: Residential area, in Hove
Communal areas: 2 lounges, dining room, conservatory, patio and garden
Accessibility: *Floors:* 3 • *Access:* Lift • *Wheelchair access:* None
Smoking: In designated area
Pets: At manager's discretion
Routines: Flexible

Room details

Single: 26
Shared: 0
En suite: 13
Facilities: TV point

Door lock: ✓
Lockable place: ✓

Services provided

Beauty services: Hairdressing
Mobile library: ✓
Religious services: ✗
Transport: Car
Activities: *Coordinator:* ✓ • *Examples:* Arts and crafts, bingo, reminiscent therapy, singing • *Outings:* ✓
Meetings: ✓

Grosvenor Park Nursing Home

Manager: Jane Smith
Owner: BUPA Care Homes Ltd
Contact: 26 Brookfield Road, Bexhill-on-Sea, East Sussex TN40 1NY
☎ 01424 213535
@ GrosvenorParkALL@BUPA.com
🖰 www.bupacarehomes.co.uk

Situated in a select residential area of Bexhill, Grosvenor Park enjoys a prime location overlooking the seafront. It is set within terraced gardens with raised flowerbeds and an ornamental fountain. The home offers a large main lounge where residents may meet to chat, play cards or entertain their guests and enjoy a drink from the licensed bar. The dining room overlooks the seafront through full-length windows. Many rooms boast spectacular sea views. Daily activities are offered, with a regular bridge club, film afternoons, crossword sessions and gardening especially popular, along with the pleasure of a stroll along the seafront.

Registered places: 53
Guide weekly rate: Undisclosed
Specialist care: Nursing, palliative care, respite, terminal care
Medical services: Podiatry, dentist, optician, physiotherapy
Qualified staff: Meets standard

Home details

Location: Residential area, 1.5 miles from Bexhill centre
Communal areas: 3 lounges, dining room, hairdressing salon, bar/café and shop, garden
Accessibility: *Floors:* 3 • *Access:* Lift • *Wheelchair access:* Good
Smoking: ✗
Pets: ✗
Routines: Flexible

Room details

Single: 48
Shared: 5
En suite: 47
Facilities: TV, telephone point

Door lock: ✗
Lockable place: ✓

Services provided

Beauty services: Hairdressing, aromatherapy
Mobile library: ✓
Religious services: ✓
Transport: ✓
Activities: *Coordinator:* ✓ • *Examples:* Exercises, quizzes, puzzles *Outings:* ✓
Meetings: ✗

Registered places: 20
Guide weekly rate: £350–£600
Specialist care: None
Medical services: Podiatry, hygienist, optician, physiotherapy
Qualified staff: Meets standard

Home details

Location: Village location, 2.5 miles from Pevensey Bay
Communal areas: Lounge, dining room, conservatory, garden
Accessibility: *Floors:* 2 • *Access:* Lift • *Wheelchair access:* Good
Smoking: ✕
Pets: ✓
Routines: Flexible

Room details

Single: 18
Shared: 1
En suite: 7
Facilities: TV point, telephone point

Door lock: ✕
Lockable place: ✓

Services provided

Beauty services: Hairdressing
Mobile library: ✓
Religious services: Monthly church services
Transport: ✕
Activities: *Coordinator:* ✓ • *Examples:* Exercise, music, quizzes
　　Outings: ✓
Meetings: ✓

Hankham Lodge

Manager: Andrew Orr
Owner: Mr and Mrs Orr
Contact: Hankham Hall Road, Westham, Pevensey, East Sussex BN24 5AG
　☎ 01323 766555

Hankham Lodge is in a small village, two miles from Pevensey and two and a half miles from the coast. There is a well-kept garden with an aviary for residents to enjoy. Currently, a sensory garden is being developed to increase the pleasantness of the garden for residents. A local dial-a-bus service means that residents are not cut off from the outside world, and have the freedom to go out on a regular basis and maintain as much of a normal lifestyle as possible. Outings are organised on a monthly basis by the activities coordinator.

Registered places: 19
Guide weekly rate: £350–£500
Specialist care: None
Medical services: Podiatry, optician
Qualified staff: Exceeds standard: 60% at NVQ Level 2

Home details

Location: Residential area, in Eastbourne
Communal areas: Lounge, dining room, garden
Accessibility: *Floors:* 4 • *Access:* Lift • *Wheelchair access:* Good
Smoking: ✕
Pets: At manager's discretion
Routines: Flexible

Room details

Single: 19
Shared: 0
En suite: 19
Facilities: TV point, telephone point

Door lock: ✕
Lockable place: ✓

Services provided

Beauty services: Hairdressing
Mobile library: ✓
Religious services: ✓
Transport: ✕
Activities: *Coordinator:* ✓ • *Examples:* Cards, darts, garden parties
　　Outings: ✕
Meetings: ✓

Hardwick House

Manager: Fiona Brittain
Owner: Margaret Goddard
Contact: 6 Hardwick Road, Eastbourne, East Sussex BN21 4NY
　☎ 01323 721230

Hardwick House is a large property set in a residential area of Eastbourne, five minutes from the seafront. It is central to all services and shops in Eastbourne town centre. The activities coordinator organises activities four days a week, including evenings. These include garden parties, barbecues, cards and quizzes. Those that are mobile also go for regular walks along the seafront accompanied by a member of staff from the home. There is an average-sized garden at the rear of the property where the residents often gather for their residents meetings or for tea with their family when visiting.

Hartfield House

Manager: Cindy Nahoor
Owner: Cindy Nahoor
Contact: 5 Hartfield Road, Eastbourne, East Sussex BN21 2AP
) 01323 731322

Hartfield House is located near Eastbourne train station and main centre where there is an abundance of shops, facilities and things to do. The home has regular visiting entertainers including locals from the community who talk about the history of the local area, magicians, live music and plays. There are also daily activities in the home to keep residents stimulated such as arts and crafts, quizzes and exercise to music. Residents are welcome to ask visitors to bring their pets to visit, which always brings a lively atmosphere, and residents benefit from a very flexible daily routine.

Registered places: 21
Guide weekly rate: £315–£450
Specialist care: None
Medical services: Podiatry
Qualified staff: Meets standard

Home details
Location: Residential area, in Eastbourne
Communal areas: Lounge, dining room, garden
Accessibility: *Floors:* Undisclosed • *Access:* Lift
Wheelchair access: Good
Smoking: ✗
Pets: ✗
Routines: Flexible

Room details
Single: 19
Shared: 1
En suite: 12
Facilities: TV point, telephone point

Door lock: ✗
Lockable place: ✓

Services provided
Beauty services: Hairdressing
Mobile library: ✓
Religious services: Monthly church services
Transport: ✓
Activities: *Coordinator:* ✗ • *Examples:* Arts and crafts, exercise, quizzes, visiting entertainers • *Outings:* ✓
Meetings: ✓

Hazlemere Nursing Home

Manager: Corinne Gadsden
Owner: Rodney and Corinne Gadsden
Contact: 9 Warwick Road, Bexhill-on-Sea, East Sussex TN39 4HG
) 01424 214988

Hazlemere Nursing Home is situated in a residential area, approximately half a mile from Bexhill town centre. The main-line station, seafront and local bus services are close by. To the rear of the home is a well-maintained garden with an ornamental fishpond. Services include hairdressing and mobile library and there are visits from a local priest and a vicar. There is an activities coordinator and although there are structured mealtimes there is a flexible routine. No pets are allowed and smoking is only permitted under supervision. Each room also has its own TV and telephone.

Registered places: 23
Guide weekly rate: £450–£650
Specialist care: Nursing, physical disability
Medical services: Podiatry, physiotherapy
Qualified staff: Exceeds standard: 60% at NVQ Level 2

Home details
Location: Residential area, 0.5 miles from Bexhill centre
Communal areas: Lounge/dining room
Accessibility: *Floors:* 2 • *Access:* Lift • *Wheelchair access:* Good
Smoking: In designated area
Pets: ✗
Routines: Flexible

Room details
Single: 15
Shared: 3
En suite: 6
Facilities: TV, telephone

Door lock: ✓
Lockable place: ✓

Services provided
Beauty services: Hairdressing
Mobile library: ✓
Religious services: Visits from local priest and vicar
Transport: ✗
Activities: *Coordinator:* ✓ • *Examples:* Games • *Outings:* ✗
Meetings: ✗

Registered places: 33
Guide weekly rate: £454–£536
Specialist care: Nursing
Medical services: Podiatry, optician
Qualified staff: Fails standard: 25% at NVQ level 2

Home details

Location: Residential area, 3 miles from Brighton centre
Communal areas: Dining room, courtyard, lounge,
    quiet lounge, garden
Accessibility: *Floors:* 1 • *Wheelchair access:* Good
Routines: Flexible
Pets: ✗
Smoking: ✗

Room details

Single: 29
Shared: 2
En suite: 31
Facilities: TV, telephone point

Door lock: ✗
Lockable place: ✓

Services provided

Beauty services: Hairdressing
Mobile library: ✗
Religious services: ✗
Transport: ✗
Activities: *Coordinator:* ✓ • *Examples:* Arts and crafts, bingo,
    wheelchair dancing • *Outings:* ✗
Meetings: ✓

Heath Hill Lodge

Manager: Vacant
Owner: Mr and Mrs Vig
Contact: Heath Hill Avenue,
Lower Bevendean, Brighton,
East Sussex BN2 4FH
☏ 01273 886788

Families and friends of residents are encouraged to participate in the activities, with a 'Heath Hill Family and Friends' group having been formed, and recently they have organised a fête. Equipment includes assisted baths, handrails in WCs, variable height beds and a selection of hoisting and moving equipment. There is a local bus service, which goes straight to near-by Brighton, which residents are able to use. All facilities are on the ground floor to serve as convenience for the residents.

Registered places: 16
Guide weekly rate: £324–£350
Specialist care: Day care, respite
Medical services: Podiatry, dentist, optician, physiotherapy
Qualified staff: Exceeds standard: 75% at NVQ Level 2

Home details

Location: Residential area, 3 miles from Hastings centre
Communal areas: 2 lounges, dining room, patio and garden
Accessibility: *Floors:* 2 • *Access:* Lift • *Wheelchair access:* Good
Smoking: ✗
Pets: At manager's discretion
Routines: Flexible

Room details

Single: 15
Shared: 1
En suite: 10
Facilities: TV point, telephone point

Door lock: ✗
Lockable place: ✓

Services provided

Beauty services: Hairdressing
Mobile library: ✓
Religious services: ✓
Transport: ✗
Activities: *Coordinator:* ✓ • *Examples:* Cooking, visiting
    entertainers • *Outings:* ✗
Meetings: ✓

Helenswood Rest Home

Manager: Jill Weeks
Owner: Graham Newton and David Grey
Contact: 195 The Ridge, Hastings,
East Sussex TN34 2AE
☏ 01424 445127
🖰 www.helenswood.co.uk

Helenswood is a large house situated in its own grounds along The Ridge on northern outskirts of Hastings. It is a mile to the nearest village where there is an array of local shops. One of the lounges has doors leading out onto a decked area, which looks out on the home's expansive gardens, giving views of Hastings and the sea. The home has a weekly activities schedule, and there is often visiting entertainment such as shows or theatre performances. Residents are also encouraged to take part in cooking lessons. The home also has a residential cat, and visitors' pets are welcome.

Highbury House Nursing Home

Manager: Benitha Siziba
Owner: Zeenat Nanji and Tasneem Osman
Contact: Steyning Road, Rottingdean, Brighton, East Sussex BN2 7GA
☎ 01273–309447

Highbury House is located in Rottingdean village with pleasant views from all rooms, and some have a sea view. The home has well-maintained gardens, which are accessible to wheelchair users. The home's activities programme is displayed on a notice board in the home. Residents are taken out for cream teas and pub lunches. Any pets that are not allowed to stay at the home can visit with family and friends.

Registered places: 30
Guide weekly rate: £350–£700
Specialist care: Nursing
Medical services: Podiatry, dentist, optician, physiotherapy
Qualified staff: Fails standard: 39% at NVQ Level 2

Home details
Location: Village location, in Rottingdean
Communal areas: Lounge, dining room, patio and garden
Accessibility: *Floors:* 2 • *Access:* Lift • *Wheelchair access:* Good
Smoking: In designated area
Pets: At manager's discretion
Routines: Flexible

Room details
Single: 27
Shared: 1
En suite: 27
Facilities: TV point, telephone point
Door lock: ✓
Lockable place: ✓

Services provided
Beauty services: Hairdressing
Mobile library: ✓
Religious services: Monthly Catholic service
Transport: ✗
Activities: *Coordinator:* ✓ • *Examples:* Horse racing, musical entertainment, wine tasting • *Outings:* ✓
Meetings: ✓

Holy Cross Priory Nursing Unit

Manager: Soley Mathai
Owner: The Grace and Compassion Benedictines
Contact: Cross-In-Hand, Heathfield, East Sussex TN21 0TS
☎ 01435 863764
@ holycrossnursingunit@tiscali.co.uk

Holy Cross Priory Nursing Unit is a purpose-built extension to The Priory Residential Care Home. The unit is attached by a corridor but is run as a separate home. Residents are able to use the facilities at The Priory if they wish and also meet with residents of The Priory, giving them more social interaction. The home is situated in Cross-in-Hand, approximately three miles from Heathfield town. The home has a large garden, and sensory garden for residents to enjoy with seating and decking for finer weather. There is also a chapel where there are frequent readings and prayer services.

Registered places: 21
Guide weekly rate: £530
Specialist care: Nursing
Medical services: Podiatry
Qualified staff: Meets standard

Home details
Location: Rural area, 3 miles from Heathfield
Communal areas: Lounge, dining room, hairdressing salon, chapel, garden
Accessibility: *Floors:* 1 • *Wheelchair access:* Good
Smoking: ✗
Pets: ✓
Routines: Flexible

Room details
Single: 21
Shared: 0
En suite: 7
Facilities: TV point, telephone point
Door lock: ✗
Lockable place: ✓

Services provided
Beauty services: Hairdressing
Mobile library: ✓
Religious services: Chapel services
Transport: ✗
Activities: *Coordinator:* ✓ • *Examples:* Bingo, games, sewing, walks • *Outings:* ✗
Meetings: ✓

Registered places: 37
Guide weekly rate: £366–£595
Specialist care: Respite
Medical services: Podiatry, dentist, optician, physiotherapy
Qualified staff: Exceeds standard: 63% at NVQ Level 2

Home details

Location: Residential area, 0.5 miles from Eastbourne centre
Communal areas: 2 lounges, dining room, conservatory and garden
Accessibility: *Floors:* Undisclosed • *Access:* Lift
    Wheelchair access: Good
Smoking: In designated area
Pets: ✓
Routines: Flexible

Room details

Single: 37
Shared: 1
En suite: 24
Facilities: TV point, telephone point

Door lock: ✗
Lockable place: ✓

Services provided

Beauty services: Hairdressing
Mobile library: ✓
Religious services: ✓
Transport: Minibus
Activities: *Coordinator:* ✓ • *Examples:* Coffee morning debates,
    seafront walks, scrabble • *Outings:* ✓
Meetings: ✓

Ingham House

Manager: Vikki Sharman
Owner: Ingham House Ltd
Contact: 10–12 Carlisle Road,
Eastbourne, East Sussex BN20 7EJ
☎ 01323 734009

Comprising of two Victorian properties linked together, Ingram House is situated close to the town's amenities and the seafront. The residents are taken out three times a week in the home's minibus on shopping trips into Hove town centre. There are also outings to Brighton Pier for fish and chips and walks along the seafront on a regular basis. There is a garden with seating for the residents to sit outside with level access.

Registered places: 54
Guide weekly rate: Undisclosed
Specialist care: Nursing, palliative care, terminal care
Medical services: Podiatry, occupational therapy, physiotherapy
Qualified staff: Undisclosed

Home details

Location: Residential area, 2 miles from Eastbourne centre
Communal areas: 4 lounges, 2 dining rooms,
    hairdressing salon, garden
Accessibility: *Floors:* 2 • *Access:* Lift • *Wheelchair access:* Good
Smoking: In designated area
Pets: ✗
Routines: Flexible

Room details

Single: 48
Shared: 3
En suite: 51
Facilities: TV, telephone point

Door lock: ✓
Lockable place: ✓

Services provided

Beauty services: Hairdressing, aromatherapy
Mobile library: ✓
Religious services: Monthly church service
Transport: ✗
Activities: *Coordinator:* 2 • *Examples:* Arts and crafts, films,
    games, music • *Outings:* ✓
Meetings: ✗

Kestrel House

Manager: Debby Potter
Owner: BUPA Care Homes Ltd
Contact: 220 Willingdon Road,
Eastbourne, East Sussex BN21 1XR
☎ 01323 431199
@ KestrelHouseEveryone@BUPA.com
🖥 www.bupacarehomes.co.uk

Kestrel House is situated close to the town centre of Eastbourne. This modern, purpose-built home has been designed to create a pleasant, well-equipped environment for elderly people and offers long-term care for those who need daily nursing and continuing care. The home has a well-maintained garden that includes a summerhouse, two water features and a gazebo where residents can sit on sunny days. Residents can also relax in one of the four comfortable lounges where activities take place. Regular activities include movement to music sessions, quizzes and art and film shows.

The Laurels Nursing Home

Manager: Vacant
Owner: The Laurels Nursing Home Ltd
Contact: 71 Old London Road,
Hastings, East Sussex TN35 5NB
☎ 01424 714258

The Laurels Nursing Home is a large detached property set back from the road at the end of a small cul-de-sac in a residential area of Hastings. A main bus route is nearby, enabling access to the shops and sea and access into Hastings centre which is approximately one and a half miles away. The home's lounge overlooks gardens that can be accessed from some bedrooms. An activities coordinator organises walks along the seafront and various games.

Registered places: 29
Guide weekly rate: £525–£735
Specialist care: Nursing, respite
Medical services: Podiatry, optician
Qualified staff: Exceeds standard: 60% at NVQ Level 2

Home details
Location: Residential area, 1.5 miles from Hastings centre
Communal areas: Lounge, 2 gardens
Accessibility: *Floors:* 2 • *Access:* Lift • *Wheelchair access:* Good
Smoking: ✗
Pets: ✗
Routines: Flexible

Room details
Single: 21
Shared: 3
En suite: 12
Facilities: TV point, telephone point

Door lock: ✓
Lockable place: ✓

Services provided
Beauty services: Hairdressing, aromatherapy, manicures
Mobile library: ✗
Religious services: ✗
Transport: ✗
Activities: *Coordinator:* ✓ • *Examples:* Bingo, games, walks
    Outings: ✓
Meetings: ✓

Lea House

Manager: Sadna Seesarun
Owner: Sadna and Baldeo Seesarun
Contact: 40 Terminus Avenue,
Bexhill-on-Sea, East Sussex TN39 3LZ
☎ 01424 220968
@ Shona2@onetel.com

Lea House is a detached property situated in a quiet residential area of Bexhill-on-Sea, near to the sea itself. The town centre with its shops and access to bus and rail services is approximately one mile away and local shops are on a short level walk. The home provides home cooking and residents can choose to have their meals in their room. There is a large garden and a conservatory. Pets are allowed and the home arranges activities such as games. The home arranges a hairdressing service for the residents and smoking is only permitted outside the building.

Registered places: 15
Guide weekly rate: £350
Specialist care: None
Medical services: Podiatry, dentist, optician
Qualified staff: Undisclosed

Home details
Location: Residential area, 1 mile from Bexhill centre
Communal areas: 2 lounges, dining room, conservatory,
    patio and garden
Accessibility: *Floors:* 2 • *Access:* Lift • *Wheelchair access:* Good
Smoking: In designated area
Pets: ✓
Routines: Flexible

Room details
Single: 13
Shared: 1
En suite: 14
Facilities: TV, telephone

Door lock: ✓
Lockable place: ✗

Services provided
Beauty services: Hairdressing
Mobile library: ✗
Religious services: ✗
Transport: ✗
Activities: *Coordinator:* ✗ • *Examples:* Music, games
    Outings: ✗
Meetings: ✗

Registered places: 34
Guide weekly rate: £450–£650
Specialist care: Nursing
Medical services: Podiatry, optician, hygienist, physiotherapy
Qualified staff: Exceeds standard: 60% at NVQ Level 2

Home details

Location: Residential area, 200 yards from St Leonards centre
Communal areas: Lounge, dining room, patio
Accessibility: *Floors:* 4 • *Access:* Lift and stair lift
   Wheelchair access: Good
Smoking: In designated area
Pets: ✓
Routines: Flexible

Room details

Single: 26   Door lock: ✓
Shared: 4   Lockable place: ✓
En suite: 30
Facilities: TV point, telephone point

Services provided

Beauty services: Hairdressing
Mobile library: ✓
Religious services: ✓
Transport: ✗
Activities: *Coordinator:* ✓ • *Examples:* Group activities
   Outings: ✓
Meetings: ✓

Leolyn Care Home

Manager: Valerie Fowler
Owner: New Century Care Ltd
Contact: 63 Pevensey Road,
St Leonards-on-Sea, East Sussex
TN38 0LE
☎ 01424 422063
@ leolyn@new-meronden.co.uk

Leolyn Care Home is a large detached property situated in a residential area of St Leonards-on-Sea. The activities coordinator publicises group outings on a notice board in the hallway. These include fish and chips on the seafront, cream teas at the local gardening centre and historical visits to local castles in Hastings. There is a large patio at the rear of the property with decking and seating which is accessible for wheelchair users. The home is also very conveniently located in terms of access to facilities. It is only 200 yards from the local shops and amenities in St Leonard's.

Registered places: 17
Guide weekly rate: £450–£525
Specialist care: None
Medical services: Podiatry, dentist, optician, physiotherapy
Qualified staff: Meets standard

Home details

Location: Rural area, 0.5 miles from Ringmer
Communal areas: Lounge, dining room, patio and garden
Accessibility: *Floors:* 2 • *Access:* Lift and stair lift
   Wheelchair access: Good
Smoking: ✓
Pets: ✗
Routines: Flexible

Room details

Single: 18   Door lock: ✓
Shared: 0   Lockable place: ✓
En suite: 9
Facilities: TV point, telephone

Services provided

Beauty services: Hairdressing
Mobile library: ✗
Religious services: ✓
Transport: ✗
Activities: *Coordinator:* ✗ • *Examples:* Bingo, games, singing
   Outings: ✓
Meetings: ✓

Lime Tree House Residential Home

Manager: Vacant
Owner: Zeenat and Salim Nanji
Contact: Lewes Road, Ringmer,
East Sussex BN8 5ES
☎ 01273 813755
@ limetree@southcarehomes.com
🖱 www.southcarehomes.com

Lime Tree House Residential Care Home is located in a rural area, only half a mile from the village of Ringmer. The home has a lounge, a dining room and a conservatory for residents to relax in, as well as a garden to enjoy in the warmer months. The home arranges religious services for the residents and there is also a varied activities programme in place. There are also outings on offer to the residents, for example to the seaside.

Longworth House

Manager: Lucy Pope
Owner: Mr and Mrs Siddiqi
Contact: 28 Eversfield Road,
Eastbourne, East Sussex BN21 2DS
☎ 01323 729700
@ Longworth.house@tiscali.co.uk

Longworth House is a converted family home. The local train station is half a mile away and the home is near a bus route. The home offers a flexible routine for the residents and an open door policy for visitors. Residents have set meal times but can choose to have their meals in their room or in the lounge. There is a portable telephone for personal calls and a mobile library which visits. The home has visiting activities coordinators who ensure that the residents partake in the activities they want. There is a large garden and good wheelchair access with a lift.

Registered places: 20
Guide weekly rate: £500–£650
Specialist care: Nursing
Medical services: Podiatry, dentist, optician, physiotherapy
Qualified staff: Fails standard: 36% at NVQ Level 2

Home details
Location: Residential area, 1 mile from Eastbourne centre
Communal areas: Lounge, dining room, conservatory, garden
Accessibility: *Floors:* 3 • *Access:* Lift • *Wheelchair access:* Good
Smoking: ✗
Pets: ✗
Routines: Flexible

Room details
Single: 12
Shared: 4
En suite: 4
Facilities: TV point, telephone point

Door lock: ✓
Lockable place: ✓

Services provided
Beauty services: Hairdressing
Mobile library: ✓
Religious services: ✗
Transport: ✗
Activities: *Coordinator:* ✓ • *Examples:* Music for health, bingo, games • *Outings:* ✗
Meetings: ✓

Lydfords Care Home

Manager: Karen Waddington
Owner: Tamaris Ltd
Contact: 23 High Street, East Hoathly,
Lewes, East Sussex BN8 6DR
☎ 01825–840259

Originally a Victorian family home, Lyfords has been extended and modified to meet the needs of all its residents. The home is situated in a semi-rural location with village shops a mere 200 yards away. A pub and church are also in close proximity to the home, however it is eight miles to Lewes where there are proper facilities. To the rear and side of the property are large natural gardens with ample seating for the residents. The there is a shopping trolley from which residents can purchase cards, toiletries, confectionary and stationary.

Registered places: 50
Guide weekly rate: £497–£695
Specialist care: Nursing
Medical services: Podiatry, optician
Qualified staff: Meets standard

Home details
Location: Rural area, 8 miles from Lewes centre
Communal areas: 3 lounges, dining room, activity room, patio
Accessibility: *Floors:* 2 • *Access:* Lift and stair lift
Wheelchair access: Good
Smoking: In designated area
Pets: ✓
Routines: Flexible

Room details
Single: 42
Shared: 4
En suite: 24
Facilities: TV point

Door lock: ✗
Lockable place: ✓

Services provided
Beauty services: Hairdressing
Mobile library: ✓
Religious services: Monthly church visits
Transport: ✗
Activities: *Coordinator:* ✓ • *Examples:* Arts and crafts, acting
Outings: ✗
Meetings: ✓

Registered places: 20
Guide weekly rate: £340–£410
Specialist care: None
Medical services: Podiatry, optician
Qualified staff: Fails standard: 40% at NVQ Level 2

Home details
Location: Village location, 5 miles from Uckfield
Communal areas: 2 lounges, conservatory, patio and garden
Accessibility: *Floors:* 3 • *Access:* Stair lift
   Wheelchair access: Limited
Smoking: In designated area
Pets: ✓
Routines: Flexible

Room details
Single: 11
Shared: 3
En suite: 8
Facilities: None

Door lock: ✗
Lockable place: ✓

Services Provided
Beauty services: Hairdressing
Mobile library: ✓
Religious services: ✓
Transport: ✓
Activities: *Coordinator:* ✓ • *Examples:* Bingo, craft, garden
   games • *Outings:* ✗
Meetings: ✓

Marlowe House

Manager: Janet Moseley
Owner: AUM Care Ltd
Contact: School Lane, Hadlow Down,
East Sussex TN22 4HY
☎ 01825 830224

Marlowe House is a detached, converted property set outside the village of Hadlow, near Uckfield town. Although it is not in close proximity to any local shops or amenities the home has its own transport which it takes residents out in regularly, for example, on weekly shopping trips. The home offers a range of activities such as cooking, karaoke, sing a longs and beauty sessions. There is a patio and garden at the rear of the property with seating for residents to enjoy.

Registered places: 17
Guide weekly rate: £337–£480
Specialist care: Respite, dementia
Medical services: Podiatry
Qualified staff: Undisclosed

Home details
Location: Residential area, in Hailsham
Communal areas: Lounge, dining room, garden
Accessibility: *Floors:* Undisclosed • *Access:* Lift
   Wheelchair access: Good
Smoking: ✗
Pets: At manager's discretion
Routines: Flexible

Room details
Single: 11
Shared: 3
En suite: 1
Facilities: TV point, telephone point

Door lock: ✓
Lockable place: ✓

Services provided
Beauty services: Hairdressing
Mobile library: ✗
Religious services: ✗
Transport: ✓
Activities: *Coordinator:* ✗ • *Examples:* Musical entertainment
   Outings: ✓
Meetings: ✗

Marshview

Manager: Maria Mapletoft
Owner: Maria Mapletoft
Contact: 77 Marshfoot Lane, Hailsham,
East Sussex BN27 2RB
☎ 01323 849207

Marshview is a large two-storey house situated in the market town of Halisham, less than one mile from its centre. While the home does not have a designated activities coordinator, care staff organise a variety of activities and the home has its own transport to take residents on outings intermittently. The home can also care for those with dementia, although it is not a nursing home.

Mountside Residential Home

Manager: Freda Steuart-Pownall
Owner: Downlands Care Ltd
Contact: 9–11 Laton Road, Hastings, East Sussex TN34 2ES
☎ 01424 424144

Mountside Residential Home is an attractive detached property, formed by the joining of two large houses. The home boasts extensive gardens to the front and rear of the property which are accessible to all residents. Residents are welcome to help maintain the garden by growing shrubbery, or planting flowerbeds. The property is situated in a residential area on the outskirts of Hastings, within close proximity to Alexandra Park. The location of the home provides easy access to Hastings town centre and public transport links.

Registered places: 38
Guide weekly rate: £322–£600
Specialist care: None
Medical services: Podiatry
Qualified staff: Exceeds standard: 65% at NVQ Level 2

Home details
Location: Residential area, 1.5 miles from Hastings centre
Communal areas: Lounge, dining room, garden
Accessibility: *Floors:* 3 • *Access:* 2 lifts and stair lift
   Wheelchair access: Good
Smoking: x
Pets: ✓
Routines: Flexible

Room details
Single: 33
Shared: 5
En suite: 16
Facilities: TV point, telephone point

Door lock: x
Lockable place: ✓

Services provided
Beauty services: Hairdressing
Mobile library: x
Religious services: Monthly church service
Transport: x
Activities: *Coordinator:* x • *Examples:* Bingo, games, music
   Outings: x
Meetings: ✓

Nightingales

Manager: Anne Lewis
Owner: Anne Lewis
Contact: 38 Western Road, Newick, East Sussex BN8 4LF
☎ 01825 721120
🖰 www.nightingalecarehome.co.uk

Nightingales care home is set in an Edwardian property which stands in one acre of land in the village of Newick. It is within walking distance of the local village shops and public houses and also from the local bus route. The communal dining and sitting room have extensive views over the gardens and farmland reaching the horizon. There is a large screen colour television in the main sitting room. A quieter area for reading, relaxing or entertaining is made available in another sitting room. Facilities are available for residents to make their own drinks and for visitors at any time of day.

Registered places: 22
Guide weekly rate: £473–£550
Specialist care: Respite
Medical services: Optician
Qualified staff: Fails standards

Home details
Location: Village location, 4.5 miles from Uckfield
Communal areas: Lounges, dining room, conservatory, garden
Accessibility: *Floors:* 2 • *Access:* Stair lift
   Wheelchair access: Limited
Smoking: In designated area
Pets: At manger's discretion
Routines: Flexible

Room details
Single: 20
Shared: 2
En suite: 0
Facilities: TV point

Door lock: x
Lockable place: ✓

Services provided
Beauty services: Hairdressing
Mobile library: x
Religious services: ✓
Transport: x
Activities: *Coordinator:* x • *Examples:* Coffee mornings, musical afternoons, jazz night, darts • *Outings:* x
Meetings: ✓

Registered places: 19
Guide weekly rate: £420–£460
Specialist care: Respite
Medical services: Podiatry, dentist, optician, physiotherapy
Qualified staff: Fails standards

Home details
Location: Residential area, in Seaford
Communal areas: Lounge, dining room, conservatory, library, garden
Accessibility: *Floors:* 3 • *Access:* Lift and stair lift
Wheelchair access: Good
Smoking: ✗
Pets: ✗
Routines: Structured

Room details
Single: 19
Shared: 0
En suite: 12
Facilities: TV point, telephone point

Door lock: ✓
Lockable place: ✗

Services provided
Beauty services: Hairdressing
Mobile library: Library facilities
Religious services: Regular Catholic visits
Transport: ✗
Activities: *Coordinator:* ✓ • *Examples:* Bingo, carpet bowles,
quizzes • *Outings:* ✓
Meetings: ✗

Nova House

Manager: Roberta Rutherford
Owner: Seaford Homes Ltd
Contact: Belgrave Road, Seaford,
East Sussex BN25 2EG
☎ 01323 896629

Nova House is a detached Edwardian property in a residential area of Seaford intending to create a 'home from home' atmosphere for its residents. Well placed only a short distance from the seafront, and with good public transport links to the town centre, the South Downs are also not far away. There is a large lounge and dining room that have views out on the well-maintained garden area. To the south and east of the house lie sun lounges and on the west there is a veranda and patio area.

Registered places: 15
Guide weekly rate: £320–£520
Specialist care: None
Medical services: Podiatry, optician
Qualified staff: Fails standard: 40% at NVQ Level 2

Home details
Location: Urban area, 1 mile from Hove centre
Communal areas: Lounge/dining room, conservatory, garden
Accessibility: *Floors:* 2 • *Access:* Lift • *Wheelchair access:* Good
Smoking: In designated area
Pets: ✗
Routines: Flexible

Room details
Single: 11
Shared: 2
En suite: 11
Facilities: TV point, telephone point

Door lock: ✗
Lockable place: ✓

Services provided
Beauty services: Hairdressing
Mobile library: ✓
Religious services: Monthly church services
Transport: ✓
Activities: *Coordinator:* ✗ • *Examples:* Bingo, afternoon tea
Outings: ✓
Meetings: ✓

Oakleigh Lodge

Manager: Lee Lockwood
Owner: Mr and Mrs Lockwood
Contact: 36 New Church Road, Hove,
East Sussex BN3 4FJ
☎ 01273 205199

Oakleigh Lodge is a large detached property situated on a main road in Hove, close to all local amenities and the seafront. There is a pleasant conservatory and garden, Which is wheelchair accessible via a ramp, and is well maintained by a visiting gardener. The home has its own transport, so residents regularly go into Hove town centre shopping. For those who are less mobile, there are activity afternoons playing scrabble, bingo and charades. Pets are welcome to come and visit residents at the home, which adds to the homely feel of this small and intimate care home.

Oakside Care Home

Manager: Barbara Clark
Owner: Peasmarsh Place Ltd
Contact: Main Street, Northiam, Rye,
East Sussex TN31 6NB
) 01797 252165
@ care@peasmarshplace.co.uk
www.peasmarshplace.co.uk

Oakside is a wooden building in the village of Northiam overlooking the village green. Village shops and local amenities are a short distance from the home. Main bus routes run close by into Rye town which is four miles away. Residents are welcome to enjoy the five acres of grounds that include an enclosed rose garden, a lake, a walled garden and tree collection, whilst walking or driving the 'house buggy'. Several pathways throughout the garden lead to the village church and more secluded areas. The home also has a resident cat from the Blue Cross Charity.

Registered places: 17
Guide weekly rate: £450–£600
Specialist care: None
Medical services: Podiatry, dentist, optician, physiotherapy
Qualified staff: Exceeds standard: 100% at NVQ Level 2

Home details
Location: Village location, 4 miles from Rye centre
Communal areas: Lounge, dining room, patio
Accessibility: *Floors:* 3 • *Access:* Stair lift
 Wheelchair access: Limited
Smoking: ✗
Pets: ✓
Routines: Flexible

Room details
Single: 7
Shared: 4
En suite: 4
Facilities: TV point, telephone point

Door lock: ✗
Lockable place: ✓

Services provided
Beauty services: Hairdressing
Mobile library: ✗
Religious services: Monthly Catholic visits
Transport: ✗
Activities: *Coordinator:* ✗ • *Examples:* Keep fit, music, coffee morning, bingo • *Outings:* ✗
Meetings: ✓

Orchardown Rest Home

Manager: Linda Clarke
Owner: Visnja Mazzoli
Contact: 4–6 Old Orchard Road,
Eastbourne, East Sussex BN21 1DB
) 01323 726829

Orchardown is a large detached Edwardian property, within walking distance of Eastbourne's town centre and railway station. The home organises regular themed events to which family and friends are welcome. Outings to local attractions, shopping, and tearooms and to the theatre are also common. The home has two lounges, one dining room and a conservatory looking out to the large rear garden that is accessible to residents. There is an interdenominational religious group which visits the home monthly. Pets are allowed in the home but smoking is not permitted.

Registered places: 17
Guide weekly rate: £346–£500
Specialist care: None
Medical services: Podiatry
Qualified staff: Exceeds standard: 90% at NVQ Level 2

Home details
Location: Residential area, 0.5 miles from Eastbourne centre
Communal areas: 2 lounges, dining room, conservatory, garden
Accessibility: *Floors:* 3 • *Access:* Lift • *Wheelchair access:* Good
Smoking: ✗
Pets: ✓
Routines: Undisclosed

Room details
Single: 17
Shared: 0
En suite: 13
Facilities: None

Door lock: ✗
Lockable place: ✓

Services provided
Beauty services: Hairdressing
Mobile library: ✗
Religious services: Monthly visits from interdenominational group
Transport: ✗
Activities: *Coordinator:* ✗ • *Examples:* Quizzes and bingo
 Outings: ✓
Meetings: Undisclosed

Registered places: 37
Guide weekly rate: £322–£450
Specialist care: None
Medical services: Podiatry, optician
Qualified staff: Undisclosed

Home details
Location: Residential area, 1 mile from Hastings centre
Communal areas: 3 lounges, dining room, garden
Accessibility: *Floors:* 3 • *Access:* Lift • *Wheelchair access:* ✓
Smoking: ✗
Pets: At manager's discretion
Routines: Flexible

Room details
Single: 33
Shared: 2
En suite: 12
Facilities: TV

Door lock: ✓
Lockable place: ✓

Services provided
Beauty services: Hairdressing
Mobile library: ✗
Religious services: ✓
Transport: ✗
Activities: *Coordinator:* ✓ • *Examples:* Exercises, games
       Outings: ✓
Meetings: ✗

The Park Beck

Manager: Vacant
Owner: Regal Care Homes Ltd
Contact: 21 Upper Maze Hill,
St Leonards-on-Sea, East Sussex
TN38 0LG
☏ 01424 445855
@ managerparkbeck@regalhomes.com
🖱 www.regalhomes.com

The Park Beck is near bus routes and Warrior Park station giving it good access for visitors. The home is well maintained and residents are able to move about the home at will with safety. The activities coordinator also takes willing residents on outings, which gives them time to bond whilst also offering time out of the home. There is no obligation for the residents to be part of the activities, so some residents simply go out or sit in the garden.

Registered places: 18
Guide weekly rate: £475–£650
Specialist care: Respite
Medical services: Podiatry, optician, physiotherapy
Qualified staff: Exceeds standard: 100% at NVQ Level 2

Home details
Location: Residential area, in Hove
Communal areas: Lounge, dining room, activities room, garden
Accessibility: *Floors:* 4 • *Access:* Lift • *Wheelchair access:* None
Smoking: In designated area
Pets: At manager's discretion
Routines: Flexible

Room details
Single: 16
Shared: 2
En suite: 18
Facilities: TV point, telephone point

Door lock: ✓
Lockable place: ✓

Services provided
Beauty services: Hairdressing, aromatherapy, manicures
Mobile library: ✓
Religious service: ✓
Transport: ✗
Activities: *Coordinator:* ✗ • *Examples:* Board games, French
       language classes, t'ai chi • *Outings:* ✓
Meetings: ✓

Pembroke Hotel for the Retired

Manager: Elaine Darby
Owner: Susan Brand
Contact: 2 Third Avenue, Hove,
East Sussex BN3 2PD
☏ 01273 326942

Pembroke Hotel is detached, Grade II listed and in a conservation area. It is very near the seafront, in the centre of Hove and near local amenities. Activities provided for the home include French language classes, board games, and a weekly session of t'ai chi. Smoking is permitted in residents' own rooms if they wish. As well as hairdressing, the home can organise aromatherapy and manicures for residents.

Pembroke Lodge

Manager: Joanne Lea
Owner: Mr and Mrs Brand
Contact: 8–10 Aymer Road, Hove,
East Sussex BN3 4GA

☎ 01273 777286

Pembroke Lodge is a residential home situated very near the seafront in the centre of Hove. Current needs of the residents are low and they have a great deal of independence. As a result there are many outings to the seafront for fish and chips, trips along Brighton Pier and historical visits to points of interest in the local area. There is a garden with seating for residents to sit out with each other or visitors in finer weather. Daily activities include knitting, bingo, scrabble and charades.

Registered places: 19
Guide weekly rate: £350–£520
Specialist care: None
Medical services: Podiatry, optician
Qualified staff: Exceeds standard: 100% at NVQ level 2

Home details
Location: Residential area, in Hove
Communal areas: 2 lounges, dining room, garden
Accessibility: *Floors:* 3 • *Access:* Lift • *Wheelchair access:* Good
Smoking: In designated area
Pets: At manager's discretion
Routines: Flexible

Room details
Single: 16
Shared: 0
En suite: 16
Facilities: TV point, telephone point
Door lock: ✓
Lockable place: ✓

Services provided
Beauty services: Hairdressing, complimentary therapies
Mobile library: ✓
Religious services: ✓
Transport: ✗
Activities: *Coordinator:* ✓ • *Examples:* Knitting, bingo, scrabbles, charades • *Outings:* ✓
Meetings: ✓

Pentlow Nursing and Summerdown

Manager: Lesley Wicks
Owner: Mr and Mrs Barry Alford
Contact: 59–63 Summerdown Road,
Eastbourne, East Sussex BN20 8DQ

☎ 01323–722245

Two separate buildings make up Pentlow Nursing Home, positioned on either side of a road. Each have been converted and adapted to provide a comfortable environment for the residents. There are lounges and separate dining rooms in each building and attractive gardens that include decking and a water feature to the rear. Staff at the home also provide community care and meals for those who wish to stay in their own home rather then move to the nursing home.

Registered places: 61
Guide weekly rate: £500–£850
Specialist care: Nursing, day care, physical disability, respite, terminal care
Medical services: Podiatry, dentist, optician, physiotherapy
Qualified staff: Exceeds standard: 62% at NVQ Level 2

Home details
Location: Residential area, 1.5 miles from Eastbourne centre
Communal areas: 3 Lounges, 2 dining room, conservatory, library, garden
Accessibility: *Floors:* 2 • *Access:* Lift • *Wheelchair access:* Good
Smoking: ✗
Pets: At manger's discretion
Routines: Flexible

Room details
Single: 48
Shared: 6
En suite: 40
Facilities: TV point, telephone point
Door lock: ✓
Lockable place: ✓

Services provided
Beauty services: Hairdressing, manicures
Mobile library: Library facilities
Religious services: Monthly Anglican service
Transport: Minibus
Activities: *Coordinator:* ✓ • *Examples:* bingo arts and craft, music *Outings:* ✓
Meetings: ✓

Registered places: 35
Guide weekly rate: £745–£834
Specialist care: Nursing, respite
Medical services: Podiatry dentist, optician, physiotherapy
Qualified staff: Meets standard

Home details

Location: Residential area, in Hove
Communal areas: Lounge/conservatory, quiet lounge,
dining room, activities room, garden
Accessibility: *Floors:* 3 • *Access:* Lift • *Wheelchair access:* Good
Smoking: ✗
Pets: At manager's discretion
Routines: Flexible

Room details

Single: 35
Shared: 0
En suite: 26
Facilities: TV point, telephone point

Door lock: ✓
Lockable place: ✓

Services provided

Beauty services: Hairdressing, diversional therapy
Mobile library: ✓
Religious services: Weekly Communion service
Transport: ✓
Activities: *Coordinator:* ✓ • *Examples:* Music, art classes,
entertainment • *Outings:* ✓
Meetings: ✓

The Pines

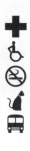

Manager: Janis Weir
Owner: Independent Age
Contact: Furze Hill, Hove, East Sussex
BN3 1PA
) 01273 820275
@ pines@independentage.org.uk
🖰 www.independentage.org.uk

The Pines is located in Hove, five minutes' walk from the seafront with good bus routes into Brighton. It is run by Independent Age, a charity devoted to helping older people stay retain their independence. The Friends of The Pines ensures excellent communication with the local community: they provide a weekly library and trolley shop service, birthday gifts, invitations to tea at their homes and chauffeured outings to the shops or seafront. The home overlooks St Anne's Well Gardens and has an entrance leading directly into it. To ensure residents' safety, residents wear a call button around their neck at all times.

Registered places: 20
Guide weekly rate: £450–£565
Specialist care: Respite
Medical services: Podiatry, optician
Qualified staff: Exceeds standard: 75% at NVQ Level 2

Home details

Location: Residential area, 3.5 miles from Brighton centre
Communal areas: Lounge, conservatory/dining room, 3 gardens
Accessibility: *Floors:* 2 • *Access:* Lift • *Wheelchair access:* Limited
Smoking: ✗
Pets: At manager's discretion
Routines: Structured

Room details

Single: 18
Shared: 1
En suite: 19
Facilities: TV, telephone point

Door lock: ✓
Lockable place: ✓

Services provided

Beauty services: Hairdressing, manicures
Mobile library: ✗
Transport: Car
Religious services: Monthly Communion service
Activities: *Coordinator:* ✗ • *Examples:* Craftwork, exercise classes,
magic shows, performers • *Outings:* ✗
Meetings: ✗

Place Farm House

Manager: Dawn Webb
Owner: Jo Tomlinson
Contact: Ladies Mile Road, Patcham,
Brighton, East Sussex BN1 8QE
) 01273 563902
@ placefarmhouse@yahoo.co.uk

Place Farm House is situated in a residential area of Brighton, with good public transport links into the centre of town. Family-run, the home intends to offer a high level of care whilst helping residents maintain independence and privacy. The home provides for residents with low mobility needs, therefore does not offer wheelchair access through the home. There is level access to small, well-maintained garden areas and many of the rooms have views of the Downs. The home offers regular social activities, ranging from magic shows and music evenings to well-being classes and craft workshops. Fees include a weekly hairdressing appointment at the home.

The Queensmead

Manager: Madeleine Marshall
Owner: Chanctonbury Healthcare Ltd
Contact: Victoria Road, Polegate,
East Sussex BN26 6BU

✆ 01323 487931

@ madeleinemarshall@hotmail.com

The Queensmead is situated in the area of Polegate, near to the town's high street, with shops and a library within walking distance. The home is approximately five miles from Eastbourne and the coast. Activities are carried out according to the needs of the resident, which emphasises that the interests of the residents come first. Mealtimes are not hurried, and there's always an alternative meal if the meal of the day does not satisfy their taste.

Registered places: 37
Guide weekly rate: £400–£560
Specialist care: None
Medical services: Podiatry, dietician, audiologist, occupational therapy, physiotherapy
Qualified staff: Undisclosed

Home details

Location: Residential area, 5 miles from Eastbourne
Communal areas: Lounge, dining room, conservatory, garden
Accessibility: *Floors:* 2 • *Access:* Lift • *Wheelchair access:* Good
Smoking: ✗
Pets: At manager's discretion
Routines: Flexible

Room details

Single: 33
Shared: 2
En suite: 35
Facilities: TV point, telephone point

Door lock: ✓
Lockable place: ✓

Services provided

Beauty services: Hairdressing
Mobile library: ✓
Religious services: ✓
Transport: ✗
Activities: *Coordinator:* ✓ • *Examples:* Arts and crafts, quizzes *Outings:* ✗
Meetings: ✗

R Janmayur Care Home

Manager: Kumarasamy Ramadas
Owner: Dr and Mr Ramadas
Contact: 15 Osmond Gardens, Osmond Road, Hove, East Sussex BN3 1TE

✆ 01273 777424

A small, family-run home that is situated in a residential area, R Janmayur is located five minutes from Brighton and there is a regular bus service. The home does not have a lift and therefore it is recommended that residents in the home are relatively mobile. There is a portable telephone which can be taken to the residents in their room. As R Janmayur is a small home the residents are given a flexible daily routine along with flexible meal times. There are regular activities such as quizzes and games and the home takes its residents on outings to the nearby seafront.

Registered places: 7
Guide weekly rate: £450
Specialist care: Respite
Medical services: Podiatry, dentist, optician, physiotherapy
Qualified staff: Undisclosed

Home details

Location: Residential area, 1 mile from Brighton centre
Communal areas: Lounge/dining room, garden
Accessibility: *Floors:* 2 • *Access:* None *Wheelchair access:* None
Smoking: ✗
Pets: ✗
Routines: Flexible

Room details

Single: 3
Shared: 4
En suite: 0
Facilities: TV

Door lock: ✓
Lockable place: ✓

Services provided

Beauty services: Hairdressing
Mobile library: ✓
Religious services: ✓
Transport: ✗
Activities: *Coordinator:* ✗ • *Examples:* Exercise, games, quizzes, crosswords • *Outings:* ✗
Meetings: ✗

Registered places: 24
Guide weekly rate: £364–£463
Specialist care: Respite
Medical services: Podiatry, optician, occupational therapy
Qualified staff: Fails standards

Home details

Location: Residential area, 1 mile from Eastbourne centre
Communal areas: Lounge, dining room, patio and garden
Accessibility: *Floors:* 3 • *Access:* Lift • *Wheelchair access:* Good
Smoking: ✗
Pets: At manager's discretion
Routines: Flexible

Room details

Single: 14
Shared: 5
En suite: 17
Facilities: TV point, telephone point

Door lock: ✓
Lockable place: ✓

Services provided

Beauty services: Hairdressing
Mobile library: ✓
Religious services: ✓
Transport: ✗
Activities: *Coordinator:* ✓ • *Examples:* Bingo, quizzes, exercises, reminiscence • *Outings:* ✓
Meetings: ✓

Ravelston Grange Care Home

Manager: Vacant
Owner: PJP Care Ltd
Contact: 10 Denton Road, Eastbourne, East Sussex BN20 7SU
☎ 01323 728528

Ravelston Grange is situated in The Meads, a peaceful residential area of Eastbourne. The home arranges seasonal outings as well as activities in house, which include board games, quizzes and reminiscence sessions. They also have visiting entertainers coming in frequently. The home can arrange for Communion to be taken privately.

Registered places: 32
Guide weekly rate: £575–£700
Specialist care: Nursing
Medical services: Podiatry, hygienist, optician, physiotherapy
Qualified staff: Fails standards

Home details

Location: Residential area, in Hove
Communal areas: Lounge, dining room, patio and garden
Accessibility: *Floors:* 3 • *Access:* Lift • *Wheelchair access:* Good
Smoking: ✗
Pets: ✗
Routines: Structured

Room details

Single: 30
Shared: 1
En suite: 31
Facilities: TV point, telephone point

Door lock: ✓
Lockable place: ✓

Services provided

Beauty services: Hairdressing
Mobile library: ✗
Religious services: ✓
Transport: ✗
Activities: *Coordinator:* ✗ • *Examples:* Bingo, themed days, quizzes *Outings:* ✓
Meetings: ✓

Regent House Nursing Home

Manager: Vanessa Farmer
Owner: Shafa Medical Services Ltd
Contact: 107–109 The Drive, Hove, East Sussex BN3 6GE
☎ 01273 220888
@ matron@impex.co.uk

Regent House Nursing Home is a detached residence converted from two houses. The home is within walking distance of local bus routes, with both Hove and Brighton town centres a short drive away. Residents can enjoy the large garden at the rear of the home, particularly in the summer season. Staff pride themselves on creating a homely atmosphere for residents to live in. Activities such as bingo and quizzes are played on a regular basis.

Rippleside Rest Home

Manager: Mr and Mrs El-Zayat
Owner: Mr and Mrs El-Zayat
Contact: 41 Jameson Road,
Bexhill-on-Sea, East Sussex TN40 1EG
☎ 01424 217092
@ sabreenelzayat@yahoo.co.uk

Rippleside is located in a quiet street close to both the seaside and town centre of Bexhill. Most of the residents at Rippleside are mobile so lead a relatively independent life, with staff enabling them to go swimming, to the shops and for walks. The home has satellite television, and a small patio garden at the front and rear of the property, which the residents are encouraged to look after. Outings involve museum trips, trips to the seafront and swimming lessons. Rippleside encourages residents to keep their independence for as long as possible.

Registered places: 8
Guide weekly rate: £485–£600
Specialist care: None
Medical services: Podiatry, dentist, optician, physiotherapy
Qualified staff: Meets standard

Home details
Location: Residential area, 1 mile from Bexhill centre
Communal areas: Lounge/dining room, lounge, garden
Accessibility: *Floors:* 3 • *Access:* Lift • *Wheelchair access:* Good
Smoking: ✗
Pets: ✗
Routines: Flexible

Room details
Single: 6
Shared: 1
En suite: 3
Facilities: TV point, television point

Door lock: ✗
Lockable place: ✓

Services provided
Beauty services: Hairdressing
Mobile library: ✗
Religious services: ✓
Transport: ✓
Activities: *Coordinator:* ✗ • *Examples:* Games, singing, bowling
    Outings: ✗
Meetings: ✓

The Roan Rest Home

Manager: Beant Vig
Owner: Joginder and Beant Vig
Contact: 27–29 Pembroke Crescent,
Hove, East Sussex BN3 5DF
☎ 01273 772927

The Roan Rest Home is situated in a residential area of Hove, within close walking distance of local shops, a library and nearby transport links. The home has a small, private rear garden, which is safe for residents to use. The home organises a film afternoon, and more lively activities such as bingo and scrabble for residents to join in. There are also regular coffee mornings, when residents sit together and discuss the morning newspapers. The home is a 10-minute walk from the seafront, which is often where residents go on outings for fish and chips or to a country pub.

Registered places: 19
Guide weekly rate: £299–£403
Specialist care: None
Medical services: Podiatry
Qualified staff: Meets standard

Home details
Location: Residential area, 1 mile from Hove centre
Communal areas: Lounge, lounge/dining rooms, garden
Accessibility: *Floors:* 3 • *Access:* Lift • *Wheelchair access:* Limited
Smoking: In designated area
Pets: ✓
Routines: Flexible

Room details
Single: 17
Shared: 1
En suite: 13
Facilities: TV point

Door lock: ✗
Lockable place: ✓

Services provided
Beauty services: Hairdressing
Mobile library: ✓
Religious services: Monthly church services
Transport: ✗
Activities: *Coordinator:* ✓ • *Examples:* Bingo, games, films
    Outings: ✗
Meetings: ✓

Registered places: 19
Guide weekly rate: £330–£380
Specialist care: None
Medical services: Podiatry, dentist, optician, physiotherapy
Qualified staff: Meets standard

Home details

Location: Residential, 6 miles from Brighton
Communal areas: Lounge, dining room, patio and garden
Accessibility: *Floors:* 2 • *Access:* Lift • *Wheelchair access:* Limited
Smoking: ✗
Pets: ✗
Routines: Flexible

Room details

Single: 13
Shared: 3
En suite: 5
Facilities: TV, telephone point

Door lock: ✓
Lockable place: ✓

Services provided

Beauty services: Hairdressing, manicures
Mobile library: ✓
Religious services: ✓
Transport: ✗
Activities: *Coordinator:* ✗ • *Examples:* Indoor games, visiting entertainers • *Outings:* ✓
Meetings: ✗

Roclyns Rest Home

Manager: Bibi Mosafeer
Owner: Mr and Mrs Mosafeer
Contact: 344 South Coast Road,
Telscombe Cliffs, East Sussex
BN10 7EW
☎ 01273 583923
@ roclynsresthome@hotmail.co.uk

Roclyns Rest Home is situated on the main South Coast Road and is near to local shops. There are good bus links to Brighton. The home has a lounge, a dining room and a garden and a patio. Services such as hairdressing are available and the home arranges religious services and visits from a mobile library. The staff arrange indoor games and other activities such as visiting entertainers and the home arranges a birthday party for each resident. There are outings for shopping and pets are allowed to visit. The residents enjoy a flexible daily routine alongside structured meal times.

Registered places: 20
Guide weekly rate: £337–£405
Specialist care: Respite
Medical services: Podiatry, dentist, optician
Qualified staff: Exceeds standard: 66% at NVQ Level 2

Home details

Location: Rural area, 7 miles from Hastings
Communal areas: Lounge, dining room, conservatory, garden
Accessibility: *Floors:* 2 • *Access:* Lift • *Wheelchair access:* Good
Smoking: ✗
Pets: ✗
Routines: Flexible

Room details

Single: 18
Shared: 1
En suite: 8
Facilities: TV point, telephone point

Door lock: ✓
Lockable place: ✓

Services provided

Beauty services: Hairdressing
Mobile library: ✓
Religious services: Monthly Anglican Communion service
Transport: ✗
Activities: *Coordinator:* ✗ • *Examples:* Music, board games
Outings: ✗
Meetings: ✗

Roselands

Manager: Sylvia Wells
Owner: Pleasantly Ltd
Contact: Cackle Street, Main Street,
Brede, Rye, East Sussex TN31 6EB
☎ 01424 882338

Roselands was formerly a guesthouse that has been adapted into a care home. The long drive makes a safe walk for residents, and the home is set in a rural location. The home has good ties to the local community; the local church choir comes monthly to sing hymns to the residents. The home is near the town of Rye and Hastings, but has limited transport links. The home aspires to create a comfortable and homely feel throughout.

Rottingdean Nursing and Care Home

Manager: Melanie Barber
Owner: Jon and Carol Breeds
Contact: 30–32 Newlands Road, Rottingdean, Brighton, East Sussex BN2 7GD
☎ 01273 308073

Rottingdean is located on a slight hill in a residential area of Rottingdean. The town centre is a short walk down hill, where there are shops, amenities and pubs. The seafront is also very near – about a five-minute walk from the home. There is a large lounge area in which various activities run by the activities coordinator take place. This includes bingo, quizzes and singalongs. There is also a garden with a seating area so residents can sit out side with one another and socialise. It is ideal in the summer for barbecues.

Registered places: 34
Guide weekly rate: £500–£550
Specialist care: Nursing
Medical services: Podiatry
Qualified staff: Meets standard

Home details
Location: Residential area, 4 miles from Brighton
Communal areas: Lounge, dining room, conservatory, garden
Accessibility: *Floors:* 3 • *Access:* Lift • *Wheelchair access:* Good
Smoking: In designated area
Pets: At manager's discretion
Routines: Flexible

Room details
Single: 28
Shared: 11
En suite: 3
Facilities: TV point

Door lock: ✓
Lockable place: ✓

Services provided
Beauty services: Hairdressing
Mobile library: ✗
Religious services: ✗
Transport: ✗
Activities: *Coordinator:* ✓ • *Examples:* Bingo, quizzes, singalongs *Outings:* ✗
Meetings: ✓

The Saffrons

Manager: Dagmar Williams
Owner: Mr and Mrs Williams
Contact: 20 Saffrons Road, Eastbourne, East Sussex BN21 1DU
☎ 01323 720430
@ dagmarwilliams@btinternet.com

The Saffrons is a three-storey building set in well-kept grounds. It is situated in a residential area close to Eastbourne town centre. Care staff organise activities for the residents, which include outings to the coast in their minibus. The home has a recently finished extension which includes four bedrooms, a large, well-lit dining room and a quiet area for those who do not wish to be in the livelier area of the main lounge.

Registered places: 24
Guide weekly rate: £350–£460
Specialist care: Respite
Medical services: Podiatry, dentistry, optician, physiotherapy
Qualified staff: Fails standards

Home details
Location: Residential area, 0.5 miles from Eastbourne centre
Communal areas: 2 lounges, dining room, garden
Accessibility: *Floors:* 3 • *Access:* Lift • *Wheelchair access:* Good
Smoking: ✗
Pets: ✓
Routines: Flexible

Room details
Single: 16
Shared: 4
En suite: 17
Facilities: TV point, telephone point

Door lock: ✓
Lockable place: ✓

Services provided
Beauty services: Hairdressing, manicures
Mobile library: ✓
Religious service: ✓
Transport: Minibus
Activities: *Coordinator:* ✗ • *Examples:* Arts and crafts, bingo, reminiscence, exercise • *Outings:* ✓
Meetings: ✗

Registered places: 24
Guide weekly rate: £323–£450
Specialist care: Day care, respite
Medical services: Podiatry, dentist, optician, physiotherapy
Qualified staff: Exceeds standard: 60% at NVQ Level 2

Home details

Location: Village location, 2.5 miles from Bexhill
Communal areas: Lounge, dining room, conservatory, garden
Accessibility: *Floors:* 2 • *Access:* Lift • *Wheelchair access:* Good
Smoking: In designated area
Pets: ✗
Routines: Flexible

Room details

Single: 20
Shared: 2
En suite: 21
Facilities: TV point, telephone point

Door lock: ✓
Lockable place: ✓

Services provided

Beauty services: Hairdressing
Mobile library: ✓
Religious services: Monthly Anglican and Catholic service
Transport: ✗
Activities: *Coordinator:* ✗ • *Examples:* Arts and crafts, exercises, motivation and music, quizzes • *Outings:* ✓
Meetings: ✓

Sandhurst Rest Home

Manager: Vicky Sharman
Owner: Cindy Nahoor
Contact: 142 Barnhorn Road,
Bexhill-on-Sea, East Sussex TN39 4QL
☏ 01424 844405
@ sandhurstcare1@aol.com

Sandhurst is a detached property found on a main road near to Little Common in Bexhill-on-Sea. The home focuses on the residents' needs and their activities are organised with this in mind. There is a wide variety of activities, from calming arts and crafts to exercises. There are also visiting entertainers for the residents to enjoy and outings to local points of interest.

Registered places: 25
Guide weekly rate: £350–£375
Specialist care: Respite
Medical services: Podiatry, optician, physiotherapy, dentist
Qualified staff: Exceeds standard: 80% at NVQ Level 2

Home details

Location: Residential area, 1 mile from Eastbourne centre
Communal areas: Lounge, dining room, conservatory and garden
Accessibility: *Floors:* 3 • *Access:* Lift • *Wheelchair access:* Good
Smoking: ✗
Pets: ✗
Routines: Flexible

Room details

Single: 25
Shared: 0
En suite: 10
Facilities: TV point, telephone point

Door lock: ✓
Lockable place: ✓

Services provided

Beauty services: Hairdressing, aromatherapy, manicures
Mobile library: ✓
Religious services: ✓
Transport: ✗
Activities: *Coordinator:* ✗ • *Examples:* Arts and crafts, bingo, singalongs, visiting entertainers • *Outings:* ✓
Meetings: ✓

Shandon House

Manager: Nicola Moss
Owner: Lindsey Bree
Contact: 3 Mill Road, Eastbourne,
East Sussex BN21 2LY
☏ 01323 723333
@ breel990@aol.com

Shandon House resides in the Ocklynge of Eastbourne. The home is a large detached three-storey house that boasts a maintained rear garden for residents to enjoy. The home has a comprehensive activities programme which includes the provision of activities in mornings and afternoons such as bingo, movement to music and singalongs. Mobile residents are encouraged to go out independently, or to participate in the home's outings, as this encourages an independent and motivated state of mind.

Southfields House Residential Care Home

Manager: David Exon
Owner: Mr and Mrs Exon
Contact: Southfields Road, Eastbourne, East Sussex BN21 1BZ

) 01323 732077
@ enquiries@southfieldshouse.com
www.southfieldshouse.com

Southfields House Residential Care Home is in a residential area of Eastbourne, within a short walk of the town centre, railway station and the public library. There is a large, attractive garden at the rear of the home. In the summer there are barbecues and al fresco meals for residents, their families, friends and neighbours to participate in. The staff aim to create a welcoming mood for residents to feel comfortable and families welcome to visit.

Registered places: 16
Guide weekly rate: £350–£500
Specialist care: Respite
Medical services: Podiatry, optician
Qualified staff: Undisclosed

Home details
Location: Residential area, 0.5 miles from Eastbourne centre
Communal areas: 2 lounges, dining room, garden
Accessibility: *Floors:* 2 • *Access:* Stair lift
    Wheelchair access: Good
Smoking: ✗
Pets: At manager's discretion
Routines: Flexible

Room details
Single: 16
Shared: 0
En suite: 13
Facilities: TV point, telephone point

Door lock: ✓
Lockable place: ✓

Services provided
Beauty services: Hairdressing
Mobile library: ✗
Religious services: Monthly Methodist service
Transport: People carrier
Activities: *Coordinator:* ✗ • *Examples:* Bingo, carpet bowls, quizzes • *Outings:* ✓
Meetings: ✓

Southlands Court

Manager: David Pollard
Owner: Southlands Court Care Ltd
Contact: 33 Hastings Road, Bexhill-on-Sea, East Sussex TN40 2HJ

) 01424 210628

Southlands Court is a hotel-style care home in well-maintained grounds in a cul-de-sac in Bexhill-on-Sea. There is one acre of garden which is wheelchair accessible. Activities are arranged frequently with something for everyone to do including computer games, bingo and quizzes. Outings are organised as well such as trips out for lunches and afternoon teas. The home has its own chef who provides a wide range of dishes on the menu. The home holds a summer fair with proceeds going to The Friends of Southlands Court and Alzheimer's Society.

Registered places: 35
Guide weekly rate: £325–£525
Specialist care: Respite, day care
Medical services: Podiatry, dentist, optician, physiotherapy
Qualified staff: Exceeds standard: 65% at NVQ Level 2

Home details
Location: Residential area, 1 mile from Bexhill centre
Communal areas: Dining room, 2 lounges, conservatory, shop, garden
Accessibility: *Floors:* 3 • *Access:* Lift • *Wheelchair access:* Good
Smoking: In designated area
Pets: At manager's discretion
Routines: Flexible

Room details
Single: 27
Shared: 4
En suite: 27
Facilities: TV point, telephone point

Door lock: ✓
Lockable place: ✓

Services provided
Beauty services: Hairdressing
Mobile library: ✓
Religious services: Communion service
Transport: ✗
Activities: *Coordinator:* ✓ • *Examples:* Bingo, computer games, jigsaws, quizzes • *Outings:* ✓
Meetings: ✓

Registered places: 60
Guide weekly rate: £470–£800
Specialist care: Nursing, dementia
Medical services: Podiatry
Qualified staff: Meets standard

Home details

Location: Residential area, 1 mile from Eastbourne
Communal areas: Lounge, dining room, garden
Accessibility: *Floors:* 2 • *Access:* Lift • *Wheelchair access:* Good
Smoking: ✗
Pets: ✗
Routines: Flexible

Room details

Single: 60
Shared: 0
En suite: 60
Facilities: TV point, telephone point

Door lock:
Lockable place:

Services provided

Beauty services: Hairdressing
Mobile library: Yes
Religious services: ✗
Transport: ✗
Activities: *Coordinator:* Yes • *Examples:* Bingo, quizzes, reminiscence sessions • *Outings:* Yes
Meetings: Yes

Sovereign Lodge Care Centre

Manager: Veronica Millen
Owner: Life Style Care Plc
Contact: Carew Road, Eastbourne, East Sussex BN21 2BF
☎ 01323 412285
@ sovereignlodge@lifestylecare.co.uk
🖥 www.lifestylecare.co.uk

Sovereign Lodge is located in a residential area, approximately one mile from Eastbourne. The home has a variety of communal areas, including a dining room and a garden. The home has its own activities coordinator who arranges daily activities such as bingo and reminiscence sessions. There are also outings for the residents, for example to a tea dance. The home has regular residents and relatives meetings to allow residents and their relatives to voice any opinions they may have.

Registered places: 12
Guide weekly rate: £417–£500
Specialist care: Nursing
Medical services: Podiatry, dentist, optician, physiotherapy
Qualified staff: Meets standard

Home details

Location: Residential area, 1 mile from Hastings
Communal areas: Lounge, dining room, conservatory, garden
Accessibility: *Floors:* 3 • *Access:* Lift, 2 stair lifts and wheelchair lift *Wheelchair access:* Good
Smoking: ✗
Pets: ✗
Routines: Flexible

Room details

Single: 7
Shared: 3
En suite: 4
Facilities: TV point

Door lock: ✓
Lockable place: ✓

Services provided

Beauty services: Hairdressing, manicures
Mobile library: ✗
Religious services: Ministers visit
Transport: ✓
Activities: *Coordinator:* ✓ • *Examples:* Bingo, games, painting *Outings:* ✓
Meetings: ✓

Springcroft

Manager: Rosemonde Samy
Owner: Mr Samy
Contact: 58 Springfield Road, St Leonards-on-Sea, East Sussex TN38 0TZ
☎ 01424 431856

Springcroft is situated in a residential area of St Leonards-on-Sea, only a short distance for amenities and shops. The home provides a small range of activities, which are sufficient to meet the needs of the residents. Such activities include outings by car. Residents are treated with dignity and respect, and there is a key worker system in place, whereby staff take responsibility for the well being of individual residents. A garden provides residents with a pleasant area to socialise and relax.

Springfields

Manager: Colleen Hutton
Owner: Mr and Mrs Vig
Contact: 11 Langdale Road, Hove, East Sussex BN3 4HQ
☎ 01273 735784

Springfields is close to the seafront in Hove. It has been converted from three houses into one property. Residents regularly enjoy outings, for example to the seafront for fish and chips or to the park. Residents are allowed to take their own belongings to the home and the routines are relatively laid back. Pets are allowed but smoking is not permitted. The home has an activities coordinator who arranges musical entertainment for the residents. The home is spread across two floors and offers a hairdressing service. The home also offers nursing care.

Registered places: 32
Guide weekly rate: £454–£550
Specialist care: Nursing
Medical services: Podiatry, physiotherapy
Qualified staff: Fails standard: 23% at NVQ Level 2

Home details
Location: Residential area, 1 mile from Hove centre
Communal areas: Lounge/dining room, garden
Accessibility: *Floors:* 2 • *Access:* Undisclosed
  Wheelchair access: Undisclosed
Smoking: ✗
Pets: At manager's discretion
Routines: Flexible

Room details
Single: 18
Shared: 7
En suite: 8
Facilities: None

Door lock: ✓
Lockable place: ✓

Services provided
Beauty services: Hairdressing
Mobile library: ✗
Religious services: ✗
Transport: ✗
Activities: *Coordinator:* ✓ • *Examples:* Musical entertainment
  Outings: ✓
Meetings: ✗

St Augustine's

Manager: Maxine Clist
Owner: St Michael's Hospice Ltd
Contact: 25 Upper Maze Hill, St Leonards-on-Sea, East Sussex TN38 0LB
☎ 01424 423000

St Augustine's was formerly run by the Augustinian nun community, now based in France, and maintain good links with them. In 2006, the home celebrated 120 years since it first opened. The home is a large property in a residential area. Its well-maintained gardens are accessible to wheelchair users. Complementary therapy is available of no extra cost to residents and includes aromatherapy and reflexology. Group activities are organised by a volunteer group who take residents shopping. Interdenominational services are held regularly and visitors are welcome to stay the night if they wish.

Registered places: 35
Guide weekly rate: From £531
Specialist care: Nursing, physically disabled, terminal care
Medical services: Podiatry, dentist, optician
Qualified staff: Exceeds standard: 75% at NVQ Level 2

Home details
Location: Residential area, in St Leonards-on-Sea
Communal areas: 4 lounges, garden room, common room, chapel, garden
Accessibility: *Floors:* 3 • *Access:* Lift • *Wheelchair access:* Good
Smoking: In designated area
Pets: ✓
Routines: Structured

Room details
Single: 32
Shared: 2
En suite: 0
Facilities: Undisclosed

Door lock: ✗
Lockable place: ✓

Services provided
Beauty services: Hairdressing, aromatherapy, reflexology
Mobile library: ✗
Religious services: ✓
Transport: ✗
Activities: *Coordinator:* ✓ • *Examples:* Craft sessions
  Outings: ✓
Meetings: ✗

Registered places: 19
Guide weekly rate: Undisclosed
Specialist care: Respite
Medical services: Podiatry, dentist, optician, physiotherapy
Qualified staff: Exceeds standard

Home details

Location: Residential area, in Hove
Communal areas: Lounge, quiet lounge, dining room,
    conservatory, patio and garden
Accessibility: *Floors:* 3 • *Access:* Stair lift
    Wheelchair access: Limited
Smoking: ✗
Pets: ✗
Routines: Flexible

Room details

Single: 13   Door lock: ✓
Shared: 2   Lockable place: ✓
En suite: 7
Facilities: TV

Services provided

Beauty services: Hairdressing, aromatherapy, manicures
Mobile library: Library facilities
Religious services: ✓
Transport: ✗
Activities: *Coordinator:* ✓ • *Examples:* Exercise classes, games,
    visiting entertainers • *Outings:* ✓
Meetings: ✓

St Christopher's Residential Home

Manager: Theresa Hounsome
Owner: Mr and Mrs Hounsome
Contact: 47–49 Rutland Gardens,
Hove, East Sussex BN3 5PD
☏ 01273 327210
@ dil@saint-christophers.com
🖰 www.saint-christophers.com

St Christopher's Residential Home is situated next to the seafront and is only a 15-minute walk to the local shops. The home offers respite care as well as residential care. The home has a lounge and a quiet lounge, a dining room, a garden with a patio area and a conservatory. Pets and smoking are not permitted in the home. The residents have regular meetings. The home has an activities coordinator who arranges exercise sessions, games and for visiting entertainers. There are also organised outings. The home has its own books and organises religious services.

Registered places: 51
Guide weekly rate: £600
Specialist care: Physical disability
Medical services: Podiatry, dentist, optician
Qualified staff: Meets standard

Home details

Location: Residential area, 0.5 miles from St Leonards-on-Sea
Communal areas: Lounge, dining room, conservatory,
    patio and garden
Accessibility: *Floors:* 3 • *Access:* Lift • *Wheelchair access:* Good
Smoking: ✗
Pets: ✗
Routines: Flexible

Room details

Single: 45   Door lock: ✗
Shared: 3   Lockable place: ✓
En suite: 45
Facilities: TV, telephone

Services provided

Beauty services: Hairdressing, aromatherapy, manicures
Mobile library: ✗
Religious services: ✓
Transport: ✗
Activities: *Coordinator:* ✓ • *Examples:* Games, exercises
    Outings: ✗
Meetings: ✓

St Dominic's Care Home

Manager: Catherine Piney
Owner: Astor Healthcare
Contact: 71 Filsham Road,
St Leonards-on-Sea, East Sussex
TN38 0PG
☏ 01424 436140

St Dominic's Care Home is a large, detached property in a residential area of St Leonards-on-Sea which offers spectacular views from the upper floor rooms to the sea and across to Eastbourne. Within easy access of local shops, the home also has good travel links provided by a bus service. The home has its own activities coordinator and a residents tenants association. The home has a lounge, a dining room, a garden, a patio and a conservatory. There are beauty facilities such as hairdressing and manicures on offer. The residents have a flexible daily routine with set meal times.

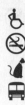

St Helen's House

Manager: Janet Holding
Owner: Gloria Williams
Contact: 3 The Ridge, Ore, Hastings,
East Sussex TN34 2AA
℡ 01424 439239
@ Sthelens@house124.wanadoo.co.uk

St Helen's House is a family-run care home on The Ridge in Hastings. Outings take place in the local area with visits to the local town for shopping and coffee mornings. The home prides itself on its spontaneous outings, seeing where the road takes them! Other activities include bingo, games, music and movement and beauty treatments. Pets are allowed at the manager's discretion. The home has a structured routine in the morning but afternoons are more flexible. The residents also have set meal times. The home is orientated around its residents and puts their needs first. The home also offers specialist respite care.

Registered places: 31
Guide weekly rate: Undisclosed
Specialist care: Respite
Medical services: Podiatry, dentist, optician
Qualified staff: Meets standard

Home details
Location: Village location, 3 miles from Hastings centre
Communal areas: 3 lounges, 2 dining rooms, patio and garden
Accessibility: *Floors:* 4 • *Access:* Lift • *Wheelchair access:* Good
Smoking: ✗
Pets: At manager's discretion
Routines: Flexible

Room details
Single: 27
Shared: 2
En suite: 21
Facilities: TV point, telephone point

Door lock: ✓
Lockable place: ✓

Services provided
Beauty services: Hairdressing, aromatherapy, manicures
Mobile library: Library facilities
Religious services: Methodist minister and Catholic priest visits
Transport: Minibus
Activities: *Coordinator:* ✓ • *Access:* Arts and crafts, bingo, games, beauty treatments • *Outings:* ✓
Meetings: ✗

St Joseph's Rest Home

Manager: Sister Noeleen Ryan
Owner: Trustees Of The Sisters Of Mercy
Contact: 3–7 Bristol Road,
Brighton, East Sussex BN2 1AP
℡ 01273 626151
@ Zen84109@zen.co.uk

St Joseph's is a detached, purpose-built property situated in the residential area of Kemp Town, Brighton. The home is run by the catholic group, the Sisters of Mercy, but admission to the home is nondenominational. There are small kitchenettes on each floor of the home, enabling residents to make their own refreshments should they choose. The home is within walking distance from local amenities and transportation. The residents also enjoy visiting musical entertainment.

Registered places: 17
Guide weekly rate: £298–£420
Specialist care: Respite
Medical services: Podiatry, hygienist, optician
Qualified staff: Exceeds standard: 69% at NVQ Level 2

Home details
Location: Residential area, 0.5 miles from Brighton centre
Communal areas: Lounge, dining room, library, chapel, kitchenettes, garden
Accessibility: *Floors:* 3 • *Access:* Lift and stair lift *Wheelchair access:* Good
Smoking: ✗
Pets: ✗
Routines: Flexible

Room details
Single: 15
Shared: 1
En suite: 16
Facilities: TV point, telephone point

Door lock: ✓
Lockable place: ✓

Services provided
Beauty services: Hairdressing
Mobile library: Library facilities
Religious services: Catholic service three times a week
Transport: ✗
Activities: *Coordinator:* ✓ • *Examples:* Bingo, painting, quizzes *Outings:* ✓
Meetings: ✓

Registered places: 17
Guide weekly rate: £320–£510
Specialist care: None
Medical services: Podiatry, optician
Qualified staff: Meets standard

Home details

Location: Residential area, 1.5 miles from Eastbourne centre
Communal areas: Lounge, dining room, garden
Accessibility: *Floors:* 3 • *Access:* 2 stair lifts
   Wheelchair access: Limited
Smoking: ✗
Pets: At manager's discretion
Routines: Flexible

Room details

Single: 11
Shared: 3
En suite: 0
Facilities: TV point

Door lock: ✗
Lockable place: ✓

Services provided

Beauty services: Hairdressing
Mobile library: ✗
Religious services: ✓
Transport: ✗
Activities: *Coordinator:* ✓ • *Examples:* Table bowling, musical
   entertainment, walks • *Outings:* ✗
Meetings: ✓

St Marguerite

Manager: Jaysen Chinapyel
Owner: Jaysen, Velaydon and Saromati Chinapyel
Contact: 10 Ashburnham Road, Eastbourne, East Sussex BN21 2HU
☏ 01323 729634
@ stmarguerite@hotmail.com

St Marguerite is a detached property located in a quiet residential area on the outskirts of Eastbourne town centre. The main lounge is split into two areas, giving residents opportunity to sit quietly. There is a well-maintained garden area with appropriate seating and is accessible to all residents. Activities are organised for the residents according to how mobile they are. Those who are very mobile may go on an afternoon walk with a member of staff, while others may play table bowling. The coordinator ensures there is time when all residents are socialising together such as quiz night or bingo night.

Registered places: 22
Guide weekly rate: £350–£700
Specialist care: Respite
Medical services: Podiatry, dentist, optician
Qualified staff: Exceeds standard: 55% at NVQ Level 2

Home details

Location: Residential area, 1 mile from Eastbourne centre
Communal areas: Lounge, dining room, garden
Accessibility: *Floors:* 2 • *Access:* Stair lifts
   Wheelchair access: Limited
Smoking: ✗
Pets: ✗
Routines: Flexible

Room details

Single: 16
Shared: 3
En suite: 11
Facilities: TV point, telephone point

Door lock: ✗
Lockable place: ✓

Services provided

Beauty services: Hairdressing
Mobile library: ✗
Religious services: Monthly Anglican service
Transport: ✓
Activities: *Coordinator:* ✗ • *Examples:* Light exercise, bowles, film
   evenings, quizzes • *Outings:* ✗
Meetings: ✓
   •

St Margarets

Manager: Teresa Howell
Owner: Total Support Solutions Ltd
Contact: 99 Carlisle Road, Eastbourne, East Sussex BN20 7TD
☏ 01323 639211
@ office@saint-margarets.co.uk
🖰 www.saint-margarets.co.uk

St Margarets is a care home in a Grade II listed building in The Meads area of Eastbourne. In an Edwardian style, the home was originally built for the Duke of Devonshire and furnished by Liberty's of London. The home has its own chef who tailors meals to individual needs. Care is provided 24 hours a day for residents' comfort. Activities include film evenings, quizzes and light exercises. There are resident meetings every two months. Pets are allowed to visit the home with friends or family but not to stay.

St Nectans Residential Care Home

Manager: Patrick Finn
Owner: St Nectans Residential Care Home Ltd
Contact: 3–9 Cantelupe Road, Bexhill-on-Sea, East Sussex TN40 1JG
☎ 01424 220030
@ plfinn@tesco.net
🖰 www.stnectans.co.uk

St Nectans is situated on a residential street a short level walk from Bexhill town centre and railway station. The home has sea views from the front and a garden at the back of the home. The building has been adapted from four adjacent properties, which are now interlinked. The home has a daily activities programme which includes movement to music, pampering treatments and visiting entertainment. The home also arranges outings to the sea, for afternoon tea and to the theatre. Smoking is permitted in a designated area outside the home. There are resident meetings every two months.

Registered places: 35
Guide weekly rate: £380–£495
Specialist care: None
Medical services: Podiatry, dentist, optician.
Qualified staff: Meets standard

Home details
Location: Residential area, in Bexhill
Communal areas: Lounge, dining room, garden
Accessibility: *Floors:* 4 • *Access:* Lift • *Wheelchair access:* Good
Smoking: In designated area
Pets: ✗
Routines: Flexible

Room details
Single: 35
Shared: 0
En suite: 35
Facilities: TV, telephone

Door lock: ✓
Lockable place: ✓

Services provided
Beauty services: Hairdressing
Mobile library: ✓
Religious services: ✓
Transport: ✗
Activities: *Coordinator:* ✗ • *Examples:* Music to movement, manicures, visiting entertainers • *Outings:* ✓
Meetings: ✓

St Paul's Care Home

Manager: Linda Anstell
Owner: New Century Care Ltd
Contact: 65 Albany Road, St Leonards-on-Sea, East Sussex TN38 0LJ
☎ 01424 425798
@ stpauls@new-meronden.co.uk
🖰 www.newcenturycare.co.uk

St Paul's Care Home is a detached property which is located half a mile from St Leonards-on-Sea. The home has recently been refurbished and has 19 single rooms and three double rooms, nine of which are en suite. The home has a large lounge and dining area, a conservatory and a garden with a patio area. The home has a daily activities programme which includes games and bingo and there are also organised visits. The home offers residents a hairdressing service and manicures are available. The home also provides care for rehabilitation and respite patients.

Registered places: 25
Guide weekly rate: Undisclosed
Specialist care: Nursing, physical disability, respite
Medical services: Podiatry, dentist, optician, physiotherapy
Qualified staff: Exceeds standard: 100% at NVQ Level 2

Home details
Location: Residential area, 0.5 miles from St Leonards-on-Sea
Communal areas: Lounge/dining room, conservatory, patio and garden
Accessibility: *Floors:* 3 • *Access:* Lift • *Wheelchair access:* Good
Smoking: ✗
Pets: ✗
Routines: Flexible

Room details
Single: 19
Shared: 3
En suite: 9
Facilities: TV, telephone

Door lock: ✓
Lockable place: ✓

Services provided
Beauty services: Hairdressing, manicures
Mobile library: ✗
Religious services: ✗
Transport: ✗
Activities: *Coordinator:* ✗ • *Examples:* Games, bingo *Outings:* ✓
Meetings: ✗

Registered places: 58
Guide weekly rate: £575–£605
Specialist care: Nursing, dementia
Medical services: Podiatry, dentist, optician, physiotherapy
Qualified staff: Fails standard

Home details

Location: Rural area, 5 miles from Haywards Heath
Communal areas: 6 lounges, 3 dining rooms, chapel, hairdressing salon, garden
Accessibility: *Floors:* 3 • *Access:* Lift • *Wheelchair access:* Good
Routines: Flexible
Pets: At manager's discretion
Smoking: In designated area

Room details

Single: 27
Shared: 15
En suite: Undisclosed
Facilities: Telephone point

Door lock: ✓
Lockable place: ✓

Services provided

Beauty services: Hairdressing
Mobile library: ✗
Religious services: Daily mass
Transport: Minibus
Activities: *Coordinator:* ✓ • *Examples:* Bingo, crafts, musical performances, walks • *Outings:* ✓
Meetings: ✓

St Raphael's Nursing Home

Manager: Sister Mary Basil
Owner: The Trustees of the Order of St Augustine of the Mercy of Jesus
Contact: Danehurst, Danehill, East Sussex RH17 7EZ
☏ 01825 790485
🖰 www.anh.org.uk

St Raphael's is a country house nursing home, specialising in caring for elderly with dementia, and run by nuns from the Order of St Augustine. Their admissions procedure is nondenominational. An enclosed garden and good access to lakes and woodland give the home ample outdoor space. The home also boasts an aviary and outside patio area. Residents have the chance to go on various outings organised by the home and have the benefit of musical entertainment from both within the home and from visitors. The management would allow fish and caged birds as pets and smoking is permitted in a designated area. The home also has its own chapel.

Registered places: 45
Guide weekly rate: £686–£854
Specialist care: Nursing, physical disability, respite
Medical services: Podiatry, hygienist, optician, physiotherapy
Qualified staff: Meets standard

Home details

Location: Residential area, 0.5 miles from Seaford
Communal areas: 3 lounges, dining room, 2 lounge/dining room, garden
Accessibility: *Floors:* 2 • *Access:* Lift • *Wheelchair access:* Good
Smoking: ✗
Pets: ✗
Routines: Structured

Room details

Single: 45
Shared: 0
En suite: 0
Facilities: TV point, telephone point

Door lock: ✓
Lockable place: ✓

Services provided

Beauty services: Hairdressing
Mobile library: ✗
Religious services: Fortnightly Communion service
Transport: ✗
Activities: *Coordinator:* ✓ • *Examples:* Musical bingo, quizzes, entertainers • *Outings:* ✓
Meetings: ✓

Threeways

Manager: Shirley Eyles
Owner: Bernard and Barbara Clarke, Caroline Mills
Contact: 40 Beacon Road, Seaford, East Sussex BN25 2LT
☏ 01323–896196

Threeways is a family-run nursing home in a residential area, close to shops and public transport links and within walking distance from the seafront and a park. Though residents are offered a structured daily routine and mealtime, those physical able are allowed to pursue a flexible lifestyle. An activities coordinator provides residents with a programme of games, musical bingo and quizzes. Entertainers also visit the home regularly.

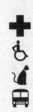

Tredegar Care Home

Manager: Sandra Barnes
Owner: New Century Care Ltd
Contact: 13 Upper Avenue, Eastbourne, East Sussex BN21 3UY
☎ 01323–412808

Tredegar is a detached property, converted and adapted into a care home in Eastbourne. The home is situated within walking distance of the main town, mainline railway station and bus routes. The seafront and a large park area are approximately a mile away. Daily activities organised for the residents include exercises, flower arranging, film night and sewing. The home has it's own transport and often residents go down to the seafront to have fish and chips, or a short walk. There is also a park near the home which more mobile residents have frequent walks to, accompanied by a carer.

Registered places: 26
Guide weekly rate: £600–£900
Specialist care: Nursing
Medical services: Podiatry, dentist, optician, physiotherapy
Qualified staff: Exceeds standard: 64% at NVQ Level 2

Home details
Location: Urban area, 1 mile from Eastbourne centre
Communal areas: 2 lounges, dining room, garden
Accessibility: *Floors:* 3 • *Access:* Lift • *Wheelchair access:* Good
Smoking: In designated area
Pets: ✓
Routines: Flexible

Room details
Single: 16
Shared: 5
En suite: 11
Facilities: TV point, telephone point

Door lock: ✗
Lockable place: ✓

Services provided
Beauty services: Hairdressing
Mobile library: ✓
Religious services: Monthly church services
Transport: ✓
Activities: *Coordinator:* ✓ • *Examples:* Exercise, flower arranging
    Outings: ✓
Meetings: ✓

Vallance Rest Home

Manager: Maria Mirza
Owner: Vallance Organisation Ltd
Contact: 7–9 Vallance Road, Hove, East Sussex BN3 2DA
☎ 01273 326053

Vallance Home consists of two converted Victorian houses. It is in a residential area of Hove within walking distance of Sussex County Cricket Ground, the public library and a museum. Staff often take residents out locally for coffee, shopping in nearby George Street or for a walk along the seafront. Furthermore, staff organise parties for residents' birthdays, to which relatives are invited. There is a Communion service every fortnight at the home.

Registered places: 19
Guide weekly rate: £268–£403
Specialist care: None
Medical services: Podiatry, dentist, optician, physiotherapy
Qualified staff: Exceeds standards

Home details
Location: Residential area, in Hove
Communal areas: 2 lounges, dining room, garden
Accessibility: *Floors:* 2 • *Access:* Lift • *Wheelchair access:* Good
Smoking: In designated area
Pets: At manager's discretion
Routines: Flexible

Room details
Single: 9
Shared: 5
En suite: 3
Facilities: TV point, telephone point

Door lock: ✓
Lockable place: ✓

Services provided
Beauty services: Hairdressing
Mobile library: ✗
Religious services: Fortnightly Communion service
Transport: ✗
Activities: *Coordinator:* ✓ • *Examples:* Artwork, bingo, exercise
    Outings: ✓
Meetings: ✓

Registered places: 29
Guide weekly rate: £475–£800
Specialist care: Respite
Medical services: Podiatry, optician, physiotherapy
Qualified staff: Meets standard

Home details
Location: Residential area, 1 mile from Crowborough centre
Communal areas: 2 lounges, dining room, conservatory,
2 terraces, summerhouse, garden
Accessibility: *Floors:* 3 • *Access:* Lift • *Wheelchair access:* Good
Smoking: ×
Pets: At manager's discretion
Routines: Flexible

Room details
Single: 26
Shared: 3
En suite: 29
Facilities: TV, telephone point

Door lock: ✓
Lockable place: ✓

Services provided
Beauty services: Hairdressing, manicures
Mobile library: ×
Religious services: Monthly Communion service
Transport: ×
Activities: *Coordinator:* ✓ • *Examples:* Darts, exercise classes,
games, quizzes, scrabble • *Outings:* ✓
Meetings: ✓

Warren Drive Residential Home

Manager: Elaine George
Owner: Bluebell Care Homes Ltd
Contact: Fielden Road, Crowborough,
East Sussex TN6 1TP
☏ 01892 654586
@ enquiries@warrendrive.com
🖳 www.warrendrive.com

Warren Drive is an attractive stone house set in two acres of mature gardens with panoramic views over Ashdown Forest. There is a separate wing providing two bed-sitting rooms with full en suite facilities and four suites with their own terraced balcony. The two-acre garden has paths through it to assure access for all residents. There is ample communal space, including a large lounge, a quiet lounge and summerhouse. There is also the annual summer barbecue and Christmas party to enjoy. Visiting entertainment visit in the form of fashion shows, musical entertainment and even mini theatre production crews.

Registered places: 25
Guide weekly rate: £535–£670
Specialist care: Physical disability
Medical services: Podiatry, dentist, optician, physiotherapy
Qualified staff: Meets standard

Home details
Location: Village location, 1 mile from Wadhurst
Communal areas: Lounge, dining room, extensive grounds
Accessibility: *Floors:* 3 • *Access:* Lift • *Wheelchair access:* Good
Smoking: In designated area
Pets: At manager's discretion
Routines: Flexible

Room details
Single: 25
Shared: 0
En suite: 25
Facilities: TV, telephone point

Door lock: ×
Lockable place: ✓

Services provided
Beauty services: Hairdressing, manicures, reflexology
Mobile library: ×
Religious services: Monthly Communion service
Transport: ×
Activities: *Coordinator:* × • *Examples:* Arts and crafts, exercises,
poetry readings • *Outings:* ✓
Meetings: ✓

Weald Hall

Manager: Louise Coppard
Owner: Crossways Trust Ltd
Contact: Mayfield Lane, Wadhurst,
East Sussex TN5 6HX
☏ 01892 782011
@ louisecoppard@crosswaystrust.org.uk
🖳 www.crosswaystrust.org.uk

Situated in Snape Valley, Weald Hall sits within a 17-acre site and gives residents attractive views of the surrounding countryside. Approximately one mile from the market town of Wadhurst, and the train station, residents at the home are encouraged to exercise independence. Wadhurst is approximately six and a half miles from Tunbridge Wells. Each private room at Weald Hall is of a good size, with its own en suite bathroom and, in many cases, a sitting room overlooking the gardens. Each room is fully furnished, including a telephone point and colour television.

Westerleigh

Manager: Carolyn Whelan
Owner: Regency Medicine
Contact: 18 Corsica Road, Seaford,
East Sussex BN25 1BD
☏ 01323 892335
🖰 www.westerleigh.info

Westerleigh is situated in a residential area close to the seafront on the western edge of Seaford and is approximately half a mile from the town centre. There is a small seating area at the rear of the home that overlooks a patio area. In addition there are two patio areas, one in the centre of the building, where some residents' rooms lead directly onto it. There are two activities organisers to provide stimulating and interesting activities, who take into account the residents' individual interests.

Registered places: 31
Guide weekly rate: £520–£730
Specialist care: Nursing, physical disability
Medical services: Podiatry
Qualified staff: Meets standard

Home details

Location: Residential area, 0.5 miles from Seaford centre
Communal areas: 3 lounges, garden, courtyard garden
Accessibility: *Floors:* 2 • *Access:* Lift • *Wheelchair access:* Good
Smoking: In designated area
Pets: ✓
Routines: Flexible

Room details

Single: 29
Shared: 1
En suite: 21
Facilities: TV point, telephone point

Door lock: ✗
Lockable place: ✓

Services provided

Beauty services: Hairdressing
Mobile library: ✓
Religious services: ✓
Transport: ✗
Activities: *Coordinator:* ✓ • *Examples:* Walks, bingo, quizzes, charades • *Outings:* ✓
Meetings: ✓

Whitegates

Manager: Alison Gates
Owner: Kathleen Courtney
Contact: Westfield Lane, Westfield,
East Sussex TN35 4SB
☏ 01424 754865
@ Whitegates.kpc@btopenworld.com
🖰 www.whitegatesretirement
home.co.uk

Whitegates is situated outside Westfield village, four and a half miles from Hastings centre. The home has its own car to aid transportation from this fairly isolated location. There are large, well-kept gardens which ground floor rooms open onto. There are organised day trips and visiting entertainers come in to perform music. There is a resident dog despite no other animals are allowed. The home's philosophy: 'more like a country hotel than a retirement home'.

Registered places: 22
Guide weekly rate: £490–£650
Specialist care: Respite
Medical services: Podiatry, dentist, optician, physiotherapy
Qualified staff: Meets standard

Home details

Location: Village location, 4.5 miles from Hastings
Communal areas: Dining room, lounge, library, patio and garden
Accessibility: *Floors:* 2 • *Access:* Lift • *Wheelchair access:* Good
Smoking: ✗
Pets: ✗
Routines: Flexible

Room details

Single: 20
Shared: 1
En suite: 21
Facilities: TV, telephone point

Door lock: ✓
Lockable place: ✓

Services provided

Beauty services: Hairdressing
Mobile library: ✓
Religious services: Monthly Anglican service
Transport: Car
Activities: *Coordinator:* ✓ • *Examples:* Bridge, bingo, exercise
Outings: ✓
Meetings: ✓

Registered places: 40
Guide weekly rate: £450–£595
Specialist care: None
Medical services: Podiatry
Qualified staff: Meets standard

Home details

Location: Village location, 1 mile from Crowborough
Communal areas: 2 lounges, dining room, conservatory, garden
Accessibility: *Floors:* 2 • *Access:* Lift • *Wheelchair access:* Good
Smoking: ✓
Pets: ✗
Routines: Flexible

Room details

Single: 36
Shared: 4
En suite: 40
Facilities: TV point, telephone point

Door lock: ✓
Lockable place: ✗

Services provided

Beauty services: Hairdressing
Mobile library: ✗
Religious services: ✓
Transport: ✗
Activities: *Coordinator:* ✓ • *Examples:* Gardening club, quizzes, bowling • *Outings:* ✓
Meetings: ✓

Windlesham Manor

Manager: Yvonne Peskett
Owner: Mr and Mrs Carey
Contact: Hurtis Hill, Crowborough, East Sussex TN6 3AA
☏ 01892 611000
🖰 www.windlesham-manor.co.uk

Windlesham Manor is a large building that has been extended. It has its own grounds that have been laid out with walkways to make it user-friendly for residents. The home is positioned on the outskirts of Ashburnham Forest, and it a mile away from the local town of Crowborough, where there are sufficient amenities. The gardening club is much encouraged for those with an interest in the environment. Residents are often taken on regular outings, a favourite of the residents being a trip into Ashburnham Forest to see local wildlife.

Abbey House Nursing Home

Manager: Susan Ann Wilson
Owner: Millennium Care Homes Ltd
Contact: 2 Abbey Hill, Netley Abbey, Southampton, Hampshire SO31 5FB
☎ 02380 454044
@ Info@abbeyhouse.org.uk
🖱 www.abbeyhouse.org.uk

Abbey House is located in a small village, three miles from Southampton centre. There are local amenities nearby as well as a park overlooking Southampton water. The home was originally a large Victorian house, but has been converted and extended. Adjacent to the home are the historic ruins of Netley Abbey. There is a varied menu of home cooked meals which allows residents to maintain any dietary requirements. There are also visits from a dog fortnightly. There is a residents meeting every six months.

Registered places: 48
Guide weekly rate: £530–£699
Specialist care: Nursing, physical disability, respite, terminal care
Medical services: Podiatry, hygienist, optician, physiotherapy
Qualified staff: Fails standard: 33% at NVQ Level 2

Home details
Location: Village location, 3 miles from Southampton
Communal areas: 4 lounges, dining room, conservatory, garden
Accessibility: *Floors:* 3 • *Access:* 3 lifts • *Wheelchair access:* Good
Smoking: ✗
Pets: ✓
Routines: Flexible

Room details
Single: 29
Shared: 7
En suite: 21
Facilities: TV, telephone

Door lock: ✓
Lockable place: ✓

Services provided
Beauty services: Hairdressing
Mobile library: ✓
Religious services: ✗
Transport: ✗
Activities: *Coordinator:* ✓ • *Examples:* Arts and crafts, reminiscence, singers • *Outings:* ✓
Meetings: ✓

Abbeygate Residential Home

Manager: Jean Benjamin
Owner: Avonpark Care Centre Ltd
Contact: 42 Quarry Road, Winchester, Hampshire SO23 0JS
☎ 01962 855056

Abbeygate is a large residential home and is part of a care homes group. It is situated on the outskirts of Winchester, approximately two miles from the town centre where there are many shop and amenities. The home is surrounded by a large, secluded garden, with patio and decking for the residents to sit outside and enjoy in better weather. Those who enjoy gardening are very much encouraged to help maintain the garden and maintain a community feel.

Registered places: 30
Guide weekly rate: £327.04–£479
Specialist care: Dementia, respite, mental disorder
Medical services: Podiatry
Qualified staff: Exceeds standard: 70% at NVQ Level 2

Home details
Location: Residential area, 1.7 miles from Winchester
Communal areas: 3 lounges, dining room, patio and garden
Accessibility: *Floors:* 2 • *Access:* Lift • *Wheelchair access:* Good
Smoking: ✗
Pets: At manager's discretion
Routines: Flexible

Room details
Single: 22
Shared: 4
En suite: 0
Facilities: TV point, telephone point

Door lock: ✗
Lockable place: ✓

Services provided
Beauty services: Hairdressing
Mobile library: ✓
Religious services: Weekly Catholic and monthly Anglican services
Activities: *Coordinator:* ✓ • *Examples:* Bingo, guitar playing, quizzes *Outings:* ✓
Meetings: ✓

Registered places: 60
Guide weekly rate: £826–£993
Specialist care: Nursing, physical disability
Medical services: Podiatry, dentist, optician, physiotherapy
Qualified staff: Fails standard: 38% at NVQ Level 2

Home details

Location: Residential area, 1.2 miles from Winchester
Communal areas: Dining room, garden
Accessibility: *Floors:* 3 • *Access:* Lift • *Wheelchair access:* Good
Smoking: ✓
Pets: ✓
Routines: Flexible

Room details

Single: 60
Shared: 0
En suite: 60
Facilities: TV point, telephone point

Door lock: ✓
Lockable place: ✓

Services provided

Beauty services: Hairdressing
Mobile library: ✗
Religious services: ✗
Transport: ✗
Activities: *Coordinator:* ✓ • *Examples:* Music club, visiting
　　entertainers • *Outings:* ✓
Meetings: ✓

Abbotts Barton Nursing Home

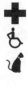

Manager: Denise Smyth
Owner: Colten Care Ltd
Contact: 40 Worthy Road, Winchester,
Hampshire SO23 7HB
　☎ 01962 626800
　@ abbotsbarton@coltoncare.co.uk
　🖰 www.coltencare.co.uk

Abbotts Barton is a purpose-built nursing
home that opened in 2001. It is situated
in a residential area within two miles of
the historic city of Winchester. Some of
the rooms offer views across to the city
and Winchester cathedral. There is a large
reception area where residents often
gather for a chat and a pre-luncheon drink.
There are several lounges overlooking the
gardens and hydrotherapy and spa baths
are available to the residents. There is a
residents meeting once a month.

Registered places: 27
Guide weekly rate: £590–£795
Specialist care: Nursing, physical disability, respite
Medical services: Podiatry, optician, physiotherapy
Qualified staff: Exceeds standard: 70% at NVQ Level 2

Home details

Location: Residential area, 11 miles from Portsmouth
Communal areas: 2 lounges, dining room, conservatory,
　　patio and garden
Accessibility: *Floors:* 2 • *Access:* Lift and stair lift
　　Wheelchair access: Good
Smoking: In designated area
Pets: ✗
Routines: Flexible

Room details

Single: 23
Shared: 2
En suite: 11
Facilities: TV point, telephone point

Door lock: ✓
Lockable place: ✓

Services provided

Beauty services: Hairdressing
Mobile library: ✗
Religious services: Monthly Anglican service
Transport: ✗
Activities: *Coordinator:* ✓ • *Examples:* Fêtes, movie afternoons,
　　visiting entertainers • *Outings:* ✓
Meetings: ✓

Acacia House Nursing Home

Manager: Linda Murray
Owner: Contemplation Homes Ltd
Contact: 33 Portsmouth Road,
Horndean, Hampshire PO8 9LN
　☎ 023 9259 4138
　@ acaciahouse@
　　　contemplation-homes.co.uk
　🖰 www.contemplation-homes.co.uk

On the outskirts of Horndean, near
Portsmouth, Acacia House offers nursing
care for 27 residents. One of the staff
acts as an activities coordinator and in
the past, residents have enjoyed fireworks
displays, theatre visits, Christmas
shopping and a visit to the home from
a mobile farm. Though pets are not
allowed there is a resident budgie. There
is an Anglican service once a month. For
those who are not Anglican the home can
arrange for all denominations to visit.

Alexandra Rose Residential Care Home

Manager: Tammy Durrant
Owner: Riva Ltd
Contact: 358 Havant Road, Farlington, Portsmouth, Hampshire PO6 1NE
) 023 9238 2944
www.alexandra-rose.co.uk

Alexandra Rose is in Farlington, a residential area of Portsmouth and has good transport links into the centre. The home aims to optimise the quality of life with freedom of choice and flexibility. The home arranges a range of activities to help the residents socialise and keep active. There is also a mobile shop for residents to purchase items including sweets, toiletries and greeting cards. The home also has a qualified cook who can cater to specific dietary requirements.

Registered places: 32
Guide weekly rate: £450–£645
Specialist care: Dementia
Medical services: Podiatry, dentist, optician, physiotherapy
Qualified staff: Exceeds standard: 90% at NVQ Level 2

Home details
Location: Residential area, 8 miles from Portsmouth
Communal areas: Lounge, dining room, 2 conservatories, garden
Accessibility: *Floors:* 2 • *Access:* Lift • *Wheelchair access:* Good
Smoking: ✗
Pets: At manager's discretion
Routines: Flexible

Room details
Single: 27
Shared: 2
En suite: 29
Facilities: TV point, telephone point
Door lock: ✓
Lockable place: ✓

Services provided
Beauty services: Hairdressing
Mobile library: ✓
Religious services: Anglican visits
Transport: ✗
Activities: *Coordinator:* ✓ • *Examples:* Entertainers, music, videos
Outings: ✓
Meetings: ✓

Allenbrook Nursing Home

Manager: John Walker
Owner: Allenbrook Care Ltd
Contact: 34 Station Road, Fordingbridge, Hampshire SP6 1JW
) 01425 656589

Allenbrook is a large Georgian-period country house situated in a residential area of Fordingbridge. The home is located half a mile from the small town of Fordingbridge, with all its amenities. There is a limited bus service from Fordingbridge to the centres of Ringwood and Salisbury. The home offers a church service every month.

Registered places: 43
Guide weekly rate: £500– £690
Specialist care: Nursing, physical disability, sensory impairment, terminal care
Medical services: Podiatry, dentist, optician, physiotherapy
Qualified staff: Exceeds standard: 55% at NVQ Level 2

Home details
Location: Residential area, 0.5 miles from Fordingbridge
Communal areas: Lounge, lounge/dining room, conservatory, garden
Accessibility: *Floors:* 3 • *Access:* Lift • *Wheelchair access:* Good
Smoking: In designated area
Pets: ✗
Routines: Flexible

Room details
Single: 35
Shared: 4
En suite: 5
Facilities: TV point, telephone point
Door lock: ✗
Lockable place: ✓

Services provided
Beauty services: Hairdressing, manicures
Mobile library: ✓
Religious services: Monthly church services
Transport: ✓
Activities: *Coordinator:* ✓ • *Examples:* Bingo, games, giant crosswords
Meetings: ✗

Registered places: 18
Guide weekly rate: Undisclosed
Specialist care: Dementia, mental disorder
Medical services: Podiatry, optician
Qualified staff: Undisclosed

Home details
Location: Village location, 0.2 miles from South Hayling
Communal areas: Lounge, dining room, garden
Accessibility: *Floors:* 2 • *Access:* Lift • *Wheelchair access:* Good
Smoking: ✗
Pets: ✗
Routines: Structured

Room details
Single: 10
Shared: 4
En suite: Undisclosed
Facilities: TV point

Door lock: ✓
Lockable place: ✗

Services provided
Beauty services: Hairdressing
Mobile library: ✗
Religious services: ✗
Transport: ✗
Activities: *Coordinator:* ✗ • *Examples:* Games, singing, Outings: ✗
Meetings: ✗

Alton House

Manager: Elaine Herridge
Owner: Alton House Partnership
Contact: 37 St Leonards Avenue, Hayling Island, Hampshire PO11 9BN
☏ 023 9246 2910

Alton House is a large, detached property set in a quiet residential area of Hayling Island a few minutes from the local village of South Hayling. The home arranges activities for residents such as singing and memory games. The home has a garden for residents to enjoy in the warmer months and there is a lounge which serves as a communal area.

Registered places: 30
Guide weekly rate: £550–£600
Specialist care: Nursing, respite, physical disability, terminal care
Medical services: Podiatry, dentist, optician, physiotherapy
Qualified staff: Exceeds standard: 58% at NVQ Level 2

Home details
Location: Residential area, 1.5 miles from Gosport
Communal areas: Lounge, dining/conservatory, patio and garden
Accessibility: *Floors:* 2 • *Access:* Lift • *Wheelchair access:* Good
Smoking: ✗
Pets: ✗
Routines: Flexible

Room details
Single: 22
Shared: 4
En suite: 12
Facilities: TV point, telephone point

Door lock: ✓
Lockable place: ✓

Services provided
Beauty services: Hairdressing
Mobile library: ✓
Religious services: Monthly Anglican Communion service
Transport: Minibus
Activities: *Coordinator:* ✓ • *Examples:* Gentle exercise, visiting musicians, quizzes • *Outings:* ✗
Meetings: ✗

Alverstoke House Nursing Home

Manager: Rosemary Cook
Owner: Janet and Andrew Hudson
Contact: Somervell Close, Alverstoke, Gosport, Hampshire PO12 2BX
☏ 023 9251 0254

Alverstoke House is a privately owned home in a residential area of Gosport. It is within easy reach of local shops and the costal area of Stokes Bay. The garden and courtyard area at the front of the house has a fountain and a fishpond. In the lounge there is a piano for those with musical inclinations. The home offers a variety of activities including visiting musicians and exercise classes. Though pets are not allowed to stay in the home they are allowed to visit with family or friends.

The Andover Nursing Home

Manager: Martin Watt
Owner: Messrs Puddepha
Contact: Weyhill Road, Andover, Hampshire SP10 3AN
) 01264 333324
@ admin@andovernursinghome.co.uk
⌂ www.andovernursinghome.co.uk

The Andover Nursing Home is situated near to the centre of Andover, one and a half miles away. The garden has been landscaped and includes a sensory garden. There are also sensory rooms in the home. The home has two activities coordinators who arrange a variety of activities including outings to the theatre. The home has visits from a mobile library and there is a designated activities room.

Registered places: 87
Guide weekly rate: Undisclosed
Specialist care: Nursing, day care, physical disability, respite
Medical services: Podiatry, dentist, optician, physiotherapy
Qualified staff: Meets standard

Home details
Location: Residential area, 1.5 miles from Andover
Communal areas: 3 lounges, 2 dining rooms, activities room, smoking room, conservatory, patio and garden
Accessibility: *Floors:* 4 • *Access:* Lift • *Wheelchair access:* Good
Smoking: In designated area
Pets: At manager's discretion
Routines: Flexible

Room details
Single: 79
Shared: 4
En suite: 87
Facilities: Undisclosed

Door lock: ✓
Lockable place: ✓

Services provided
Beauty services: Hairdressing
Mobile library: ✓
Religious services: ✓
Transport: ✗
Activities: *Coordinators:* ✓ • *Examples:* Bingo, crosswords, visiting entertainers • *Outings:* ✓
Meetings: ✓

Anglesey Court

Manager: Anne Margaret O'Gorman
Owner: Anglesey Court Ltd
Contact: 26 Crescent Road, Alverstoke, Gosport, Hampshire PO12 2DJ
) 023 9258 2322

Anglesey Court, a large detached property, is situated in the village of Alverstoke. It is opposite a public park and the beach is a short distance away. There is a communal lounge and dining room, as well as seating areas on each floor. Though pets are not allowed to stay in the home they can visit. There is a shop, post office, bank, bus stop and pub within a quarter of a mile.

Registered places: 20
Guide weekly rate: £336–£377
Specialist care: Respite
Medical services: Podiatry, dentist, optician
Qualified staff: Exceeds standard: 75% at NVQ Level 2

Home details
Location: Village location, 1.8 miles from Gosport
Communal areas: Lounge, dining room, garden
Accessibility: *Floors:* 3 • *Access:* Lift and stair lift *Wheelchair access:* Good
Smoking: ✗
Pets: ✗
Routines: Flexible

Room details
Single: 9
Shared: 5
En suite: 0
Facilities: TV

Door lock: ✓
Lockable place: ✓

Services provided
Beauty services: Hairdressing
Mobile library: ✗
Religious services: Monthly Catholic Communion service
Transport: ✗
Activities: *Coordinator:* ✗ • *Examples:* Craftwork, exercises, nostalgia chats • *Outings:* ✗
Meetings: ✓

Registered places: 19
Guide weekly rate: £335–£600
Specialist care: Dementia, respite
Medical services: Podiatry, optician, physiotherapy
Qualified staff: Exceeds standard: 75% at NVQ Level 2

Home details

Location: Residential area, 0.4 miles to Bramley
Communal areas: 2 lounges, dining room, conservatory, garden
Accessibility: *Floors:* 2 • *Access:* Lift and stair lift
    Wheelchair access: Good
Smoking: In designated area
Pets: At manager's discretion
Routines: Flexible

Room details

Single: 13	Door lock: ✓
Shared: 6	Lockable place: ✓
En suite: 2	

Facilities: TV point, telephone point

Services provided

Beauty services: Hairdressing, manicures, aromatherapy
Mobile library: ✓
Religious services: Fortnightly visits
Transport: Minibus
Activities: *Coordinator:* ✗ • *Examples:* Arts and crafts, bingo, karaoke • *Outings:* ✓
Meetings: ✓

Applewood Care Home

Manager: Natalie Betsworth
Owner: Milkwood Residential Care Ltd
Contact: Coopers Lane, Bramley, Basingstoke, Hampshire RG26 5BZ
☎ 01730 895485
🖱 www.elderlycare.co.uk

Applewood is a large, detached property which is currently undergoing a major change in layout. An extension is also being planned for additional rooms with en suite facilities. The home is situated in a quiet residential area in the village of Bramley, Hampshire. There are residents' meetings every three to six months and religious visits every two weeks. Staff create a homely, family-like atmosphere for residents, providing a friendly level of care for all residents. Activities are provided by the home, such as arts and crafts and bingo. Outings are also made via the home's own minibus.

Registered places: 17
Guide weekly rate: £460–£475
Specialist care: Dementia, mental disorder
Medical services: Undisclosed
Qualified staff: Fails standard: 25% at NVQ Level 2

Home details

Location: Residential area, 0.6 miles from Southsea
Communal areas: Lounge/dining room, conservatory, garden
Accessibility: *Floors:* 3 • *Access:* Stair lifts
    Wheelchair access: None
Smoking: In designated area
Pets: Undisclosed
Routines: Undisclosed

Room details

Single: 5	Door lock: Undisclosed
Shared: 6	Lockable place: Undisclosed
En suite: Undisclosed	

Services provided

Beauty services: Undisclosed
Mobile library: ✗
Religious services: ✗
Transport: ✗
Activities: *Coordinator:* ✓ • *Examples:* Bingo, games, puzzles, reminiscence • *Outings:* ✓
Meetings: ✓

Arborough House

Manager: Francesca Kitching
Owner: Sally-Ann Biggs
Contact: 7 Yarborough Road, Southsea, Hampshire PO5 3DZ
☎ 023 9282 1181
@ kitchingc@btconnect.com

Arborough House residential home is a care home specialising in providing care for those with age related mental health problems and general age frailty. The home is situated in a residential area of Southsea, Portsmouth, close to the shopping centre. Access to the garden is provided by a ramp with rails. Two members of staff run activities specially designed for those with dementia, such as reminiscence therapy. Regular outings are made to the theatre, on walks and to local attractions such as the zoo. Smoking is permitted in a designated area and but pets are not allowed.

Ashlett Dale Rest Home

Manager: Collette Willis
Owner: Frederick and Maureen Liddington
Contact: Stonehills, Fawley, Southampton, Hampshire SO45 1DU
☎ 023 8089 2075

Ashlett Dale specialises in giving care to the elderly, those with dementia, mental illness or physical disabilities. It is situated on the outskirts of the New Forest, approximately one mile from Fawley. The home has a garden with seating areas and fruit trees growing. There is a cook who can cater for specialist dietary requirement and also bakes a fresh cake every day. The home offers a range of activities, with something for everyone including colouring and walks.

Registered places: 14
Guide weekly rate: £395–£410
Specialist care: Day care, dementia, learning disability, mental disorder, physical disability
Medical services: Podiatry, dentist, optician, physiotherapy
Qualified staff: Exceeds standard: 100% at NVQ Level 2

Home details

Location: Rural area, 0.8 miles from Fawley
Communal areas: Lounge, Dining room, garden
Accessibility: *Floors:* 2 • *Access:* Stair lift
  Wheelchair access: Good
Smoking: In designated area
Pets: Only budgies
Routines: Flexible

Room details

Single: 14
Shared: 0
En suite: 14
Facilities: TV point

Door lock: ✓
Lockable place: ✓

Services provided

Beauty services: Hairdressing, manicures
Mobile library: ✓
Religious services: Monthly Communion service
Transport: ✗
Activities: *Coordinator:* ✓ • *Examples:* Bingo, games, walks
  Outings: ✓
Meetings: ✗

Ashley Arnewood Manor

Manager: S Rawlins
Owner: SCOFIL Ltd
Contact: 32 Ashley Road, New Milton, Hampshire BH25 6BB
☎ 01425 611 453

Ashley Arnewood Manor is a privately owned and run care home set in a residential area close to amenities and New Milton town centre. Though only cats are allowed in the home there is a Pets As Therapy scheme. The home also brings in visiting entertainment for residents to enjoy. There are residents meetings every three months allowing residents to discuss any issues they may have.

Registered places: 20
Guide weekly rate: From £440
Specialist care: Dementia, respite
Medical services: Podiatry, dentist, optician, physiotherapy
Qualified staff: Fails standard: 16% at NVQ Level 2

Home details

Location: Residential area, 1.7 miles from New Milton
Communal areas: Lounge, dining room, patio and garden
Accessibility: *Floors:* 2 • *Access:* Stair lift
  Wheelchair access: Limited
Smoking: ✗
Pets: At manager's discretion
Routines: Flexible

Room details

Single: 18
Shared: 1
En suite: 2
Facilities: None

Door lock: ✓
Lockable place: ✓

Services provided

Beauty services: Hairdressing, aromatherapy
Mobile library: ✓
Religious services: Monthly Anglican visits
Transport: ✗
Activities: *Coordinator:* ✗ • *Examples:* Bingo, gentle exercise, visiting entertainers • *Outings:* ✓
Meetings: ✓

Registered places: 34
Guide weekly rate: £533.96
Specialist care: Dementia, mental disorder
Medical services: Podiatry, optician, physiotherapy
Qualified staff: Exceeds standard: 80% at NVQ Level 2

Home details
Location: Residential area, 1 mile from Bordon
Communal areas: 5 Lounges, dining room, pub, garden
Accessibility: *Floors:* 2 • *Access:* Lift • *Wheelchair access:* Good
Smoking: In designated area
Pets: At manager's discretion
Routines: Flexible

Room details
Single: 34
Shared: 0
En suite: 34
Facilities: TV point, telephone point

Door lock: ✓
Lockable place: ✓

Services provided
Beauty services: Hairdressing, manicures
Mobile library: ✗
Religious services: Fortnightly church visits
Transport: ✗
Activities: *Coordinator:* ✓ • *Examples:* Arts and crafts, baking
   Outings: ✓
Meetings: ✓

Ashley House

Manager: Margaret Powel
Owner: Sanctuary Care Ltd
Contact: 56 Forest Road, Bordon,
Hampshire GU35 0XT
) 01420 489877
@ Margaret.powel@
   sanctury-housing.co.uk

Ashley House is a purpose-built home that is sub-divided into six clusters of accommodation each with a small lounge and kitchenette area. Residents also have a communal dining area which leads onto a garden filled with shrubs and plants. Residents are actively involved in one-to-one activities with a coordinator, such as the make up of a resident's history album using old photographs. The home boasts an in-house 'pub' that residents use as a social venue for building bonds with fellow residents. There are residents meetings twice a month.

Registered places: 77
Guide weekly rate: Undisclosed
Specialist care: Nursing, dementia, physical disability, terminal care, respite
Medical services: Podiatry, occupational therapy, physiotherapy
Qualified staff: Undisclosed

Home details
Location: Rural area, 1.5 miles from New Milton
Communal areas: 6 lounges, 3 dining rooms, kitchenette, hairdressing salon, garden
Accessibility: *Floors:* 2 • *Access:* 2 lifts • *Wheelchair access:* Good
Smoking: ✗
Pets: ✗
Routines: Flexible

Room details
Single: 77
Shared: 0
En suite: 73
Facilities: TV, telephone point

Door lock: ✓
Lockable place: ✗

Services provided
Beauty services: Hairdressing, aromatherapy
Mobile library: ✓
Religious services: ✓
Transport: ✓
Activities: *Coordinator:* ✓ • *Examples:* Arts and crafts, gardening
   and board games • *Outings:* ✓
Meetings: ✓

Ashley Lodge Residential and Nursing Home

Manager: Joanna Collins
Owner: BUPA Care Homes Ltd
Contact: Golden Hill, Ashley Lane, Ashley, New Milton, Hampshire BH25 5AH
) 01425 611334
@ AshleyLodgeALL@BUPA.com
🖰 www.bupacarehomes.co.uk

Originally a private house, Ashley Lodge is set in two acres of land in the countryside, close to New Milton. It has undergone an extensive refurbishment and extension programme which was completed in January 2008. Local shops are within walking distance and it is on a local bus route. The home consists of two separate houses. The Forest suite offers care to dementia residents. Daily activities include arts and crafts, gardening and board games, as well as trips to local places of interest. Ashley Lodge also offers care to older people with physical disabilities and to those requiring palliative or terminal care.

Ashley Manor Nursing and Residential Care Home

Manager: Rosamund Heath

Owner: Theresa Andrews

Contact: Winchester Road, Shedfield, Hampshire SO32 2JF

) 01329 833810

@ info@ashleymanorhome.co.uk

^ www.ashleymanorhome.co.uk

Ashley Manor is set in two acres countryside with well-maintained gardens containing raised flowerbeds and paved areas allowing wheelchair access. The activities coordinator organises a range of activities for residents including special celebrations for birthdays and Christmas. There are also monthly themed parties on topical events such as a tropical beach party, 4th July celebrations and Halloween.

Registered places: 45

Guide weekly rate: £637–£724

Specialist care: Nursing, respite, physical disability

Medical services: Podiatry

Qualified staff: Fails standard

Home details

Location: Village location, 10 miles to Southampton

Communal areas: Lounge, dining room, conservatory, hairdressing salon, garden

Accessibility: *Floors:* 3 • *Access:* Lift • *Wheelchair access:* Good

Smoking: In designated area

Pets: ✗

Routines: Flexible

Room details

Single: 35

Shared: 5

En suite: 25

Facilities: TV point

Door lock: ✓

Lockable place: ✓

Services provided

Beauty services: Hairdressing, manicures.

Mobile library: ✗

Religious services: Monthly Anglican service

Transport: ✗

Activities: *Coordinator:* ✓ • *Examples:* Crafts, parties, visiting musicians • *Outings:* ✗

Meetings: ✓

Avon Park

Manager: Janine Haynes

Owner: A Nethersole

Contact: 66 Southampton Road, Park Gate, Hampshire SO31 6AF

) 01489 574616

@ alexandernethersole@btinternet.com

^ www.avonparkresidential carehome.co.uk

Avon Park is located in a quiet residential area of Park Gate, close to shops and local amenities. The home arranges meetings often for residents to take part in and voice any concerns. The garden is wheelchair accessible. There are also frequent outings including trips to the sea in fine weather and afternoon trips out to local points of interest and shopping. They have strong links with the local church, who come for Communion and also arrange the Christmas carol service and summer songs of praise. They also invite all residents to attend their summer fête and other exciting events.

Registered places: 30

Guide weekly rate: Undisclosed

Specialist care: Physical disability, respite

Medical services: Podiatry, dentist, optician, physiotherapy

Qualified staff: Meets standard

Home details

Location: Residential area, 1.2 miles from Lockheath

Communal areas: 2 lounges, dining room, garden

Accessibility: *Floors:* 2 • *Access:* Lift • *Wheelchair access:* Good

Smoking: ✗

Pets: At manager's discretion

Routines: Flexible

Room details

Single: 28

Shared: 1

En suite: 29

Facilities: TV point, telephone point

Door lock: ✓

Lockable place: ✓

Services provided

Beauty services: Hairdressing

Mobile library: ✓

Religious services: Monthly Communion service

Transport: ✗

Activities: *Coordinator:* ✓ • *Examples:* Arts and crafts, bingo, music to movement • *Outings:* ✓

Meetings: ✓

Registered places: 14
Guide weekly rate: £375–£500
Specialist care: Dementia, mental disorder
Medical services: Podiatry, dentist, optician
Qualified staff: Exceeds standard: 78% at NVQ Level 2

Home details

Location: Village location, 8 miles from Southampton
Communal areas: Lounge, dining room, garden
Accessibility: *Floors:* 2 • *Access:* Lift • *Wheelchair access:* Good
Smoking: ✗
Pets: ✗
Routines: Flexible

Room details

Single: 12
Shared: 1
En suite: 10
Facilities: TV point, telephone point

Door lock: ✗
Lockable place: ✓

Services provided

Beauty services: Hairdressing
Mobile library: ✗
Religious services: Weekly church service
Transport: ✗
Activities: *Coordinator:* ✓ • *Examples:* Arts and crafts, reminiscence, puzzles • *Outings:* ✗
Meetings: ✓

Avondale Lodge Care Home

Manager: Wendy Osman
Owner: Wendy and Gary Osman
Contact: Hythe Road, Marchwood, Southampton, Hampshire SO40 4WT
☏ 023 8066 6534

Avondale Lodge is a small family-run home where one of the proprietors doubles as the manager. The building is one of the oldest buildings in the village. The home's activities coordinator arranges activities including reminiscence sessions and arts and crafts. There is also a church service once a week. The home gives residents training in independent living. There are regular outings and trips to get residents out of the house such as tours of the local area. The home is not near local shops, however it is very near to the Marchwood bypass which leads into Southampton.

Registered places: 25
Guide weekly rate: £325– £450
Specialist care: Dementia, respite
Medical services: Podiatry, dentist, optician
Qualified staff: Meets standard

Home details

Location: Residential area, 11 miles from Southampton
Communal areas: 3 lounges, 2 dining rooms, garden
Accessibility: *Floors:* 2 • *Access:* Stair lift
    Wheelchair access: Good
Smoking: In designated area
Pets: Undisclosed
Routines: Flexible

Room details

Single: 21
Shared: 2
En suite: 0
Facilities: TV point, telephone point

Door lock: ✓
Lockable place: ✓

Services provided

Beauty services: Hairdressing
Mobile library: ✗
Religious services: Monthly church service
Transport: ✗
Activities: *Coordinator:* ✗ • *Examples:* Art classes, DVD nights *Outings:* ✓
Meetings: ✗

Badgers Holt

Manager: Gina Rayner
Owner: Teresa Rayner
Contact: Butts Ash Lane, Hythe, Southampton, Hampshire SO45 3QY
☏ 023 8084 9310
@ info@badgersholtresidential.co.uk
🖰 www.badgersholtresidential.co.uk

On the edge of the New Forest, close to the small villages of Dibden Purlieu and Hythe, Badgers Holt is located 11 miles from Southampton town centre. The area is very scenic, with views including beaches, the sea and forests. The home aims to have an activity every weekday, including exercise with music, outings, DVDs and art classes. The monthly church service sees Methodist, Anglican and Catholic ministers alternating each month.

Baroda Care Home for the Elderly

Manager: Joan Vijayanathan
Owner: Branksome Care Ltd
Contact: 34 Merdon Avenue, Chandlers Ford, Eastleigh, Hampshire SO53 1EP
☎ 023 8025 2643

Baroda Care Home is located in a residential area of Chandlers Ford, Eastleigh, half a mile from the town centre where there is an abundance of shops and facilities. The home is set in a spacious landscaped garden, which can be accessed via the main lounge. Two of the first floor bedrooms have balconies overlooking the garden. Regular daily activities include armchair exercises, card games and regular visiting entertainers who give talks, sing live or do magic.

Registered places: 12
Guide weekly rate: £468–£520
Specialist care: None
Medical services: Podiatry, dentist, optician, physiotherapy
Qualified staff: Undisclosed

Home details
Location: Residential area, 0.5 miles from Eastleigh
Communal areas: 2 lounges, dining room
Accessibility: *Floors:* 2 • *Access:* Stair lift
  Wheelchair access: Good
Smoking: In designated area
Pets: ✗
Routines: Flexible

Room details
Single: 12
Shared: 0
En suite: 10
Facilities: TV point, telephone point

Door lock: ✓
Lockable place: ✗

Services provided
Beauty services: Hairdressing
Mobile library: ✗
Religious services: Weekly church visits
Transport: ✗
Activities: *Coordinator.* ✗ • *Examples:* Armchair aerobics, card games, visiting entertainers • *Outings:* ✗
Meetings: ✓

Barton Lodge Residential Retirement Care

Manager: Pamela Torr
Owner: Manucourt Ltd
Contact: Barton Common Road, Barton-on-Sea, Hampshire BH25 5PR
☎ 01425 617111
🖰 www.lovingcare-matters.co.uk

Barton Lodge is set in a rural area, on the edge of Barton Common, with views over a golf course and overlooking the Solvent and the Isle of Wight. Residents are taken on regular outings to the duck pond at New Milton, the ice-cream parlour at Barton-on-Sea and out shopping. The home has developed a system of 'mapping' each resident's likes and dislikes, to tailor activities accordingly. All bedrooms have views over the golf course, Solvent or gardens and some bedrooms have their own balcony.

Registered places: 39
Guide weekly rate: £850–£950
Specialist care: Dementia, respite, physical disability
Medical services: Podiatry, physiotherapy
Qualified staff: Meets standard

Home details
Location: Rural area, 1 mile from Barton-on-Sea
Communal areas: 2 lounges, dining room, conservatory, garden
Accessibility: *Floors:* 2 • *Access:* Lift • *Wheelchair access:* Good
Smoking: ✗
Pets: ✗
Routines: Flexible

Room details
Single: 23
Shared: 7
En suite: 24
Facilities: TV point, telephone point

Door lock: ✓
Lockable place: ✓

Services provided
Beauty services: Hairdressing, massage
Mobile library: ✓
Religious services: Monthly Anglican and Catholic service
Transport: ✗
Activities: *Coordinator.* ✗ • *Examples:* Games, visiting entertainers • *Outings:* ✓
Meetings: ✓

Registered places: 12
Guide weekly rate: £420– £460
Specialist care: Day care, dementia, mental disorder, respite
Medical services: Podiatry, dentist, optician, physiotherapy
Qualified staff: Exceeds standard: 90% at NVQ Level 2

Home details

Location: Residential area, 2.5 miles from Waterlooville
Communal areas: Lounge, lounge/dining room,
    conservatory, garden
Accessibility: *Floors:* 2 • *Access:* Stair lift
    Wheelchair access: Limited
Smoking: In designated area
Pets: At manager's discretion
Routines: Flexible

Room details

Single: 8
Shared: 2
En suite: 1
Facilities: TV point, telephone point

Door lock: ✓
Lockable place: ✓

Services provided

Beauty services: Hairdressing
Mobile library: ✓
Religious services: Monthly Anglican service
Transport: ✗
Activities: *Coordinator:* ✓ • *Examples:* Bingo, chair exercises,
    creative memories • *Outings:* ✓
Meetings: ✓

Bayith Rest Home

Manager: Jane Giles
Owner: C Parker and Jane Giles
Contact: 18–20 Bevan Road, Lovedean,
Waterlooville, Hampshire PO8 9QH
☎ 023 9259 7388
@ janegiles@ntlworld.com

Bayith Rest Home is located close to local amenities, bus and rail links are in easy reach. Someone comes in once a week to partake in activities with the residents and local school children regularly write letters and talk with them. The home sends out questionnaires for residents to fill out and on their return there is a meeting for all issues to be discussed. Though there are no formal meetings there are coffee mornings where the residents and their families can talk with the manager about concerns or issues.

Registered places: 7
Guide weekly rate: £395–£495
Specialist care: Dementia, mental disorder, respite
Medical services: Podiatry, hygienist, optician, physiotherapy
Qualified staff: Exceeds standard: 75% at NVQ Level 2

Home details

Location: Residential area, 2.8 miles from New Milton
Communal areas: Lounge/dining room, garden
Accessibility: *Floors:* 2 • *Access:* Lift • *Wheelchair access:* Good
Smoking: ✗
Pets: ✗
Routines: Flexible

Room details

Single: 5
Shared: 1
En suite: 1
Facilities: TV point

Door lock: ✓
Lockable place: ✗

Services provided

Beauty services: Hairdressing, aromatherapy, manicures
Mobile library: ✗
Religious services: ✓
Transport: ✗
Activities: *Coordinator:* ✗ • *Examples:* Gardening, board games
    Outings: ✗
Meetings: ✗

Beach Crest

Manager: Vallabhdas Faldu
Owner: Vallabhdas and Shobhna Faldu
Contact: Marine Drive East,
Barton-on-Sea, New Milton,
Hampshire BH25 7DX
☎ 01425 612506
@ beachrest@hotmail.co.uk

Beach Crest is situated on the seafront, offering views of the Isle of Wight. The home is located in a residential area close to local amenities and approximately three miles from New Milton. It is a small home offering a family style environment to the residents. Residents regularly help in the garden, play board games and cards as activities.

Beacon House

Manager: J Deaville
Owner: Wilton Rest Homes Ltd
Contact: Victoria Hill Road, Fleet,
Hampshire GU51 4LG
☎ 01252 615035
@ JanetDeaville@aol.com

Beacon Home is located on the outskirts of Fleet and is within access of local shops and other amenities. Residents enjoy the views of the large, highly maintained garden. Programmes of daily activities for residents are implemented, such as cinema trips and board games. The home also provides many outings to places of interest, such as garden centres, Brighton beach and Bournemouth.

Registered places: 20
Guide weekly rate: £560–£620
Specialist care: Dementia, respite
Medical services: Podiatry, dentistry, optician, physiotherapy
Qualified staff: Exceeds standard: 95% at NVQ Level 2

Home details
Location: Urban area, 1 mile from Fleet
Communal areas: 2 Lounges, dining room, garden
Accessibility: *Floors:* 2 • *Access:* Lift • *Wheelchair access:* Good
Smoking: In designated area
Pets: At manager's discretion
Routines: Flexible

Room details
Single: 20
Shared: 0
En suite: Undisclosed
Facilities: TV point, telephone point

Door lock: ✓
Lockable place: ✓

Services provided
Beauty services: Hairdressing, manicures
Mobile library: ✗
Religious services: Monthly church service
Transport: ✗
Activities: *Coordinator:* ✗ • *Examples:* Board games, visiting musicians • *Outings:* ✓
Meetings: ✓

Bedhampton Nursing Home

Manager: Lindsey Janet Gurney
Owner: Cheer Health Ltd
Contact: 55 Hulbert Road, Bedhampton,
Havant, Hampshire PO9 3TB
☎ 023 9247 5125

Bedhampton Nursing Home is situated approximately one mile from Havant, in a residential area close to local amenities. There is a mature garden at the back of the home. The home arranges a variety of activities for residents including baking and arts and crafts, allowing residents to continue previous hobbies or begin new ones.

Registered places: 30
Guide weekly rate: £600–£895
Specialist care: Nursing, dementia, physical disability, respite, terminal care
Medical services: Podiatry, dentist, optician
Qualified staff: Meets standard

Home details
Location: Residential area, 1.3 miles from Havant
Communal areas: Lounge, dining room, garden
Accessibility: *Floors:* 2 • *Access:* Lift • *Wheelchair access:* Good
Smoking: ✗
Pets: At manager's discretion
Routines: Flexible

Room details
Single: 24
Shared: 3
En suite: 12
Facilities: TV point

Door lock: ✓
Lockable place: ✓

Services provided
Beauty services: Hairdressing
Mobile library: ✓
Religious services: Clergy visits
Transport: ✗
Activities: *Coordinator:* ✓ • *Examples:* Arts and crafts, baking, music and movement • *Outings:* ✗
Meetings: ✓

Registered places: 25
Guide weekly rate: £604–£709
Specialist care: Nursing, physical disability, respite, terminal care
Medical services: Podiatry, physiotherapy, dentist, optician
Qualified staff: Meets standard

Home details

Location: Residential area, 1 mile from Gosport
Communal areas: 2 lounges, dining room, patio and garden
Accessibility: *Floors:* 2 • *Access:* Lift • *Wheelchair access:* Good
Smoking: ✗
Pets: At matron's discretion
Routines: Flexible

Room details

Single: 19
Shared: 3
En suite: 14
Facilities: TV

Door lock: ✓
Lockable place: ✓

Services provided

Beauty services: Hairdressing, aromatherapy, manicures
Mobile library: ✓
Religious services: ✓
Transport: ✗
Activities: *Coordinator:* ✓ • *Examples:* Gardening, horse racing, poetry reading • *Outings:* ✓
Meetings: ✓

Beechcroft Green Nursing Home

Manager: Rebecca Metelko
Owner: Contemplation Homes Ltd
Contact: 1 Anglesey Road, Alverstoke, Gosport, Hampshire PO12 2EG
☎ 023 9258 5512
@ beechcroftgreen@
    contemplation-homes.co.uk
🖱 www.contemplation-homes.co.uk

Beechcroft Green Nursing Home was formerly a rectory and family home and is found in a residential area of Gosport, close to shops and with good transport links. The home employs an activities coordinator who organises a range of activities, from poetry readings to visiting entertainers. A copy of the weekly activities is put in each resident's bedroom. There are regular residents meetings and the home also organises for a mobile library to visit. The home also offers respite care.

Registered places: 30
Guide weekly rate: £604–£709
Specialist care: Nursing, physical disability, respite, terminal care
Medical services: Podiatry, dentist, optician, physiotherapy
Qualified staff: Exceeds standard: 63% at NVQ Level 2

Home details

Location: Residential area, 1.2 miles from Gosport
Communal areas: 2 lounge/dining rooms, conservatory, garden
Accessibility: *Floors:* 3 • *Access:* Lift • *Wheelchair access:* Good
Smoking: ✗
Pets: At matron's discretion
Routines: Flexible

Room details

Single: 8
Shared: 22
En suite: 3
Facilities: TV

Door lock: ✓
Lockable place: ✓

Services provided

Beauty services: Hairdressing, aromatherapy, manicures
Mobile library: ✓
Religious services: ✓
Transport: ✗
Activities: *Coordinator:* ✓ • *Examples:* Bingo, visiting entertainers, skittles • *Outings:* ✓
Meetings: ✓

Beechcroft Manor Nursing Home

Manager: Dawn Swift
Owner: Contemplation Homes Ltd
Contact: 1 Beechcroft Road, Alverstoke, Gosport, Hampshire PO12 2EP
☎ 023 9258 3908
@ beechcroftmanor@
    contemplation-homes.co.uk
🖱 www.contemplation-homes.co.uk

Beechcroft Manor is a large detached property, in a residential area of Gosport. There are local bus links to the town centre. The home provides nursing and respite care for 30 residents. Three of the single rooms in the home have en suite facilities. The home has an activities coordinator who arranges daily activities as well as outings for the residents. The residents each receive a copy of the weekly activities programme. There are regular meetings to give residents the opportunity to voice their opinions.

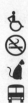

Belford House Care Home

Manager: Michael Curtis
Owner: Belford Care Ltd
Contact: Lymington Bottom, Four Marks, Alton, Hampshire GU34 5AH
☏ 01962 773588
@ belfordhouse@aol.com

Belford House Care Home is a family-run home located in the village of Four Marks. The home is set in three acres of ground and has a lounge as well as large gardens with a patio area. The home arranges a variety of activities for residents including dancing, games and exercise sessions. There are regular visits from Catholic and Anglican clergy and there are also outings organised for the residents.

Registered places: 30
Guide weekly rate: £400–£550
Specialist care: Dementia, day care, mental disorder, respite
Medical services: Podiatry, dentist, optician
Qualified staff: Meets standard

Home details
Location: Village location, 6 miles from Alton
Communal areas: Lounge, patio and garden
Accessibility: *Floors:* • Undisclosed *Access:* Lift
    Wheelchair access: Good
Smoking: ✗
Pets: ✓
Routines: Flexible

Room details
Single: 24
Shared: 3
En suite: 3
Facilities: TV, telephone

Door lock: ✓
Lockable place: ✓

Services provided
Beauty services: Hairdressing
Mobile library: ✓
Religious services: Anglican and Catholic clergy visits
Transport: ✓
Activities: *Coordinator:* ✓ • *Examples:* Dancing, games, exercise • *Outings:* ✓
Meetings: ✓

Belmont Castle

Manager: Michelle Shann
Owner: London Residential Healthcare Ltd
Contact: Portsdown Hill Road, Bedhampton, Hampshire PO9 3JW
☏ 023 9247 5624
@ info@lrh-homes.com
🖰 www.lrh-homes.com

Belmont Castle is situated in three acres of landscaped, well-maintained gardens. It is located in a quiet, residential area with views of Portsmouth and the Solvent. The home has budgies and fish in residence for residents to enjoy. The home goes on monthly outings in the summer months and offers some creative and interesting activities. The home can cater to special dietary requirements and there is a library service that brings large print books and talking books.

Registered places: 40
Guide weekly rate: £400– £640
Specialist care: Dementia, physical disability, respite
Medical services: Podiatry, dentist, optician, physiotherapy
Qualified staff: Meets standard

Home details
Location: Residential area, 1 mile from Havant
Communal areas: 2 lounges, 2 dining rooms, library, garden
Accessibility: *Floors:* 3 • *Access:* Lift • *Wheelchair access:* Good
Smoking: ✗
Pets: ✗
Routines: Flexible

Room details
Single: 30
Shared: 5
En suite: Undisclosed
Facilities: TV point

Door lock: ✓
Lockable place: ✓

Services provided
Beauty services: Hairdressing
Mobile library: ✓
Religious services: Monthly Anglican Communion service
Transport: ✗
Activities: *Coordinator:* ✓ • *Examples:* Arts and crafts, bingo
    Outings: ✓
Meetings: ✗

Registered places: 55
Guide weekly rate: £705– £935
Specialist care: Nursing , physical disability, terminal care
Medical services: Podiatry, hygienist, optician, physiotherapy
Qualified staff: Meets standard

Home details

Location: Residential area, 0.5 miles from Lymington
Communal areas: 4 lounges, dining room, garden
Accessibility: *Floors:* 3 • *Access:* Lift • *Wheelchair access:* Good
Smoking: x
Pets: x
Routines: Flexible

Room details

Single: 55
Shared: 0
En suite: 55
Facilities: TV point, telephone point

Door lock: ✓
Lockable place: ✓

Services provided

Beauty services: Hairdressing, aromatherapy, manicures
Mobile library: ✓
Religious services: Weekly
Transport: x
Activities: *Coordinator:* ✓ • *Examples:* Exercise classes, entertainment, quizzes • *Outings:* ✓
Meetings: ✓

Belmore Lodge Nursing and Residential Home

Manager: Karen Maidment
Owner: Colten Care Ltd
Contact: 20–22 Milford Road, Lymington, Hampshire SO41 9HL
☎ 01590 674700
@ enquiries@coltencare.co.uk
🖰 www.coltencare.co.uk

Belmore Lodge is purpose built and is located in a residential area and on a bus route. It is very close to the historic market town of Lymington. The home has a large, well-maintained garden area which is accessible to residents. Residents are offered nutritious meals and have the option to invite guests. The home provides a range of activities and also arranges outings for the residents.

Registered places: 56
Guide weekly rate: £759–£850
Specialist care: Nursing, dementia, mental disorder, respite
Medical services: Podiatry, optician, physiotherapy
Qualified staff: Undisclosed

Home details

Location: Residential area, 1 mile from Winchester centre
Communal areas: 4 lounges, 3 dining rooms, hairdressing salon, garden
Accessibility: *Floors:* 2 • *Access:* lift • *Wheelchair access:* Good
Smoking: x
Pets: At manager's discretion
Routines: Fexible

Room details

Single: 54
Shared: 0
En suite: 9
Facilities: TV point

Door lock: ✓
Lockable place: x

Services provided

Beauty services: Hairdressing
Mobile library: ✓
Religious services: Monthly church service
Transport: ✓
Activities: *Coordinator:* ✓ • *Examples:* Cookery, scrapbooks *Outings:* ✓
Meetings: ✓

Bereweeke Court

Manager: Tracey Hillier
Owner: BUPA Care Homes Ltd
Contact: Bereweeke Road, Winchester, Hampshire SO22 6AN
☎ 01962 878999
@ BereweekeCourtALL@BUPA.com
🖰 www.bupacarehomes.co.uk

Bereweeke Court is situated in a residential area of Winchester, 10 minutes outside the town centre. Local shops are within walking distance and the home is on a local bus route. Bereweeke Court provides specialist dementia nursing care. The home has a small garden and patio area safe for residents to use, and the majority of the bedrooms are for single occupancy. Daily activities are arranged and personal interests are encouraged. The house also has a resident cat and every week Pets As Therapy visits.

Bethany

Manager: Margaret Murray
Owner: Bethany Care Trust
Contact: Pamber Heath Road, Tadley, Basingstoke, Hampshire RG26 3TH

) 0118 9701710

@ bethanycaretrust@btconnect.com

 www.bethanycaretrust.org.uk

Bethany is a large, detached property, set in spacious grounds. It is a Christian home with the Local Assembly within walking distance. A separate room is available for residents to entertain guests in privacy, in addition to the communal areas. The home has been under construction to create an adjoining coffee shop. There is also Bethany Oak which is an independent living village with landscaped gardens and a pond. The home arranges a range of activities including missionary classes and video sessions. The home doesn't have a residents association but there are residents meetings twice a year to quarterly.

Registered places: 37
Guide weekly rate: £490–£595
Specialist care: Respite
Medical services: Podiatry, dentist, optician, physiotherapy
Qualified staff: Meets standard

Home details
Location: Village location, 10 miles from Basingstoke
Communal areas: 2 lounges, dining room, writing room, hairdressing salon, coffee shop, garden
Accessibility: *Floors:* 3 • *Access:* Lift • *Wheelchair access:* Good
Smoking: ✗
Pets: At manager's discretion
Routines: Flexible

Room details
Single: 23
Shared: 7
En suite: 30
Facilities: TV point, telephone

Door lock: ✓
Lockable place: ✓

Services provided
Beauty services: Hairdressing
Mobile library: ✗
Religious services: Nondenominational service
Transport: Minibus
Activities: *Coordinator:* ✗ • *Examples:* Puzzles, videos, handwork *Outings:* ✓
Meetings: ✗

Bethel House

Manager: Linda Wilson
Owner: Aspa Ltd
Contact: 28 Beach Avenue, Barton-on-Sea, Hampshire BH25 7EJ

) 01425 610453

Bethel House is situated close to the cliff tops at Barton-on-Sea. The home is purpose built and some of the bedrooms have French doors leading into the garden. The home is family run and residents have a lot of contact with the manager and staff. The manager also keeps in close contact with the families to hear any issues or requests personally. The home has an 'Extend' tutor, visiting the home three times a week to run a variety of activities. Residents are also encouraged to attend social groups in the community, such as the Women's Institute. The home has its own cat.

Registered places: 31
Guide weekly rate: £475– £550
Specialist care: Day care, dementia, mental disorder, respite
Medical services: Podiatry, dentist, optician, physiotherapy
Qualified staff: Exceeds standard: 60% at NVQ Level 2

Home details
Location: Urban area, 0.5 miles from Barton-on-Sea
Communal areas: 2 lounges, quiet lounge, dining room, day room, garden
Accessibility: *Floors:* 2 • *Access:* Lift • *Wheelchair access:* Good
Smoking: ✗
Pets: ✗
Routines: Flexible

Room details
Single: 31
Shared: 0
En suite: 29
Facilities: TV point, telephone point

Door lock: ✓
Lockable place: ✓

Services provided
Beauty services: Hairdressing
Mobile library: ✓
Religious services: Weekly Catholic Communion, monthly Anglican Communion service
Transport: ✗
Activities: *Coordinator:* ✗ • *Examples:* Arts and crafts, music and movement, quizzes • *Outings:* ✓
Meetings: ✗

Registered places: 21
Guide weekly rate: £420–£700
Specialist care: Nursing, physical disability, terminal care
Medical services: Podiatry, hygienist, optician, physiotherapy
Qualified staff: Exceeds standard: 90% at NVQ Level 2

Home details

Location: Residential area, 1 mile from Totton
Communal areas: Lounge, dining room, garden
Accessibility: *Floors:* 2 • *Access:* Lift • *Wheelchair access:* Good
Smoking: ✗
Pets: ✗
Routines: Flexible

Room details

Single: 9
Shared: 6
En suite: 15
Facilities: TV point

Door lock: ✗
Lockable place: ✓

Services provided

Beauty services: Hairdressing
Mobile library: ✓
Religious services: Monthly Communion service
Transport: ✗
Activities: *Coordinator:* ✗ • *Examples:* Bingo, quizzes, carpet bowls consense *Outings:* ✓
Meetings: ✗

The Birches Nursing Home

Manager: Lesley Kay Head
Owner: Harcare Ltd
Contact: 239 Water Lane, Totton, Southampton, Hampshire SO40 3GE
☏ 023 8066 7141

The home is situated in a residential area of Totton, approximately one mile from the town centre. To the rear and side of the home is a small but pleasant garden area with a patio. This can be accessed via the newly extended, spacious lounge. Daily activities include bingo, quizzes, walks, skittles and carpet. The residents are also taken on walks and the home arranges a Communion service once a month.

Registered places: 50
Guide weekly rate: £565
Specialist care: Nursing, dementia, physical disability, terminal care
Medical services: Podiatry, dentist, optician, physiotherapy
Qualified staff: Meets standard

Home details

Location: Urban area, 1 mile from Southsea
Communal areas: 1 TV lounge, one quiet room, aviary, garden
Accessibility: *Floors:* 3 • *Access:* 3 lifts
     Wheelchair access: Good
Smoking: In designated area
Pets: ✓
Routines: Flexible

Room details

Single: 38
Shared: 6
En suite: Undisclosed
Facilities: TV

Door lock: ✓
Lockable place: ✓

Services provided

Beauty services: Hairdressing
Mobile library: ✗
Religious services: ✓
Transport: 6-seater vehicle
Activities: *Coordinator:* ✗ • *Examples:* Bingo, visiting entertainers *Outings:* ✓
Meetings: ✗

Bluebell Nursing Home

Manager: Ian Smith
Owner: Techscheme Ltd
Contact: 45–53 St Ronan's Road, Southsea, Hampshire PO4 0PP
☏ 023 9282 3104
🖥 www.bluebellcarehome.com

Bluebell Nursing Home is situated in Southsea, a short walk from Southsea Pier, a predominant feature of the area, which is well serviced by local bus companies. The home aims to stimulate and care for the needs of elderly patients, including those who are mentally ill, through activities such as visits to the nearby seafront. The nursing home is comprised of five period town houses combined to create a single building. Smoking is only allowed outside under supervision. Residents can have a lock on their room but carers would require access for dementia patients.

Bowood House

Manager: Puspavadee Peedoly
Owner: N Peedoly
Contact: 1 Lansdowne Road, Aldershot, Hampshire GU11 3ER
☏ 01252 323 834

A small home that resides five minutes from local shops and amenities in Aldershot, Bowood House has facilities for 10 residents. The home has its own transport and arranges for a hairdressing service and for the use of a mobile library. The residents can have either a flexible or a structured routine depending on their needs and meal times are flexible. Daily activities include bingo, card games and newspaper reading. The home prides itself on being family orientated.

Registered places: 10
Guide weekly rate: From £285
Specialist care: Dementia
Medical services: None
Qualified staff: Fails standard

Home details
Location: Urban area, 0.1 miles from Aldershot
Communal areas: Lounge, dining room, garden
Accessibility: *Floors:* 2 • *Access:* Stair lift
　　　Wheelchair access: None
Smoking: In designated area
Pets: At manager's discretion
Routines: Flexible

Room details
Single: 2	**Door lock:** ✓
Shared: 4	**Lockable place:** ✓
En suite: 0	
Facilities: TV	

Services provided
Beauty services: Hairdressing
Mobile library: ✓
Religious services: ✗
Transport: ✓
Activities: *Coordinator:* ✗ • *Examples:* Bingo, cards
　　　Outings: ✗
Meetings: ✗

Brackenlea Care Home

Manager: Jacqueline Coles
Owner: Shawford Healthcare Ltd
Contact: Pearson Lane, Shawford, Winchester, Hampshire SO21 2AG
☏ 01962 713242

Brackenlea is situated three miles south of Winchester in the village of Shawford. The home is approximately 20 minutes from a train station, post office and bus stop.

The home has a mature garden with seating areas that are enjoyable when the home puts on garden parties. Outings include trips to the ice cream parlour and various clubs and Brackenlea also has two budgies. Though the home does not have its own transport, one member of staff is insured to take residents out in their car.

Registered places: 25
Guide weekly rate: £440–£475
Specialist care: Dementia, respite
Medical services: Podiatry, dentist, optician, physiotherapy
Qualified staff: Exceeds standard: 56% at NVQ Level 2

Home details
Location: Rural area, 3 miles from Winchester
Communal areas: Lounge, dining room, conservatory, garden
Accessibility: *Floors:* 2 • *Access:* Lift • *Wheelchair access:* Limited
Smoking: ✗
Pets: At manager's discretion
Routines: Flexible

Room details
Single: 25	**Door lock:** ✓
Shared: 0	**Lockable place:** ✓
En suite: 12	
Facilities: TV point, telephone point	

Services provided
Beauty services: Hairdressing
Mobile library: ✓
Religious services: Monthly Communion service
Transport: ✗
Activities: *Coordinator:* ✓ • *Examples:* Arts and crafts, exercise, visiting entertainers • *Outings:* ✓
Meetings: ✓

Registered places: 25
Guide weekly rate: £285–£425
Specialist care: Dementia
Medical services: Podiatry
Qualified staff: Exceeds standard: 60% at NVQ Level 2

Home details
Location: Urban area, 0.5 miles from Locks Heath
Communal areas: 2 lounges, dining room, conservatory, hairdressing salon, library, patio and garden
Accessibility: *Floors:* 3 • *Access:* Stair lift
   Wheelchair access: Good
Smoking: In designated area
Pets: ✓
Routines: Flexible

Room details
Single: 21
Shared: 2
En suite: 14
Facilities: Telephone point

Door lock: ✓
Lockable place: ✓

Services provided
Beauty services: Hairdressing
Mobile library: Library facilities
Religious services: Monthly Anglican and Catholic services
Transport: ✗
Activities: *Coordinator:* ✗ • *Examples:* Arts and crafts, bingo, exercise • *Outings:* ✓
Meetings: ✗

Brook Lane Rest Home

Manager: Helen Dibdin
Owner: Norman Ratcliffe
Contact: 290–292 Brook Lane, Sarisbury Green, Southampton, Hampshire SO31 7DP
☎ 01489 576010

Brook Lane is located in the residential area of Sarisbury Green and is near local amenities. The home is half a mile from the town centre of Locks Heath. The home has a large garden with patio area at the rear for residents' use. The home has its own cat that the residents enjoy caring for. The home arranges monthly religious services for both Anglican and Catholic denominations.

Registered places: 22
Guide weekly rate: £408–£535
Specialist care: Day care, dementia, mental disorder, respite
Medical services: Podiatry, hygienist, optician, physiotherapy
Qualified staff: Undisclosed

Home details
Location: Residential area, 1 mile from Eastleigh
Communal areas: 3 Lounges, dining room, patio and garden
Accessibility: *Floors:* 2 • *Access:* Stair lift
   Wheelchair Access: Good
Smoking: ✗
Pets: At manager's discretion
Routines: Flexible

Room details
Single: 12
Shared: 5
En suite: 15
Facilities: TV, telephone point

Door lock: ✓
Lockable place: ✓

Services provided
Beauty services: Hairdressing
Mobile library: ✓
Religious services: ✓
Transport: Car
Activities: *Coordinator:* ✓ • *Examples:* Arts and crafts, cross-stitching, movement to music • *Outings:* ✓
Meetings: ✗

Brookdale House Residential Home

Manager: Lesley Cairnduff
Owner: Ronald and Lesley Cairnduff
Contact: 31 Hursley Road, Chandlers Ford, Eastleigh, Hampshire SO53 2FS
☎ 023 8026 1987
@ info@brookdalehouse.co.uk
🖰 www.brookdalehouse.co.uk

Brookdale House has a part-time activities coordinator, responsible for arranging entertainment and activities for the residents three days a week, suitable for both the active and less active participants. The home is close to local amenities and has strong ties to the local community including the schools and church choirs. The home will also take residents to any local church they may choose. The home also supports the Duke of Edinburgh and work experience schemes.

Brookfield

Manager: J Filsell
Owner: J Filsell
Contact: 1 Clayhall Road, Alverstoke, Gosport, Hampshire PO12 2BY
☎ 023 9258 1103
@ j.a.filsall@tinyworld.co.uk
🖥 www.brookfieldcarehome.co.uk

Brookfield is a care home set in a residential area with views of Stoke Lake. The home has ample grounds, accessible to residents, with a sensory garden. Social events at the home are held on a regular basis, and friends and family are invited. A programme of activities provides residents with arts and crafts sessions, reminiscence and reading sessions. The home emphasises the need for.

Registered places: 29
Guide weekly rate: £395–£430
Specialist care: Dementia, mental disorder
Medical services: Podiatry, dental, optician, physiotherapy
Qualified staff: Meets standard

Home details

Location: Residential area, 0.5 miles from Alverstoke
Communal areas: 4 Lounges, dining room, 2 conservatories, patio and garden
Accessibility: *Floors:* 3 • *Access:* None *Wheelchair access:* Limited
Smoking: ✗
Pets: ✓
Routines: Flexible

Room details

Single: 29
Shared: 0
En suite: 25
Facilities: TV point, telephone point
Door lock: ✓
Lockable place: ✓

Services provided

Beauty services: Hairdressing, aromatherapy, manicures
Mobile library: ✗
Religious services: Monthly Communion service
Transport: ✓
Activities: *Coordinator:* ✗ • *Examples:* Arts and crafts, ball games, reminiscence • *Outings:* ✗
Meetings: ✓

Brookvale Lawn

Manager: E Raison
Owner: Brookvale Homes Ltd
Contact: 15 Lawn Road, Portswood, Southampton, Hampshire SO17 2EX
☎ 023 8057 7786

Brookvale Lawn is situated in a residential area of Southampton, and is within walking distance of the amenities of Portswood. The River Itchen is approximately a mile from the home and Southampton Airport is three miles from the home. Each floor has its own spacious lounge and the home also has its own chapel and hairdressing salon.

Registered places: 30
Guide weekly rate: £310–£360
Specialist care: Dementia, respite
Medical services: Podiatry, dentist, optician
Qualified staff: Exceeds standard: 70% at NVQ Level 2

Home details

Location: Residential area, 2.2 miles from Southampton
Communal areas: Lounge, lounge/dining room, hairdressing salon, chapel, library, patio
Accessibility: *Floors:* 3 • *Access:* Lift • *Wheelchair access:* Good
Smoking: ✗
Pets: ✗
Routines: Flexible

Room details

Single: 30
Shared: 0
En suite: Undisclosed
Facilities: TV point, telephone point
Door lock: ✓
Lockable place: ✓

Services provided

Beauty Services: Hairdressing
Mobile library: ✗
Religious services: ✗
Transport: 7-seater vehicle
Activities: *Coordinator:* ✓ • *Examples:* Arts and crafts, board games *Outings:* ✓
Meetings: ✓

Registered places: 35
Guide weekly rate: £328–£420
Specialist care: Dementia, mental disorder, physical disability
Medical services: Podiatry, optician
Qualified staff: Fails standard: 43% at NVQ Level 2

Home details
Location: Residential area, 2.3 miles from Southampton
Communal areas: Dining room, patio and garden
Accessibility: *Floors:* 2 • *Access:* Lift • *Wheelchair access:* Good
Smoking: x
Pets: x
Routines: Flexible

Room details
Single: 23
Shared: 6
En suite: 23
Facilities: TV point, telephone point

Door lock: x
Lockable place: ✓

Services provided
Beauty services: Hairdressing
Mobile library: ✓
Religious services: Monthly
Transport: x
Activities: *Coordinator:* x • *Examples:* Arts and crafts, bingo, visiting entertainers • *Outings:* ✓
Meetings: ✓

Brookvale House

Manager: H Ward
Owner: Brookvale Homes Ltd
Contact: 4 Brookvale Road, Portswood, Southampton, Hampshire SO17 1QL
☎ 023 8032 2541

Brookvale House provides care for those with age-related mental health problems and illnesses associated with dementia. The home is situated near the local amenities at Portswood, in a residential area of Southampton, approximately two and a half miles from the town centre. The home organises meetings for the residents every two months. Patio doors lead out onto the garden where there is seating for residents to sit out and enjoy the fresh air. If residents enjoy gardening, they are welcome to help maintain the garden and do flower arranging and weeding.

Registered places: 51
Guide weekly rate: £450–£734
Specialist care: Nursing, physical disability, respite, terminal care
Medical services: Podiatry, hygienist, optician, physiotherapy
Qualified staff: Meets standard

Home details
Location: Urban area, 2 miles from Fareham
Communal areas: 4 lounges, dining room, conservatory, patio and garden
Accessibility: *Floors:* 2 • *Access:* Lift • *Wheelchair access:* Good
Smoking: Undisclosed
Pets: x
Routines: Flexible

Room details
Single: 51
Shared: 0
En suite: Undisclosed
Facilities: TV point, telephone point

Door lock: x
Lockable place: ✓

Services provided
Beauty services: Hairdressing
Mobile library: ✓
Religious services: Monthly Communion service
Transport: Shared minibus
Activities: *Coordinator:* ✓ • *Examples:* Arts and crafts, movement to music • *Outings:* ✓
Meetings: ✓

Cams Ridge Nursing and Residential Care Home

Manager: David McLaughlan
Owner: Southern Cross Healthcare Ltd
Contact: 7 Charlemont Drive, Cams Hill, Fareham, Hampshire PO16 8RT
☎ 01329 238156
@ camsridge2@schealthcare.co.uk
🖰 www.ashbournesl.co.uk

Cams Ridge is located in an urban area, two miles from Fareham town centre. The activities coordinator at Cams Ridge ensures there are a variety of activities for residents to participate in if they wish, such as themed days like St George's day. Pets are allowed to visit and the home aims for a flexible and homely atmosphere. Residents are encouraged to be active and continue their own individual lifestyles.

Canford Manor Nursing Home

Manager: Vacant
Owner: Christopher and Kathryn Imonikhe
Contact: 38 Manor Way,
Lee-on-the-Solent, Hampshire
PO13 9JH
) 023 9255 0437

Canford Manor is situated in a quiet residential area of Lee-on-the-Solent, close to local amenities, shops and public transport links. There is a large lounge/dining room and a smaller lounge as well as a garden, accessible to residents. Activities include visiting entertainers such as musicians and a visiting Pets As Therapy dog.

Registered places: 24
Guide weekly rate: Up to £650
Specialist care: Nursing, physical disability, terminal care
Medical services: Podiatry
Qualified staff: Meets standard

Home details
Location: Residential area, 0.3 miles from Lee-on-the-Solent
Communal areas: Lounge, lounge/dining room, garden
Accessibility: *Floors:* 2 • *Access:* Lift • *Wheelchair access:* Good
Smoking: Undisclosed
Pets: Undisclosed
Routines: Flexible

Room details
Single: 24
Shared: 0
En suite: 24
Facilities: Undisclosed

Door lock: Undisclosed
Lockable place: Undisclosed

Services provided
Beauty services: Hairdressing
Mobile library: ✗
Religious services: ✗
Transport: ✗
Activities: *Coordinator:* ✓ • *Examples:* Baking, films, Pets As Therapy • *Outings:* ✗
Meetings: Undisclosed

Carleen Nursing and Residential Care Home

Manager: Joyce Dawson
Owner: Serincourt Ltd
Contact: 38 Portchester Road, Fareham, Hampshire PO16 8PT
) 01329 232418

Carleen is a large house, in a residential area of Fareham, close to local amenities. The home has well-tended front and rear gardens which are easily accessible to residents. An activities coordinator organises painting sessions, music and games, exercise and reminiscence. Residents are also encouraged to attend community groups.

Registered places: 36
Guide weekly rate: £525–£625
Specialist care: Nursing, physical disability, respite, terminal care
Medical services: Podiatry, hygienist, optician
Qualified staff: Exceeds standard: 70% at NVQ Level 2

Home details
Location: Residential area, 1.5 miles from Fareham
Communal areas: 2 lounges, dining room, garden
Accessibility: *Floors:* 2 • *Access:* Lift • *Wheelchair access:* Good
Smoking: ✗
Pets: ✗
Routines: Flexible

Room details
Single: 24
Shared: 6
En suite: 13
Facilities: TV point telephone point

Door lock: ✓
Lockable place: ✓

Services provided
Beauty services: Hairdressing
Mobile library: ✓
Religious services: ✓
Transport: ✗
Activities: *Coordinator:* ✓ • *Examples:* Games, music, painting *Outings:* ✓
Meetings: ✗

Registered places: 33
Guide weekly rate: £395–£575
Specialist care: Day care, dementia, mental disorder, respite
Medical services: Podiatry, hygienist, optician, physiotherapy
Qualified staff: Exceeds standard: 65% at NVQ Level 2

Home details

Location: Residential area, 1.8 miles from New Milton
Communal areas: 3 lounges, dining room, library,
    patio and garden
Accessibility: *Floors:* 3 • *Access:* Lift • *Wheelchair access:* Good
Smoking: In designated area
Pets: At manager's discretion
Routines: Flexible

Room details

Single: 33 | Door lock: ✓
Shared: 0 | Lockable place: ✓
En suite: 22
Facilities: TV point, telephone point

Services provided

Beauty services: Hairdressing
Mobile library: ✓
Religious services: Anglican minister and Catholic priest visit
Transport: ✗
Activities: *Coordinator:* ✓ • *Examples:* Exercise classes,
    weekly entertainers • *Outings:* ✓
Meetings: ✗

Carlton House Rest Home

Manager: Caroline Herridge
Owner: Caroline Herridge
Contact: 15 Barton Court Road,
New Milton, Hampshire BH25 6NN
☎ 01425 612218
@ herridge19@hotmail.com

Originally a hotel, the building was converted into a care home some years ago. Carlton House is a large detached building located in a residential area, close to the town centre of New Milton. Emphasis is placed on independence, and there are a number of activities for residents to enjoy, including exercise classes and theatre trips. Members from the local college also come in every week to run a craft session with the residents. There is a pleasant garden with a bird aviary and the home has strong local ties.

Registered places: 30
Guide weekly rate: £514–£800
Specialist care: Nursing, physical disability
Medical services: None
Qualified staff: Fails standard: 45% at NVQ Level 2

Home details

Location: Residential area, 1.4 miles from Romsey
Communal areas: 2 lounges, lounge/dining room, garden
Accessibility: *Floors:* 2 • *Access:* Lift • *Wheelchair access:* Good
Smoking: Undisclosed
Pets: Undisclosed
Routines: Undisclosed

Room details

Single: 22 | Door lock: Undisclosed
Shared: 4 | Lockable place: Undisclosed
En suite: 22
Facilities: Undisclosed

Services provided

Beauty services: Hairdressing
Mobile library: ✓
Religious services: ✓
Transport: Minibus
Activities: *Coordinator:* ✓ • *Examples:* Arts and crafts,
    music and movement, visiting entertainers • *Outings:* ✓
Meetings: Undisclosed

Cedar Lawn Nursing Home

Manager: Sheila Hewitt
Owner: Sentinel Health Care Ltd
Contact: Woodley Court, Braishfield,
Romsey, Hampshire SO51 7PA
☎ 01794 523300

A former manor house, Cedar Lawn is located in a residential area, on the outskirts of Romsey, a small market town. As well as offering nursing care, the home also cares for those who are terminal care. Staff at the home organise theme days, such as St Patrick's Day, an Indian theme day and celebrations for Burns Night. Residents can also take afternoon classes in association with a local college.

Challoner House

Manager: Lorraine Dent-Magnusson
Owner: Barchester Healthcare Ltd
Contact: 175 Winchester Road,
Chandlers Ford, Eastleigh,
Hampshire SO53 2DU
☎ 023 8026 6036
🖥 www.barchester.com

Challoner House is in a residential area of Chandlers Ford, close to local shops. The home has five communal areas for residents to socialise and enjoy activities, as well as a well-maintained garden. Hairdressing is also offering by the home on a regular basis. Activities such as cards, themed events and bingo are enjoyed by residents on a weekly programme. The home also offers residents with a changing weekly menu system to add a variety of nutritious meals.

Registered places: 49
Guide weekly rate: Undisclosed
Specialist care: Nursing, physical disability, respite, terminal care
Medical services: Podiatry, physiotherapy
Qualified staff: Meets standard

Home details
Location: Residential area, 1 mile from Eastleigh
Communal areas: 2 lounges, dining room, conservatory
Accessibility: *Floors:* 3 • *Access:* Lift • *Wheelchair access:* Good
Smoking: ✗
Pets: ✗
Routines: Flexible

Room details
Single: 43
Shared: 3
En suite: 46
Facilities: TV point, telephone point

Door lock: ✓
Lockable place: ✓

Services provided
Beauty services: Hairdressing
Mobile library: ✗
Religious services: Once a month
Transport: ✗
Activities: *Coordinator:* ✓ • *Examples:* Cards, themed events, knitting • *Outings:* ✗
Meetings: ✓

Chandlers Ford Christian Nursing Home

Manager: Sharon Griffin
Owner: Trinity Care Homes Ltd
Contact: Winchester Road,
Chandlers Ford, Eastleigh,
Hampshire SO53 2GJ
☎ 023 8026 7963
@ chandlersford@schealthcare.co.uk
🖥 www.schealthcare.co.uk

Chandlers Ford Christian Nursing Home is situated in Chandlers Ford on the same site as the Methodist church and is close to shops, pubs and other amenities. The home has a strong Christian ethos and meets regularly with the church group. The home is backed by woodland, and has a pleasant garden to the rear of the building, which has seating for residents. The home organises regular outings in the local area for country walks or pub lunches.

Registered places: 45
Guide weekly rate: £500– £700
Specialist care: Nursing, physical disability
Medical services: Podiatry, optician, physiotherapy
Qualified staff: Exceeds standard: 70% at NVQ Level 2

Home details
Location: Urban area, 0.5 miles from Eastleigh
Communal areas: Lounge, dining room, garden
Accessibility: *Floors:* 2 • *Access:* Lift • *Wheelchair access:* Good
Smoking: In designated area
Pets: At manager's discretion
Routines: Structured

Room details
Single: 39
Shared: 3
En suite: 23
Facilities: TV point

Door lock: ✗
Lockable place: ✓

Services provided
Beauty services: Hairdressing
Mobile library: ✓
Religious services: Weekly church services
Transport: ✗
Activities: *Coordinator:* ✓ • *Examples:* Games • *Outings:* ✓
Meetings: ✗

Registered places: 24
Guide weekly rate: £450– £650
Specialist care: Nursing, physical disability
Medical services: Undisclosed
Qualified staff: Exceeds standard: 60% at NVQ Level 2

Home details

Location: Rural area, 2 miles from Liss
Communal areas: 2 lounges, conservatory, patio and garden
Accessibility: *Floors:* Undisclosed • *Access:* Undisclosed
    Wheelchair access: Undisclosed
Smoking: x
Pets: x
Routines: Flexible

Room details

Single: 13
Shared: 5
En suite: 9
Facilities: Undisclosed

Door lock: x
Lockable place: x

Services provided

Beauty services: None
Mobile library: x
Religious services: Monthly visit from vicar
Transport: x
Activities: *Coordinator:* x • *Examples:* Exercise, karaoke, organist
    sessions • *Outings:* x
Meetings: x

Chatterwood Nursing Home

Manager: Joyce Gilfroy
Owner: Milkwood Care Ltd
Contact: Huntsbottom Lane, Hillbrow,
Liss, Hampshire GU33 7PA
☎ 01730 895485

Chatterwood Nursing Home is located in a rural area and the shops at Liss are accessible by public transport. There are two lounges in which activities including karaoke, exercise and crafts take place, as well as visiting musicians. There is a patio area that leads from the conservatory but some parts of the garden are sloped, making it hard for some residents to access. The home receives a visit from a vicar every month.

Registered places: 25
Guide weekly rate: £450– £475
Specialist care: Day care, dementia, respite
Medical services: Podiatry, dentist, optician
Qualified staff: Exceeds standard: 60% at NVQ Level 2

Home details

Location: Residential area, 1.7 miles from New Milton
Communal areas: Lounge, 2 dining rooms, hairdressing salon,
    patio and garden
Accessibility: *Floors:* 2 • *Access:* Lift • *Wheelchair access:* Good
Smoking: In designated area
Pets: At manager's discretion
Routines: Flexible

Room details

Single: 23
Shared: 1
En suite: 24
Facilities: TV point, telephone point

Door lock: ✓
Lockable place: ✓

Services provided

Beauty services: Hairdressing
Mobile library: ✓
Religious services: Monthly Anglican service
Transport: x
Activities: *Coordinator:* ✓ • *Examples:* Arts and crafts,
    entertainers, exercise • *Outings:* ✓
Meetings: x

Chestnut Court Rest Home

Manager: Patricia Harrison
Owner: Goldenpride Ltd
Contact: 9 Copse Road, New Milton,
Hampshire BH25 6ES
☎ 01425 620000

Chestnut Court is a large building, close to the amenities of New Milton. The town centre of approximately two miles away. There is a large garden with patio area and a gazebo for residents to enjoy. As the home has an activities organiser there are a lot of activities on offer, for those who wish for a more active or restful lifestyle there is something for everyone. The home also has two pantomimes a year – one at Christmas and one in the summer.

Clarendon Care Home

Manager: Silvia Paton
Owner: Alice Dunbar
Contact: 64–66 Clarendon Road, Southsea, Hampshire PO5 2JZ
☎ 023 9282 4644

Clarendon is a large property situated within one mile of the town centre of Southsea, and close to the seafront and pier. Recent outings have included fish and chips on the seafront, trips to the local gardening centre and a trip to the New Forest for afternoon tea. The activities coordinator plans group activities weekly, however she also sees residents on a one-to-one basis to play individual games if the residents wish. There is a good-sized garden which is well kept and has lots of local wildlife at the rear of the property, with seating for residents.

Registered places: 20
Guide weekly rate: £395
Specialist care: Dementia
Medical services: Podiatry, dentist, optician, physiotherapy
Qualified staff: Exceeds standard: 80% at NVQ Level 2

Home details
Location: Urban area, 0.5 miles from Southsea
Communal areas: 2 lounges, dining room, patio and garden
Accessibility: *Floors:* Undisclosed • *Access:* Lift *Wheelchair access:* Good
Smoking: In designated area
Pets: ✓
Routines: Flexible

Room details
Single: 8
Shared: 6
En suite: 5
Facilities: TV point

Door lock: ✓
Lockable place: ✓

Services provided
Beauty services: Hairdressing
Mobile library: ✓
Religious services: Monthly
Transport: ✓ .
Activities: *Coordinator:* ✓ • *Examples:* Bingo, individual games *Outings:* ✓
Meetings: ✓

Clifford House

Manager: Alwyn Brenchley
Owner: Alwyn Brenchley
Contact: 11 Alexandra Road, Andover, Hampshire SP10 3AD
☎ 01264 324571
@ alwynbrenchley@ cliffordhouse.co.uk
🖥 www.cliffordhouse.co.uk

Clifford House is situated in a quiet residential area of Andover, one mile from the town centre. Entertainment is organised by Age Concern for the home, and there is an entertainment night once a month. The home follows Christian values, though it is not a strictly Christian home and access to a Catholic church is within 50 yards. There is also a monthly Anglican Communion service.

Registered places: 21
Guide weekly rate: £415–£539
Specialist care: Day care, dementia, respite
Medical services: Podiatry, hygienist, optician, physiotherapy
Qualified staff: Exceeds standard: 87% at NVQ Level 2

Home details
Location: Residential area, 1 mile from Andover
Communal areas: Lounge/dining room, patio and garden
Accessibility: *Floors:* 2 • *Access:* Lift • *Wheelchair access:* Good
Smoking: ✗
Pets: ✗
Routines: Flexible

Room details
Single: 19
Shared: 1
En suite: 7
Facilities: None

Door lock: ✓
Lockable place: ✓

Services provided
Beauty services: Hairdressing
Mobile library: ✓
Religious services: Monthly Anglican Communion service
Transport: ✗
Activities: *Coordinator:* ✗ • *Examples:* Bingo, entertainment *Outings:* ✓
Meetings: ✗

Registered places: 6
Guide weekly rate: £495–£520
Specialist care: None
Medical services: Podiatry, dentist, optician
Qualified staff: Meets standard

Home details

Location: Residential area, 0.5 miles from Basingstoke
Communal areas: Lounge, dining room, patio and garden
Accessibility: *Floors:* 2 • *Access:* Stair lift
    Wheelchair access: Limited
Smoking: ✗
Pets: At manager's discretion
Routines: Flexible

Room details

Single: 6
Shared: 0
En suite: 6
Facilities: TV point, telephone point

Door lock: ✓
Lockable place: ✓

Services provided

Beauty services: Hairdressing
Mobile library: ✓
Religious services: Monthly nondenominational
    Communion service
Transport: Car
Activities: *Coordinator:* ✗ • *Examples:* Film nights, knitting circle
    Outings: ✓
Meetings: ✗

Clifton Court Residential Home

Manager: Sarah Yarney
Owner: Clifton Court Ltd
Contact: 23 Richmond Road,
Basingstoke, Hampshire RG21 2NX
☎ 01256 325715

Clifton Court is a large, detached house in a residential area of Basingstoke. The home is close to the town centre and local transport links. The back of the home has a small, lawned garden with a patio area. There are a lot of activities to choose from with film nights every week and knitting circles as well as board games. As the home is small the residents have a say in what activities are offered and also when they would like their mealtimes to take place.

Registered places: 17
Guide weekly rate: £385–£446
Specialist care: Dementia, mental disorder, respite
Medical services: Podiatry dentist
Qualified staff: Exceeds standard: 60% at NVQ Level 2

Home details

Location: Residential area, 1 mile from Milford-on-Sea
Communal areas: 2 lounges, dining room, conservatory, garden
Accessibility: *Floors:* 3 • *Access:* Stair lift
    Wheelchair access: Limited
Smoking: ✗
Pets: ✗
Routines: Flexible

Room details

Single: 9
Shared: 4
En suite: 3
Facilities: TV point

Door lock: ✓
Lockable place: ✓

Services provided

Beauty services: Hairdressing
Mobile library: ✓
Religious services: Monthly Anglican service
Transport: ✓
Activities: *Coordinator:* ✓ • *Examples:* Arts and craft, cooking
    Outings: ✓
Meetings: ✓

The Coach House

Manager: Donna Fry
Owner: Donna Fry
Contact: 67 Keyhaven Road,
Milford-on-Sea, Lymington,
Hampshire SO41 0QX
☎ 01590 642581

The Coach House is situated in a quiet residential area, approximately one mile from Milford-on-Sea. The nearest amenities are located within Lymington town centre, which is approximately two miles from the home. The staff provide activities for the residents including visiting entertainers and pet therapy sessions. The home has a very relaxed atmosphere with the residents having the freedom of choice over their daily routines. The home arranges an Anglican service once a month.

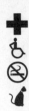

Colbury House Nursing and Residential Home

Manager: Margaret Collins
Owner: Jeffrey and Margaret Collins
Contact: Hill Street, Totton, Southampton, Hampshire SO40 2RX
☎ 023 8086 9876
@ Margaret@colbury.com
🖱 www.colbury.com

Colbury House Nursing Home is situated in Totton, in a quiet lane close to the New Forest. The home has four and a half acres of land and is approximately two miles from Totton town centre. The home's lounge has views over the countryside and there are two separate dining rooms and two lounges. Residents can choose their own meal times and where they wish to have their meals. Small pets are allowed and outings are arranged to the theatre. Nine residents are accommodated in the Coach House, a separate building with its own lounge and dining room.

Registered places: 51
Guide weekly rate: £327–£700
Specialist care: Nursing, dementia, physical disability, respite
Medical services: Podiatry, dentist, optician, physiotherapy
Qualified staff: Meets standard

Home details
Location: Rural area, 2.2 miles from Totton
Communal areas: 2 lounges, 2 dining rooms, garden
Accessibility: *Floors:* 2 • *Access:* Lift and stair lift
　Wheelchair access: Good
Smoking: ✗
Pets: ✓
Routines: Flexible

Room details
Single: 39 　　　　**Door lock:** ✓
Shared: 12 　　　　**Lockable place:** ✓
En suite: 51
Facilities: TV point, telephone point

Services provided
Beauty services: Hairdressing, aromatherapy, manicures
Mobile library: ✗
Religious services: ✗
Transport: ✗
Activities: *Coordinator:* ✗ • *Examples:* Arts and crafts, reminiscing, movement to music • *Outings:* ✓
Meetings: ✗

Coombe Grange Residential Home

Manager: Vacant
Owner: BML Healthcare
Contact: Coombe Lane, Slay, Lymington, Hampshire SO41 6BP
☎ 01590 682519
@ coombegrange@
　bmlhealthcare.co.uk
🖱 www.coombegrange-rh.co.uk

Coombe Grange is set in a rural location on the outskirts of the village of Sway, in the New Forest between Brocklehurst and Milton. There are large, accessible gardens around the home. The home has two lounges and five quiet seating areas and a dining room. The rooms in the home are single occupancy but there are four double rooms available for married couples. The rooms all have en suite facilities and walk-in showers have recently been installed. The home arranges also outings for example to the nearby forest or for cream tea. The home has its own cat.

Registered places: 40
Guide weekly rate: £425–£650
Specialist care: Dementia, mental disorder
Medical services: Podiatry, dentist, optician
Qualified staff: Exceeds standard: 70% at NVQ Level 2

Home details
Location: Rural area, 3.6 miles from Lymington
Communal areas: 2 lounges, dining room, garden
Accessibility: *Floors:* 3 • *Access:* 2 lifts • *Wheelchair Access:* Good
Smoking: In designated area
Pets: ✗
Routines: Flexible

Room details
Single: 32 　　　　**Door lock:** ✓
Shared: 4 　　　　　**Lockable place:** ✓
En suite: 20
Facilities: TV, telephone point

Services provided
Beauty services: Hairdressing
Mobile library: ✓
Religious services: ✓
Transport: ✗
Activities: *Coordinator:* • *Examples:* Games, music, relaxation *Outings:* ✓
Meetings: ✓

Registered places: 30
Guide weekly rate: £525
Specialist care: Dementia
Medical services: Podiatry, dentist, optician
Qualified staff: Exceeds standard: 59% at NVQ Level 2

Home details
Location: Residential area, 8.5 miles from Portsmouth
Communal areas: Lounge, dining room, patio and garden
Accessibility: *Floors:* 3 • *Access:* Lift • *Wheelchair access:* Good
Smoking: In designated area
Pets: ✗
Routines: Flexible

Room details
Single: 26
Shared: 2
En suite: 30
Facilities: TV point, telephone

Door lock: ✓
Lockable place: ✓

Services provided
Beauty services: Hairdressing, manicures, massage
Mobile library: ✓
Religious services: ✗
Transport: ✗
Activities: *Coordinator:* ✗ • *Examples:* Exercise, music, visiting entertainers • *Outings:* ✓
Meetings: ✗

Cornelia House

Manager: A Hardingham
Owner: Stephen Geach
Contact: 134 Portchester Road, Fareham, Hampshire PO16 8QP
☎ 01329 233603

Set back from the main Porchester Road, approximately nine miles from Portsmouth, Cornelia House is situated near to a train station and bus service. There is a mobile library which visits and religious services can be arranged. The home has an activities programme which includes visiting entertainers and games as well as visits from an exercise instructor. Outings are arranged to the local theatre and to the local pub. Pets are not allowed but smoking is permitted outside. The organisation that owns the home also owns an employment agency that provides temporary staff and training to care homes.

Registered places: 47
Guide weekly rate: £440–£470
Specialist care: Nursing, physical disability, respite, terminal care
Medical services: Podiatry, optician
Qualified staff: Exceeds standard: 61% at NVQ Level 2

Home details
Location: Residential area, 5 miles from Portsmouth
Communal areas: Lounge, dining room, conservatory, patio
Accessibility: *Floors:* 2 • *Access:* Lift • *Wheelchair access:* Good
Smoking: In designated area
Pets: ✗
Routines: Flexible

Room details
Single: 43
Shared: 2
En suite: 0
Facilities: TV point, telephone point

Door lock: ✗
Lockable place: ✓

Services provided
Beauty services: None
Mobile library: ✗
Religious services: ✗
Transport: ✗
Activities: *Coordinator:* ✓ • *Examples:* Arts and crafts, scrabble, gardening • *Outings:* ✗
Meetings: ✓

Cosham Court Nursing Home

Manager: Anne Hazeldine
Owner: Masum Gulamhusein
Contact: 2–4 Albert Road, Cosham, Portsmouth, Hampshire PO6 3DD
☎ 023 92 324301

Cosham Court is five miles from Portsmouth, situated in a residential area. There is no garden at the home, but there is a courtyard area with a pond and a conservatory. This area contains flowerbeds which have been planted by residents themselves. The home's activities programme is advertised on a newssheet which is displayed around the home. This includes activities such as arts and crafts, clothes shows, gardening activities and barbecues. There is also a variety of languages spoken at the home such as English, Afrikaans, Punjabi and Hindi.

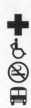

Court Lodge Nursing and Residential Home

Manager: Alison Fearnley
Owner: Colten Care Ltd
Contact: Court Close, Ridgeway Lane, Lymington, Hampshire SO41 8NQ
☏ 01590 673956
@ courtlodge@coltencare.co.uk
🖰 www.coltencare.co.uk

Court Lodge Nursing Home is on the outskirts of Lymington, one mile from the town centre. The home has well-maintained gardens and courtyard areas. Seating is available in the garden and it is wheelchair accessible. There is an activities coordinator who organises a range of activities including arts and crafts, skittles and memory box. There is a chef who can cater to those with dietary requirements.

Registered places: 41
Guide weekly rate: £566–£853
Specialist care: Nursing, dementia, physical disability, respite, terminal care
Medical services: Podiatry, dentist, optician
Qualified staff: Fails standard: 48% at NVQ Level 2

Home details
Location: Residential area, 1 mile from Lymington
Communal areas: 2 lounges, dining room, library, hairdressing salon, garden
Accessibility: *Floors:* 2 • *Access:* 2 lifts • *Wheelchair access:* Good
Smoking: ✗
Pets: ✗
Routines: Flexible

Room details
Single: 39
Shared: 1
En suite: 40
Facilities: TV, telephone point

Door lock: ✓
Lockable place: ✓

Services provided
Beauty services: Hairdressing
Mobile library: ✓
Religious services: Fortnightly visit from vicar
Transport: Minibus
Activities: *Coordinator:* ✓ • *Examples:* Exercise classes, quizzes, yoga • *Outings:* ✓
Meetings: ✓

Croft Manor Residential Care Home

Manager: Dawn McInnes
Owner: Heathfield Care Homes Ltd
Contact: 38 Osborn Road, Fareham, Hampshire PO16 7DS
☏ 01329 233593

Croft Manor is a privately owned and run care home situated within easy walking distance of Fareham town centre, approximately half a mile away. The home's location allows residents to enjoy a degree of independence in visiting shops and services near by. The home takes residents on walks and also arranges a varied activities programme. There are also regular residents meetings.

Registered places: 20
Guide weekly rate: £425
Specialist care: Dementia, respite, mental disorder
Medical services: Podiatry, dentist, hygienist, optician, physiotherapy
Qualified staff: Exceeds standard: 75% at NVQ Level 2

Home details
Location: Residential area, 0.7 miles from Fareham
Communal areas: 2 lounges, dining room, conservatory, garden
Accessibility: *Floors:* 3 • *Access:* Lift • *Wheelchair access:* Good
Smoking: ✗
Pets: ✓
Routines: Flexible

Room details
Single: 18
Shared: 2
En suite: 20
Facilities: TV point, telephone point

Door lock: ✓
Lockable place: ✓

Services provided
Beauty services: Hairdressing
Mobile library: ✗
Religious services: Monthly
Transport: ✗
Activities: *Coordinator:* ✓ • *Examples:* Art class, armchair exercise *Outings:* ✓
Meetings: ✓

Registered places: 30
Guide weekly rate: £590–£630
Specialist care: Respite
Medical services: Podiatry, dentist, optician, physiotherapy
Qualified staff: Meets standard

Home details

Location: Residential area, 1 mile from Fleet
Communal areas: Lounge/conservatory, dining room, library, hairdressing salon, garden
Accessibility: *Floors:* 3 • *Access:* Lift and stair lift
  Wheelchair access: Good
Smoking: ✗
Pets: At manager's discretion
Routines: Flexible

Room details

Single: 30
Shared: 0
En suite: 30
Facilities: TV point, telephone point

Door lock: ✓
Lockable place: ✓

Services provided

Services: Hairdressing, aromatherapy
Mobile library: ✓
Religious services: Weekly Catholic service, monthly Anglican
Transport: ✗
Activities: *Coordinator:* ✓ • *Examples:* Bridge clubs, music to movement, visiting singers • *Outings:* ✓
Meetings: ✓

Derriford House

Manager: Carolyn Lunn
Owner: Derriford House Ltd
Contact: Pinewood Hill, Fleet, Hampshire, GU51 3AW
  ☎ 01252 627364
  @ derrifordhouse@farthingscare.co.uk
  🖰 www.farthingscare.co.uk

Derriford House is located in the north Hampshire town of Fleet, one mile from the town centre. The home is adjacent to public transport links and local amenities. The home is family run and aims to create an atmosphere where the residents have the most privacy and are able to enjoy a special diets and requirements catered for by their chef. The home also retains strong links with the community and trips to local points of interest can be arranged. The home organises residents meetings once a month.

Registered places: 43
Guide weekly rate: £895–£1,055
Specialist care: Nursing, physical disability, terminal care
Medical services: Podiatry, hygienist, optician, physiotherapy
Qualified staff: Exceeds standard: 72% at NVQ Level 2

Home details

Location: Village location, 2 miles from Winchester
Communal areas: Dining room, library area, hairdressing salon, physiotherapy room, garden
Accessibility: *Floors:* 2 • *Access:* Lift • *Wheelchair access:* Good
Smoking: ✗
Pets: ✗
Routines: Flexible

Room details

Single: 43
Shared: 0
En suite: 43
Facilities: TV point, telephone point

Door lock: ✗
Lockable place: ✓

Services provided

Beauty services: Hairdressing
Mobile library: ✗
Religious services: ✓
Transport: ✗
Activities: *Coordinator:* ✓ • *Examples:* Bowls, tea afternoons *Outings:* ✓
Meetings: ✓

The Dower House Nursing Home

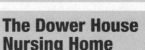

Manager: Mary Ann Crutchfield
Owner: Judith Lywood
Contact: Springvale Road, Headbourne Worthy, Winchester, Hampshire SO23 7LD
  ☎ 01962 882848

The Dower House is situated, in Headbourne Worthy, approximately two miles from Winchester. The home boasts large, well-maintained gardens and views of the surrounding countryside. There is level access in most areas of the grounds and seating areas for the residents. The majority of bedrooms are on ground level and lead directly into the garden via French doors. The activities coordinator organises daily activities to keep residents stimulated such as newspaper reading afternoons, walks in the grounds, bowls and collective activities such as afternoon tea.

Downham Lodge

Manager: Balamanee Lingaloo
Owner: Narain and Balamanee Lingaloo
Contact: 29 St Edward's Road,
Southsea, Hampshire PO5 3DH
☎ 023 9283 9816

Downham Lodge is a detached building located in a residential area of Southsea close to Southsea Common. There is a large lounge which leads out on to the home's courtyard garden and also a quiet lounge for those wishing to sit quietly. The home encourages visitors to get involved, sitting in on meetings and attending the summer events of barbecues and garden parties. They also celebrate residents' birthdays with cake and a party. For those who wish to see the sea it is only a five-minute walk, where the home takes them on outings.

Registered places: 12
Guide weekly rate: £375–£425
Specialist care: Dementia, mental disorder, respite.
Medical services: Podiatry, hygienist, optician, physiotherapy
Qualified staff: Fails standard: 30% at NVQ Level 2

Home details
Location: Residential area, 0.5 miles from Southsea
Communal areas: Lounge, quiet lounge, dining room, garden
Accessibility: *Floors:* 2 • *Access:* Lift • *Wheelchair access:* None
Smoking: ✗
Pets: ✗
Routines: Flexible

Room details
Single: 4	**Door lock:** ✓
Shared: 4	**Lockable place:** ✓
En suite: 7	
Facilities: TV point	

Services provided
Beauty services: Hairdressing
Mobile library: ✓
Religious services: Weekly Catholic Communion service
Transport: ✗
Activities: *Coordinator:* ✓ • *Examples:* Arts and crafts, board
  Outings: ✓
Meetings: ✓

The Downs House

Manager: Paul Rogers
Owner: Western Health Care Ltd
Contact: Reservoir Lane, Petersfield,
Hampshire GU32 2HX
☎ 01730 261474
@ info@downshouse.co.uk
🖰 www.downshouse.co.uk

The Downs House is situated on a quiet road, one mile outside the bustling market town of Petersfield. There is an activities programme and two or three activities are organised per day, including a weekly outing and a happy hour each Sunday, when residents get pre-lunch drinks in the lounge. Other activities include video afternoon, birthday parties, board games and bridge. There are also extensive grounds around the home, which are well maintained and residents are welcome to wander round. There is level access in most parts.

Registered places: 37
Guide weekly rate: £480–£610
Specialist care: None
Medical services: Podiatry, dentist, optician
Qualified staff: Exceeds standard: 72% at NVQ Level 2

Home details
Location: Residential area, 1 mile from Petersfield
Communal areas: 2 lounges, dining room, conservatory, garden
Accessibility: *Floors:* 3 • *Access:* Lift • *Wheelchair access:* Good
Smoking: In designated area
Pets: At manager's discretion
Routines: Flexible

Room details
Single: 31	**Door lock:** ✗
Shared: 3	**Lockable place:** ✓
En suite: 34	
Facilities: TV point, telephone point	

Services provided
Beauty services: Hairdressing, masseuse
Mobile library: ✗
Religious services: ✓
Transport: Minibus
Activities: *Coordinator:* ✓ • *Examples:* Exercise classes,
  gardening, yoga • *Outings:* ✓
Meetings: ✓

Registered places: 33
Guide weekly rate: £513–£681
Specialist care: Nursing, dementia, physical disability
Medical services: Podiatry, optician
Qualified staff: Meets standard

Home details

Location: Village location, 10 miles from Southampton
Communal areas: Lounge, dining room, garden
Accessibility: *Floors:* 2 • *Access:* Lift • *Wheelchair access:* Good
Smoking: ✗
Pets: At manager's discretion
Routines: Flexible

Room details

Single: 23
Shared: 5
En suite: 0
Facilities: TV point

Door lock: ✗
Lockable place: ✓

Services provided

Beauty services: Hairdressing, aromatherapy
Mobile library: ✓
Religious services: ✓
Activities: *Coordinator:* ✓ • *Examples:* Gardening, knitting, singing
   Outings: ✗
Meetings: ✓

Durban House Nursing Home

Manager: Perpetual Chikuyo-Mafunga
Owner: J Sai Group Ltd
Contact: Woodley Lane, Romsey, Hampshire SO51 7JL
) 01794 512332

Durban House is situated in the village of Romsey, 10 miles from Southampton. The home has developed an activities programme, run by a coordinator, which involves organising activities to keep residents busy and involved. This includes singing, knitting and gardening as well as outings. Residents have a flexible routine choosing their own bed times, however, mealtimes are structured because it is seen as a sociable time when all residents sit together in the dining room.

Registered places: 34
Guide weekly rate: £383–£740
Specialist care: None
Medical services: Podiatry, hygienist, optician, physiotherapy
Qualified staff: Exceeds standard: 57% at NVQ Level 2

Home details

Location: Village location, 5 miles from Petersfield
Communal areas: Lounge, 2 dining rooms, hairdressing salon, library, garden
Accessibility: *Floors:* 3 • *Access:* Lift • *Wheelchair access:* Good
Smoking: ✓
Pets: At manager's discretion
Routines: Flexible

Room details

Single: 34
Shared: 0
En suite: 22
Facilities: None

Door lock: ✗
Lockable place: ✓

Services provided

Beauty services: Hairdressing
Mobile library: ✓
Religious services: ✓
Transport: ✓
Activities: *Coordinator:* ✓ • *Examples:* Arts and crafts, exercise, quizzes • *Outings:* ✓
Meetings: ✓

East Hill House Residential Care Home

Manager: Priscilla Le Pla
Owner: East Hill Ltd
Contact: East Hill Drive, Hillbrow Road, Liss, Hampshire GU33 7RR
) 01206 828290

East Hill House is a large old house on the outskirts of the village of Liss which overlooks the West Downs. Although it has been modernised substantially, the home retains much of its period features. The home is set in three acres of land, which is maintained by a gardener who comes weekly. There is a terraced seating area where views of the West Downs can be seen from outside the house. In the summer the garden is used for regular barbecues and summer parties.

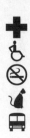

Eastfield Nursing and Residential Care Home

Manager: Dennis Anthony Greenwood
Owner: Wenham Holt Homes Ltd
Contact: Hillbrow Road, Liss, Hampshire GU33 7PB
) 01730 892268

Eastfield Nursing Home is situated on a main road a short distance from Liss where there are local facilities and shops. The home is set in landscaped gardens. There are decking areas and seating area for residents so they can sit outside and socialise. In the summer months there are often afternoon tea parties or barbecues in the garden. Residents also have access to a therapy pool with a wave machine, which aims to relax the residents and keep them comfortable. Residents can attend two trips out a week, for shopping, to the local garden centre and walking trips.

Registered places: 37
Guide weekly rate: Undisclosed
Specialist care: Nursing, dementia, physical disability, terminal care
Medical services: Podiatry, optician, hygienist, physiotherapy
Qualified staff: Exceeds standard: 55% at NVQ Level 2

Home details
Location: Village location, 4 miles from Petersfield
Communal areas: Lounge, lounge/dining room, conservatory, garden
Accessibility: *Floors:* 2 • *Access:* Lift • *Wheelchair access:* Good
Smoking: x
Pets: At manager's discretion
Routines: Flexible

Room details
Single: 29
Shared: 4
En suite: 31
Facilities: TV point, telephone point

Door lock: x
Lockable place: ✓

Services provided
Beauty services: Hairdressing
Mobile library: x
Religious services: ✓
Transport: ✓
Activities: *Coordinator:* x • *Examples:* Arts and crafts, exercise, musical afternoons • *Outings:* ✓
Meetings: ✓

Elingfield House

Manager: Susan Hollingworth
Owner: Susan Hollingworth
Contact: 26 High Street, Totton, Hampshire SO40 9HN
) 023 8066 3363

Elingfield House is located in the centre of Old Totton, a small town near Southampton and the New Forest. It is an old building, retaining much of its character. There is a garden for residents to enjoy, and pets are very welcome as the home is a member of the Cinnamon Trust. Social carers also come in on a weekly basis and have a one-to-one with each of the residents and take them out for the day or simply sit with them for company.

Registered places: 14
Guide weekly rate: £375–£500
Specialist care: Dementia, respite
Medical services: Podiatry, dentist, holistic massage, optician, physiotherapy
Qualified staff: Exceeds standard: 60% at NVQ Level 2

Home details
Location: Urban area, 0.7 miles from Totton
Communal areas: Lounge, dining room, patio and garden
Accessibility: *Floors:* 2 • *Access:* 2 stair lifts *Wheelchair access:* Good
Smoking: x
Pets: ✓
Routines: Flexible

Room details
Single: 4
Shared: 5
En suite: 1
Facilities: TV point, telephone point

Door lock: ✓
Lockable place: ✓

Services provided
Beauty services: x
Mobile library: x
Religious services: Monthly Communion service
Transport: x
Activities: *Coordinator:* x • *Examples:* Entertainers, reminiscence therapy, tea parties • *Outings:* ✓
Meetings: x

Registered places: 31
Guide weekly rate: £550–£650
Specialist care: Day care, dementia, respite
Medical services: Podiatry, dentistry
Qualified staff: Exceeds standard: 85% at NVQ Level 2

Home details

Location: Residential area, 2.5 miles from New Milton
Communal areas: 3 lounges, dining room, patio and garden
Accessibility: *Floors:* 2 • *Access:* Lift • *Wheelchair access:* Good
Smoking: ✗
Pets: At manager's discretion
Routines: Flexible

Room details

Single: 25
Shared: 3
En suite: 27
Facilities: TV point, telephone point

Door lock: ✓
Lockable place: ✓

Services provided

Beauty services: Hairdressing
Mobile library: ✗
Religious services: Weekly Communion service
Transport: ✓
Activities: *Coordinator:* ✓ • *Examples:* Painting, musical exercise
     Outings: ✓
Meetings: ✗

Engleburn

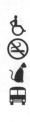

Manager: Tracey Holland
Owner: Maureen Grey
Contact: Milford Road, Barton-on-Sea, Hampshire BH25 5PN
✆ 01425 610865
@ engleburn@aol.com

Engleberg is a large, detached property set in its own grounds, two and a half miles from New Milton. Some rooms have balconies over the garden and others on the ground floor have patio doors that open on to the garden. Engleberg boasts a seven-acre garden spread for residents to enjoy, particularly in the warmer months. Engleberg is visited monthly by a church choir who sing hymns for residents to enjoy. There are also outings to art exhibitions.

Registered places: 40 places
Guide weekly rate: £320–£600
Specialist care: Dementia, mental disorder,
     physical disability, respite
Medical services: Podiatry, hygienist, optician, physiotherapy
Qualified staff: Exceeds standard: 60% at NVQ Level 2

Home details

Location: Residential area, 2.5 miles from Fareham
Communal areas: 2 lounges, dining room, conservatory, garden
Accessibility: *Floors:* Undisclosed • *Access:* Lift
     Wheelchair access: Good
Smoking: ✗
Pets: ✓
Routines: Flexible

Room details

Single: 32
Shared: 4
En suite: 34
Facilities: TV point, telephone point

Door lock: ✗
Lockable place: ✓

Services provided

Beauty services: Hairdressing
Mobile library: ✓
Religious services: Weekly Catholic service,
     fortnightly Anglican service
Transport: ✓
Activities: *Coordinator:* ✓ • *Examples:* Darts, gardening, skittles
     Outings: ✓
Meetings: ✓

Farehaven Lodge

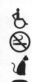

Manager: Theresa Thompson
Owner: Fareham Court Ltd
Contact: 8 Nashe Close, Hill Park, Fareham, Hampshire PO15 6LT
✆ 01329 846765

Fareham Lodge is located in a quiet residential area of Fareham, two and a half miles from the town centre. The home has its own private minibus to take residents on day trips or simply into Fareham to do some shopping. The home is set in grounds which are well maintained and there are seating area for residents to sit outside. The conservatory is currently being extended to create another lounge which will overlook the grounds. There are scenic walks around the home for those who are mobile.

Farmhouse Rest Home

Manager: Jean Hunt
Owner: Richard Kitchen
Contact: 87 Water Lane, Totton, Southampton, Hampshire SO40 3DJ
☏ 023 8086 8895

Farmhouse Rest Home is situated in a residential area, less than a mile from Totton town centre. Local shops and amenities are a short walk away and public transport is easily accessible. The home often organises singalongs and sherry parties that are held on the patio at the rear of the building. The residents also partake in excursions and outings every Wednesday to various local attractions. The home organises Catholic, Methodist and Anglican services every month.

Registered places: 20
Guide weekly rate: £385–£420
Specialist care: Dementia, respite, day care
Medical services: Podiatry, dentist, optician, physiotherapy
Qualified staff: Exceeds standard: 60% at NVQ Level 2

Home details
Location: Residential area, 0.3 miles from Totton
Communal areas: 2 lounges, dining room, patio
Accessibility: *Floors:* 2 • *Access:* 2 stair lifts
    Wheelchair access: Good
Smoking: In designated area
Pets: At manager's discretion
Routines: Flexible

Room details
Single: 10
Shared: 5
En suite: 15
Facilities: TV, telephone

Door lock: ✓
Lockable place: ✓

Services provided
Beauty services: Hairdressing
Mobile library: ✗
Religious services: Monthly Catholic, Methodist and Anglican services
Transport: ✗
Activities: *Coordinator:* ✓ • *Examples:* Exercise, games, reminiscence sessions • *Outings:* ✓
Meetings: ✗

Ferndale Residential Care Home

Manager: Kathy Greenfield
Owner: Sussex Training Services Ltd
Contact: 8 Stein Road, Southbourne, Emsworth, Hampshire PO10 8LD
☏ 01243 371841
@ kathy.greenfield@btopenworld.com

Ferndale is a privately owned, three-storey detached Victorian property, situated in a residential area, one and a half miles from Emsworth. It is approximately one mile from the seafront. Residents regularly go on outings to garden centres, pubs, shops and walks. The garden is safe for residents, with raised flowerbeds that residents can help with. The home has an ongoing programme of refurbishment and two bathrooms are being presently refurbished to meet the needs of the residents.

Registered places: 17
Guide weekly rate: £375–£560
Specialist care: Dementia
Medical services: Podiatry, dentist, optician
Qualified staff: Meets standard

Home details
Location: Residential area, 1.5 miles from Emsworth
Communal areas: Lounge, dining room, conservatory, patio and garden
Accessibility: *Floors:* 2 • *Access:* Undisclosed
    Wheelchair access: Good
Smoking: ✗
Pets: ✗
Routines: Flexible

Room details
Single: 17
Shared: 0
En suite: 4
Facilities: TV point, telephone point

Door lock: ✓
Lockable place: ✓

Services provided
Beauty services: Hairdressing
Mobile library: ✗
Religious services: Catholic priest visits
Transport: ✗
Activities: *Coordinator:* ✓ • *Examples:* Bowls, gardening, music therapy • *Outings:* ✓
Meetings: ✗

Registered places: 39
Guide weekly rate: £520–£763
Specialist care: Nursing, physical disability, respite, terminal care
Medical services: Podiatry, dentist, optician, physiotherapy
Qualified staff: Meets standard

Home details

Location: Residential area, 2 miles from Waterlooville
Communal areas: 3 lounges, dining room, sensory room,
    patio and garden
Accessibility: *Floors:* 2 • *Access:* Lift • *Wheelchair access:* Good
Smoking: ✗
Pets: At manager's discretion
Routines: Flexible

Room details

Single: 7
Shared: 16
En suite: 0
Facilities: TV point

Door lock: ✓
Lockable place: ✓

Services provided

Beauty services: Hairdressing, aromatherapy
Mobile library: ✗
Religious services: ✗
Transport: ✗
Activities: *Coordinator:* ✓ • *Examples:* Bingo, exercise, quizzes
    Outings: ✗
Meetings: ✗

Fieldgate Nursing Home

Manager: Muriel Emery
Owner: Extraservices Ltd
Contact: 153 Portsmouth Road,
Horndean, Hampshire PO8 9LG
☏ 023 9259 3352

The home is situated in a residential area of Horndean, approximately two miles from Waterlooville. The home has a sensory room that contains soft lighting, slides and music. There is a spacious garden with a seating area and sun lounges for residents to use in fine weather. The staff organise summer and Christmas fêtes for the residents and visitors.

Registered places: 22
Guide weekly rate: Undisclosed
Specialist care: Dementia, learning disability, respite
Medical services: Podiatry, dentist, optician
Qualified staff: Meets standard

Home details

Location: Residential area, 0.5 miles from Locks Heath
Communal areas: Lounge, dining room, patio
Accessibility: *Floors:* 2 • *Access:* Lift • *Wheelchair access:* Good
Smoking: ✗
Pets: ✗
Routines: Flexible

Room details

Single: 16
Shared: 3
En suite: 22
Facilities: TV, telephone

Door lock: ✓
Lockable place: ✓

Services provided

Beauty services: Hairdressing, manicures
Mobile library: ✗
Religious services: Weekly church service
Transport: ✗
Activities: *Coordinator:* ✗ • *Examples:* Arts and crafts, visiting
    entertainers • *Outings:* ✗
Meetings: ✓

The Firs

Manager: I Caldwell
Owner: Caldwell Care Ltd
Contact: 83 Church Road, Locks Heath,
Southampton, Hampshire SO31 6LS
☏ 01489 574624

The Firs is situated in Locks Heath, seven and a half miles from Southampton. The home has places for 20 permanent residents and two places for respite care. The home has two large lounge and a connecting dining room. There is a large patio area for residents to enjoy in good weather in the garden. The home offers a weekly church service and beauty therapies such as hairdressing and manicures. The home has an exercise coordinator and an activities programme which includes visiting entertainers and arts and crafts.

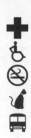

Flowerdown Nursing Home

Manager: Carol Taylor
Owner: Tamhealth Ltd
Contact: Harestock Road,
Winchester, Hampshire SO22 6NT
☏ 01962 881060

Flowerdown Nursing Home is situated in a semi rural area on the outskirts of Winchester, Hampshire, two and a half miles from the town centre. The home has recently completed an extensive programme of redecoration and refurbishment. The home also has large well-maintained gardens with seating areas for the residents' use. The home organises an interdenominational church service once a month.

Registered places: 53
Guide weekly rate: £650–£800
Specialist care: Nursing, respite
Medical services: Podiatry, dentist, optician, physiotherapy
Qualified staff: Meets standard

Home details

Location: Residential area, 2.5 miles from Winchester
Communal areas: 2 lounges, 2 dining rooms, patio and garden
Accessibility: *Floors:* 2 • *Access:* 2 lifts
   Wheelchair access: Good
Smoking: ✗
Pets: At manager's discretion
Routines: Flexible

Room details

Single: 48
Shared: 1
En suite: 49
Facilities: TV point, and telephone point

Door lock: ✓
Lockable place: ✓

Services provided

Beauty services: Hairdressing
Mobile library: ✗
Religious services: Monthly interdenominational service
Transport: Minibus
Activities: *Coordinator:* ✓ • *Examples:* Games, quizzes
   Outings: ✓
Meetings: ✗

Forest Brow Care Home

Manager: Susan Makhzangi
Owner: BRIJ Care Ltd
Contact: 63 Forest Road, Liss,
Hampshire GU33 7BL
☏ 01730 893342
@ sue@forestbrow.wannadoo.co.uk

Forest Brow is in a semi-rural location, in the small village of Liss, approximately seven miles from Petersfield. The home has a one and a half acre garden with a large patio and seating area for residents to relax in. The home displays each month's activities clearly on a wall, and activities are designed to benefit those with dementia. Two parties are held each year, a Pimm's party in summer and a Christmas festive event, to which friends and family are invited. Pets can visit but are not permitted to stay.

Registered places: 30
Guide weekly rate: £396–£660
Specialist care: Dementia, physical disability
Medical services: Podiatry, optician, physiotherapy
Qualified staff: Exceeds standard: 80% at NVQ Level 2

Home details

Location: Village location, 7 miles from Petersfield
Communal areas: Lounge, dining room, conservatory,
   patio and garden
Accessibility: *Floors:* 3 • *Access:* Lift • *Wheelchair access:* Good
Smoking: ✗
Pets: ✗
Routines: Flexible

Room details

Single: 18
Shared: 6
En suite: 20
Facilities: TV point

Door lock: ✓
Lockable place: ✓

Services provided

Beauty services: Hairdressing, massage
Mobile library: ✓
Religious services: Weekly Catholic Communion service
Transport: ✗
Activities: *Coordinator:* ✗ • *Examples:* Music and movement,
   reminiscence • *Outings:* ✓
Meetings: ✗

Registered places: 22
Guide weekly rate: From £425
Specialist care: Dementia, mental disorder
Medical services: Podiatry, dentist, optician
Qualified staff: Exceeds standard: 99% at NVQ Level 2

Home details

Location: Rural area, 4 miles from Totton
Communal areas: Lounge, dining room, conservatory, garden
Accessibility: *Floors:* 2 • *Access:* Lift • *Wheelchair access:* Good
Smoking: In designated area
Pets: x
Routines: Structured

Room details

Single: 22
Shared: 0
En suite: 22
Facilities: TV point, telephone point

Door lock: ✓
Lockable place: ✓

Services provided

Beauty services: Hairdressing
Mobile library: ✓
Religious service: Monthly
Transport: x
Activities: *Coordinator:* ✓ • *Examples:* Games, painting, reading
    Outings: x
Meetings: x

Forest Edge Rest Home

Manager: Linda Parker
Owner: John and Linda Hughes
Contact: Southampton Road,
Cadnam, Hampshire SO40 2NF
) 023 8081 3334
@ Forest.edge@btinternet.com

Forest Edge is a 22-bed home found on the outskirts at Cadna, four miles from Totton town centre. It is opposite a garden centre. The home is located near the New Forest, giving residents the opportunity to visit the forest. Activities are used to encourage sociality and include games and reading. The activities coordinator comes to the home once a fortnight and the staff have activities training. Residents have set mealtimes but can choose to have their meal in their room. Smoking is permitted outside.

Registered places: 46
Guide weekly rate: £360–£673
Specialist care: Nursing
Medical services: Podiatry, dentist
Qualified staff: Meets standard

Home details

Location: Residential area, 0.5 miles from Brockenhurst
Communal areas: Lounge, dining room, garden
Accessibility: *Floors:* 3 • *Access:* Lift • *Wheelchair access:* Good
Smoking: In designated area
Pets: x
Routines: Flexible

Room details

Single: 46
Shared: 0
En suite: 42
Facilities: TV point, telephone point

Door lock: ✓
Lockable place: x

Services provided

Beauty services: Hairdressing, manicures
Mobile library: x
Religious services: Monthly Communion service
Transport: x
Activities: *Coordinator:* x • *Examples:* Exercise, painting, videos
    Outings: ✓
Meetings: ✓

Forest Oaks Home for the Elderly

Manager: Glynis Garmen
Owner: The Wilverley Association Ltd
Contact: The Rise, Brockenhurst,
Hampshire SO42 7SJ
) 01590 622424

Forest Oaks is a purpose-built home surrounded by private gardens. It is near Brockenhurst town, half a mile from the town centre. The staff at the home organise trips twice a year for the residents, which involves a boat trip up the river with drinks and snacks. There are other outings throughout the year for pub lunches or to museums in the local area. Painting afternoon and video evenings are just two of the activities that the home organises for residents on a weekly basis.

Foxes' Moon Residential Home

Manager: Mrs Ramsey
Owner: Mrs Ramsey and Mrs Lubbock
Contact: 40 Ringwood Road, St Ives, Ringwood, Hampshire BH24 2NY
☏ 01425 474347
@ foxesmoon@btconnect.com

A beautiful house situated in of St Ives and not far from Ringwood and the New Forest, Foxes' Moon is in an attractive location. Foxes Moon is focused heavily on those residents with dementia or Alzheimer's. Residents are gently encouraged to take part in activities while a rear patio and enclosed gardens – with potted plants and flowers – provide a peaceful refuge outside the home. Due to the nature of most of the clients' mental health, there are resident and relative meetings in place of a resident tenants association.

Registered places: 31
Guide weekly rate: £600–£700
Specialist care: Day care, mental disorder, respite
Medical services: Podiatry, dentist, optician
Qualified staff: Undisclosed

Home details
Location: Village of St Ives
Communal areas: 2 lounges, conservatory, patio and garden
Accessibility: *Floors:* 2 • *Access:* Lift • *Wheelchair access:* Good
Smoking: ✗
Pets: ✗
Routines: Flexible

Room details
Single: 31
Shared: 0
En suite: 13
Facilities: TV point, telephone point

Door lock: ✓
Lockable place: ✗

Services provided
Beauty services: Hairdressing
Mobile library: ✗
Religious: Fortnightly Communion service
Transport: ✗
Activities: *Coordinator:* ✓ • *Examples:* Games, music sessions
　　　Outings: ✗
Meetings: ✓

Fraryhurst

Manager: Dawn Davie
Owner: Springfield Health Services Ltd
Contact: Prinsted Lane, Prinsted, Emsworth, Hampshire PO10 8HR
☏ 01243 372024
@ mantroness@
　　　springfieldnursing.co.uk
🖰 www.springfieldnursing.co.uk

Fraryhurst is a large, detached, extended building set in its own grounds in the village of Southbourne. Situated in a residential area, the home is within close to local shops, with good public transport links to travel into the local town of Engleburn. The home's outings include trips to beauty spots, garden centres and local pubs. Residents are not obliged to attend all activities and can retire to their room if preferred.

Registered places: 27
Guide weekly rate: £600–£700
Specialist care: Nursing, respite
Medical services: Podiatry, optician, physiotherapy
Qualified staff: Exceeds standard: 96% at NVQ Level 2

Home details
Location: Residential area, 1.2 miles from Emsworth
Communal areas: Lounge, dining room, patio and garden
Accessibility: *Floors:* 2 • *Access:* Lift • *Wheelchair access:* Good
Smoking: ✗
Pets: ✗
Routines: Flexible

Room details
Single: 19
Shared: 4
En suite: Undisclosed
Facilities: TV point, telephone point

Door lock: ✓
Lockable place: ✓

Services provided
Beauty services: Hairdressing, reflexology
Mobile library: ✗
Religious services: Fortnightly Communion service
Transport: ✗
Activities: *Coordinator:* ✗ • *Examples:* Arts and crafts, gentle
　　　exercise, music sessions • *Outings:* ✓
Meetings: ✗

Registered places: 17
Guide weekly rate: £395–£550
Specialist care: Day care, dementia, respite
Medical services: Podiatry, dentist, optician, physiotherapy
Qualified staff: Fails standard: 45% at NVQ Level 2

Home details

Location: Residential area, 1 mile from Lymington
Communal areas: Lounge/dining room, library, quiet lounge,
2 patios and garden
Accessibility: *Floors:* 2 • *Access:* Lift • *Wheelchair access:* Good
Smoking: ×
Pets: ×
Routines: Flexible

Room details

Single: 13
Shared: 2
En suite: 6
Facilities: Telephone point

Door lock: ✓
Lockable place: ✓

Services provided

Beauty services: Hairdressing
Mobile library: ✓
Religious services: Monthly Anglican Communion service
Transport: ×
Activities: *Coordinator:* × • *Examples:* Knitting, exercises,
reminiscence • *Outings:* ✓
Meetings: ✓

Freegrove

Manager: Angela Andrews
Owner: Charlotte Duffin
Contact: 60 Milford Road, Pennington,
Lymington, Hampshire SO41 8DU
☏ 01590 673168

Freegrove is set in a residential area, on the outskirts of the town Lymington, one mile from the town centre. There is a large garden to the front of the property and an enclosed garden behind. The home specialises in caring for residents with dementia. Trips are taken regularly to the New Forest. The manager had been working at the home for 25 years. Though pets are not allowed to stay at the home they can visit. There are monthly residents meetings.

Registered places: 24
Guide weekly rate: £385–£406
Specialist care: Dementia, respite
Medical services: Podiatry, hygienist, optician, physiotherapy
Qualified staff: Exceeds standard: 57% at NVQ Level 2

Home details

Location: Residential area, 3.5 miles from Southampton
Communal areas: Lounge, dining room, conservatory,
patio and garden
Accessibility: *Floors:* 2 • *Access:* Lift and stair lift
Wheelchair access: Limited
Smoking: ×
Pets: At manager's discretion
Routines: Flexible

Room details

Single: 14
Shared: 5
En suite: 8
Facilities: TV

Door lock: ✓
Lockable place: ✓

Services provided

Beauty services: Hairdressing
Mobile library: ✓
Monthly church service: ✓
Transport: Minibus
Activities: *Coordinator:* ✓ • *Examples:* Barbecues, exercise to
music, reminiscence sessions • *Outings:* ✓
Meetings: ✓

The Gables

Manager: Karen Edney
Owner: David and Thelma Jackson
Contact: 13 St Mary's Road,
Netley Abbey, Southampton, Hampshire
SO31 5AT
☏ 023 8045 2324

The Gables is located in a quiet residential area of Netley, approximately three and a half miles from Southampton. The home puts on seasonal events for its residents, such as a summer barbecue, a Halloween party, or a trip to the local garden centre to see the Christmas decorations. The home's lounge has a good selection of books and an electric organ. The garden is enclosed, and suitable for residents to use. There is a resident cat and other pets would be allowed at the manager's discretion. There is a residents meeting every month.

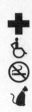

Glen Heathers Nursing and Residential Care Home

Manager: John Perkins
Owner: Saffronland Homes
Contact: 48 Milvil Road,
Lee-on-the-Solent, Hampshire
PO13 9LX

☎ 023 9236 6666
@ glenheathers@saffronland.co.uk
🖰 www.saffronland.co.uk

Glen Heathers is located in the costal town of Lee-on-the-Solent, half a mile from the town centre. There is a separate wing for seven residents with dementia, with its own lounge area. Each month, an external entertainer visits the home. This has included a brass band, miniature farm and musicians. During the Christmas season, residents are invited to attend a pantomime and a bazaar was organised at the home. Religious services can be arranged if requested.

Registered places: 53
Guide weekly rate: £500–£650
Specialist care: Nursing, dementia, respite, terminal care
Medical services: Podiatry, optician
Qualified staff: Meets standard

Home details
Location: Residential area, 0.5 miles from Lee-on-the-Solvent
Communal areas: 2 lounges, dining room, patio and garden
Accessibility: *Floors:* 2 • *Access:* Lift and stair lift
   Wheelchair access: Good
Smoking: ✗
Pets: At manager's discretion
Routines: Flexible

Room details
Single: 33
Shared: 10
En suite: 43
Facilities: TV, telephone point

Door lock: ✓
Lockable place: ✓

Services provided
Beauty services: Hairdressing
Mobile library: ✓
Religious services: ✓
Transport: ✗
Activities: *Coordinator:* ✗ • *Examples:* Bingo, exercises, visiting entertainers • *Outings:* ✗
Meetings: ✗

Glen Lyn

Manager: Joy Leach
Owner: Saffronland Homes Group
Contact: 16 Glen Road, Sarisbury Green, Southampton, Hampshire SO31 7FD
☎ 01489 602222

Glen Lyn is located in a rural area, approximately six miles from Southampton town centre. The home has a dining room as well as a large garden with a seating area. There are a range of activities on offer including music sessions, table football games and an indoor putting set. The home also arranges outings for residents.

Registered places: 43
Guide weekly rate: Undisclosed
Specialist care: Dementia, respite
Medical services: Podiatry, optician
Qualified staff: Meets standard

Home details
Location: Rural area, 6 miles from Southampton
Communal areas: Dining room, garden
Accessibility: *Floors:* 2 • *Access:* Lift and stair lift
   Wheelchair access: Good
Smoking: ✗
Pets: ✗
Routines: Flexible

Room details
Single: 19
Shared: 12
En suite: 31
Facilities: TV

Door lock: ✓
Lockable place: ✓

Services provided
Beauty services: Hairdressing
Mobile library: ✗
Religious services: ✓
Transport: ✗
Activities: *Coordinator:* ✗ • *Examples:* Music, table football
   Outings: ✓
Meetings: ✗

Registered places: 37
Guide weekly rate: £530–£850
Specialist care: Physical disability, respite, terminal care
Medical services: Podiatry, holistic therapy, physiotherapy, psychiatry
Qualified staff: Exceeds standard: 68% at NVQ Level 2

Home details
Location: Village location, 4 miles from Ringwood
Communal areas: 2 lounges, 3 dining rooms, library, conservatory, patio and garden
Accessibility: *Floors:* 2 • *Access:* Lift • *Wheelchair access:* Good
Smoking: In designated area
Pets: ✓
Routines: Flexible

Room details
Single: 26
Shared: 5
En suite: 21
Facilities: TV point, telephone point

Door lock: ✓
Lockable place: ✓

Services provided
Beauty services: Hairdressing, manicures, reflexology
Mobile library: ✗
Religious services: Monthly Communion service
Transport: Minibus
Activities: *Coordinator:* ✓ • *Examples:* Arts and crafts, exercise, entertainers • *Outings:* ✓
Meetings: ✗

Gorselands Nursing Home

Manager: Patricia Vinycomb
Owner: Gorselands in the Forest Ltd
Contact: Coach Hill Lane, Burley Street, Ringwood, Hampshire
BH24 4HN
☎ 01425 402316
@ gorselands@btconnect.com

Gorselands has landscaped gardens with views over the New Forest. A new wing has been added to the home providing an additional 10 en suite bedrooms. A sensory garden is also planned. The main dining room overlooks the gardens. During the warmer months, the home's minibus allows for one-to-one trips to be made, for example, just before Christmas residents were taken shopping to buy Christmas presents. Every effort made to accommodate cultural or religious interests, a monthly Communion services is arranged.

Registered places: 25
Guide weekly rate: £670–£728
Specialist care: Nursing, physical disability
Medical services: Podiatry, dentist, optician, physiotherapy
Qualified staff: Exceeds standard: 77% at NVQ Level 2

Home details
Location: Village location, 5 miles from Basingstoke
Communal areas: Lounge/conservatory, quiet lounge, dining room, patio and garden
Accessibility: *Floors:* 2 • *Access:* lift • *Wheelchair access:* Good
Smoking: In designated area
Pets: At manager's discretion
Routines: Flexible

Room details
Single: 23
Shared: 1
En suite: 1
Facilities: TV point, telephone point

Door lock: ✓
Lockable place: ✓

Services provided
Beauty services: Hairdressing
Mobile library: ✓
Religious services: Monthly Communion service, monthly Salvation Army service
Transport: ✗
Activities: *Coordinator:* ✓ • *Examples:* Crosswords, discussion *Outings:* ✓
Meetings: ✗

The Grange Nursing Home

Manager: Maureen Rowsell
Owner: Britaniascheme Ltd
Contact: Vyne Road, Sherborne St John, Basingstoke, Hampshire RG24 9HX
☎ 01256 851191

The Grange Nursing Home is set in large gardens, in a semi-rural area of Basingstoke. The home is a large converted farmhouse and the dining room extends onto the patio. Many of the rooms have pleasant views over the countryside. The activities coordinator has attended a training course in therapeutic activities and is qualified to provide Reiki and massage. There are also visits from musicians and theme days as part of the activities programme. There is a resident cat and a Pets As Therapy scheme in place here for residents to enjoy.

The Grange Nursing Home

Manager: Carolyn Ryves
Owner: Angela, Roy and Heather Northover
Contact: 72 Upper Northam Road, Hedge End, Southampton, Hampshire SO30 4EB
☎ 01489 790177
@ Carolyn.ryves@zen.co.uk

The Grange is a nursing home on the outskirts of Southampton, five miles from the town centre. It is a two-storey residential property converted for use as a home. The home has a lounge, a dining room and there is a large, well-maintained garden accessible to residents. The residents have a flexible daily routine and a varied activities programme including a charitable business venture in which they make their own soap. The home also organises special meals with relatives. Pets are not allowed but there are visits from a Pets As Therapy dog.

Registered places: 43
Guide weekly rate: £550–£770
Specialist care: Nursing, physical disability, terminal care
Medical services: Podiatry, dentist, optician
Qualified staff: Exceeds standard: 100% at NVQ Level 2

Home details
Location: Residential area, 5 miles from Southampton
Communal areas: Lounge, dining room, patio and garden
Accessibility: *Floors:* 2 • *Access:* 2 lifts
  Wheelchair access: Good
Smoking: ✗
Pets: ✗
Routines: Flexible

Room details
Single: 29	**Door lock:** ✓
Shared: 7	**Lockable place:** ✓
En suite: 31	
Facilities: TV	

Services provided
Beauty services: Hairdressing, aromatherapy, manicures
Mobile library: ✗
Religious services: Monthly Communion service
Transport: ✗
Activities: *Coordinator:* ✓ • *Examples:* Crafts, poetry, quizzes
  Outings: ✓
Meetings: ✓

Grasmere House

Manager: Mrs Ramtohal
Owner: Mrs Ramtohal
Contact: 33 Cargate Avenue, Aldershot, Hampshire GU11 3EW
☎ 01252 328 052
🖥 www.grasmerehouse.co.uk

Grasmere House is a large house in a residential area of Aldershot, half a mile from the town centre. The home is close to the local shops and to the main shopping centre of Aldershot. Newspapers are delivered to the home daily. There are large gardens to the front and back of the home, with paved seating areas for the residents. The home offers a hairdressing service once a week. Residents have daily delivery of their chosen newspaper, and often karaoke is a favourite activity in the evening.

Registered places: 9
Guide weekly rate: £395–£550
Specialist care: Dementia, mental disorder, respite
Medical services: Podiatry, hygienist, optician, physiotherapy
Qualified staff: Exceeds standard: 75% at NVQ Level 2

Home details
Location: Residential area, 0.5 miles from Aldershot
Communal areas: Lounge, dining room, garden
Accessibility: *Floors:* 3 • *Access:* Stair lift
  Wheelchair access: Good
Smoking: In designated area
Pets: At manager's discretion
Routines: Flexible

Room details
Single: 7	**Door lock:** ✓
Shared: 1	**Lockable place:** ✓
En suite: 3	
Facilities: TV point, telephone point	

Services provided
Beauty services: Hairdressing
Mobile library: ✗
Religious services: Weekly church visits
Transport: ✗
Activities: *Coordinator:* ✓ • *Examples:* Crosswords, jigsaws, karaoke • *Outings:* ✗
Meetings: ✗

Registered places: 38
Guide weekly rate: £583–£700
Specialist care: Nursing, dementia, respite
Medical services: Podiatry, dentist, optician
Qualified staff: Exceeds standard: 60% at NVQ Level 2

Home details

Location: Village location, 1 mile from Hindhead
Communal areas: Lounge, dining room, patio and garden
Accessibility: *Floors:* 3 • *Access:* Lift • *Wheelchair access:* Good
Smoking: ✗
Pets: ✗
Routines: Flexible

Room details

Single: 8
Shared: 15
En suite: 0
Facilities: TV point, telephone point

Door lock: ✗
Lockable place: ✓

Services provided

Beauty services: Hairdressing, aromatherapy, manicures
Mobile library: ✗
Religious services: Monthly interdenominational service
Transport: ✗
Activities: *Coordinator:* ✓ • *Examples:* Ball games, cookery, music
   Outings: ✓
Meetings: ✓

Green Gables Nursing Home

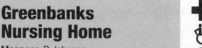

Manager: Margaret Lydon
Owner: Downing Ltd
Contact: Church Lane, Grayshott,
Hampshire GU26 6LY
✆ 01428 604220

Green Gables is situated in the village of Grayshott on the border of Hampshire and Surrey. The home focuses on independent care while also creating a caring and friendly environment. An activities programme is published monthly. This programme includes Pets As Therapy visits, cookery, flower arranging and crafts. Outings take place several times a month, going to the local shops, and to cafés and to have afternoon tea in the community.

Registered places: 30
Guide weekly rate: £506–£700
Specialist care: Nursing, dementia, physical disability
Medical services: Podiatry
Qualified staff: Meets standard

Home details

Location: Residential area, 0.5 miles from Liphook
Communal areas: Lounge, dining room, garden
Accessibility: *Floors:* Undisclosed • *Access:* Undisclosed
   Wheelchair access: Good
Smoking: ✗
Pets: ✓
Routines: Flexible

Room details

Single: 20
Shared: 5
En suite: 21
Facilities: TV point

Door lock: ✓
Lockable place: ✓

Services provided

Beauty services: Hairdressing
Mobile library: ✓
Religious services: Weekly Communion service
Transport: ✗
Activities: *Coordinator:* ✓ • *Examples:* Bingo, flower arranging,
   movement to music • *Outings:* ✗
Meetings: ✓

Greenbanks Nursing Home

Manager: P Johnson
Owner: Buckland Care Ltd
Contact: 29 London Road, Liphook,
Hampshire GU30 7AP
✆ 01428 727343
@ greenbanks29@aol.com
🖥 www.bucklandscare.co.uk

Formerly a Victorian home, Greenbanks was converted into a nursing home in 1990. It is situated half a mile from the centre of Liphook, a small village between Petersfield and Farnham. The surrounding countryside is noted for its natural beauty and provides many unspoilt walks and places to visit. The dining room is attractively decorated with well-presented tables. Residents are encouraged to meet here and linger over varied, tasty and well-balanced meals. Special diets are happily catered for and meals can be served in residents' rooms when required.

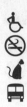

Greensleeves Residential Care Home

Manager: Maria Sebastianpillai
Owner: Greensleeves Residential Care Home Ltd
Contact: 8 Westwood Road, Portswood, Southampton, Hampshire SO17 1DN
☏ 023 8031 5777

Greensleeves Residential Care Home is situated two miles from Southampton and has access to a local bus service. There are two lounges, a dining room and a garden and the home has its own transport. The home has its own activities coordinator and activities include films, games and knitting. There are also outings in the summer months to the nearby common. The residents have a flexible routine with set meal times. Pets are allowed and smoking is not permitted. There is a resident tenants association which meets regularly to discuss any issues the residents may have.

Registered places: 21
Guide weekly rate: £420
Specialist care: Dementia
Medical services: Podiatry, dentist, optician
Qualified staff: Exceeds standard: 99% at NVQ Level 2

Home details
Location: Residential area, 2 miles from Southampton
Communal areas: 2 lounges, dining room, garden
Accessibility: *Floors:* 2 • *Access:* Stair lift
 Wheelchair access: Good
Smoking: ✗
Pets: ✓
Routines: Flexible

Room details
Single: 19   **Door lock:** ✓
Shared: 2   **Lockable place:** ✓
En suite: Undisclosed
Facilities: Undisclosed

Services provided
Beauty services: Hairdressing, manicures
Mobile library: ✓
Religious services: ✓
Transport: ✓
Activities: *Coordinator:* ✓ • *Examples:* Films, games, knitting
 Outings: ✓
Meetings: ✓

Grey Gables

Manager: Mohamed Haniff
Owner: Mohamed Haniff
Contact: 29 Kennard Road, New Milton, Hampshire BH25 5JR
☏ 01425 610144

Grey Gables is set in a residential area on the outskirts of New Milton, half a mile from the town centre. There is a well-maintained garden to the rear and side of the property for residents to enjoy in better weather. The home arranges reminiscence sessions for the residents, when they have quiet one-to-one time with a carer to reflect. The home is unusual in that as well as catering for the elderly and those with dementia; it also treats those who are dependent on drugs.

Registered places: 24
Guide weekly rate: £400–£550
Specialist care: Dementia
Medical services: Podiatry, optician
Qualified staff: Undisclosed

Home details
Location: Residential area, 0.5 miles from New Milton
Communal areas: Lounge, dining room, garden
Accessibility: *Floors:* 2 • *Access:* Lift • *Wheelchair access:* Good
Smoking: ✗
Pets: ✗
Routines: Flexible

Room details
Single: 24   **Door lock:** ✗
Shared: 0   **Lockable place:** ✓
En suite: 11
Facilities: TV point, telephone point

Services provided
Beauty services: Hairdressing
Mobile library: ✓
Religious services: Monthly church visits
Transport: ✓
Activities: *Coordinator:* ✗ • *Examples:* Arts and craft, music, reminiscence • *Outings:* ✗
Meetings: ✓

Registered places: 9
Guide weekly rate: £390–£474
Specialist care: Residential
Medical services: Podiatry, hygienist, optician, physiotherapy
Qualified staff: Meets standard

Home details

Location: Residential area, 0.5 miles from Lyndhurst
Communal areas: 2 lounges, dining room, garden
Accessibility: *Floors:* 2 • *Access:* Stair lift
   Wheelchair access: Limited
Smoking: ✗
Pets: At manager's discretion
Routines: Flexible

Room details

Single: 8   Door lock: ✓
Shared: 1   Lockable place: ✓
En suite: 9
Facilities: TV point, telephone point

Services provided

Beauty services: Hairdressing
Mobile library: ✗
Religious services: Monthly church service
Transport: ✗
Activities: *Coordinator:* ✗ • *Examples:* Exercises • *Outings:* ✓
Meetings: ✗

Hansa Rest Home

Manager: Vacant
Owner: Peter and Ann Colato
Contact: 9 Empress Road, Lyndhurst, Hampshire SO43 7AE
☎ 023 8028 2298

Hansa Rest Home is a detached house on a quiet residential road close to the centre of Lyndhurst and the new forest. The home is half a mile from the town centre and is run privately by a parent and daughter team. The carers regularly take residents for walks around the village. The home has a computer for residents to keep in touch with residents over email if they wish.

Registered places: 20
Guide weekly rate: £380–£442
Specialist care: Day care, dementia, respite
Medical services: Podiatry, hygienist, optician, physiotherapy
Qualified staff: Meets standard.

Home details

Location: Residential area, 6 miles from Portsmouth
Communal areas: 2 Lounges, 2 dining rooms, patio and 2 gardens
Accessibility: *Floors:* 2 • *Access:* Lift • *Wheelchair access:* Good
Smoking: In designated area
Pets: ✗
Routines: Flexible

Room details

Single: 18   Door lock: ✓
Shared: 1   Lockable place: ✓
En suite: 19
Facilities: TV point, telephone point

Services provided

Beauty services: Hairdressing, aromatherapy, manicures
Mobile library: ✓
Religious services: ✓
Transport: ✗
Activities: *Coordinator:* ✓ • *Examples:* Arts and crafts, exercise, visiting musicians • *Outings:* ✓
Meetings: ✓

The Haven

Manager: T Hall
Owner: S Spencer
Contact: 191 Havant Road, Drayton, Portsmouth, Hampshire PO6 1EE
☎ 023 9237 2356
@ the_haven_resthome@ btopenworld.com

The Haven is set in a quiet residential suburb of Portsmouth, six miles from the town centre. The home organises regular entertainment from visiting musicians and maintains links with the local community. Any resident who wishes to have any religious service from any denomination will be accommodated. The home also arranges outings and there are residents meetings once a month.

Haven Rose Rest Home

Manager: Dionne Campbell
Owner: Haven Rose Rest Home Ltd
Contact: 33 Languard Road, Shirley,
Southampton, Hampshire SO15 5DL
✆ 023 80 322999
@ haven.rose@tiscali.co.uk

Situated in the suburb of Shirley, two and a half miles from Southampton, Haven Rose Rest Home is a home whose philosophy it is to maintain and encourage independence. The home has its own library, with a wide selection of books on different topical areas. There is a large garden with seating at the rear of the property for residents to enjoy, and activities such as bingo and games are organised on a daily basis to keep residents motivated. There is a smoking room for those who choose to smoke, and resident's pets are welcome to come and visit.

Registered places: 16
Guide weekly rate: £327–£388
Specialist care: Dementia, mental disorder
Medical services: Podiatry, dentist, optician
Qualified staff: Meets standard

Home details

Location: Residential area, 2.5 miles from Southampton
Communal areas: Lounge, dining room, smoking room, conservatory, library, garden
Accessibility: *Floors:* 3 • *Access:* Stair lift
 Wheelchair access: Good
Smoking: In designated area
Pets: ✓
Routines: Flexible

Room details

Single: 8
Shared: 4
En suite: 4
Facilities: TV point, telephone point

Door lock: ✓
Lockable place: ✓

Services provided

Beauty services: Hairdressing
Mobile library: Library facilities
Religious services: Every 6 weeks
Transport: ✗
Activities: *Coordinator:* ✗ • *Examples:* Bingo, games, visiting entertainers • *Outings:* ✗
Meetings: ✓

Hazeldene Residential Care Home

Manager: James Hartley
Owner: James Hartley
Contact: 20 Bury Road, Gosport,
Hampshire PO12 3UD
✆ 023 9252 7153

Hazeldene Residential Care Home is approximately one mile from Gosport Town Centre where there are many shops, facilities and public transport links. One of the lounges in the home is allocated as the 'quiet lounge' while the other has a computer with internet access which residents may use. The activities coordinator organises puzzle night, carpet bowls and cream tea afternoons, which is a time for residents to socialise.

Registered places: 26
Guide weekly rate: £385–£415
Specialist care: Dementia, respite
Medical services: Dementia
Qualified staff: Meets standard

Home details

Location: Residential area, 1.2 miles from Gosport
Communal areas: 2 lounges, dining room, computer facilities, conservatory, garden
Accessibility: *Floors:* 2 • *Access:* Lift • *Wheelchair access:* Good
Smoking: ✗
Pets: ✗
Routines: Flexible

Room details

Single: 24
Shared: 1
En suite: 22
Facilities: TV point, telephone point

Door lock: ✗
Lockable place: ✓

Services provided

Beauty services: Hairdressing
Mobile library: ✓
Religious service: Communion service
Transport: ✗
Activities: *Coordinator:* ✓ • *Examples:* Bowls, cream tea, puzzles *Outings:* ✓
Meetings: ✓

Registered places: 31
Guide weekly rate: £350–£850
Specialist care: Nursing, physical disability
Medical services: Podiatry
Qualified staff: Fails standard: 25% at NVQ Level 2

Home details
Location: Rural area, 4 miles from Petersfield
Communal areas: 3 lounges, dining room, conservatory,
    patio and garden
Accessibility: *Floors:* 3 • *Access:* Lift • *Wheelchair access:* Good
Smoking: In designated area
Pets: At manager's discretion
Routines: Flexible

Room details
Single: 21
Shared: 5
En suite: 25
Facilities: TV point, telephone point

Door lock: ✗
Lockable place: ✓

Services provided
Beauty services: Hairdressing
Mobile library: ✗
Religious services: ✗
Transport: Minibus
Activities: *Coordinator:* ✓ • *Examples:* Arts and crafts,
    cream teas, walks • *Outings:* ✓
Meetings: ✓

Heathmount Nursing and Residential Care Home

Manager: Vacant
Owner: Southern Cross Healthcare Ltd
Contact: Rake, Liss, Hampshire GU33 7PG
☏ 01730 894485
@ heathmount@
    ashbournehealthcare.co.uk

Heathmount is a three-storey Victorian building set in 30 acres of its own grounds with views towards the South Downs. The centre is situated four miles from the market town of Petersfield. The gardens are landscaped and offer views of the hills of the South Downs. The activities coordinator often organises cream tea evenings for residents to 'catch-up' with each other, as well as more active activities such as country walks and outings.

Registered places: 34
Guide weekly rate: £319–£473
Specialist care: Respite
Medical services: Podiatry, optician, occupational therapy
Qualified staff: Exceeds standard: 60% at NVQ Level 2

Home details
Location: Rural area, 5 miles from Basingstoke
Communal areas: Lounge, dining room, conservatory,
    patio and garden
Accessibility: *Floors:* 2 • *Access:* Lift • *Wheelchair access:* Good
Smoking: ✗
Pets: At manager's discretion
Routines: Flexible

Room details
Single: 32
Shared: 1
En suite: 28
Facilities: TV point, telephone point

Door lock: ✓
Lockable place: ✓

Services provided
Beauty services: Hairdressing, aromatherapy
Mobile library: ✓
Religious services: Monthly Anglican service,
    Catholic Communion service
Transport: ✗
Activities: *Coordinator:* ✓ • *Examples:* Dancing, gentle exercise,
    reminiscence sessions • *Outings:* ✓
Meetings: ✗

Heatherside Rest Home

Manager: Siobhan Mary Phillips
Owner: Pearl Care Ltd
Contact: Scures Hill, Nately Scures, Basingstoke, Hampshire RG27 9JR
☏ 01256 762233
@ heathersideresthome@tiscali.co.uk

Heatherside is a large, converted Edwardian property set in two acres of well-maintained gardens, which some rooms have views of. The home is in a residential area, in a small village five miles from Basingstoke. Though the monthly religious service is Anglican, the nuns can visit for Catholic Communion service if required. The home organises an activities programme for the residents which includes gentle exercise and reminiscence sessions.

Hillyfield Rest Home

Manager: Jane Harmer-Manning
Owner: Hillyfield Rest Home Ltd
Contact: Barnes Lane, Milford-on-Sea, Lymington, Hampshire SO41 ORP
📞 01590 642121
@ hillyfieldresthome@tesco.net

Hillyfield Rest Home is located in a residential area of Milford-on-Sea within walking distance of the village shops and approximately one mile from the town centre. It has recently added a conservatory onto its lounge, creating a large, light space and a new plasma TV has been purchased. A landscaped garden is found to the rear of the property. Visiting entertainers come to the home on a weekly basis as part of the activities programme. There are also quizzes and outings organised for the residents. The home has its own minibus.

Registered places: 16
Guide weekly rate: £490–£677
Specialist care: Undisclosed
Medical services: Dentist, optician
Qualified staff: Meets standard

Home details
Location: Residential area, 1 mile from Milford–on-Sea
Communal areas: Lounge/conservatory, garden
Accessibility: *Floors:* 2 • *Access:* Lift • *Wheelchair access:* Good
Smoking: ✗
Pets: ✗
Routines: Flexible

Room details
Single: 16
Shared: 0
En suite: 16
Facilities: None

Door lock: ✗
Lockable place: ✓

Services provided
Beauty services: ✗
Mobile library: ✗
Religious services:
Transport: Minibus
Activities: *Coordinator:* ✗ • *Examples:* Quizzes, visiting entertainers *Outings:* ✓
Meetings: Undisclosed

Hollybank Rest Home

Manager: Marilyn Pusey
Owner: Marilyn Pusey
Contact: 41 Winchester Street, Botley, Southampton, Hampshire SO30 2EB
📞 01489 784 144

Hollybank is situated in a village, seven miles from Southampton, with good access to shops, amenities and public transport. The home has a well-tended and accessible garden. The home maintains an open relationship with the residents and they are regularly sent questionnaires to fill out. Though only an Anglican service is held the home can arrange for a Catholic service if requested. The home has a decking area for residents to enjoy in the garden. While there is good wheelchair access it should be noted that some rooms are accessed by a small staircase.

Registered places: 17
Guide weekly rate: £480–£575
Specialist care: Dementia, physical disability, day care, respite
Medical services: Podiatry, dentist, optician
Qualified staff: Exceeds standard: 75% at NVQ Level 2

Home details
Location: Village location, 7 miles from Southampton
Communal areas: Lounge, dining room, library, patio and garden
Accessibility: *Floors:* 2 • *Access:* Lift • *Wheelchair access:* Good
Smoking: In designated area
Pets: At manager's discretion
Routines: Flexible

Room details
Single: 11
Shared: 3
En suite: 2
Facilities: TV point

Door lock: ✓
Lockable place: ✓

Services provided
Beauty services: Hairdressing
Mobile library: ✓
Religious services: Monthly Communion service
Transport: ✗
Activities: *Coordinator:* ✗ • *Examples:* Garden parties, movement to music, reminiscence • *Outings:* ✗
Meetings: ✓

Registered places: 10
Guide weekly rate: £550–£600
Specialist care: Dementia, respite
Medical services: Podiatry, dentist, optician, physiotherapy
Qualified staff: Meets standard

Home details

Location: Village location, 4 miles from Romsey
Communal areas: Lounge, dining room, garden
Accessibility: *Floors:* 2 • *Access:* Stair lift
  Wheelchair access: Good
Smoking: x
Pets: At manager's discretion
Routines: Flexible

Room details

Single: 6
Shared: 2
En suite: 1
Facilities: TV

Door lock: ✓
Lockable place: x

Services provided

Beauty services: Hairdressing
Mobile library: ✓
Religious services: ✓
Transport: x
Activities: *Coordinator:* x • *Examples:* Games, knitting
  Outings: x
Meetings: x

Kents Oak Residential Care Home

Manager: S Burbridge
Owner: Mr and Mrs Burbridge
Contact: Awbridge, Romsey,
Hampshire SO51 0HH
☎ 01794 341 212

This home is set in a small village four miles to the nearest town of Romsey. Due to its small size, the home has a 'family' feel to it and the residents have real independence. The home organises board games for the residents and can arrange religious services. Pets would be allowed at the manager's discretion but smoking is not permitted. The home has a pleasant garden with the possibility of a conservatory being built in the future. There are two floors with a stair lift and the home has good wheelchair access.

Registered places: 20
Guide weekly rate: £450
Specialist care: Dementia
Medical services: Podiatry, dentist, optician
Qualified staff: Meets standard

Home details

Location: Residential area, 1 mile from Fareham
Communal areas: Lounge, dining room, garden
Accessibility: *Floors:* Undisclosed • *Access:* Lift
  Wheelchair access: Good
Smoking: In designated area
Pets: x
Routines: Flexible

Room details

Single: 14
Shared: 3
En suite: 6
Facilities: TV point, telephone point

Door lock: x
Lockable place: ✓

Services provided

Beauty services: Hairdressing
Mobile library: x
Religious services: Monthly church service
Transport: x
Activities: *Coordinator:* x • *Examples:* Bingo, games, movement
  to music • *Outings:* ✓
Meetings: x

Kiln Lodge

Manager: Rosemary Kingdon
Owner: Mark and Steven Cowling
Contact: 66 Kiln Road, Fareham,
Hampshire PO16 7UG
☎ 01329 233808

Situated in a residential area and set back from the main Kiln Road, Kiln Lodge primarily cares for those older individuals with mild to moderate dementia. The staff try to organise activities to keep the residents stimulated such as movement to music and visiting entertainers. The home is one mile Fareham town centre. There is a garden at the rear of the property that residents can enjoy, and there are also caterers who cater for specific dietary requirements.

Kinross Residential Home

Manager: Vacant
Owner: Peter Wride
Contact: 201 Havant Road, Drayton, Portsmouth, Hampshire PO6 1EG
) 023 9238 6934

Kinross Residential Home is situated close to local shops, and opposite a surgery and chemist. It is situated in Cosham, approximately five miles from Portsmouth town centre. Residents enjoy the home's Victorian features and well-established garden, particularly during the summer months. The home offers a range of activities organised by a coordinator, such as quizzes, entertainers, hand massages and exercises. Outings are also arranged for residents.
Registered places: 31

Guide weekly rate: £375–£570
Specialist care: Dementia, mental disorder, physical disability, respite
Medical services: Podiatry, dentist, optician, physiotherapy
Qualified staff: Meets standard

Home details
Location: Residential area, 5 miles from Portsmouth centre
Communal areas: 2 lounges, dining room, conservatory, patio and garden
Accessibility: *Floors:* 3 • *Access:* Lift • *Wheelchair access:* Good
Smoking: ✗
Pets: ✗
Routines: Flexible

Room details
Single: 21
Shared: 5
En suite: 26
Facilities: TV point, telephone point

Door lock: ✓
Lockable place: ✓

Services provided
Beauty services: Hairdressing, manicures, massages
Mobile library: ✓
Religious services: Monthly Anglican service
Transport: ✗
Activities: *Coordinator:* ✓ • *Examples:* Armchair exercises, quizzes, visiting entertainers • *Outings:* ✓
Meetings: ✗

Knellwood

Manager: Janet Gover
Owner: Farnborough Housing Society Ltd
Contact: 83 Canterbury Road, Farnborough, Hampshire GU14 6QN
) 01252 542169
@ knellwood@aol.com
⌂ www.knellwood.co.uk

Knellwood is a large Victorian property, with extensive grounds, situated in Farnborough, with good access to local shops and transport. The home always has a service of remembrance in the main hall, which is attended by civic dignitaries and members of the British Legion. Outings include trips to the theatre and concerts, visiting garden centres, museums and the coast. There are two electric organs and one piano in the lounge, available for anyone to play. Crafts made by the residents, such as soap, cards and rugs are sold at the home's fêtes to fund activities in the home.

Registered places: 52
Guide weekly rate: £380–£442
Specialist care: Dementia, respite
Medical services: Podiatry, physiotherapy
Qualified staff: Exceeds standard: 60% at NVQ Level 2

Home details
Location: Residential area, 1 mile from Farnborough
Communal areas: Lounge, quiet lounge, 2 dining rooms, conservatory, 3 kitchenettes, hairdressing salon, patio and garden
Accessibility: *Floors:* 3 • *Access:* Lift • *Wheelchair access:* Good
Smoking: ✗
Pets: ✗
Routines: Flexible

Room details
Single: 52
Shared: 0
En suite: 52
Facilities: TV point, telephone point

Door lock: ✓
Lockable place: ✓

Services provided
Beauty services: Hairdressing, manicures
Mobile library: ✓
Religious services: Monthly Methodist and Anglican services
Transport: ✗
Activities: *Coordinator:* ✓ • *Examples:* Bingo, crafts, scrabble • *Outings:* ✓
Meetings: ✗

Registered places: 22
Guide weekly rate: £400–£500
Specialist care: Physical disability
Medical services: Podiatry
Qualified staff: Exceeds standard: 88% at NVQ Level 2.

Home details
Location: Residential area, 0.5 miles from Emsworth
Communal areas: Lounge, dining room, conservatory, garden
Accessibility: *Floors:* 2 • *Access:* Lift • *Wheelchair access:* Good
Smoking: ✗
Pets: ✓
Routines: Flexible

Room details
Single: 22
Shared: 0
En suite: 0
Facilities: TV point, telephone point

Door lock: ✗
Lockable place: ✓

Services provided
Beauty services: Hairdressing
Mobile library: ✗
Religious services: Fortnightly Communion service
Transport: ✗
Activities: *Coordinator:* ✓ • *Examples:* Games, puzzles, walks
    Outings: ✓
Meetings: ✓

Lane End House

Manager: Balkrishna Ramaya-Untiah
Owner: Caromar Care Ltd
Contact: Lane End Drive, Emsworth,
Hampshire PO10 7JH
☏ 01243 373046

Lane End House is situated in secluded grounds at the end of a cul-de-sac in a residential area of Emsworth. The home is half a mile from the town centre. The home provides a variety of age-related activities for residents to participate in. Residents have a lot of freedom to organise their own activities such as walks to local shops. The home is also relatively near to the river which the residents often visit on outings. There is also a rear well-kept garden for residents to enjoy with seating and enjoyable views.

Registered places: 3
Guide weekly rate: £575–£650
Specialist care: Nursing, physical disability, terminal care
Medical services: Podiatry, dentist, optician, physiotherapy
Qualified staff: Meets standard

Home details
Location: Residential area, 1.5 miles from Gosport
Communal areas: Lounge, 2 dining rooms, patio and garden
Accessibility: *Floors:* 2 • *Access:* Lift • *Wheelchair access:* Good
Smoking: In designated area
Pets: ✗
Routines: Flexible

Room details
Single: 25
Shared: 5
En suite: 17
Facilities: TV point

Door lock: ✓
Lockable place: ✓

Services provided
Beauty services: Hairdressing
Mobile library: ✓
Religious services: Quarterly Anglican and Catholic services
Transport: ✗
Activities: *Coordinator:* ✓ • *Examples:* Bingo, crafts, quizzes
    Outings: ✓
Meetings: ✓

Langdale Nursing Home

Manager: Rebecca McBride
Owner: Ruby and Bethney-Jane Kelly and Rebecca McBride
Contact: 11 The Avenue, Alverstoke, Gosport, Hampshire PO12 2JS
☏ 023 9258 1754

Langdale Nursing Home has been converted from an old house and is situated in a residential area of Gosport. The home is one and a half miles from the town centre. The home offers a broad range of activities and takes the residents out on trips. The home is also close to local shops and public transport. Quarterly services from the Catholic and Anglican church are arranged for the residents. The home also arranges for a mobile library to visit.

Lansdowne Retirement Home

Manager: Nicola Withers
Owner: Mr and Mrs Withers
Contact: 35 Liphook Road, Lindford, Bordon, Hampshire GU35 0PT
☎ 01420 475448

Lansdowne is situated in the village of Lindford near Borden and close to public transport routes and amenities. The home is one and a half miles from the town centre. The home has a pleasant enclosed garden and provides a friendly atmosphere. Recently a woman celebrated her 100th birthday at Lansdowne, and this was reported in the local newspaper. The home arranges activities on an ad hoc basis allowing residents to choose. Activities have included ball games and there are also organised outings.

Registered places: 17
Guide weekly rate: £379–£650
Specialist care: ✗
Medical services: Podiatry, dentist, optician
Qualified staff: Exceeds standard: 100% at NVQ Level 2

Home details

Location: Village location, 1.5 miles from Bordon
Communal areas: Lounge, dining room, garden
Accessibility: *Floors:* 2 • *Access:* Undisclosed
　　Wheelchair access: Good
Smoking: ✗
Pets: ✗
Routines: Flexible

Room details

Single: 17
Shared: 0
En suite: 17
Facilities: TV point

Door lock: ✓
Lockable place: ✓

Services provided

Beauty services: Hairdressing
Mobile library: Monthly
Religious services: ✗
Transport: ✗
Activities: *Coordinator:* ✓ • *Examples:* Ball games • *Outings:* ✓
Meetings: ✓

Latham Lodge Nursing and Residential Home

Manager: Shaun Morrissey
Owner: Latham Lodge Ltd
Contact: 137–139 Stakes Road, Purbrook, Hampshire PO7 5PD
☎ 023 9225 4175
@ latham@caringhomes.org
🖥 www.caringhomes.org

Latham Lodge is based a 10-minute walk from Purbrook where there is an array of shops and amenities. The home is one and a half miles from Waterlooville. The activities cooordinator develops a weekly recreational programme that provides both mental and social stimulation for residents. Activity programmes include reminiscence games, board games, bingo and crafts. Home cooking and baking, combined with flexible meal times, allows the residents a nutritious diet. The cook prepares home-style meals with the emphasis on choice and personal preferences at the forefront of menu planning.

Registered places: 40
Guide weekly rate: £370–£690
Specialist care: Nursing, physical disability, terminal care
Medical services: Podiatry, dentist, optician, physiotherapy
Qualified staff: Meets standard

Home details

Location: Residential area, 1.5 miles from Waterlooville
Communal areas: 2 lounges, dining room, garden
Accessibility: *Floors:* 2 • *Access:* Lift • *Wheelchair access:* Good
Smoking: ✗
Pets: ✓
Routines: Flexible

Room details

Single: 26
Shared: 7
En suite: 13
Facilities: TV point, telephone point

Door lock: ✗
Lockable place: ✓

Services provided

Beauty services: Hairdressing
Mobile library: ✓
Religious services: Monthly church service
Transport: ✗
Activities: *Coordinator:* ✓ • *Examples:* Bridge, gardening, sewing
　　Outings: ✓
Meetings: ✓

Registered places: 68
Guide weekly rate: £500–£825
Specialist care: Nursing, dementia
Medical services: Podiatry, dentist, optician, physiotherapy
Qualified staff: Meets standard

Home details

Location: Residential area, 1.5 miles from Farnborough
Communal areas: Lounge, dining room, patio
Accessibility: *Floors:* 3 • *Access:* Lift • *Wheelchair access:* Good
Smoking: In designated area
Pets: At manager's discretion
Routines: Flexible

Room details

Single: 68
Shared: 0
En suite: 68
Facilities: TV point

Door lock: ✗
Lockable place: ✓

Services provided

Beauty services: Hairdressing, aromatherapy
Mobile library: ✗
Religious services: Monthly
Transport: ✗
Activities: *Coordinator:* ✓ • *Examples:* Arts and crafts, quizzes, visiting entertainers • *Outings:* ✓
Meetings: ✓

Lavender Lodge Nursing Home

Manager: Joseph Ramtohal
Owner: Southern Cross Healthcare Ltd
Contact: Bruntile Close, Farnborough, Hampshire GU14 6PR
✆ 01252 517569
@ Lavenderlodge@highfield.care.com
🖰 www.schealthcare.co.uk

Situated in a residential area Lavender Lodge Nursing Home is one and a half miles outside the centre of Farnborough. The home has a self-contained dementia unit as well as a separate 'old age' unit. The home offers an aromatherapy treatment on a weekly basis to help residents relax. Activities are run on a weekly basis and the programme includes arts and craft lessons, bingo and quizzes. There are also visiting entertainers that come in on a monthly basis and there are outings once a month to a point of interest in the local area.

Registered places: 9
Guide weekly rate: £385–£387
Specialist care: Dementia, mental disorder
Medical services: Podiatry, dentist, optician, physiotherapy
Qualified staff: Meets standard

Home details

Location: Residential area, 1 mile from Netley
Communal areas: Lounge, dining room, patio and garden
Accessibility: *Floors:* 3 • *Access:* Lift • *Wheelchair access:* Good
Smoking: In designated area
Pets: ✓
Routines: Flexible

Room details

Single: 1
Shared: 4
En suite: 1
Facilities: TV point, telephone point

Door lock: ✓
Lockable place: ✓

Services provided

Beauty services: Hairdressing, manicures
Mobile library: ✗
Religious services: ✗
Transport: ✗
Activities: *Coordinator:* ✗ • *Examples:* Bingo, games,music
Outings: ✓
Meetings: ✗

Leigh Grange

Manager: Patricia Axson
Owner: Patricia Axson
Contact: 21 St Marys Road, Netley Abbey, Southampton, Hampshire SO31 5AU
✆ 023 8045 5812

Leigh Grange is situated in a residential area, one mile from Netley. The home is located close to local amenities such as shops, the library, local pub and to local areas of interest such as Victoria Country Park, Hamble village and the Hamble River. The home happily accepts residents who wish to bring pets with them, and the home itself owns two dogs. Outings are often organised by the staff which can include tea dances and pub lunches.

Linden House

Manager: Mark Baker
Owner: Rita and Mark Baker
Contact: 44–46 Station Road, Sholing, Southampton, Hampshire SO19 8HH
) 023 8044 1472

Linden House benefits from a scenic enclosed garden with ample seating for resident's to enjoy during the warmer months. There are good transport links to the city centre, which offers a range of social, recreational and historical interests. Local health and shopping facilities are equally accessible. The home is located in a residential area, one and a half miles from Southampton. While there is a stair lift providing access to the residents it only reaches the first floor, meaning that wheelchair access is limited.

Registered places: 21
Guide weekly rate: £245–£295
Specialist care: Dementia, mental disorder
Medical services: Podiatry, optician
Qualified staff: Meets standard

Home details
Location: Residential area, 1.5 miles from Southampton
Communal areas: Lounge, dining room, quiet area, conservatory
Accessibility: *Floors:* 3 • *Access:* Stair lift
    Wheelchair access: Limited
Smoking: ✗
Pets: At manager's discretion
Routines: Flexible

Room details
Single: 13
Shared: 4
En suite: 1
Facilities: Telephone point

Door lock: ✗
Lockable place: ✓

Services provided
Beauty services: Hairdressing
Mobile library: ✓
Religious services: ✓
Transport: ✓
Activities: *Coordinator:* ✓ • *Examples:* Ball games, darts, knitting
    Outings: ✗
Meetings: ✓

Little Brook House

Manager: Janet Cooper
Owner: Little Brook House Ltd
Contact: 101 Brook Lane, Warsash, Hampshire SO31 9FE
) 01489 582821
@ team@littlebrookhouse.co.uk
🖰 www.littlebrookhouse.co.uk

Little Brook House is located in the rural area of Warsash, Hampshire. The 300-year-old building was formerly a farmhouse and gets its name from the brook that runs through the grounds of the home. The gardens are landscaped. The home is a listed building and contains a lot of steps. While stair lifts are provided, the home cannot accommodate wheelchair users, as there is no lift. The home has good bus links and arranges a variety of activities such as flower arranging and visits to the forest. There are regular residents meetings and the home has its own library facilities.

Registered places: 20
Guide weekly rate: £550–£675
Specialist care: Nursing, day care, dementia, mental disorder, respite
Medical services: Podiatry, dentist, optician, physiotherapy
Qualified staff: Exceeds standard: 100% at NVQ Level 2

Home details
Location: Rural area, 7 miles from Southampton
Communal areas: Lounge, dining room, 2 conservatories, garden
Accessibility: *Floors:* 2 • *Access:* Stair lift
    Wheelchair access: None
Smoking: In designated area
Pets: At manager's discretion
Routines: Flexible

Room details
Single: 20
Shared: 0
En suite: 20
Facilities: TV

Door lock: ✗
Lockable place: ✓

Services provided
Beauty services: Hairdressing, manicures
Mobile library: Library facilities
Religious services: ✓
Transport: ✗
Activities: *Coordinator:* ✗ • *Examples:* Exercise classes, flower arranging • *Outings:* ✓
Meetings: ✓

Single: 120   Door lock: ✓
Shared: 0   Lockable place: ✗
En suite: 120
Facilities: TV point, telephone point

Registered places: 16
Guide weekly rate: £400
Specialist care: Respite
Medical services: Podiatry, hygienist, optician, physiotherapy
Qualified staff: Exceeds standard: 78% at NVQ Level 2

Home details
Location: Residential area, 3.5 miles from Hayling Island
Communal areas: Lounge/conservatory, quiet lounge, dining room, library, patio and garden
Accessibility: *Floors:* 2 • *Access:* Lift • *Wheelchair access:* Good
Smoking: ✗
Pets: At manager's discretion
Routines: Flexible

Room details
Single: 16
Shared: 0
En suite: 14
Facilities: TV point, telephone point

Door lock: ✓
Lockable place: ✓

Services provided
Beauty services: Hairdressing
Mobile Library: ✓
Religious services: Monthly Communion services
Transport: ✗
Activities: *Coordinator:* ✓ • *Examples:* Art courses, exercise to music, visiting entertainers • *Outings:* ✓
Meetings: ✓

The Wedge

Manager: John Macey
Owner: Monica and John Macey
Contact: 8 Park Road, Hayling Island, Hampshire PO11 0HU
📞 023 9246 5225
@ maceyjoanna@aol.com
🖱 www.thewedgeonhayling.co.uk

The Wedge is a large detached building set in a quiet residential area of Hayling Island. A well-maintained garden has various seating areas for residents to enjoy. This family-owned home, offers many different activities such as arts courses and exercise sessions. Residents are asked through surveys and meetings which activities they would like to take part in. During the week there are visiting pets for the residents to enjoy as well as interesting outings.

Registered places: 46
Guide weekly rate: £430–£630
Specialist care: Dementia, physical disability, palliative care, terminal care
Medical services: Podiatry, hygienist, optician, physiotherapy
Qualified staff: Meets standard

Home details
Location: Rural area, 2 miles from Liss
Communal areas: Lounge, dining room, garden
Accessibility: *Floors:* Undisclosed • *Access:* Lift *Wheelchair access:* Good
Smoking: In designated area
Pets: ✗
Routines: Flexible

Room details
Single: 22
Shared: 12
En suite: 16
Facilities: TV point

Door lock: ✗
Lockable place: ✓

Services provided
Beauty services: Hairdressing, aromatherapy, massage
Mobile library: ✓
Religious services: ✓
Transport: ✓
Activities: *Coordinator:* ✓ • *Examples:* Arts and crafts, bingo, music and movement • *Outings:* ✓
Meetings: ✓

Wenham Holt Nursing and Residential Care Home

Manager: Rosemary Gorvin
Owner: Wenham Holt Homes Ltd
Contact: Hillbrow, Liss, Hampshire GU33 7PB
📞 01730 895125

Wenham Holt is a family-run home situated in a rural area, approximately two miles from Liss. It is purpose built and 16 beds in the home are designated for continuing care. These work in conjunction with the local NHS Primary Care Trust. The large garden with seating areas is in the process of being landscaped and made more accessible to wheelchair users. There is a residents meeting once a month and the home has its own transport for outings.

Wessex Lodge

Manager: Veronica Bovill
Owner: Hestia Care Ltd
Contact: Jobson Close, Newbury Road, Whitchurch, Hampshire RG28 7DX
☎ 01256 895982

Wessex Lodge is located half a mile from the village of Whitchurch. The residents have an extensive choice of entertainment, including excursions such as pub lunches and shopping trips. There are also a lot of daily activities based inside the home such as arts and crafts, bingo, movement to music and bridge. There is a garden with seating and level access for residents to sit outside and socialise with other residents, or take their visitors for a slice of tea and cake.

Registered places: 40
Guide weekly rate: £520–£850
Specialist care: Nursing, dementia
Medical services: Podiatry, optician
Qualified staff: Meets standard

Home details
Location: Residential area, 0.5 miles from Whitchurch
Communal areas: 3 lounges, dining room, patio and garden
Accessibility: *Floors:* 3 • *Access:* Lift • *Wheelchair access:* Good
Smoking: In designated area
Pets: ✗
Routines: Flexible

Room details
Single: 40	**Door lock:** ✓
Shared: 0	**Lockable place:** ✓
En suite: 40	

Facilities: TV point, telephone point

Services provided
Beauty services: Hairdressing, aromatherapy
Mobile library: ✓
Religious services: Monthly church service
Transport: ✗
Activities: *Coordinator:* ✓ • *Examples:* Arts and crafts, games, music and movement • *Outings:* ✓
Meetings: ✗

Westacre Nursing Home

Manager: Polly Foxwell
Owner: Nursing Home Services ltd
Contact: Sleepers Hill, Winchester, Hampshire SO22 4NE
☎ 01962 855188
@ watson.sue@btconnect.com

Westacre Nursing Home is located in a quiet residential area, close to the centre of Winchester. The home has a large garden, which residents can enjoy safely. The home has a total of six communal areas, and ample space for residents to sit quietly. There are two activities coordinators who create weekly activities, such as art groups and flower arranging. The daily routine is structured, with room for residents' choice.

Registered places: 53
Guide weekly rate: £800–£900
Specialist care: Nursing, dementia
Medical services: Podiatry, dentist, optician, physiotherapy
Qualified staff: Meets standard

Home details
Location: Residential area, 2 miles from Winchester
Communal areas: 2 lounges, 1 dining room, conservatory, quiet room, patio and garden
Accessibility: *Floors:* 3 • *Access:* 2 lifts • *Wheelchair access:* Good
Smoking: ✗
Pets: ✗
Routines: Structured

Room details
Single: 47	**Door lock:** ✓
Shared: 3	**Lockable place:** ✓
En suite: 50	

Facilities: TV, telephone

Services provided
Beauty services: Hairdressing
Mobile library: ✓
Religious services: Monthly Communion
Transport: ✗
Activities: *Coordinator:* ✓ • *Examples:* Art groups, flower arranging, movement to music • *Outings:* ✗
Meetings: ✗

Registered places: 33
Guide weekly rate: £327–£560
Specialist care: Day care, dementia, respite
Medical services: Podiatry, dentist, optician, massage
Qualified staff: Exceeds standard: 86% at NVQ Level 2

Home details

Location: Rural area, 6 miles from Alton
Communal areas: Lounge, quiet lounge/dining room,
  dining room, conservatory
Accessibility: *Floors:* 2 • *Access:* Lift and stair lift
  Wheelchair access: Good
Smoking: In designated area
Pets: At manager's discretion
Routines: Flexible

Room details

Single: 33
Shared: 0
En suite: 33
Facilities: TV point, telephone point

Door lock: ✓
Lockable place: ✓

Services provided

Beauty services: Hairdressing, beautician, therapeutic massage
Mobile library: ✓
Religious services: Monthly Anglican and Catholic service
Transport: ✗
Activities: *Coordinator:* ✓ • *Examples:* Dancing, exercise, games
  Outings: ✓
Meetings: ✗

Westlands House

Manager: Lesley Tagima
Owner: Lesley Tagima and Anthony Daly
Contact: Headmoor Lane, Alton,
Hampshire GU34 3EP
☎ 01420 588 412

Westlands Home is a family-run home, located in a rural area six miles from Alton. The home offers a range of activities with massage and manicures on a regular basis as well as dancing, exercise and classic board games. The home also has a regular wine tasting evening and a tuck shop. There are also outings arranged including visiting a farm and going on country walks. Home-cooked food is freshly prepared on site with a nutritious menu for residents to choose from.

Registered places: 42
Guide weekly rate: £530–£762
Specialist care: Dementia, day care, mental disorder, respite
Medical services: Podiatry, hygienist, optician, physiotherapy
Qualified staff: Exceeds standard: 80% at NVQ Level 2

Home details

Location: Rural area, 7.5 miles from Southampton
Communal areas: 10 lounges/dining rooms, courtyard garden
Accessibility: *Floors:* 2 • *Access:* Lift • *Wheelchair access:* Good
Smoking: In designated area
Pets: ✓
Routines: Flexible

Room details

Single: 36
Shared: 3
En suite: 25
Facilities: ✗

Door lock: ✓
Lockable place: ✓

Services provided

Beauty services: Hairdressing
Mobile library: ✗
Religious services: Monthly Anglican service
Transport: Minibus
Activities: *Coordinator:* ✓ • *Examples:* Visiting entertainers
  Outings: ✓
Meetings: ✗

The White House Residential Home

Manager: Emma Hampton
Owner: The White House Ltd
Contact: Vicarage Lane, Curdridge,
Hampshire SO32 2DP
☎ 01489 786 633
@ julietwh@aol.com
🖰 www.whitehouseresidential
  home.co.uk

The White House is located in 18 acres of land, in a rural setting, seven and a half miles from Southampton. Their extensive gardens are home to animals such as pot-bellied pigs, pygmy goats, wallabies and peacocks. In the past, residents have been on trips to the local pub, a mystery tour, the seaside the New Forest and garden centres. There is ample communal space and three activities coordinators who entertain the residents.

White Lodge Rest Home

Manager: Michael Foot
Owner: Michael Foot
Contact: 79–83 Alma Road,
Portswood, Southampton, Hampshire
SO14 6UQ

☎ 023 8055 4478

@ oakmountresidentialhome@
hotmail.com

🖱 www.whiteoakcare.com

Whitelodge is located close to Southampton, less than one mile from Portswood. There is a garden and patio area accessible to residents at the back of the home. The home has two floors with a lift but cannot cater for wheelchair users. The home arranges activities which include arts and crafts every fortnight, chair exercises and visiting entertainers. The residents have a flexible daily routine with set meal times. The home has its own transport and also arranges regular religious services.

Registered places: 28
Guide weekly rate: £359–£410
Specialist care: Dementia, mental disorder
Medical services: Podiatry, dentist, optician
Qualified staff: Meets standard

Home details

Location: Residential area, 0.5 miles from Portswood
Communal areas: 2 lounges, 2 dining rooms, conservatory, patio and garden
Accessibility: Floors: 2 • Access: Stair lift
    Wheelchair access: None
Smoking: Allowed in designated area
Pets: At manager's discretion
Routines: Flexible

Room details

Single: 20
Shared: 4
En suite: 2
Facilities: TV, telephone

Door lock: ✓
Lockable place: ✓

Services provided

Beauty services: Hairdressing, manicures
Mobile library: ✓
Religious services: ✓
Transport: ✓
Activities: Coordinator: ✗ • Examples: Arts and crafts, bingo, chair exercises, quizzes • Outings: ✗
Meetings: ✗

Whitegates Care Home

Manager: Kay Chapman
Owner: Jean and Adele Dubois
Contact: Gravel Lane, Ringwood,
Hampshire BH24 1LL

☎ 01425 472302

@ jean_jacquesdubois@btconnect.com

Whitegates is situated in a quiet residential area, half a mile from Ringwood town centre. At the home fluent French is spoken to cater for any French residents, which brings a multi-cultural feel to the home. The residents are encouraged to take part in light exercise classes to keep them agile. The home also organises visiting entertainers to come in once a month and this includes singers, actors and historians. There is a garden at the rear of the home for the residents to enjoy, most parts with level access.

Registered places: 21
Guide weekly rate: £544–£650
Specialist care: Physical disability
Medical services: Podiatry, dentist, optician
Qualified staff: Exceeds standard: 69% at NVQ Level 2

Home details

Location: Residential area, 0.5 miles from Ringwood
Communal areas: 3 lounges, dining room, garden
Accessibility: Floors: 2 • Access: Lift • Wheelchair access: Good
Smoking: ✗
Pets: ✗
Routines: Flexible

Room details

Single: 21
Shared: 0
En suite: 5
Facilities: TV point, telephone point

Door lock: ✗
Lockable place: ✓

Services provided

Beauty services: Hairdressing
Mobile library: ✓
Religious services: Monthly church service
Transport: ✗
Activities: Coordinator: ✗ • Examples: Crafts, exercise classes, quizzes • Outings: ✗
Meetings: ✓

Registered places: 25
Guide weekly rate: £375–£450
Specialist care: Respite
Medical services: Podiatry, dentist, optician
Qualified staff: Exceeds standard: 75% at NVQ Level 2

Home details

Location: Residential area, 1 mile from Fareham
Communal areas: 2 lounges, dining room, conservatory, garden
Accessibility: *Floors:* 2 • *Access:* Lift • *Wheelchair access:* None
Smoking: ✗
Pets: ✗
Routines: Flexible

Room details

Single: 15
Shared: 5
En suite: 20
Facilities: TV point, telephone point

Door lock: ✓
Lockable place: ✓

Services provided

Beauty services: Hairdressing
Mobile library: ✓
Religious services: Visiting Anglican minister
Transport: Car
Activities: *Coordinator:* ✓ • *Examples:* Arts and crafts, singalongs, music for health • *Outings:* ✓
Meetings: ✗

Whiteoaks

Manager: Mrs Panchalingathurai
Owner: Mr and Mrs Panchalingathurai
Contact: 56–58 The Avenue, Fareham, Hampshire PO14 1NZ
☎ 01329 232860

Whiteoaks is a large detached property in Fareham, one mile from the town centre. There is ample space for residents to sit in communal areas, as well as a smaller upstairs lounge which residents can request to sit privately if they wish. A range of activities and outings are offered, including a Valentines Day dinner, countryside trips and visits to beaches. There are also in house singalongs and arts and crafts. Barbecues and visiting entertainment take place regularly.

Registered places: 18
Guide weekly rate: £450
Specialist care: Day care, dementia, respite
Medical services: Podiatry
Qualified staff: Exceeds standard: 100% at NVQ Level 2

Home details

Location: Residential area, 1 mile from Farnborough
Communal areas: 2 lounges, dining room, garden
Accessibility: *Floors:* 2 • *Access:* Lift • *Wheelchair access:* Good
Smoking: ✗
Pets: At manager's discretion
Routines: Flexible

Room details

Single: 10
Shared: 4
En suite: 0
Facilities: TV point

Door lock: ✓
Lockable place: ✓

Services provided

Beauty services: Hairdressing
Mobile library: Library facilities
Religious services: Monthly Catholic and Anglican Communion service
Transport: ✗
Activities: *Coordinator:* ✗ • *Examples:* Bingo, games, visiting entertainers • *Outings:* ✓
Meetings: ✓

Willow House

Manager: Lynne Cotterell
Owner: Willow Residential Care Ltd
Contact: 2 Reading Road, Farnborough, Hampshire GU14 6NA
☎ 01252 522596
@ lynnecotterell@talktalk.net

Willow House is a family run home situated in a residential area. The home has two lounges, one of which is a quiet room. The home also has a new entertainment system for residents. There is also a dining room and a garden for residents to relax in. The home arranges religious services as well as visiting entertainers to come to the home on a monthly basis. There are daily activities held in the home such as bingo and games.

Winton Nursing Home

Manager: Elaine Phelps
Owner: Evelyn Cornelius-Reid
Contact: Wallop House, Nether Wallop,
Nr Salisbury, Hampshire
SO20 8HE
☎ 01264 781366

Set in the village of Nether Wallop, Winton Nursing Home is within easy reach of local amenities at Stockbridge and Andover. Residents enjoy a regularly changing menu for meals that accommodate their own preferences. An activities coordinator also organises daily entertainment such as music nights, exercise lessons and games night. There are monthly visits from the church choir who sing live for the residents, and there are also seasonal pantomime visits. The house is set in gardens, which are well maintained and stretch over two acres. If residents are interested, they are welcome to take part in gardening activities.

Registered places: 45
Guide weekly rate: £525–£850
Specialist care: Nursing, dementia, respite
Medical services: Podiatry, optician, physiotherapy
Qualified staff: Fails standard: 33% at NVQ Level 2

Home details
Location: Village location, 4 miles from Stockbridge
Communal areas: Lounges, dining room, garden
Accessibility: *Floors:* 2 • *Access:* Lift and stair lift
Wheelchair access: Good
Smoking: ✗
Pets: ✗
Routines: Flexible

Room details
Single: 35
Shared: 5
En suite: 40
Facilities: TV point, telephone point
Door lock: ✗
Lockable place: ✓

Services provided
Beauty services: Hairdressing
Library: ✓
Religious services: Fortnightly church service
Transport: ✗
Activities: *Coordinator:* ✓ • *Examples:* Music and movement, plays
Outings: ✗
Meetings: ✓

Wisteria Lodge Residential Home

Manager: Rosa White
Owner: Rosa White
Contact: 82 London Road, Horndean,
Hampshire PO8 0BU
☎ 023 9259 8074
@ info@wisterialodge.co.uk
🖥 www.wisterialodge.co.uk

Wisteria Lodge is a family-run home and aims to fulfil all the residents' needs and wishes. There are frequently organised outings and in house entertainment. There are ample communal facilities, with a TV lounge, quiet lounge, conservatory, dining room and a large courtyard area outside for residents to sit outside in comfort, as well as walking in the terraced garden. The home also organises Anglican services once a month.

Registered places: 19
Guide weekly rate: Undisclosed
Specialist care: Day care, dementia, mental disorder, respite
Medical services: Podiatry, dentist, optician, physiotherapy, speech therapy
Qualified staff: Exceeds standard: 85% at NVQ Level 2

Home details
Location: village location, 3.5 miles from Waterlooville
Communal areas: Lounge, quiet lounge, dining room, conservatory, patio and garden
Accessibility: *Floors:* 2 • *Access:* Stair lift
Wheelchair access: Good
Smoking: ✗
Pets: At manager's discretion
Routines: Flexible

Room details
Single: 15
Shared: 2
En suite: 14
Facilities: TV point, telephone point
Door lock: ✓
Lockable place: ✓

Services provided
Beauty services: Hairdressing
Mobile library:
Religious services: Monthly Anglican and Catholic service.
Transport: Car
Activities: *Coordinator:* ✓ • *Examples:* Arts and crafts, exercise to music, summer parties • *Outings:* ✓
Meetings: ✗

Registered places: 40
Guide weekly rate: £432–£600
Specialist care: Dementia, respite
Medical services: Podiatry, dentist, optician
Qualified staff: Meets standard

Home details

Location: Rural area, 3 miles from Totton
Communal areas: 2 lounges, 2 dining rooms, library,
    garden room, garden
Accessibility: *Floors:* 2 • *Access:* Undisclosed
    Wheelchair access: Undisclosed
Smoking: ✗
Pets: At manager's discretion
Routines: Flexible

Room details

Single: 32
Shared: 2
En suite: 34
Facilities: TV point, telephone point

Door lock: ✗
Lockable place: ✓

Services provided

Beauty services: Hairdressing, manicures
Mobile library: ✗
Religious services: ✗
Transport: ✗
Activities: *Coordinator:* ✓ • *Examples:* Arts and crafts,
    flower arranging, film afternoons • *Outings:* ✓
Meetings: ✓

Woodlands House

Manager: Terry Whayman
Owner: H W Group Ltd
Contact: 205 Woodlands Road,
Woodlands, Southampton, Hampshire
SO40 7GL
☎ 023 8029 2213
@ woodlands@compuserve.co.uk

Woodlands House is a detached property, set in extensive grounds on the edge of the New Forest. The home is three miles from Totton town centre. The grounds of the home are ideal for residents to take walks in and provide views from the house. Activities in the home include a summer barbecue, a concert, a footwear sale, and outings to a local tea dance and bowls club. The home can facilitate private family get-togethers and meals in the library for special events.

Registered places: 24
Guide weekly rate: £603–£767
Specialist care: Nursing, physical disability, respite
Medical services: Podiatry, optician, hygienist, physiotherapy
Qualified staff: Exceeds standard: 80% at NVQ Level 2

Home details

Location: Rural area, 7 miles from Southampton
Communal areas: Lounge, dining room, garden
Accessibility: *Floors:* 2 • *Access:* Lift • *Wheelchair access:* Good
Smoking: In designated area
Pets: ✗
Routines: Flexible

Room details

Single: 19
Shared: 5
En suite: Undisclosed
Facilities: TV point, telephone point

Door lock: ✓
Lockable place: ✓

Services provided

Beauty services: Hairdressing
Mobile library services: ✓
Religious services: ✓
Transport: ✗
Activities: *Coordinator:* ✗ • *Examples:* Bingo, cards, quizzes
    Outings: ✓
Meetings: ✓

Woodlands Ridge Nursing Home

Manager: Julie Sutherland
Owner: Contemplation Homes Ltd
Contact: 191 Woodlands Road,
Woodlands, Southampton, Hampshire
SO40 7GL
☎ 023 8029 2475
@ woodlandsridge@
    contemplation-homes.co.uk
🖥 www.contemplation-homes.co.uk

Situated in Woodlands on the outskirts of Southampton city, Woodlands Ridge Nursing Home benefits from easy access to the New Forest. Residents have the opportunity to participate in daily activities, such as bingo, quizzes and playing cards. The home caters for personal trips for residents who wish to make shopping trips or visit certain events. The home arranges regular religious services and there is a residents meeting once a month.

Woodpeckers Nursing and Residential Home

Manager: Jacqueline Reddell
Owner: Colten Care Ltd
Contact: Sway Road, Brockenhurst, Hampshire SO42 7RX

☎ 01590 623280
@ woodpeckers@coltencare.co.uk
🖰 www.coltoncare.co.uk

Originally a very large farmhouse, Woodpeckers is located in Brockenhurst, a large village in the centre of the New Forest. The town of Lymington is six miles away, and it is four miles to Lyndhurst. The garden has several patio areas and a path that is wheelchair accessible. As well as an activities coordinator, who organises a wide variety of activities, the home employs a social carer, who spends time individually with residents. There is a residents meeting held every three months.

Registered places: 41
Guide weekly rate: £580–£900
Specialist care: Nursing, dementia, physical disability, respite, terminal care
Medical services: Podiatry, physiotherapy, dentist, optician
Qualified staff: Meets standard

Home details

Location: Rural area, 0.5 miles from Brockenhurst
Communal areas: 3 lounges, dining room, patio and garden
Accessibility: *Floors:* 3 • *Access:* 2 lifts • *Wheelchair access:* Good
Smoking: x
Pets: x
Routines: Flexible

Room details

Single: 37
Shared: 2
En suite: 32
Facilities: TV, telephone point

Door lock: ✓
Lockable place: ✓

Services provided

Beauty services: Hairdressing
Mobile library: ✓
Religious services: Monthly Communion service
Transport: Shared minibus
Activities: *Coordinator:* ✓ • *Examples:* Arts and crafts, painting, quizzes • *Outings:* ✓
Meetings: ✓

Registered places: 12
Guide weekly rate: £350–£450
Specialist care: Day care, dementia, physical disability, respite
Medical services: Podiatry, dentist, optician, physiotherapy
Qualified staff: Exceeds standard: 60% at NVQ Level 2

Home details

Location: Residential area, in Shanklin
Communal areas: Dining room, lounge, garden
Accessibility: *Floors:* 2 • *Access:* Stair lift
    Wheelchair access: Limited
Smoking: ✗
Pets: ✗
Routines: Flexible

Room details

Single: 10
Shared: 2
En suite: 1
Facilities: TV point, telephone point

Door lock: ✓
Lockable place: ✓

Services provided

Beauty services: Hairdressing, beautician
Mobile library: ✗
Religious services: ✗
Transport:
Activities: *Coordinator:* ✓ • *Examples:* Arts and crafts, games,
    music, quizzes • *Outings:* ✓
Meetings: ✓

Acacia

Manager: Georgina Doughty
Owner: Jeremy and Georgina Doughty
Contact: 1 Arthurs Hill, Shanklin,
Isle of Wight PO37 6EW
☎ 01983 863845
@ ninadoughty@aol.com

Acacia is a large two-storey Edwardian House close to the centre of Shanklin town. Shops and amenities are only a few minutes' walk away. Tree-lined gardens surround the home, and there is a gazebo for residents to sit comfortably in. A hairdresser, beautician and independent entertainer all visit the home on a regular basis. Age Concern also comes in to take residents out on organised trips. Activities in the home include games, memory club and quizzes.

Registered places: 50
Guide weekly rate: £435–£525
Specialist care: Physical disability, respite
Medical services: Podiatry, dentist, optician
Qualified staff: Exceeds standard: 56% at NVQ Level 2

Home details

Location: Village location, 1.5 miles from Newport centre
Communal areas: 5 lounges, dining room, conservatory, library,
    patio and garden
Accessibility: *Floors:* 3 • *Access:* Lift • *Wheelchair access:* Good
Smoking: ✗
Pets: ✗
Routines: Flexible

Room details

Single: 50
Shared: 0
En suite: 50
Facilities: TV point, telephone point

Door lock: ✓
Lockable place: ✓

Services provided

Beauty services: Hairdressing
Mobile library: ✓
Religious services: Monthly Anglican visits
Transport: ✗
Activities: *Coordinator:* ✓ • *Examples:* Bingo, crafts, music,
    quizzes • *Outings:* ✓
Meetings: ✓

Blackwater Mill

Manager: Patricia Flux
Owner: Richard Key
Contact: Blackwater, Newport,
Isle of Wight PO30 3BJ
☎ 01983 520539
@ admin@blackwatermill.co.uk
⌂ www.blackwatermill.co.uk

As its name suggests, Blackwater Mill is an old mill house; a substantial property set in approximately five acres of land. Close to a large lake which is home to ducks and wildlife, the home permits attractive views for the many residents whose bedrooms which overlook it. The residential home is located in rural Blackwater just short of two miles from Newport town centre where there are shops and other amenities. The closet shop is approximately one mile away though the home also offers a weekly residents' shop. A comprehensive activities programme includes fêtes and barbecues in the summer.

Brighstone Grange

Manager: Wendy Dickson
Owner: Brighstone Care Ltd
Contact: Brighstone Grange,
Brighstone, Isle of Wight PO30 4DZ

☎ 01983 740236
@ Wendydickson_bcl@hotmail.com
🖰 www.brighstonegrange.co.uk

Brighstone Grange is large country house, set within its own substantial grounds with beautiful views over the English Channel. It is near to the village of Brighstone and is seven miles from Totland town. Activities, birthdays and festive events are programmed monthly, which include a bonfire and firework party, fully available for residents to view inside and as well as out. The home also offers to take residents out or to go shopping on a one-to-one basis which allows a more personal level of social interaction to take place.

Registered places: 23
Guide weekly rate: £420–£450
Specialist care: Dementia, respite
Medical services: Podiatry
Qualified staff: Exceeds standard

Home details
Location: Rural area, 7 miles from Totland
Communal areas: Lounge, dining room, patio and garden
Accessibility: *Floors:* 3 • *Access:* Stair lift
  Wheelchair access: Good
Smoking: ✗
Pets: ✓
Routines: Flexible

Room details
Single: 18	**Door lock:** ✓
Shared: 2	**Lockable place:** ✓
En suite: 15	

Facilities: TV point, telephone point

Services provided
Beauty services: Hairdressing
Mobile library: ✗
Religious services: ✓
Transport: ✓
Activities: *Coordinator:* ✗ • *Examples:* Gentle exercise, reminiscence, singalongs • *Outings:* ✓
Meetings: ✓

Capri

Manager: Christine Basham
Owner: Isle of Wight Care Ltd
Contact: 48 St Johns Road, Sandown,
Isle of Wight PO36 8HE

☎ 01983 402314

Capri care home is a small care home where staff accommodation is built into the property and located on the third floor. A five-minute walk from the seafront, Capri is situated in a very picturesque location with views across the channel. It is situated a five-minute stroll to local shops and is close to Sandown high street where there are all necessary amenities. There is also a garden for residents to enjoy, and those who enjoy gardening and are mobile are encouraged to help maintain the garden.

Registered places: 9
Guide weekly rate: £230–£260
Specialist care: Dementia
Medical services: Podiatry, optician, physiotherapy
Qualified staff: Fails standards

Home details
Location: Residential area, in Sandown
Communal areas: Lounge, dining room, garden
Accessibility: *Floors:* 2 • *Access:* Stair lift
  Wheelchair access: Limited
Smoking: ✗
Pets: At manager's discretion
Routines: Flexible

Room details
Single: 7	**Door lock:** ✗
Shared: 1	**Lockable place:** ✓
En suite: 6	

Facilities: TV point, telephone point

Services provided
Beauty services: Hairdressing
Mobile library: ✗
Religious services: ✓
Transport: ✓
Activities: *Coordinator:* ✗ • *Examples:* Games, quizzes, walks *Outings:* ✓
Meetings: ✓

Registered places: 35
Guide weekly rate: £366–£460
Specialist care: Day care, mental disorder, respite
Medical services: Podiatry, dentist, optician, physiotherapy
Qualified staff: Exceeds standard: 68% at NVQ Level 2

Home details

Location: Residential area, 0.5 miles from Cowes centre
Communal areas: Dining room, lounge, patio and garden
Accessibility: *Floors:* 2 • *Access:* Lift • *Wheelchair access:* Good
Smoking: In designated area
Pets: At manager's discretion
Routines: Flexible

Room details

Single: 35
Shared: 0
En suite: 33
Facilities: TV

Door lock: ✓
Lockable place: ✓

Services provided

Beauty services: Hairdressing
Mobile library: ✗
Religious services: Monthly visit from priest
Transport: Car
Activities: *Coordinator:* ✓ • *Examples:* Bell ringing, exercises, singalongs • *Outings:* ✓
Meetings: ✓

Cherry Blossom

Manager: Judith Dawkins
Owner: Islandcare Ltd
Contact: 252–257 Arctic Road, Cowes, Isle of Wight PO31 7PJ
☎ 01983 293849

Cherry Blossom care home overlooks the River Medina, half a mile from Cowes town centre. It consists of a large two-storey purpose-built building and an older property, which has been incorporated. In the town centre, which is only half a mile away, there are shops, ferry and bus terminals. An external company, Independent Arts, provides the entertainment and this includes visiting entertainers. There are outings such as a trip to Haven Street, a steam railway. The staff aim to create a friendly and caring environment for residents and visiting relatives to enjoy.

Registered places: 25
Guide weekly rate: From £420
Specialist care: Mental disorder, physical disability
Medical services: Podiatry, optician
Qualified staff: Meets standard

Home details

Location: Residential area, 0.5 miles from Cowes centre
Communal areas: Lounge, lounge/dining room, garden
Accessibility: *Floors:* 2 • *Access:* Lift • *Wheelchair access:* Limited
Smoking: In designated area
Pets: ✓
Routines: Flexible

Room details

Single: 25
Shared: 0
En suite: 21
Facilities: Telephone point

Door lock: ✓
Lockable place: ✓

Services provided

Beauty services: Hairdressing
Mobile library: Library facilities
Religious services: Monthly visit from Anglican
Transport: Car
Activities: *Coordinator:* ✗ • *Examples:* Exercise, games, musical performers • *Outings:* ✓
Meetings: ✓

Cherry Trees Care Home

Manager: Shirley Carley
Owner: Mr and Mrs Gustar
Contact: 149 Park Road, Cowes, Isle of Wight PO31 7NQ
☎ 01983 299731

Cherry Trees is within 10 minutes' walking distance of Cowes centre and the Southampton Red Jet, which is very useful for visitors. There is also a regular bus service from outside the home for the less able. It is set within its own gardens and erects a gazebo in the summer for residents to enjoy the outdoors. Set on two floors, each has its own communal room with TV which double as a dining room. Cherry Trees provides care for the physically disabled and elderly suffering from mental disorders besides dementia. It prides itself on its friendly atmosphere, regarding the atmosphere as a 'family' home.

Cornelia Heights

Manager: Marion Hilton
Owner: Bryn Jones and Stephen Geach
Contact: 93 George Street, Ryde,
Isle of Wight PO33 2JE
) 01983 567265

Cornelia Heights is in the centre of Ryde town, close to shops and next door to the library in a Grade II listed building. The home has good links with the local community, organising summer fêtes, bonfire nights and Christmas parties. Activities are organised by a designated coordinator and there are fortnightly outings. The garden is not accessible for those with mobility problems without the help of a member of staff.

Registered places: 23
Guide weekly rate: £365–£495
Specialist care: Dementia, physical disability, respite
Medical services: Podiatry, dentist, optician
Qualified staff: Fails standard: 40% at NVQ Level 2

Home details
Location: Residential area, in Ryde
Communal areas: 2 lounges, dining room, garden
Accessibility: *Floors:* 2 • *Access:* Lift and stair lift
 Wheelchair access: Good
Smoking: In designated area
Pets: ✗
Routines: Flexible

Room details
Single: 19 | **Door lock:** ✓
Shared: 2 | **Lockable place:** ✓
En suite: 12
Facilities: TV point, telephone point

Services provided
Beauty services: Hairdressing
Mobile library: Library facilities
Religious services: Weekly Catholic visits, fortnightly Anglican visits
Transport: ✗
Activities: *Coordinator:* ✓ • *Examples:* Bingo, exercise to music, skittles • *Outings:* ✓
Meetings: ✓

Cornelia Manor

Manager: Robert Francey
Owner: Bryn Jones and Stephen Geach
Contact: 60 Watergate Road, Newport,
Isle of Wight PO30 1XP
) 01983 522964

Cornelia Manor is a detached period residence situated in a quiet residential area on the outskirts of Newport. Residents have access to a well-tended garden at the front of the property that is enjoyed in the warmer seasons. An activities programme is displayed around the home. External entertainers visit the home around twice weekly. The home provides residents with supported access to external activities, for example, visits to town for shopping or coffee. Flexible daily routines allow residents to partake in activities of their own choice, and are not obliged to participate in the home's activities.

Registered places: 34
Guide weekly rate: £429–£495
Specialist care: Day care, dementia, physical disability
Medical services: Podiatry, hygienist, optician, physiotherapy
Qualified staff: Fails standards

Home details
Location: Residential area, 0.5 miles from Newport centre
Communal areas: 2 lounges, dining room, garden
Accessibility: *Floors:* 2 • *Access:* Lift • *Wheelchair access:* Good
Smoking: ✗
Pets: ✗
Routines: Flexible

Room details
Single: 34 | **Door lock:** ✓
Shared: 0 | **Lockable place:** ✓
En suite: 34
Facilities: TV point, telephone point

Services provided
Beauty services: Hairdressing
Mobile library: ✗
Religious services: Monthly Communion service
Transport: ✗
Activities: *Coordinator:* ✗ • *Examples:* Arts and crafts, entertainers, singalongs • *Outings:* ✓
Meetings: ✓

Registered places: 48
Guide weekly rate: Undisclosed
Specialist care: Nursing, dementia, physical disability, terminal care
Medical services: Podiatry, physiotherapy
Qualified staff: Exceeds standard: 61% at NVQ Level 2

Home details

Location: Residential area, in Bembridge
Communal areas: 2 lounges, dining room conservatory, patio and garden
Accessibility: *Floors:* 3 • *Access:* Lift • *Wheelchair access:* Good
Smoking: In designated area.
Pets: ✗
Routines: Flexible

Room details

Single: 48
Shared: 0
En suite: 48
Facilities: TV point, telephone point

Door lock: ✓
Lockable place: ✓

Services provided

Beauty services: Hairdressing, aromatherapy, manicures
Mobile library: ✗
Religious services: ✓
Transport: Minibus
Activities: *Coordinator:* ✗ • *Examples:* Games, poetry readings, visiting entertainers • *Outings:* ✓
Meetings: ✗

The Elms Nursing Home

Manager: Elizabeth Pearson
Owner: Scio Healthcare Ltd
Contact: Swains Road, Bembridge, Isle of Wight PO35 5XS
) 01983 872248
@ info@sciohealthcare.co.uk
www.sciohealthcare.co.uk

The Elms is within walking distance of Bembridge in a quiet area with good transport links: the ferry port from Portsmouth is only seven miles away. Local shops and amenities are nearby as is the beach. The home has a landscaped garden with a fountain and a conservatory. The home has its own minibus and there are a range of activities going on for both individuals and groups. Pets are allowed to visit and the home arranges outings to the seafront and local garden centres. There are two lounges: one quiet room and one TV room.

Registered places: 21
Guide weekly rate: £362–£422
Specialist care: Dementia, respite, physical disability
Medical services: Podiatry, optician
Qualified staff: Exceeds standard: 96% at NVQ Level 2

Home details

Location: Residential area, in Oakfield
Communal areas: Lounge, dining room, garden
Accessibility: *Floors:* 3 • *Access:* Lift • *Wheelchair access:* Good
Smoking: In designated area
Pets: At manger's discretion
Routines: Flexible

Room details

Single: 21
Shared: 0
En suite: 1
Facilities: TV point

Door lock: ✗
Lockable place: ✓

Services provided

Beauty services: Hairdressing
Mobile library: ✓
Religious services: Monthly church service
Transport: ✓
Activities: *Coordinator:* ✓ • *Examples:* Films, quizzes, singalongs • *Outings:* ✓
Meetings: ✓

Fallowfield

Manager: Carol Montague
Owner: Keith and Jennifer Betteley
Contact: 14 Great Preston Road, Ryde, Isle of Wight PO33 1DR
) 01983 611531

Formerly a Victoria residence, Fallowfield has been converted to provide care services for the frail, those suffering from dementia or those with a physical disability. There is wheelchair access throughout. The home is located in a residential area of Ryde, with no near local shops, however Ryde train station is a short walk from the home. A range of activities are provided on a weekly basis including shopping trips, singalongs and outings. The coordinators try and arrange the activities to suit the residents in the home at the time, to keep them interested and stimulated. There is a large garden for residents to enjoy with seating.

Firbank

Manager: Angela Hodgson
Owner: Georgia Rose Residential
Care Ltd
Contact: 8 Crescent Road, Shanklin,
Isle of Wight PO37 6DH
☎ 01983 862522
@ firbank@btconnect.com

Formerly a hotel, Firbank is located on a quiet, tree-lined road in Shanklin close to local amenities, shops and public transport. There are extensive sea views from the home and residents can go on cliff top walks and minibus outings to the coast. In-house activities organised by an activities coordinator include bingo, quizzes, games and a visiting singer. A residents meeting is held every Monday with sherry and refreshments, where views are sought and details of the week's activities are given.

Registered places: 26
Guide weekly rate: £366–£460
Specialist care: Day care, dementia, learning disability, physical disability
Medical services: Podiatry, optician, physiotherapy
Qualified staff: Exceeds standard: 75% at NVQ Level 2

Home details
Location: Residential area, in Shanklin
Communal areas: Lounges, dining room, conservatory, patio, garden
Accessibility: *Floors:* 3 • *Access:* Lift • *Wheelchair access:* Good
Routines: Flexible
Pets: At manager's discretion
Smoking: ✗

Room details
Single: 15
Shared: 6
En suite: 2
Facilities: TV point

Door lock: ✓
Lockable place: ✓

Services provided
Beauty services: Hairdressing
Mobile library: ✗
Religious services: ✓
Transport: ✗
Activities: *Coordinator:* ✓ • *Examples:* Bingo, quizzes, visiting singer, games • *Outings:* ✓
Meetings: ✓

Greyfriars

Manager: Ann Cable
Owner: David and Ann Cable
Contact: 26 Clarence Gardens, Shanklin,
Isle of Wight PO37 6HA
☎ 01983 864361

Greyfriars is a small, detached property situated in a quiet residential area of Shanklin, approximately one mile from the town centre and its amenities. There is a small garden to the front of the property. The area has a lawn, various flowers and shrubs and a patio with seating. The home and residents enjoy organising annual garden parties and all residents' birthdays are celebrated. The home is a five-minute stroll from the seafront, making it a regular outing for residents, with a fish and chip stop along the way.

Registered places: 9
Guide weekly rate: £349–£420
Specialist care: Dementia
Medical services: Podiatry, hygienist, optician
Qualified staff: Meets standard

Home details
Location: Residential area, 0.5 miles from Shanklin centre
Communal areas: Lounge, dining room, patio and garden
Accessibility: *Floors:* 2 • *Access:* Stair lift
Wheelchair access: Limited
Smoking: In designated area
Pets: ✓
Routines: Flexible

Room details
Single: 9
Shared: 0
En suite: 0
Facilities: TV point

Door lock: ✗
Lockable place: ✓

Services provided
Beauty services: Hairdressing
Mobile library: ✓
Religious services: ✓
Transport: ✗
Activities: *Coordinator:* ✗ • *Examples:* Bingo, cards, scrabble
Outings: ✗
Meetings: ✓

Registered places: 23
Guide weekly rate: £425–£500
Specialist care: Day care, dementia, physical disability
Medical services: Podiatry
Qualified staff: Fails standard: 40% at NVQ Level 2

Home details

Location: Residential area, in Shanklin
Communal areas: Lounge, dining room, patio and garden
Accessibility: *Floors:* 2 • *Access:* Lift • *Wheelchair access:* Good
Smoking: In designated area
Pets: ✓
Routines: Flexible

Room details

Single: 23	Door lock: ✗
Shared: 0	Lockable place: ✓
En suite: 0	
Facilities: TV point	

Services provided

Beauty services: Hairdressing
Mobile library: ✗
Religious services: ✗
Transport: ✗
Activities: *Coordinator:* ✓ • *Examples:* Arts and crafts, t'ai chi,
    quizzes • *Outings:* ✓
Meetings: ✗

Highfield House

Manager: Teresa Cornelius
Owner: Island Healthcare Ltd
Contact: 4 Highfield Road, Shanklin,
Isle of Wight PO37 6PP
☏ 01983 862195

Highfield House is located on a quiet residential street situated off Victoria Road, which leads down to the seafront at Shanklin. The property is a large Victorian house that has been extended and adapted to meet the requirements of the residents. The modifications are in keeping with the periodic features of the home. The home provides a secure rear garden with an attractive seating area for residents' use. There are frequent walks along the seafront for fish and chips, and weekly activities such as arts and crafts afternoon, t'ai chi and a quiz evening.

Registered places: 31
Guide weekly rate: Up to £462
Specialist care: Dementia, physical disability
Medical services: Podiatry, dentist, optician
Qualified staff: Meets standard

Home details

Location: Village location, 3 miles from Ryde
Communal areas: Lounge, dining room, patio and garden
Accessibility: *Floors:* 3 • *Access:* Lift and stair lift
    Wheelchair access: Limited
Smoking: In designated area
Pets: ✗
Routines: Flexible

Room details

Single: 23	Door lock: ✓
Shared: 2	Lockable place: ✓
En suite: 12	
Facilities: Telephone point	

Services provided

Beauty services: Hairdressing
Mobile library: Library facilities
Religious services: Anglican and Catholic services
Transport: Shared minibus
Activities: *Coordinator:* ✓ • *Examples:* Bingo, music, quizzes,
    visiting entertainers • *Outings:* ✓
Meetings: ✗

Holmdale House

Manager: Michael Smyth
Owner: Michael and Mahin Smyth
Contact: Main Road, Havenstreet, Ryde,
Isle of Wight PO33 4DP
☏ 01983 882002
@ Holmdale.iow@btinternet.com

Holmdale House is a large detached property in the village of Havenstreet. Residents are encouraged to be as mobile as possible. Some rooms have views of the local countryside. Residents have a say in all of their activities except for two days when professional performers come to visit. Outings and eating out are organised frequently. Residents can voice any inquires at any time to staff rather than having a meeting once a month. Staff will try to meet all requests including trips to local churches. Volunteers also come in to the home to play cards and read to the residents.

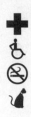

Inglefield Nursing Home

Manager: Gaynor Pitman
Owner: Buckland Care Ltd
Contact: Madeira Road, Totland,
Isle of Wight PO39 0BJ
☎ 01983 754949
🖳 www.bucklandcare.co.uk

Inglefield Nursing Home was built before the turn of the century as Lord Beaverbrooks' Isle of Wight home. Standing in its own grounds, it is a fine example of Victorian architecture, the style of which has been maintained in the recent extension. The home is situated in Totland with Totland Bay but a few minutes' walk away with its picturesque promenade and pier. Inglefield has recently been completely refurbished, extended and tastefully decorated to provide 36 single and two double rooms all with en suite facilities. Many of the rooms have balconies and enjoy country views.

Registered places: 40
Guide weekly rate: Undisclosed
Specialist care: Nursing
Medical services: None
Qualified staff: Exceeds standard: 87% at NVQ Level 2

Home details
Location: Village location, in Totland
Communal areas: 4 lounges, dining room, patio and garden
Accessibility: *Floors:* 3 • *Access:* Lift • *Wheelchair access:* Good
Smoking: ✗
Pets: ✓
Routines: Flexible

Room details
Single: 36
Shared: 2
En suite: 38
Facilities: TV point, telephone point

Door lock: ✗
Lockable place: ✓

Services provided
Beauty services: Hairdressing
Mobile library: ✗
Religious services: ✓
Transport: ✗
Activities: *Coordinator:* ✗ • *Examples:* Arts and crafts, games, singalongs • *Outings:* ✓
Meetings: ✓

Kite Hill Nursing Home

Manager: Margaret Groves
Owner: Colville Care Ltd
Contact: Kite Hill, Wootton Bridge,
Isle of Wight PO33 4LE
☎ 01983 882874

Kite Hill Nursing Home is a period property that has been modified and extended to ensure all the resident's needs are met. The home is situated in Wootton Bridge, on a main road between Newport and Ryde. Public transport to and from the home is available as a local bus service routinely passes the home. Activities include arts and crafts afternoons, knitting, cards and walks for those who are more mobile. There is also a large garden to the rear with seating and decking to sit outside as well as views over the river from the secure balcony.

Registered places: 31
Guide weekly rate: £510–£650
Specialist care: Nursing, dementia, physical disability
Medical services: Podiatry, hygienist, optician, physiotherapy
Qualified staff: Exceeds standard: 65% at NVQ Level 2

Home details
Location: Village location, in Wootten Bridge
Communal areas: Lounge/dining room, garden
Accessibility: *Floors:* 2 • *Access:* Lift • *Wheelchair access:* Good
Smoking: In designated area
Pets: At manager's discretion
Routines: Flexible

Room details
Single: 31
Shared: 0
En suite: 21
Facilities: TV point, telephone point

Door lock: ✗
Lockable place: ✓

Services provided
Beauty services: Hairdressing, manicures
Mobile library: ✓
Religious services: ✓
Transport: ✗
Activities: *Coordinator:* ✓ • *Examples:* Arts and crafts, walks, knitting • *Outings:* ✓
Meetings: ✓

Registered places: 32
Guide weekly rate: £369–£453
Specialist care: Dementia, physically disabled
Medical services: Podiatry
Qualified staff: Meets standard

Home details

Location: Residential area, in East Cowes
Communal areas: 2 lounges, dining room, conservatory,
    patio and garden
Accessibility: *Floors:* 2 • *Access:* Lift • *Wheelchair access:* Good
Smoking: In designated area
Pets: At manager's discretion
Routines: Structured

Room details

Single: 32
Shared: 0
En suite: 23
Facilities: TV point, telephone point

Door lock: ✓
Lockable place: ✓

Services provided

Beauty services: Hairdressing
Mobile library: ✗
Religious services: ✗
Transport: Minibus
Activities: *Coordinator:* ✓ • *Examples:* Arts and crafts,
    board games, music and movement • *Outings:* ✓
Meetings: ✓

Kynance

Manager: Corinne Lovejoy
Owner: Mentfade Ltd
Contact: 97 York Avenue, East Cowes,
Isle of Wight PO32 6BP
☎ 01983 297885

Kynance is on a main road in a residential area of East Cowes. The home offers daily activities to keep residents active and twice-weekly outings in the home's minibus. The location is good for relatives who live on the mainland due to its close proximity to the ferry. Residents can also gain easy access to local amenities through the minibus or walking. There is also a maintenance man who ensures problems are fixed quickly.

Registered places: 32
Guide weekly rate: £434–£485
Specialist care: Dementia, physical disability
Medical services: Podiatry, hygienist, optician, physiotherapy
Qualified staff: Exceeds standard: 70% at NVQ Level 2

Home details

Location: Village location, in Bembridge
Communal areas: 2 lounges, dining room, conservatory, garden
Accessibility: *Floors:* 3 • *Access:* Lift • *Wheelchair access:* Limited
Smoking: In designated area
Pets: ✗
Routines: Structured

Room details

Single: 32
Shared: 0
En suite: 32
Facilities: Undisclosed

Door lock: ✓
Lockable place: ✓

Services provided

Beauty services: Hairdressing, manicures
Mobile library: ✗
Religious services: Catholic and Anglican visits
Transport: Minibus
Activities: *Coordinator:* ✗ • *Examples:* Exercise, reminiscence,
    singalongs • *Outings:* ✓
Meetings: ✗

The Limes

Manager: Lynne Preston
Owner: Susan Betteridge and
Alison Neve-Dewen
Contact: 43 Foreland Road, Bembridge,
Isle of Wight PO35 5XN
☎ 01983 873655
@ the.limes@btconnect.com

The Limes is a care home in Bembridge village, a few minutes' walk from the local shops and beach. There is an enclosed garden to the rear of the house, accessible to residents. While the home has a passenger lift to its three floors, four of the rooms are on a mezzanine level and can only be accessed by able residents. The home offers views of the Downs, and occasionally there are ice cream outings for residents. The home has its own minibus, fitted with a hydraulic lift.

Little Hayes

Manager: Amanda Sanders
Owner: David Burn and
Christopher James
Contact: Church Hill, Totland,
Isle of Wight PO39 0EX
) 01983 752378

Little Hayes is well situated on the outskirts of Totland, within walking distance to shops and the sea. There is also a bus route right outside the home. A number of rooms have sea views and also views of the landscaped garden. Local newspapers are available free of charge. Musical entertainment visits as well as many other activities such as exercises. There are also two budgies in the living room.

Registered places: 26
Guide weekly rate: Undisclosed
Specialist care: Dementia, physical disability
Medical services: Podiatry, hygienist, optician, physiotherapy
Qualified staff: Exceeds standard: 60% at NVQ Level 2

Home details
Location: Residential area, in Totland
Communal areas: Lounge, dining room, patio and garden
Accessibility: *Floors:* 2 • *Access:* 2 lifts
   Wheelchair access: Good
Smoking: ✕
Pets: At manager's discretion
Routines: Flexible

Room details
Single: 60
Shared: 0
En suite: 21
Facilities: TV point, telephone point

Door lock: ✓
Lockable place: ✓

Services provided
Beauty services: Hairdressing, manicures
Mobile library: ✕
Religious services: Monthly Anglican and Catholic visits
Transport: ✕
Activities: *Coordinator:* ✓ • *Examples:* Exercises, readings and musical performances • *Outings:* ✕
Meetings: ✓

Merrydale

Manager: Patricia Cluett
Owner: Mr and Mrs Pryer
Contact: Spencer Road, Ryde,
Isle of Wight PO33 3AL
) 01983 563017

The owners of Merrydale acquired the home in 2004. It is in a quiet, private road within walking distance of the town centre. The day care facility is in a purpose-built extension with a separate entrance. Pets are welcome and the home already has two cats and one dog. The home focuses on a homely atmosphere and aids residents in remaining as active as possible. The home has two cars which are used for trips into town and outings.

Registered places: 16
Guide weekly rate: £385–£525
Specialist care: Day care, respite
Medical services: Podiatry, dentist, optician, physiotherapy
Qualified staff: Exceeds standard: 75% at NVQ Level 2

Home details
Location: Residential area, in Ryde
Communal areas: Lounge, 2 dining rooms, patio and garden
Accessibility: *Floors:* 2 • *Access:* Stair lift
   Wheelchair access: Good
Smoking: ✕
Pets: ✓
Routines: Flexible

Room details
Single: 16
Shared: 0
En suite: 10
Facilities: TV point, telephone point

Door lock: ✓
Lockable place: ✓

Services provided
Beauty services: Hairdressing
Mobile library: ✕
Religious services: Weekly visits from all denominations
Transport: 2 cars
Activities: *Coordinator:* ✓ • *Examples:* Arts and crafts, bridge club, music • *Outings:* ✓
Meetings: ✓

Registered places: 25
Guide weekly rate: Undisclosed
Specialist care: Dementia, physical disability
Medical services: Podiatry, optician, physiotherapy
Qualified staff: Exceeds standard: 87% at NVQ level 2

Home details

Location: Residential area, 0.75 miles from Cowes centre
Communal areas: Lounge, dining room, conservatory, garden
Accessibility: *Floors:* 3 • *Access:* Lift • *Wheelchair access:* Good
Smoking: ✗
Pets: ✓
Routines: Flexible

Room details

Single: 23
Shared: 2
En suite: 25
Facilities: TV point, telephone point

Door lock: ✓
Lockable place: ✓

Services provided

Beauty services: Hairdressing, massages
Mobile library: ✗
Religious services: Monthly Communion service
Transport: ✗
Activities: *Coordinator:* ✓ • *Examples:* Bingo, happy hour,
   exercise, quizzes • *Outings:* ✓
Meetings: ✓

The Moorings

Manager: Dawn Richards
Owner: Janet Holmes
Contact: Egypt Hill, Cowes, Isle of Wight
PO31 8BP
☎ 01983 297129
@ office@themooringscare.demon.co.uk

The Moorings is an attractive period
house set in its own grounds and close to
Cowes seafront. The amenities of Cowes
centre are less than half a mile away.
The home offers residents with good
views of the Solent from some of the first
floor windows. The home offers a weekly
programme of activities, such as bingo,
happy hour and quizzes.

Registered places: 40
Guide weekly rate: £575–£710
Specialist care: Nursing, dementia, physical disability,
   terminal care
Medical services: Podiatry
Qualified staff: Exceeds standard: 60% at NVQ Level 2

Home details

Location: Village location, 4 miles from Ryde
Communal areas: 2 lounges, 2 dining rooms, patio and garden
Accessibility: *Floors:* 2 • *Access:* 2 lifts • *Wheelchair access:* Good
Smoking: ✗
Pets: At manager's discretion
Routines: Flexible

Room details

Single: 40
Shared: 0
En suite: 40
Facilities: Undisclosed

Door lock: ✓
Lockable place: ✓

Services provided

Beauty services: Hairdressing
Mobile library
Religious: ✗
Transport: Wheelchair-accessible vehicle
Activities: *Coordinator:* ✓ • *Examples:* Games, reminiscence,
   t'ai chi • *Outings:* ✗
Meetings: ✓

Northbrooke House

Manager: Sally Jolliffe
Owner: Island Healthcare Ltd
Contact: Main Road, Havenstreet,
Isle of Wight PO33 4DR
☎ 01983 882236

Northbrook House provides nursing care
for 40 people, and is a converted period
house set in extensive grounds with
panoramic views across the countryside.
The grounds are landscaped in some
areas. The home also has a patio, as well
as a balcony on the first floor. The home
is situated in the village of Havenstreet,
and there is a post office, bus stop and
pub all within a quarter of a mile. There
is a shop, chemist, library, GP surgery,
bank, shopping centre and train station
all within three miles. The activities
coordinator organises weekly activities for
the residents such as t'ai chi and yoga.

Northfield

Manager: Melanie Paterson
Owner: Anthony and Pauline Obeyesekere
Contact: 85 George Street, Ryde, Isle of Wight PO33 2JE
) 01983 562064

Northfields is located close to the centre of Ryde and within 10 minutes of the seafront, ferry, rail links and shops. Here, an emphasis is put on the clients, and the day is structured around their needs. The activities coordinator is at hand to keep the residents active and trips out for tea are regularly organised.

Registered places: 24
Guide weekly rate: £340–£360
Specialist care: Nursing, dementia, mental disorder, physical disability
Medical services: Podiatry, optician
Qualified staff: Fails standard: 46% at NVQ level 2

Home details
Location: Residential area, in Ryde
Communal areas: Lounge, dining room, conservatory, garden
Accessibility: *Floors:* 4 • *Access:* Lift • *Wheelchair access:* Good
Smoking: In designated area
Pets: At manager's discretion
Routines: Flexible

Room details
Single: 16	Door lock: ✓
Shared: 4	Lockable place: ✓
En suite: 2	
Facilities: TV point	

Services provided
Beauty services: Hairdressing
Mobile library: ✗
Religious services: ✗
Transport: ✗
Activities: *Coordinator:* ✓ • *Examples:* Bingo, quizzes
  Outings: ✓
Meetings: ✗

Palissy House

Manager: Shirley Irving
Owner: Shirley Irving
Contact: 37 Clatterford Road, Carisbrooke, Isle of Wight, PO30 1PA
) 01983 524378

Palissy House is located in a residential area, one and a half miles from the town centre of Newport, close to local amenities. The home has a lounge, a dining room and a garden with a patio area. The home has a varied activities programme, which includes games, and there are also regular outings in the local area. The home also holds residents meetings.

Registered places: 24
Guide weekly rate: From £370
Specialist care: None
Medical services: Podiatry, dentist, optician
Qualified staff: Meets standard

Home details
Location: Residential area, 1.5 miles from Newport
Communal areas: Lounge, dining room, patio and garden
Accessibility: *Floors:* 3 • *Access:* Lift • *Wheelchair access:* Limited
Smoking: ✗
Pets: At manager's discretion
Routines: Flexible

Room details
Single: 22	Door lock: ✓
Shared: 1	Lockable place: ✓
En suite: 6	
Facilities: TV point	

Services provided
Beauty services: Hairdressing
Mobile library: ✗
Religious services: ✗
Transport: ✓
Activities: *Coordinator:* ✗ • *Examples:* Games • *Outings:* ✓
Meetings: ✓

Registered places: 39
Guide weekly rate: £586–£650
Specialist care: Nursing
Medical services: Podiatry, dentist, optician, physiotherapy
Qualified staff: Exceeds standard: 75% at NVQ level 2

Home details

Location: Residential area, in Sandown
Communal areas: Lounge, dining room, conservatory
Accessibility: *Floors:* 2 • *Access:* Lift • *Wheelchair access:* Good
Smoking: ✗
Pets: ✓
Routines: Flexible

Room details

Single: 35
Shared: 2
En suite: 11
Facilities: TV point, telephone point

Door lock: ✗
Lockable place: ✓

Services provided

Beauty services: Hairdressing
Mobile library: ✗
Religious services: Monthly church service
Transport: ✗
Activities: *Coordinator:* ✗ • *Examples:* Arts group, bingo, scrabble, walks • *Outings:* ✗
Meetings: ✗

Sandown Nursing Home

Manager: Teresa Riley
Owner: Belinda, Richard and Elizabeth Davies
Contact: 28 Grove Road, Sandown, Isle of Wight PO36 9BE
☏ 01983 402946
@ admin@sandownnursinghome.co.uk
🖰 www.sandownnursinghome.co.uk

Sandown Nursing Home is situated in a prominent and easily accessible position on the corner of Broadway and Grove Road and comprises of an attractive detached Victorian house that has been extended to provide 33 bedrooms. The home is situated within easy reach of the railway station, high street, esplanade and sandy beaches. The current owners have planned and implemented extensive refurbishment and improvements to the home since they purchased it in May 2001.

Registered places: 25
Guide weekly rate: From £480
Specialist care: Day care, dementia, physical disability, respite
Medical services: Podiatry, dentist, optician, physiotherapy
Qualified staff: Exceeds standard: 80% at NVQ Level 2

Home details

Location: Village location, 1 mile from Totland centre
Communal areas: Lounge, dining room, reading room, library, garden
Accessibility: *Floors:* 3 • *Access:* Lift • *Wheelchair access:* Limited
Smoking: ✗
Pets: ✓
Routines: Flexible

Room details

Single: 22
Shared: 3
En suite: 25
Facilities: TV point, telephone point.

Door lock: ✓
Lockable place: ✓

Services provided

Beauty services: Hairdressing, aromatherapy, manicures
Mobile library: Library facilities
Religious services: Every other month nondenominational service
Transport: ✗
Activities: *Coordinator:* ✓ • *Examples:* Exercise class, slide shows *Outings:* ✗
Meetings: ✓

Seven Gables Rest Home

Manager: John Bush
Owner: Anthony Leeson
Contact: Seven Gables, York Lane, Totland Bay, Isle of Wight PO39 0ER
☏ 01983 754765
@ sevengablescare@aol.com

Seven Gables is a period building situated in its own grounds on the outskirts of Totland. The home is down a country lane and buses stop at end of lane but are relatively infrequent. Parties and fêtes are held each year, with staff keen to consult residents for ideas. Staff focus on stimulating the residents with theme nights and many activities available on a regular basis. These have included a 1940s re-enactment day. The manager lives on site and is personally involved in the residents' care.

Solent Grange

Manager: Angela Clarke
Owner: London Residential
Healthcare Ltd
Contact: Staplers Road, Wootton,
Isle of Wight PO33 4RW
☎ 01983 882382
@ solent@lrh-homes.com
🖥 www.lrh-homes.com

Solent Grange, on the outskirts of Newport, is undergoing an extension to build a new care centre. This will include a refurbishment of the original building. The home currently has two floors with two lifts and good wheelchair access. There are 34 single rooms and three double rooms but this number will increase. There is a full list of the home's activities, including visiting entertainers, displayed in reception. Activities include croquet, bingo, craft, games and exercises. *The Solent Grange Messenger*, a quarterly newsletter, has been set up to increase communication between the home, residents and their relatives.

Registered places: 40
Guide weekly rate: £420–£450
Specialist care: Dementia
Medical services: Podiatry, dentist, optician
Qualified staff: Exceeds standard: 72% at NVQ Level 2

Home details
Location: Rural area, 3.5 miles from the centre of Newport
Communal areas: 2 lounges, 2 dining rooms
Accessibility: *Floors:* 2 • *Access:* 2 lifts • *Wheelchair access:* Good
Smoking: ✗
Pets: ✗
Routines: Flexible

Room details
Single: 34
Shared: 3
En suite: 19
Facilities: TV, telephone point

Door lock: ✓
Lockable place: ✓

Services provided
Beauty services: Hairdressing
Mobile library: ✗
Religious services: ✓
Transport: ✗
Activities: *Coordinator:* ✓ • *Examples:* Arts and crafts, cooking, films, visiting entertainers • *Outings:* ✗
Meetings: ✗

Solent View

Manager: David Elliott
Owner: Lynne Knight
Contact: 43 Victoria Grove, East Cowes,
Isle of Wight PO32 6DL
☎ 01983 290348

Solent View is a two-storey Victorian property situated on a residential road outside of East Cowes, opposite a recreational ground. The home's minibus provides transport for residents to go on day trips or to take them shopping into East Cowes. Recent outings include trips to the local pub and to the Havenstreet Railway's 1940s weekend. Often mobile residents wander down to the seafront for exercise, which is about 15 minutes' walk away. There is a designated smoking area in the porch of the home to accommodate smokers.

Registered places: 19
Guide weekly rate: £360–£460
Specialist care: Dementia, physical disability
Medical services: Podiatry, optician, physiotherapy
Qualified staff: Meets standard

Home details
Location: Residential area, 1 mile from East Cowes centre
Communal areas: Lounge, dining room, garden
Accessibility: *Floors:* 2 • *Access:* Lift • *Wheelchair access:* Good
Smoking: In designated area
Pets: ✓
Routines: Flexible

Room details
Single: 15
Shared: 2
En suite: 16
Facilities: TV point, telephone point

Door lock: ✗
Lockable place: ✓

Services provided
Beauty services: Hairdressing
Mobile library: ✓
Religious services: ✓
Transport: Minibus
Activities: *Coordinator:* ✓ • *Examples:* Debates, games, puzzles *Outings:* ✓
Meetings: ✓

Registered places: 44
Guide weekly rate: Undisclosed
Specialist care: Nursing, dementia, physical disability, terminal care
Medical services: Podiatry, dentist, optician, physiotherapy
Qualified staff: Exceeds standard: 100% at NVQ Level 2

Home details

Location: Residential area, 0.5 miles from Shanklin centre
Communal areas: 3 lounges, dining room, garden
Accessibility: *Floors:* 2 • *Access:* 3 lifts • *Wheelchair access:* Good
Smoking: In designated area
Pets: x
Routines: Flexible

Room details

Single: 44
Shared: 0
En suite: 44
Facilities: TV, telephone

Door lock: ✓
Lockable place: ✓

Services provided

Beauty services: Hairdressing
Mobile library: x
Religious services: Monthly church services
Transport: x
Activities: *Coordinator:* ✓ • *Examples:* Arts and crafts, painting,
   quizzes • *Outings:* ✓
Meetings: x

Springfield Nursing Home

Manager: Lisa Newnham
Owner: Scio Healthcare Ltd
Contact: 26 Arthur's Hill, Shanklin,
Isle of Wight PO37 6EX
℡ 01983 862934
@ Lisa.newnham@sciohealthcare.co.uk
🖰 www.sciohealthcare.co.uk

Springfield is an extended, older property in its own grounds. The original building has been extended several times. The property is very close to the beach, with sea views. The home is within half a mile of local shops and is situated on the main road so is easily accessible. All the rooms are single with en suite facilities. The home has a garden, a quiet room, a TV room and an ICT lounge. Pets are allowed to visit and the home has an activities coordinator who arranges activities such as table games, bingo and arts and crafts.

Registered places: 27
Guide weekly rate: £380–£474
Specialist care: Day care, dementia, physical disability, respite
Medical services: Podiatry, dentist, optician, physiotherapy
Qualified staff: Meets standard

Home details

Location: Residential area, in Sandown
Communal areas: 3 lounges, dining room, library,
   patio and garden
Accessibility: *Floors:* 2 • *Access:* Lift • *Wheelchair access:* Good
Smoking: In designated area
Pets: x
Routines: Flexible

Room details

Single: 27
Shared: 0
En suite: Undisclosed
Facilities: TV point, telephone point

Door lock: ✓
Lockable place: ✓

Services provided

Beauty services: Hairdressing
Mobile library: x
Religious services: Monthly Communion service
Transport: x
Activities: *Coordinator:* ✓ • *Examples:* Board games,
   movement to music, quizzes • *Outings:* ✓
Meetings: ✓

Stonehaven

Manager: Margaret Cowen
Owner: Raymond and Margaret Cowen
Contact: 23 Carter Street, Sandown,
Isle of Wight PO36 8DG
℡ 01983 402213
@ rayslegs@aol.com

Stonehaven is in Sandown, close to the seafront and opposite a parish church.
   There is an enclosed flat garden with ramp access from a decking area in front of the lounge. The residents of the home go on various trips out and there is a choice of activities for them to choose from. Pets are allowed to visit but not to stay in the home. There are meetings with residents every two months to discuss the daily life of the home.

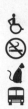

Sunnycliffe Cottage

Manager: Sarah-Jane Collins
Owner: Shantina Niles
Contact: 20–22 Broadway, Sandown, Isle of Wight PO36 9DQ
✆ 01983 403844

Sunnycliffe Cottage is a large, detached property, situated on the main road to Sandown. It is located a five-minute walk from the seafront and is within walking distance of Sandown train station. The home is undergoing a large extension to give 15 more rooms all of which will be en suite. The home has a large, well-maintained garden with seating areas for residents to socialise. Some of the daily activities involve gardening or flower arranging. Others involve film afternoon, quizzes and outings to the seafront.

Registered places: 31
Guide weekly rate: £448–£482
Specialist care: Dementia, physical disability
Medical services: Podiatry, hygienist, optician
Qualified staff: Exceeds standard: 85% at NVQ Level 2

Home details
Location: Residential area in Sandown
Communal areas: 2 lounges, dining room, library, garden
Accessibility: *Floors:* 3 • *Access:* Lift • *Wheelchair access:* Good
Smoking: ✗
Pets: At manager's discretion
Routines: Flexible

Room details
Single: 25
Shared: 3
En suite: 9
Facilities: TV point, telephone point

Door lock: ✓
Lockable place: ✓

Services provided
Beauty services: Hairdressing
Mobile library: Library facilities
Religious services: ✓
Transport: ✓
Activities: *Coordinator:* ✗ • *Examples:* Films, flower arranging, visiting entertainers • *Outings:* ✓
Meetings: ✓

Tile House

Manager: Catherine Leather
Owner: Island Healthcare Ltd
Contact: Tile House, 34 Victoria Avenue, Shanklin, Isle of Wight PO37 6LS
✆ 01983 862762
@ tileilh@btconnect.com

Tile House is a residential home providing care and accommodation for 17 residents, some with dementia. It is a period town house situated near Shanklin, and is on a regular bus route. There are three floors with an upstairs flat. There is a stair lift and good wheelchair access. There are shops a few yards away from the home. The home has its own activities coordinator and an activities programme is in place, including, quizzes, bingo and various outings for shopping and cream tea.

Registered places: 17
Guide weekly rate: £480–£500
Specialist care: Dementia
Medical services: Podiatry, dentist, optician, physiotherapy
Qualified staff: Exceeds standard: 54% at NVQ Level 2

Home details
Location: Residential area, in Shanklin
Communal areas: Lounge, dining room, conservatory, library, patio and garden
Accessibility: *Floors:* 3 • *Access:* Stair lifts *Wheelchair access:* Good
Smoking: In designated area.
Pets: At manager's discretion
Routines: Flexible

Room details
Single: 17
Shared: 0
En suite: 13
Facilities: TV

Door lock: ✓
Lockable place: ✗

Services provided
Beauty services: Hairdressing, manicures
Mobile library: Library facilities
Religious services: ✓
Transport: ✓
Activities: *Coordinator:* ✓ • *Examples:* Gentle exercises, reminiscence sessions, visiting musicians • *Outings:* ✓
Meetings: ✓

Registered places: 23
Guide weekly rate: £700
Specialist care: Nursing, dementia, physical disability, respite
Medical services: Podiatry, dentist, optician
Qualified staff: Undisclosed

Home details

Location: Residential area, in Ventnor
Communal areas: Lounge, dining room, garden
Accessibility: *Floors:* 4 • *Access:* Lift • *Wheelchair access:* Good
Smoking: ✗
Pets: Manager's discretion
Routines: Structured

Room details

Single: 13
Shared: 5
En suite: Undisclosed
Facilities: TV point, telephone point

Door lock: ✗
Lockable place: ✗

Services provided

Beauty services: Hairdressing
Mobile library: ✗
Religious services: ✓
Transport: ✗
Activities: *Coordinator:* ✗ • *Examples:* Reminiscence sessions, visiting entertainers • *Outings:* ✗
Meetings: ✗

Ward House Nursing Home

Manager: Susan Davies
Owner: Ward House Ltd
Contact: 21–23 Alpine Road, Ventnor, Isle of Wight PO38 1BT
☎ 01983 854122
@ Matron.whl@btconnect.com

Comprised of two older properties, Ward House Nursing Home provides appropriate communal space and enjoys the features of an enclosed rear garden that overlooks the sea. It is situated in Ventnor, to the south of the island. A number of the bedrooms have sea views, as well as views of the home's garden. Visiting entertainers occasionally visit as part of the home's activities programme. On residents' birthdays, the home specially bakes cakes for all residents to enjoy.

Registered places: 20
Guide weekly rate: £443
Specialist care: Physical disability, respite
Medical services: Podiatry, optician
Qualified staff: Exceeds standard

Home details

Location: Residential area, 0.5 miles from Oakfield
Communal areas: 2 Lounges, dining room, conservatory, garden
Accessibility: *Floors:* 2 • *Access:* Lift • *Wheelchair access:* Good
Smoking: In designated area
Pets: At manager's discretion
Routines: Flexible

Room details

Single: 19
Shared: 1
En suite: Undisclosed
Facilities: TV point, telephone point

Door lock: ✓
Lockable place: ✓

Services provided

Beauty services: Hairdressing
Mobile library: ✗
Religious services: Monthly Communion service
Transport: Minibus
Activities: *Coordinator:* ✗ • *Examples:* Gentle exercise, board games, quizzes • *Outings:* ✓
Meetings: ✓

Waxham House

Manager: Jamie Bunter
Owner: Mr and Mrs Ramdany
Contact: 1 High Park Road, Ryde, Isle of Wight PO33 1BP
☎ 01983 564326

Waxham House is a large, period house that has been adapted as a care home. Situated within a residential area of Hyde, the home is approximately half a mile from Oakfield. A social activities programme is displayed in the home, which involves board games, bingo, quizzes and gentle chair exercises. Hairdressing is also available for residents, and a visiting manicurist regularly comes to the home. There is a residents meeting every three months.

Whiteley Bank House

Manager: Daphne Hayles
Owner: Daphne Hayles
Contact: Canteen Road, White Bank, Ventroi, Isle of Wight PO38 3AF

☎ 01983 867541

@ daphnehayles@btinternet.com

An older property situated in the village, Whiteley Bank House is a former coach house that resides in substantial grounds. Access to local amenities can be found in Shanklin. The home is two miles from the village of Godshill which is a popular tourist destination. The home hosts barbecues in garden and a patio in the summer. The residents have a flexible daily routine with set meal times. Pets are allowed and the home has adopted its own cat. There is a TV in each room and the residents can set up their own phone line if they wish.

Registered places: 12
Guide weekly rate: Undisclosed
Specialist care: Dementia, physical disability
Medical services: Podiatry, dentist, optician
Qualified staff: Meets standard

Home details

Location: Village location, 2.5 miles from Shanklin
Communal areas: Lounge, dining room, patio and garden
Accessibility: *Floors:* 2 • *Access:* Lift • *Wheelchair access:* Good
Smoking: In designated area
Pets: ✓
Routines: Flexible

Room details

Single: 6
Shared: 3
En suite: 1
Facilities: TV, telephone point

Door lock: ✓
Lockable place: ✓

Services provided

Beauty services: Hairdressing, manicures
Mobile library: ✗
Religious services: ✓
Transport: ✓
Activities: *Coordinator:* ✗ • *Examples:* Exercise, slide shows, visiting entertainers • *Outings:* ✓
Meetings: ✗

Registered places: 22
Guide weekly rate: £565–£700
Specialist care: Nursing, physical disability, respite
Medical services: Podiatry, dentist, optician
Qualified staff: Undisclosed

Home details

Location: Residential area, 1 mile from West Kingsdown
Communal areas: Lounge, dining room, garden
Accessibility: *Floors:* 2 • *Access:* Lift • *Wheelchair access:* Good
Smoking: In designated area
Pets: ✗
Routines: Flexible

Room details

Single: 16
Shared: 3
En suite: 8
Facilities: TV point

Door lock: ✓
Lockable place: ✓

Services provided

Beauty services: Hairdressing
Mobile library: ✗
Religious services: ✓
Transport: ✗
Activities: *Coordinator:* ✓ • *Examples:* Bingo, exercises,
    flower arranging • *Outings:* ✗
Meetings: ✗

Abbey Court Nursing Home

Manager: Rohini Persand
Owner: Abbey Court Nursing Home Ltd
Contact: School Lane, West Kingsdown,
Kent TN15 6JB
☎ 01474 854136

Abbey Court Nursing Home is purpose built and is located in a residential area, approximately one mile from West Kingsdown. The home has a pleasant garden for residents to enjoy in the finer weather and a variety of activities, such as bingo and flower arranging. Religious services are offered from the local church and visits from other religious leaders can be organised on request.

Registered places: 18
Guide weekly rate: £318–£460
Specialist care: None
Medical services: Podiatry, dentist, optician
Qualified staff: Meets standard

Home details

Location: Residential area, 1 mile from Hythe
Communal areas: 2 lounges, dining room, library, conservatory,
    patio and garden
Accessibility: *Floors:* 3 • *Access:* Lift and stair lift
    Wheelchair access: Good
Smoking: ✗
Pets: ✗
Routines: Flexible

Room details

Single: 16
Shared: 1
En suite: 14
Facilities: TV point

Door lock: ✗
Lockable place: ✓

Services provided

Beauty services: Hairdressing, reflexology
Mobile library: ✓
Religious services: ✗
Transport: ✗
Activities: *Coordinator:* ✗ • *Examples:* Coffee mornings,
    exercise to music, games • *Outings:* ✓
Meetings: ✓

Abbey Lodge Residential Care Home

Manager: Elizabeth Brown
Owner: Abbey Lodge Ltd
Contact: 91 Seabrook Road,
Hythe, Kent CT21 5QP
☎ 01303 265175
@ mail@abbeyresthome.co.uk
🖱 www.abbeyresthome.co.uk

Abbey Lodge is a family-run home on the outskirts of Hythe in Kent, one mile from the town centre. There are sea views that can be enjoyed from the garden. The daily activities programme includes games afternoons, reminiscence afternoons, parties, coffee mornings and an extensive library. The home also has a visiting local access library with large print books available on loan. The home celebrates all residents' birthdays with a home-made cake and a tea party, and on summer evenings, a barbecue in the garden.

Abbeyfield Rogers House

Manager: Lucy Dixon
Owner: Abbeyfield Society Ltd
Contact: Drewery Drive, Rainham, Gillingham, Kent ME8 0NX
☎ 01634 262266

Abbeyfield Rogers House is a modern purpose-built home located in a residential area in Rainham, within easy walking distance of local shops. The home boasts a sensory garden with bright, pleasant-smelling flowers which evokes the senses. There is a seating area for residents to sit in warm weather. There are also daily activities organised, such as morning newspaper discussions where residents voice their thoughts and opinions, giant crossword and bingo evening.

Registered places: 43
Guide weekly rate: £465
Specialist care: Respite
Medical services: Podiatry, optician
Qualified staff: Meets standard

Home details
Location: Residential area, 2 miles from Rainham
Communal areas: 2 lounges, dining room, garden
Accessibility: *Floors:* 3 • *Access:* Lift • *Wheelchair access:* Good
Smoking: ✗
Pets: ✗
Routines: Flexible

Room details
Single: 37
Shared: 2
En suite: 39
Facilities: TV point, telephone point

Door lock: ✗
Lockable place: ✓

Services provided
Beauty services: Hairdressing
Mobile library: ✓
Religious services: Monthly
Transport: ✓
Activities: *Coordinator:* ✓ • *Examples:* Giant crossword, newspaper discussions • *Outings:* ✗
Meetings: ✓

Abbeyrose House

Manager: Heather Maulayah
Owner: Ramaul Ltd
Contact: 1 St Michaels Road, Maidstone, Kent ME16 8BS
☎ 01622 762369

Established in 1989, Abbeyrose House is a former vicarage converted to its present use as a care home. The home has a large secluded and mature garden to the rear of the property for residents to enjoy. The home is situated in a residential area, one mile from Maidstone. This small, family-run business provides activities such as arts and crafts, and old DVD film showings. There are religious services organised as well as residents meetings.

Registered places: 23
Guide weekly rate: £240–£260
Specialist care: Respite
Medical services: Podiatry, optician, physiotherapy
Qualified staff: Meets standard

Home details
Location: Residential area, 1 mile from Maidstone
Communal areas: 3 lounges, dining room, library, garden
Accessibility: *Floors:* 2 • *Access:* Lift • *Wheelchair access:* Limited
Smoking: ✗
Pets: ✓
Routines: Flexible

Room details
Single: 23
Shared: 0
En suite: 0
Facilities: TV point, telephone point

Door lock: ✓
Lockable place: ✓

Services provided
Beauty services: Hairdressing, manicures
Mobile library: ✗
Religious services: ✓
Transport: ✗
Activities: *Coordinator:* ✗ • *Examples:* Arts and crafts, film shows *Outings:* ✓
Meetings: ✓

Registered places: 120
Guide weekly rate: Undisclosed
Specialist care: Nursing, dementia, respite
Medical services: Podiatry, physiotherapy
Qualified staff: Undisclosed

Home details

Location: Residential area, 1 mile from Sidcup centre
Communal areas: 8 lounges, 8 dining rooms,
   hairdressing salon, garden
Accessibility: *Floors:* 2 • *Access:* lift • *Wheelchair access:* Good
Smoking: ✗
Pets: ✗
Routines: Flexible

Room details

Single: 120
Shared: 0
En suite: 120
Facilities: TV point, telephone point

Door lock: ✓
Lockable place: ✗

Services provided

Beauty services: Hairdressing, aromatherapy
Mobile library: ✓
Religious services: Fortnightly church service
Transport: ✓
Activities: *Coordinator:* ✓ • *Examples:* Musical entertainment,
   painting, gardening • *Outings:* ✓
Meetings: ✗

Abbotsleigh Mews Nursing Home

Manager: Tracey Cheeseman
Owner: BUPA Care Homes Ltd
Contact: Old Farm Road East,
Sidcup, Kent DA15 8AY
☎ 020 8308 9590
@ Abbotsleighmewsall@BUPA.com
🖰 www.bupacarehomes.co.uk

Situated in a residential area of Sidcup, Abbotsleigh Mews is five minutes from Sidcup station and on a local bus route. This purpose-built redbrick home consists of four houses: two provide nursing care, one provides residential care, and one offers residential dementia care. There are also landscaped gardens and sensory areas for residents to sit outside. Many bedrooms enjoy garden views and all offer en suite facilities. Daily activities are offered including cookery, games, quizzes and crafts, as well as trips to local places of interest. There are also overnight facilities for guests.

Registered places: 76
Guide weekly rate: £467–£762
Specialist care: Nursing, dementia
Medical services: Podiatry, dentist, optician
Qualified staff: Meets standard

Home details

Location: Residential area, 0.5 miles from Bexleyheath
Communal areas: Hairdressing salon, garden
Accessibility: *Floors:* 2 • *Access:* Undisclosed
   Wheelchair access: Undisclosed
Smoking: Undisclosed
Pets: Undisclosed
Routines: Flexible

Room details

Single: 76
Shared: 0
En suite: 76
Facilities: Undisclosed

Door lock: ✗
Lockable place: ✗

Services provided

Beauty services: Undisclosed
Mobile library: Undisclosed
Religious services: Undisclosed
Transport: Undisclosed
Activities: *Coordinator:* ✓ • *Examples:* Bingo, card games
   Outings: ✗
Meetings: Undisclosed

Adelaide Nursing and Residential Care Home

Manager: Vacant
Owner: Southern Cross Healthcare Ltd
Contact: 35 West Street,
Bexleyheath, Kent DA7 4RE
☎ 020 8304 3303
🖰 www.schealthcare.co.uk

The Adelaide Care Home is a purpose-built property, half a mile from Bexleyheath. The home is separated into four units, for different care needs including dementia. There is an enclosed garden to the rear of the property. The home has an activities coordinator who arranges card games and bingo for the residents. The home also has a hairdressing salon and a garden for residents to enjoy in warmer months.

Admiral House

Manager: Diana Simmons
Owner: Vinod and Santosh Gupta
Contact: 5–6 Lennard Road,
Folkestone, Kent CT20 1PD
- ☎ 01303 254898
- @ admiralhouse@hotmail.co.uk
- 🖱 www.admiralhouse.org

Admiral House is a large, late-Victorian building situated in a residential area of Folkestone, close to the harbour and local shops. The home is also near to the station and the town centre. The home also a lounge with a TV, a dining room, a quiet lounge, as well as a garden. The activities coordinator organises a range of activities including games, puzzles, karaoke, and arts and crafts. There are also organised outings to the harbour and for tea. The home has its own transport for these outings. The home also arranges a regular religious service.

Registered places: 41
Guide weekly rate: £312–£471
Specialist care: Dementia, respite
Medical services: Podiatry, dentist, optician
Qualified staff: Exceeds standard: 75% at NVQ Level 2

Home details
Location: Residential area, 1.2 miles from Folkstone
Communal areas: Lounge, dining room, quiet room, garden
Accessibility: *Floors:* 3 • *Access:* Lift • *Wheelchair access:* Good
Smoking: In designated area
Pets: ✗
Routines: Flexible

Room details
Single: 41	**Door lock:** ✓
Shared: 0	**Lockable place:** ✓
En suite: 30	

Facilities: TV point, telephone point

Services provided
Beauty services: Hairdressing
Mobile library: ✗
Religious services: Weekly church service
Transport: ✓
Activities: *Coordinator:* ✓ • *Examples:* Games, karaoke, puzzles
   Outings: ✓
Meetings: ✓

Agape House

Manager: Nanthini Paramasivam
Owner: Nanthini Paramasivam
Contact: 45 Maidstone Road,
Chatham, Kent ME4 6DG
- ☎ 01634 841002

Agape House is a detached Victorian home situated in a residential area less than a mile from Chatham railway station and town centre. The home is also located on a main bus route and local shops including a post office are within walking distance. The home has attractive front and rear gardens with seating. There are also two double rooms for married couples. Residents are offered activities such as bowling and sing alongs, however there is also a quiet lounge if residents prefer not to participate.

Registered places: 20
Guide weekly rate: £370–£415
Specialist care: Nursing, dementia
Medical services: Podiatry, dentist, physiotherapy
Qualified staff: Meets standard

Home details
Location: Residential area, 0.5 miles from Chatham
Communal areas: Lounge, quiet lounge, hairdressing salon,
   patio and garden
Accessibility: *Floors:* 2 • *Access:* Lift • *Wheelchair access:* Good
Smoking: ✗
Pets: ✓
Routines: Flexible

Room details
Single: 18	**Door lock:** ✓
Shared: 2	**Lockable place:** ✓
En suite: 0	

Facilities: TV point, telephone point

Services provided
Beauty services: Hairdressing
Mobile library: ✗
Religious services: Monthly Anglican and Catholic visits
Transport: ✗
Activities: *Coordinator:* ✓ • *Examples:* Bingo, cards, scrabble
   Outings: ✗
Meetings: ✓

Registered places: 32
Guide weekly rate: £314–£411
Specialist care: Residential, respite, day care
Medical services: Podiatry, dentist, optician
Qualified staff: Exceeds standard: 70% at NVQ level 2

Home details
Location: Residential area, 0.5 miles from Whitfield
Communal areas: 2 lounges, dining room, conservatory, garden
Accessibility: *Floors:* 2 • *Access:* Lift • *Wheelchair access:* Good
Smoking: In designated area
Pets: At manager's discretion
Routines: Structured

Room details
Single: 30
Shared: 1
En suite: 5
Facilities: TV point, telephone point

Door lock: ✓
Lockable place: ✓

Services provided
Beauty services: Hairdressing
Mobile library: ✓
Religious services: ✓
Transport: ✗
Activities: *Coordinator:* ✓ • *Examples:* Arts and crafts, exercise
   Outings: ✓
Meetings: ✗

Alandale

Manager: Paul Maple
Owner: Paul Maple
Contact: 9 The Drove, Whitfield, Dover, Kent CT16 3JB
☏ 01304 824904
@ alandaleresidentialhome@ ntlword.com

In a semi-rural setting five minutes' walk from the local pub and 10 minutes' walk from the village shops, Alandale is an extended detached home that boasts a raised pond in its maintained garden. The home is family run, and activities are carried out by a dedicated coordinator, such as exercise, arts and crafts and monthly outings. There are also religious services arranged.

Registered places: 31
Guide weekly rate: £500–£570
Specialist care: Dementia
Medical services: Podiatry, dentist, hygienist, optician, physiotherapy
Qualified staff: Undisclosed

Home details
Location: Residential area, 1 mile from Chislehurst
Communal areas: 2 lounges, dining room, library, chapel, garden
Accessibility: *Floors:* 2 • *Access:* Lift • *Wheelchair access:* Good
Smoking: In designated area
Pets: ✗
Routines: Flexible

Room details
Single: 31
Shared: 0
En suite: 0
Facilities: TV, telephone point

Door lock: ✗
Lockable place: ✗

Services provided
Beauty services: Hairdressing
Mobile library: ✓
Religious services: Twice-weekly Catholic service
Transport: ✗
Activities: *Coordinator:* ✓ • *Examples:* Barbecues, concerts, exercise to music, games • *Outings:* ✗
Meetings: ✗

Antokol

Manager: Alina Gaskin
Owner: Polish Citizens' Committee Housing Association Ltd
Contact: 45 Holbrook Lane, Chislehurst, Kent BR7 6PE
☏ 020 8467 8102
@ antokolhome@btconnect.com
⌂ www.antokol.co.uk

Antokol is a large, Edwardian detached house situated in a rural area that cares for Polish residents. The home maintains the Polish traditions and communication frequently takes place in Polish as well as English. There is a Catholic service twice a week as well as a chapel within the home. The home also has a garden, two lounges and library facilities.

Applecroft Care Home

Manager: Steven Rowley
Owner: Festival Care Management Ltd
Contact: Sanctuary Close, off Chilton Way, Dover, Kent CT17 0ER
☏ 01304 821331

Applecroft is a large, detached, purpose-built care home, situated in a quiet residential cul-de-sac in River, Dover. The home has an activities coordinator and a part-time activities assistant. Weekly activities are displayed on notice boards on each floor. Effort is made to ensure there are activities suited to every person, from group games to personal attention. Pets such as guinea pigs, hamsters and budgies visit the home. A weekly shopping trolley makes the rounds, and residents are offered sherry and beer off the weekly drinks trolley.

Registered places: 75
Guide weekly rate: £400–£750
Specialist care: Nursing, dementia, respite
Medical services: Podiatry, dentist, optician
Qualified staff: Fails standard: 38% at NVQ Level 2

Home details
Location: Residential area, 3 miles from Dover
Communal areas: Lounge, dining room, activities room, smoking room, garden
Accessibility: *Floors:* 2 • *Access:* lift • *Wheelchair access:* Good
Smoking: In designated area
Pets: At manager's discretion
Routines: Flexible

Room details
Single: 75
Shared: 0
En suite: 75
Facilities: TV point, telephone point

Door lock: ✗
Lockable place: ✓

Services provided
Beauty services: Hairdressing
Mobile library: ✓
Religious services: ✗
Transport: ✗
Activities: *Coordinator:* ✓ • *Examples:* Armchair exercises, cooking, karaoke • *Outings:* ✗
Meetings: ✓

Ashcroft

Manager: Stella Barnes
Owner: Care Providers Ltd
Contact: 48–50 London Lane, Bromley, Kent BR1 4HE
☏ 020 8460 0424
@ suemaloney@care-providers.co.uk
🖰 www.care-providers.co.uk

Ashcroft is a detached, older property. It is a family-run business situated in a residential area, one mile from Bromley. With a part-time activities organiser there are regular activities on offer, such as bingo and quizzes. There are also regular outings and the home arranges Communion once a week.

Registered places: 22
Guide weekly rate: £600–£950
Specialist care: Nursing
Medical services: Podiatry, dentist, optician, physiotherapy
Qualified staff: Exceeds standard: 82% at NVQ Level 2

Home details
Location: Residential area, 1 mile from Bromley
Communal areas: Lounge, dining room, patio and garden
Accessibility: *Floors:* 3 • *Access:* Lift • *Wheelchair access:* Good
Smoking: ✗
Pets: At manager's discretion
Routines: Flexible

Room details
Single: 9
Shared: 5
En suite: 0
Facilities: TV point, telephone point

Door lock: ✓
Lockable place: ✓

Services provided
Beauty services: Hairdressing
Mobile library: ✓
Religious services: Weekly Communion, monthly service
Transport: ✗
Activities: *Coordinator:* ✓ • *Examples:* Bingo, singing, quizzes *Outings:* ✓
Meetings: ✓

Registered places: 82
Guide weekly rate: £874
Specialist care: Nursing, dementia, respite
Medical services: Podiatry, dentist, optician, physiotherapy
Qualified staff: Exceeds standard: 75% at NVQ Level 2

Home details

Location: Residential area, 2 miles from Ashford
Communal areas: 4 communal rooms, conservatory
Accessibility: *Floors:* 3 • *Access:* 2 lifts • *Wheelchair access:* Good
Smoking: Outside in designated area
Pets: ✗
Routines: Flexible

Room details

Single: 82
Shared: 0
En suite: 82
Facilities: TV

Door lock: ✓
Lockable place: ✓

Services provided

Beauty services: Hairdressing, massage
Mobile library: ✓
Religious services: Monthly
Transport: ✓
Activities: *Coordinator:* ✓ • *Examples:* Communal crosswords, movement to music • *Outings:* ✗
Meetings: ✓

The Ashford Nursing Home and Brabourne Care Centre

Manager: Vacant
Owner: Opus Care Ltd
Contact: Hythe Road, Ashford, Kent TN24 0QJ
☏ 01233 643555
@ ashfordnursinghome@mail.com

A new purpose-built home that is set on the main Hythe Brabourne Care Centre is set in its own grounds close to its sister home, The Ashford Nursing Home. Each floor has an allocated quiet area as well as a lounge for residents to enjoy. The ground floor boasts the largest room which is used for entertainment alongside the conservatory. The home aims to create a 'homely' feel whilst enjoying modern features such as two lifts and a secure entry system. The home has a hair and beauty salon and offers activities including communal crosswords and movement to music.

Registered places: 15
Guide weekly rate: £378–£575
Specialist care: Respite
Medical services: Podiatry, hygienist, optician
Qualified staff: Meets standard

Home details

Location: Residential area, 1 mile from Bickley
Communal areas: Lounge, conservatory, garden
Accessibility: *Floors:* 3 • *Access:* Lift • *Wheelchair access:* Good
Smoking: ✗
Pets: ✗
Routines: Flexible

Room details

Single: 9
Shared: 3
En suite: 0
Facilities: TV point, telephone point

Door lock: ✓
Lockable place. ✗

Services provided

Beauty services: Hairdressing, manicures, hand massage
Mobile library: ✓
Religious services: ✗
Transport: ✗
Activities: *Coordinator:* ✓ • *Examples:* Quizzes, singalongs *Outings:* ✓
Meetings: ✓

Ashglade Rest Home

Manager: Denise Gill
Owner: Chislehurst Care Ltd
Contact: 178 Southborough Road, Bickley, Bromley, Kent BR2 8AL
☏ 020 8467 0640
@ ashgladecare@tiscali.co.uk

Ashglade is a detached Edwardian house located on a bus route between Petts Wood and Bromley. There is a garden at the rear of the home accessed by a ramp.

The activities programme is displayed every month in the home. The activities coordinator organises various outings, such as a trip to the local garden centre or shopping at Bromley shopping centre as well as in-house activities. These include singalongs and quizzes. The home also arranges for a mobile library to visit.

Ashling Lodge

Manager: Sally Perry
Owner: Chislehurst Care Ltd
Contact: 20 Station Road,
Orpington, Kent BR6 0SA
) 01689 877946
@ aslinglodge@ciscali.co.uk

Ashling Lodge is within a half a mile of Orpington town centre which offers a range of shops, leisure facilities, and public transport links. A church is situated across the road from the home which residents can attend. The vicar also occasionally visits the home. The home often arranges cream teas and garden parties with other local care and nursing homes for the residents to enjoy. The home also offers hairdressing and manicures to the residents.

Registered places: 13
Guide weekly rate: £358–£540
Specialist care: Respite
Medical services: Podiatry, Dentist, optician, physiotherapy
Qualified staff: Fails standard: 30% at NVQ Level 2

Home details
Location: Residential area, 0.5 miles from Orpington
Communal areas: Lounge, dining room, conservatory, garden
Accessibility: *Floors:* 2 • *Access:* Stair lift
   Wheelchair access: Good
Smoking: ✗
Pets: At manager's discretion
Routines: Flexible

Room details
Single: 12
Shared: 1
En suite: 1
Facilities: TV point, telephone point

Door lock: ✓
Lockable place: ✓

Services provided
Beauty services: Hairdressing, manicures
Mobile library: ✗
Religious services: ✓
Transport: ✗
Activities: *Coordinator:* ✗ • *Examples:* Bingo, film evenings, visiting entertainers • *Outings:* ✗
Meetings: ✓

Ashton Lodge

Manager: Manoon Ramasawmy
Owner: Mr and Mrs Ramasawmy
Contact: 22 St Michaels Road,
Maidstone, Kent ME16 8BS
) 01622 677149

Ashton Lodge is a large house that has been converted into a rest home. The home is approximately half a mile from Maidstone where there are shops, a post office, and a pub. The home goes on small outings and the daily activities programme includes bingo and exercise sessions. The vicar visits the home regularly.

Registered places: 12
Guide weekly rate: £350–£400
Specialist care: Respite
Medical services: Podiatry, dentist, optician
Qualified staff: Meets standard

Home details
Location: Residential area, 0.5 miles from Maidstone
Communal areas: Lounge, dining room, garden
Accessibility: *Floors:* 2 • *Access:* Lift • *Wheelchair access:* Good
Smoking: ✗
Pets: ✗
Routines: Flexible

Room details
Single: 10
Shared: 1
En suite: 0
Facilities: TV point, telephone point

Door lock: ✓
Lockable place: ✓

Services provided
Beauty services: Hairdressing
Mobile library: ✗
Religious services: Vicar visits regularly
Transport: ✗
Activities: *Coordinator:* ✗ • *Examples:* Bingo, crosswords, exercise • *Outings:* ✓
Meetings: ✗

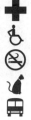

Ashurst Park Care Home

Manager: Anne Trigg
Owner: Four Seasons Healthcare Ltd
Contact: Fordcombe Road, Fordcombe, Tunbridge Wells, Kent TN3 0RD
) 01892 709000
www.fshc.co.uk

Ashurst Park Care Home is half a mile from the village of Fordcombe and can be easily accessed by bus. Situated in large gardens, the home has a large lounge and separate dining room on the ground floor as well as a small bar. Some of the rooms have patio access to the grounds. There are also library facilities and a physiotherapy room. The home has its own minibus and runs a fortnightly nondenominational church service. The activities coordinator runs a fitness programme for residents and there are also arranged outings.

Registered places: 53
Guide weekly rate: £750–£850
Specialist care: Nursing
Medical services: Podiatry, optician, physiotherapy
Qualified staff: Fails standard

Home details
Location: Village location, 0.5 mile from Fordcombe
Communal areas: Lounge, dining room, lounge/kitchen, physiotherapy room, patio and garden
Accessibility: *Floors:* 2 • *Access:* Lift • *Wheelchair access:* Good
Smoking: ✗
Pets: ✓
Routines: Flexible

Room details
Single: 42
Shared: 2
En suite: 35
Facilities: TV, telephone point
Door lock: ✓
Lockable place: ✗

Services provided
Beauty services: Hairdressing
Mobile library: Library facilities
Religious services: Fortnightly nondenominational church service
Transport: Minibus
Activities: *Coordinator:* ✓ • *Examples:* Fitness programme, games *Outings:* ✓
Meetings: ✗

Ashurst Place

Manager: Paul Iles
Owner: Louise and Julia Watts
Contact: Lampington Row, Langton Green, Tunbridge Wells, Kent TN3 0JG
) 01892 863661

The home is in a rural location, approximately three miles from Tunbridge Wells. The home aims to create a comfortable place for residents to feel at home. They have a variety of activities such as quizzes and music and movement. There are also outings available for the residents. Each month there are visits from Anglican and Catholic clergy. The home has its own library facilities and a garden for residents to enjoy.

Registered places: 37
Guide weekly rate: £400–£700
Specialist care: Respite
Medical services: Podiatry, dentist, optician
Qualified staff: Exceeds standard: 60% at NVQ Level 2

Home details
Location: Village location, 3 miles from Tunbridge Wells
Communal areas: Lounge, dining room, conservatory, library, garden
Accessibility: *Floors:* 2 • *Access:* Lift • *Wheelchair access:* Good
Smoking: In designated area
Pets: At manager's discretion
Routines: Flexible

Room details
Single: 30
Shared: 3
En suite: 7
Facilities: TV point, telephone point
Door lock: ✓
Lockable place: ✓

Services provided
Beauty services: Hairdressing
Mobile library: Library facilities
Religious services: Monthly Catholic and Anglican visits
Transport: ✗
Activities: *Coordinator:* ✓ • *Examples:* Bingo, music and movement, quizzes • *Outings:* ✓
Meetings: ✗

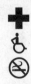

Balgowan Nursing Home

Manager: Penelope Selby
Owner: Premium Healthcare Ltd
Contact: 46 Bartholomew Lane, Hythe, Kent CT21 4BX
☎ 01303 266782
@ balgowan@premiumhealthcare.co.uk
🖰 www.premiumhealthcare.co.uk

Balgowan Nursing Home is a large, detached two-storey house situated in a rural area, one mile from Hythe. Regular outings are organised to the local pub and the activities coordinator takes residents out for walks. The daily activities programme includes arts and crafts and games, as well as exercise sessions.

Registered places: 33
Guide weekly rate: £600–£700
Specialist care: Nursing
Medical services: Podiatry, physiotherapy
Qualified staff: Meets standard

Home details
Location: Rural area, 1 mile from Hythe
Communal areas: Lounge, dining room, garden
Accessibility: *Floors:* 2 • *Access:* Lift and stair lift *Wheelchair access:* Good
Smoking: ✗
Pets: ✗
Routines: Flexible

Room details
Single: 25
Shared: 4
En suite: 4
Facilities: TV point

Door lock: ✗
Lockable place: ✓

Services provided
Beauty services: Hairdressing
Mobile library: ✗
Religious services: ✗
Transport: ✗
Activities: *Coordinator:* ✓ • *Examples:* Arts and crafts, games, exercise • *Outings:* ✓
Meetings: ✗

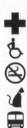

Barham House Nursing Home

Manager: Sheralyn Kelly
Owner: Arj Shandandaqumar
Contact: The Street, Barham, Canterbury, Kent CT4 6PA
☎ 01227 833400

Barham House is a Grade II listed Georgian House in its own grounds, approximately eight miles from Canterbury. The home has a lounge and a garden for residents to socialise and there are regular activities and outings. These include arts and crafts and quiz sessions. The home has its own transport for outings. The home also arranges for Anglican ministers to visit the home once a week. There are residents meetings every six months to enable residents to voice their opinions.

Registered places: 23
Guide weekly rate: £470–£600
Specialist care: Nursing
Medical services: Podiatry, dentist, optician.
Qualified staff: Meets standard

Home details
Location: Village location, 8 miles from Canterbury
Communal areas: Lounge, dining room, garden
Accessibility: *Floors:* 3 • *Access:* Lift • *Wheelchair access:* Good
Smoking: ✗
Pets: At manager's discretion
Routines: Flexible

Room details
Single: 13
Shared: 6
En suite: 9
Facilities: TV point, telephone point

Door lock: ✓
Lockable place: ✓

Services provided
Beauty services: Hairdressing
Mobile library: ✗
Religious services: Weekly Anglican visits
Transport: ✓
Activities: *Coordinator:* ✓ • *Examples:* Arts and crafts, bingo, quizzes • *Outings:* ✓
Meetings: ✓

Registered places: 9
Guide weekly rate: From £425
Specialist care: Day care
Medical services: Podiatry, dentist, optician, physiotherapy
Qualified staff: Exceeds standard: 100% at NVQ Level 2

Home details
Location: Rural area, 5 miles from Sittingbourne
Communal areas: Lounge, dining room, 2 patios and garden
Accessibility: *Floors:* 1 • *Wheelchair access:* Good
Smoking: ✗
Pets: At manager's discretion
Routines: Flexible

Room details
Single: 7   Door lock: ✓
Shared: 1   Lockable place: ✓
En suite: 8
Facilities: TV point, telephone point

Services provided
Beauty services: Hairdressing, aromatherapy
Mobile library: ✓
Religious services: Monthly Communion service
Transport: Car
Activities: *Coordinator:* ✗ • *Examples:* Art therapy, flower
    arranging, quizzes • *Outings:* ✓
Meetings: ✓

Beechfields

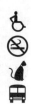

Manager: Dorothy Saffrey
Owner: Mr and Mrs Saffrey
Contact: Conyer Road, Teynham,
Sittingbourne, Kent ME9 9ET
☎ 01795 520580

Beechfields is a purpose-built home, five miles from Sittingbourne. The home is on one level with several seating areas set around the outside the building. There are countryside views from most of the windows. The home aims for residents to live as independently and actively as possible. The home can cater to all denominations with links to local churches. The daily activities programme includes art therapy sessions and quizzes. The home also arranges outings for the residents.

Registered places: 54
Guide weekly rate: £487–£624
Specialist care: Day care, dementia, mental disorder
Medical services: Podiatry, dentist, optician, physiotherapy
Qualified staff: Exceeds standard: 68% at NVQ level 2

Home details
Location: Residential area, 1 mile from St Paul's Cray
Communal areas: 3 communal areas, quiet room, 2 gardens
Accessibility: *Floors:* 2 • *Access:* Lift • *Wheelchair access:* Good
Smoking: In designated area
Pets: ✓
Routines: Flexible

Room details
Single: 54   Door lock: ✗
Shared: 0   Lockable place: ✓
En suite: 0
Facilities: TV point

Services provided
Beauty services: Hairdressing, aromatherapy
Mobile library: ✓
Religious services: ✓
Transport: ✗
Activities: *Coordinator:* ✓ • *Examples:* Bingo, quizzes
    Outings: ✓
Meetings: ✓

Belle Grove

Manager: Margaret Rolls
Owner: Shaw Healthcare Ltd
Contact: 100 Mickleham Road, St Pauls
Cray, Orpington, Kent BR5 2RJ
☎ 020 8300 0108
@ bellegrove@shaw.co.uk

Located in a residential area, Bellegrove is a purpose-built home that is one mile from St Paul's Cray. The home is situated opposite the local library, next to the primary care trust centre and close to shops. The home has an open door policy allowing residents to come and go as they please. The home arranges a range of activities and outings and there are large-scale board games for communal play. There is a residents committee which meets every month and a relatives committee which meets every quarter.

Benedict House Nursing Home

Manager: Izzy Hitcham
Owner: Sunglade Care Ltd
Contact: 63 Copers Cope Road, Beckenham, Kent BR3 1NJ
☎ 020 8663 3954

Benedict House is a large detached building situated in a residential area, one mile from Beckenham. The home has an activities coordinator who arranges music to movement sessions for the residents. The home also employs a handyman who deals all maintenance issues. He also checks safety issues. The home has a conservatory and garden for residents to enjoy.

Registered places: 48
Guide weekly rate: Undisclosed
Specialist care: Nursing
Medical services: None
Qualified staff: Exceeds standard: 100% at NVQ level 2

Home details
Location: Residential area, 1 mile from Beckenham
Communal areas: Lounge, dining room, conservatory, garden
Accessibility: *Floors:* 4 • *Access:* Lift • *Wheelchair access:* Good
Smoking: ✗
Pets: Undisclosed
Routines: Flexible

Room details
Single: 48
Shared: 0
En suite: Undisclosed
Facilities: TV

Door lock: ✓
Lockable place: ✓

Services provided
Beauty services: Hairdressing
Mobile library: ✗
Religious services: ✗
Transport: ✗
Activities: *Coordinator:* ✓ • *Examples:* Music to movement
    Outings: ✗
Meetings: ✗

Berengrove Park Nursing Home

Manager: Carole Godden
Owner: Berengrove Ltd
Contact: 43–45 Park Avenue, Gillingham, Kent ME7 4AH
☎ 01634 850411

Berengrove Park is located on a residential area approximately one mile from Gillingham. As it is an older building many of the rooms are of a generous size and are shared rooms. Most of the residents tend to eat their meals in their rooms. The home offers a range of activities including exercises to help keep the residents active such as exercise sessions and music therapy. There are also frequent trips to local points of interest.

Registered places: 36
Guide weekly rate: £496–£581
Specialist care: Nursing, dementia, respite
Medical services: Podiatry, dentist, optician, physiotherapy
Qualified staff: Exceeds standard: 60% at NVQ Level 2

Home details
Location: Residential area, 1 mile from Gillingham
Communal areas: 3 lounges, dining room, patio and garden
Accessibility: *Floors:* 2 • *Access:* Lift • *Wheelchair access:* Good
Smoking: ✗
Pets: ✗
Routines: Flexible

Room details
Single: 18
Shared: 9
En suite: Undisclosed
Facilities: TV point

Door lock: ✓
Lockable place: ✓

Services provided
Beauty services: Hairdressing
Mobile library: ✓
Religious services: Monthly Anglican service
Transport: ✗
Activities: *Coordinator:* ✓ • *Examples:* Light therapy, music therapy
    Outings: ✓
Meetings: ✗

Registered places: 38
Guide weekly rate: £475–£700
Specialist care: None
Medical services: Podiatry, dentist, optician, physiotherapy
Qualified staff: Meets standard

Home details

Location: Rural area, 3.5 miles from Tunbridge Wells
Communal areas: 3 lounges, dining room, conservatory, garden
Accessibility: *Floors:* 4 • *Access:* Lift • *Wheelchair access:* Good
Smoking: In designated area
Pets: ✓
Routines: Flexible

Room details

Single: 38
Shared: 0
En suite: 38
Facilities: TV point, telephone point

Door lock: ✗
Lockable place: ✓

Services provided

Beauty services: Hairdressing
Mobile library: ✓
Religious services: Monthly
Transport: ✓
Activities: *Coordinator:* ✗ • *Examples:* Coffee mornings, gardening
       Outings: ✓
Meetings: ✓

Birchwood House Rest Home

Manager: Janice Collins
Owner: Malvirt Ltd
Contact: Stockland Green Road,
Speldhurst, Tunbridge Wells,
Kent TN3 0TU
☏ 01892 863559

Birchwood House is a detached property standing in its own grounds. The garden provides a safe walking area with pretty views overlooking the local countryside. There are regular activities organised for residents such as walks round local woodland, flower arranging, bingo and coffee mornings. There are frequent outings as the home has its own minibus. There are shopping trips into town weekly and outings to local points of interest.

Registered places: 17
Guide weekly rate: £570–£700
Specialist care: Nursing
Medical services: Podiatry, dentist, optician, physiotherapy
Qualified staff: Exceeds standard: 100% at NVQ level 2

Home details

Location: Residential area, 0.5 miles from Bromley
Communal areas: TV lounge, dining room, patio and garden
Accessibility: *Floors:* 2 • *Access:* Lift • *Wheelchair access:* Good
Smoking: In designated area
Pets: ✗
Routines: Flexible

Room details

Single: 1
Shared: 16
En suite: Undisclosed
Facilities: TV

Door lock: ✗
Lockable place: ✓

Services provided

Beauty services: Hairdressing
Mobile library: ✓
Religious services: ✓
Transport: ✗
Activities: *Coordinator:* ✗ • *Examples:* Bingo, reminiscence sessions
       Outings: ✓
Meetings: ✗

Blyth House

Manager: Rhona Robinson
Owner: Chislehurst Care Ltd
Contact: 16 Blyth Road,
Bromley, Kent BR1 3RX
☏ 020 8460 3070
@ blythhouse@tiscali.co.uk

Blyth House has been purpose built and is located approximately half a mile from Bromley. Once a month, a visiting entertainer comes into the home and there is an activities programme displayed in the lounge. There is a lounge/dining room on the ground floor of the home and a secluded garden and patio area with garden furniture. The home offers a variety of religious services for different denominations. The home also arranges a variety of outings including a pantomime at Christmas. Smoking is permitted outside under supervision and pets are allowed to visit.

Bracknell House

Manager: Vindoo Jaunky
Owner: Bidianund and Vindoo Jaunky
Contact: 34 Helena Road,
Capel-le-Ferne, Folkestone, Kent
CT18 7LQ
☎ 01303 254496
@ bracknellhouse@btconnect.com

Bracknell House is found in a residential area of Dover, five miles from the town centre. The home has several small lounges as well as a conservatory and a garden. The home has a daily activities programme and organises special events for residents' birthdays. There are also regular residents meetings and outings in the local area.

Registered places: 20
Guide weekly rate: £312–£360
Specialist care: Day care, respite
Medical services: Podiatry, dentist, optician
Qualified staff: Meets standard

Home details
Location: Residential area, 5 miles from Dover
Communal areas: Lounges, conservatory, garden
Accessibility: *Floors:* 2 • *Access:* Stair lift
Wheelchair access: Good
Smoking: ✗
Pets: ✓
Routines: Flexible

Room details
Single: 14
Shared: 3
En suite: 10
Facilities: TV, telephone

Door lock: ✓
Lockable place: ✓

Services provided
Beauty services: Hairdressing
Mobile library: ✗
Religious services: ✓
Transport: ✗
Activities: *Coordinator:* ✓ • *Examples:* Bingo, birthday parties
Outings: ✓
Meetings: ✓

Bradfield Residential Home

Manager: Brenda Johnson
Owner: David and Brenda Johnson
Contact: Hawksdown Road,
Walmer, Deal, Kent CT14 7PW
☎ 01304 360960

Bradfield Residential Home is a family-run home set in a quiet area approximately half a mile from Walmer village and its amenities, including Walmer Castle. The home is also approximately seven miles from Dover. The seafront is within walking distance from the home with some top-floor bedrooms permitting sea views. The home arranges a residents meeting once a fortnight and religious services once a month.

Registered places: 21
Guide weekly rate: £303–£425
Specialist care: None
Medical services: Podiatry, dentist, optician, physiotherapy
Qualified staff: Exceeds standard: 75% at NVQ Level 2

Home details
Location: Village location, 7 miles from Dover
Communal areas: 3 lounges, dining room, conservatories, garden
Accessibility: *Floors:* 3 • *Access:* Lift • *Wheelchair access:* Good
Smoking: ✗
Pets: At manager's discretion
Routines: Flexible

Room details
Single: 21
Shared: 0
En suite: 19
Facilities: TV point, telephone point

Door lock: ✓
Lockable place: ✓

Services provided
Beauty services: Hairdressing, manicures
Mobile library: ✗
Religious services: Monthly Communion service,
monthly Anglican service
Transport: Minibus
Activities: *Coordinator:* ✓ • *Examples:* Barbecues, bingo, games
Outings: ✓
Meetings: ✓

Registered places: 18
Guide weekly rate: Undisclosed
Specialist care: Day care, respite
Medical services: Podiatry, dentist, optician
Qualified staff: Undisclosed

Home details

Location: Village location, 6.5 miles from Ashford
Communal areas: 2 lounges, dining room, conservatory, patio and garden
Accessibility: *Floors:* 2 • *Access:* Lift • *Wheelchair access:* Good
Smoking: ✗
Pets: At manager's discretion
Routines: Flexible

Room details

Single: 18
Shared: 0
En suite: 8
Facilities: TV point, telephone point

Door lock: ✓
Lockable place: ✓

Services provided

Beauty services: Hairdressing
Mobile library: ✓
Religious services: Regular visits from local clergy
Transport: Cars
Activities: *Coordinator:* ✗ • *Examples:* Board games, garden parties, pantomimes • *Outings:* ✓
Meetings: ✓

Brambles

Manager: Arnold Parker
Owner: Arnold, Kevin and Jean Parker
Contact: Bramble Lane,
Wye, Ashford, Kent TN25 5EW
☎ 01233 813217
@ info@bramblescare.co.uk

Brambles is situated in a village location, six and a half miles from Ashford. A bus stop and train station are nearby. In summer, the garden is used for outdoor eating, parties and fêtes. There is also a greenhouse for the use of any residents who enjoy gardening. The home has two budgies and a fish tank. Residents are treated as part of the local community and are invited to events in the village hall.

An 11-bed extension to the home is in the process of construction.

Registered places: 20
Guide weekly rate: From £377
Specialist care: Day care, dementia respite
Medical services: Podiatry, dentist, optician
Qualified staff: Exceeds standard: 80% at NVQ Level 2

Home details

Location: Rural area, 9 miles from Dover
Communal areas: Lounge, lounge/dining room, conservatory, patio and garden
Accessibility: *Floors:* 2 • *Access:* Lift • *Wheelchair access:* Good
Smoking: In designated area
Pets: At manager's discretion
Routines: Structured

Room details

Single: 16
Shared: 2
En suite: 2
Facilities: TV point

Door lock: ✓
Lockable place: ✓

Services provided

Beauty services: Hairdressing, aromatherapy
Mobile library: ✗
Religious services: Monthly Communion service
Transport: ✗
Activities: *Coordinator:* ✓ • *Examples:* Animal therapy, bingo *Outings:* ✗
Meetings: ✓

Brambling House

Manager: Lalitha Kumar
Owner: Kanagaratnam Rajaseelan
Contact: 46 Eythorne Road,
Shepherdswell, Dover, Kent CT15 7PG
☎ 01304 830276
@ bramblinghouse@firstchoicehomes.co.uk

Brambling House is an extended detached property located in the quiet and rural village of Shepherdswell, nine miles from Dover. The local area is served by a public bus service, but the village has a train station with direct mainline access. There is a landscaped garden to the rear of the property, along with a patio area that provides tables and chairs for residents to enjoy during good weather. The home arranges a residents meeting once every three months and there is Communion on a monthly basis.

The Bramblings Residential Home

Manager: Bernadette Ramsey
Owner: Bramblings Ltd
Contact: Hartley Road,
Longfield, Kent DA3 7PE
☏ 01474 702332

The Bramblings Residential Home is located in the village of Longfield, five and a half miles from Gravesend. The capacity of the home is being increased with 22 new rooms to be registered in July 2007. All of these rooms will be en suite. Residents tend to eat their meals in their own rooms. There are outings for groups going to the theatre, garden centres and the beach during good weather. The home also arranges some in house activities including beauty therapy afternoons and music and movement.

Registered places: 26
Guide weekly rate: £322–£396
Specialist care: Day care, learning disability
Medical services: Podiatry, hygienist, optician, physiotherapy
Qualified staff: Exceeds standard: 90% at NVQ Level 2

Home details
Location: Village location, 5.5 miles from Gravesend
Communal areas: Lounge, dining room, garden
Accessibility: *Floors:* 2 • *Access:* Lift • *Wheelchair access:* Good
Smoking: ✗
Pets: At manager's discretion
Routines: Flexible

Room details
Single: 26
Shared: 0
En suite: 26
Facilities: TV point, telephone point

Door lock: ✓
Lockable place: ✓

Services provided
Beauty services: Hairdressing
Mobile library: ✓
Religious services: Fortnightly Anglican service
Transport: ✗
Activities: *Coordinator:* ✗ • *Examples:* Arts and crafts, beauty therapy, music and movement • *Outings:* ✓
Meetings: ✗

Brampton Lodge

Manager: Claire Ebbs
Owner: Nickolls Care Ltd
Contact: 4 Dixwell Road,
Folkestone, Kent CT20 2LG
☏ 01303 258 227
🖱 www.bramptonlodge.com

Brampton Lodge is a large, detached property, one and a half miles from Folkstone. The home employs a qualified chef and food is of a high standard. The home offers a variety of activities including music and movement. The home has its own transport for outings and also arranges an Anglican service to take place once a month.

Registered places: 18
Guide weekly rate: £507–£599
Specialist care: Respite
Medical services: Podiatry
Qualified staff: Meets standard

Home details
Location: Residential area, 1.5 miles from Folkstone
Communal areas: Lounge, dining room, patio and garden
Accessibility: *Floors:* 2 • *Access:* Lift • *Wheelchair access:* Good
Smoking: In designated area
Pets: At manager's discretion
Routines: Flexible

Room details
Single: 18
Shared: 0
En suite: 18
Facilities: TV, telephone

Door lock: ✓
Lockable place: ✓

Services provided
Beauty services: Hairdressing, aromatherapy
Mobile library: ✗
Religious services: Monthly Anglican service
Transport: Car
Activities: *Coordinator:* ✓ • *Examples:* Quizzes, armchair exercises, music and movement • *Outings:* ✓
Meetings: ✗

Registered places: 42
Guide weekly rate: Undisclosed
Specialist care: Nursing, respite
Medical services: Podiatry, physiotherapy, occupational therapy
Qualified staff: Undisclosed

Home details

Location: Rural area, 2.5 miles from Dartford
Communal areas: 3 lounges, dining room,
hairdressing salon, garden
Accessibility: *Floors:* 2 • *Access:* Lift and stair lift
Wheelchair access: Good
Smoking: ✗
Pets: ✓
Routines: Flexible

Room details

Single: 42
Shared: 0
En suite: 42
Facilities: TV point

Door lock: ✓
Lockable place: ✗

Services provided

Beauty services: Hairdressing, aromatherapy
Mobile library: ✓
Religious services: Weekly Communion service
Transport: ✓
Activities: *Coordinator:* ✓ • *Examples:* Arts and crafts, gardening,
games • *Outings:* ✓
Meetings: ✓

Broad Oak Manor Nursing Home

Manager: Sandra Nevard
Owner: BUPA Care Homes Ltd
Contact: Broad Oak Close,
Arnolds Lane, Sutton-at-Hone,
Dartford, Kent DA4 9HF
☏ 01322 223591
@ BroadOakManorALL@BUPA.com
🖰 www.bupacarehomes.co.uk

Originally a private house, Broad Oak Manor has been converted into a nursing home. Situated in the small village of Sutton-at-Hone, it is on a local bus route and shops are within easy reach. The dining room overlooks the garden and patio area, which offers a pleasant sunny afternoon with its views over the Darenth Valley. All the bedrooms are for single occupancy and have en suite facilities. Daily activities offered include arts and crafts, gardening, games, quizzes and trips to local places of interest.

Registered places: 10
Guide weekly rate: £339–£400
Specialist care: None
Medical services: Podiatry, dentist, optician, physiotherapy
Qualified staff: Meets standard

Home details

Location: Residential area, 2.5 miles from Sheerness
Communal areas: Lounge, dining room, patio and garden
Accessibility: *Floors:* 2 • *Access:* Lift • *Wheelchair access:* None
Smoking: ✗
Pets: ✗
Routines: Structured

Room details

Single: 10
Shared: 0
En suite: 8
Facilities: TV point, telephone point

Door lock: ✓
Lockable place: ✓

Services provided

Beauty services: Hairdressing
Mobile library: ✗
Religious services: ✓
Transport: ✗
Activities: *Coordinator:* ✗ • *Examples:* Bingo, dominoes
Outings: ✓
Meetings: ✗

Bromfield House Residential Care Home Ltd

Manager: Teresa Oakey
Owner: Malcom Jackman
Contact: 316 Minster Road,
Minster-on-Sea, Sheerness,
Kent ME12 3NR
☏ 01795 873018

Bromfield House is located in a residential area, approximately two and a half miles from Sheerness. Although outings are offered, the residents do not always take them up. The home can offer religious services on request. For the residents' birthdays, an entertainer is brought in. The home also a daily activities programme which includes bingo and dominoes. There is a garden with a patio area for residents to enjoy in the warmer months.

Byron Lodge Residential Nursing Home

Manager: Margaret Spurgeon
Owner: Dr and Mrs Jana
Contact: 105–107 Rock Avenue, Gillingham, Kent ME7 5PX
☏ 01634 855136

Byron Lodge is a purpose-built care home, half a mile from Gillingham. The staff aim to make the residents as comfortable as possible and bring in large print books, audio books and DVDs. They also have parties for residents' birthdays, and recently, a diamond wedding celebration. There are good views from all the rooms and the home is close to local amenities. The daily activities offered to residents include painting and drawing, bingo and large floor games. There are also visits from an Anglican vicar several times a year.

Registered places: 28
Guide weekly rate: £496–£525
Specialist care: Nursing
Medical services: Podiatry, optician, physiotherapy
Qualified staff: Exceeds standard: 75% at NVQ Level 2

Home details
Location: Residential area, 0.5 miles from Gillingham
Communal areas: Lounge, dining room, patio and garden
Accessibility: *Floors:* 3 • *Access:* Lift • *Wheelchair access:* Good
Smoking: ✗
Pets: ✗
Routines: Flexible

Room details
Single: 22	Door lock: ✓
Shared: 3	Lockable place: ✓
En suite: 12	
Facilities: TV point, telephone point	

Services provided
Beauty services: Hairdressing
Mobile library: ✗
Religious services: Visits from Anglican vicar
Transport: ✗
Activities: *Coordinator:* ✓ • *Examples:* Bingo, painting
    Outings: ✓
Meetings: ✓

Capel Grange

Manager: Sara Grist
Owner: Safequarter Ltd
Contact: Maidstone Road, Five Oak Green, Tunbridge, Kent TN12 6QY
☏ 01892 834225
@ care@capelgrange.co.uk
🖥 www.capelgrange.co.uk

Capel Grange has been a care home since 1981 and is a converted country house with a purpose-built two-storey extension. The home stands in three and a half acres of gardens with paved areas and a lake. The home goes on a range of outings, to the pantomime, choral services and local places of interest. There are also in house activities such as bingo and card games. There are Anglican and Catholic services twice a week in the home.

Registered places: 38
Guide weekly rate: £496–£600
Specialist care: Respite
Medical services: Podiatry, dentist, optician, physiotherapy
Qualified staff: Exceeds standard: 100% at NVQ Level 2

Home details
Location: Village location, 6 miles from Tunbridge Wells
Communal areas: Lounge, dining room, 2 conservatories, patio and garden
Accessibility: *Floors:* 2 • *Access:* 2 lifts • *Wheelchair access:* Good
Smoking: ✗
Pets: ✗
Routines: Flexible

Room details
Single: 30	Door lock: ✓
Shared: 5	Lockable place: ✓
En suite: 31	
Facilities: TV point, telephone point	

Services provided
Beauty services: Hairdressing
Mobile library: Library facilities
Religious services: Twice weekly Anglican and Catholic services
Transport: ✗
Activities: *Coordinator:* ✓ • *Examples:* Bingo, board games, music
    Outings: ✓
Meetings: ✓

Registered places: 28
Guide weekly rate: £595
Specialist care: Nursing, respite
Medical services: Podiatry, physiotherapy
Qualified staff: Exceeds standard: 60% at NVQ Level 2

Home details

Location: Residential area, 8.5 miles from Dover
Communal areas: 3 lounges, dining room, patio and garden
Accessibility: *Floors:* 3 • *Access:* Lift and stair lift
    Wheelchair access: Good
Smoking: In designated area
Pets: x
Routines: Flexible

Room details

Single: 8	Door lock: ✓
Shared: 7	Lockable place: ✓
En suite: 12	

Facilities: TV point, telephone point

Services provided

Beauty services: Hairdressing
Mobile library: x
Religious services: x
Transport: x
Activities: *Coordinator:* x • *Examples:* Bingo, exercises, quizzes
    Outings: x
Meetings: ✓

The Carleton Nursing Home

Manager: Christine Follett
Owner: Seawind Care Services Ltd
Contact: 70 London Road, Deal, Kent CT14 9TR
☏ 01304 360218

The Carleton Nursing Home is a large detached building, situated in a residential area of Deal. The home is within walking distance to the town centre, and is therefore within easy reach of the town facilities, the seafront, and Deal Castle. The home arranges various activities for its residents including bingo and exercise sessions and also organises residents meetings to take place once a month. There are three lounges for residents to relax in as well as a garden with a patio area.

Registered places: 43
Guide weekly rate: £317–£437
Specialist care: Respite, day care
Medical services: Podiatry, hygienist, opticians, physiotherapy
Qualified staff: Exceeds standard: 60% at NVQ Level 2

Home details

Location: Residential area, 1 mile from Faversham
Communal areas: 4 lounge/dining rooms, 2 gardens
Accessibility: *Floors:* 3 • *Access:* Lift and stair lift
    Wheelchair access: Good
Smoking: x
Pets: At manager's discretion
Routines Flexible

Room details

Single: 24	Door lock: ✓
Shared: 7	Lockable place: ✓
En suite: 20	

Facilities: TV point, telephone point

Services provided

Beauty services: Hairdressing, aromatherapy
Mobile library: x
Religious services: Weekly Catholic Communion, monthly Anglican visits
Transport: Minibus
Activities: *Coordinator:* ✓ • *Examples:* Games, music, quizzes
    Outings: ✓
Meetings: ✓

Carnalea Residential Home

Manager: Karina Carter-Pope
Owner: Betty Wake
Contact: 5–9 London Road, Faversham, Kent ME13 8TA
☏ 01795 532629
@ eldercare@carnalea.com
⌂ www.carnalea.com

Carnalea Residential Home is a converted Victorian building with two extensions at ground and first-floor level. The grounds include a large, attractive walled garden with a seating area at the rear. The home is situated, one mile from Faversham town centre and train station. Local shops are within walking distance. The home often organises various outings for the residents, including trips to the beach and strawberry teas. There are weekly visits from a Catholic priest who offers Communion and an Anglican minister visits once a month.

Cedar House Residential Care Home

Manager: Christine Ransley
Owner: Cedar House Ltd
Contact: 93 Seabrook Road,
Hythe, Kent CT21 5QP
☎ 01303 267065

Cedar House is approximately one mile from Hythe, and five minutes' drive into the centre of town, Seabrooke, where there is an abundance of shops and facilities. The home has a large garden with a summerhouse, where residents can sit and enjoy the weather. Staff also try to arrange a range of activities such as orientation tasks, as well as newspaper discussion which stimulated debate and keep residents aware of current affairs.

Registered places: 29
Guide weekly rate: £303–£520
Specialist care: Respite
Medical services: Podiatry, optician, physiotherapy
Qualified staff: Meets standard

Home details
Location: Residential area, 1 mile from Hythe
Communal areas: 2 lounges, dining room, garden
Accessibility: *Floors:* 2 • *Access:* Lift • *Wheelchair access:* Good
Smoking: In designated area
Pets: ✗
Routines: Flexible

Room details
Single: 22
Shared: 3
En suite: 25
Facilities: TV point, telephone point

Door lock: ✗
Lockable place: ✓

Services provided
Beauty services: Hairdressing
Mobile library: ✗
Religious services: Weekly Communion service
Transport: ✗
Activities: *Coordinator:* ✗ • *Examples:* Orientation, newspaper discussions, skittles • *Outings:* ✗
Meetings: ✓

The Chestnuts

Manager: Michael Banks
Owner: Michael and Patricia Banks
Contact: Wrotham Road,
Meopham, Gravesend, Kent DA13 9AH
☎ 01474 812152
@ PatMikeRestHome@aol.com

Sitting in its own grounds, The Chestnuts is located on a bus route and is a five-minute walk from the village's facilities which include shops and a train station with services to London. It is a family-run home, and is set in three quarters of an acre with well maintained gardens and seating areas for residents to enjoy. The home provides a visitor's bedroom with en suite facilities for relatives to stay if necessary. Activities are organised for residents on a daily basis, such as music nights, cards, darts and skittles.

Registered places: 29
Guide weekly rate: £380–£456
Specialist care: Respite
Medical services: Podiatry, optician, physiotherapy
Qualified staff: Meets standard

Home details
Location: Village location, 4.3 miles from Gravesend
Communal areas: 3 lounges, hairdressing salon, dining room, garden
Accessibility: *Floors:* 2 • *Access:* Lift and stair lift *Wheelchair access:* Good
Smoking: ✗
Pets: ✗
Routines: Flexible

Room details
Single: 22
Shared: 3
En suite: 22
Facilities: TV point

Door lock: ✓
Lockable place: ✓

Services provided
Beauty services: Hairdressing
Mobile library: ✓
Religious services: ✗
Transport: ✗
Activities: *Coordinator:* ✗ • *Examples:* Cards, darts, music nights *Outings:* ✓
Meetings: ✓

Registered places: 29
Guide weekly rate: £336–£410
Specialist care: Day care, respite
Medical services: Podiatry, dentist, optician
Qualified staff: Meets standard

Home details
Location: Village location, 5 miles from Rochester
Communal areas: 2 lounges, dining room, patio and garden
Accessibility: *Floors:* 2 • *Access:* Lift • *Wheelchair access:* Good
Smoking: ✗
Pets: At manager's discretion
Routines: Flexible

Room details
Single: 29
Shared: 0
En suite: 0
Facilities: TV, telephone point

Door lock: ✓
Lockable place: ✗

Services provided
Beauty services: Hairdressing, manicures
Mobile library: ✗
Religious services: ✗
Transport: ✗
Activities: *Coordinator:* ✗ • *Examples:* Visiting entertainers
 Outings: ✗
Meetings: ✓

Chimnies Residential Care Home

Manager: Kim San Ong
Owner: Kim San Ong
Contact: Stoke Road, Allhallows, Rochester, Kent ME3 9BL
☎ 01634 270119

Set in a rural area of Rochester, five miles from the town centre, Chimnies Residential Care Home enjoys extensive views across the countryside. Originally the church rectory, Chimnies is also situated a few minutes' walk from the local church. The home has two lounges, a separate dining room and a garden with a patio area. The home arranges for visiting entertainers to come to the home as part of the activities programme.

Registered places: 30
Guide weekly rate: From £800
Specialist care: Nursing, terminal care
Medical services: Podiatry, dentist, optician, physiotherapy
Qualified staff: Meets standard

Home details
Location: Residential area, 1 mile from Bromley
Communal areas: 3 lounges, dining room, garden
Accessibility: *Floors:* 2 • *Access:* Lift • *Wheelchair access:* Good
Smoking: In designated area
Pets: At manager's discretion
Routines: Flexible

Room details
Single: 20
Shared: 4
En suite: 24
Facilities: TV point, telephone point

Door lock: ✓
Lockable place: ✓

Services provided
Beauty services: Hairdressing
Mobile library: ✓
Religious services: Fortnightly Anglican service
Transport: Estate car
Activities: *Coordinator:* ✓ • *Examples:* Baking, light exercises,
 planting • *Outings:* ✗
Meetings: ✓

Clairleigh Nursing Home

Manager: Mercian Courtney
Owner: Palmgrange Ltd
Contact: 104 Plaistow Lane, Bromley, Kent BR1 3AS
☎ 020 8460 1527

The home is situated one mile from Bromley town centre with a wealth of entertainment and shops for residents to visit. The grounds are well kept, with cut lawns and flowerbeds and places to sit in the shade. There is a monthly library delivery from Bromley library, including large print book and talking books. A variety of activities are offered including baking and gardening. The home offers monthly meetings for residents to take part in.

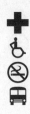

Cornford House

Manager: Linda Wenham
Owner: Cornford House Ltd
Contact: Cornford Lane, Pembury,
Tunbridge Wells, Kent TN2 4QS
☎ 01892 822079
@ Enquiries@cornfordhouse.co.uk
🖱 www.cornfordhouse.co.uk

Cornford House is a detached property, set in 10 acres of land in Pembury, near Tunbridge Wells. A new building project is underway, in which the existing house will be knocked down and rebuilt with 80 places. The home was originally opened to meet the needs of retired missionaries, and still has a Christian focus. There is a library with many large print books. Residents enjoy the home cooked, nutritious meals that meet their dietary meals. The home has its own transport for outings and an activities programme which includes exercise sessions and quizzes.

Registered places: 32
Guide weekly rate: £500–£895
Specialist care: Nursing
Medical services: Podiatry, dentist, optician, occupational therapy
Qualified staff: Exceeds standard: 75% at NVQ Level 2

Home details
Location: Residential area, 1 mile from Tunbridge Wells
Communal areas: 5 lounges, 2 dining rooms, library, garden
Accessibility: *Floors:* 2 • *Access:* Lift • *Wheelchair access:* Good
Smoking: ✗
Pets: ✗
Routines: Flexible

Room details
Single: 32
Shared: 0
En suite: 32
Facilities: TV point, computer point

Door lock: ✓
Lockable place: ✓

Services provided
Beauty services: Hairdressing, manicures
Mobile library: Library facilities
Religious services: Communion service
Transport: ✓
Activities: *Coordinator:* ✗ • *Examples:* Arts and craft, exercises, quizzes • *Outings:* ✓
Meetings: ✓

Creedy House

Manager: Shirley Brooke
Owner: Charing Healthcare
Contact: Nether Avenue,
Littlestone-on-Sea, New Romney,
Kent TN28 8NB
☎ 01797 362248

Creedy House is a large detached building in the small town of Littlestone, within walking distance to the sea, local shops and other amenities. There is a large garden for residents to sit outside, and there are regular outings to the seafront. There is also the occasional leisurely pub lunch. Pets are welcome to come and visit the home. Weekly activities include gardening, walks, arts and craft and bingo.

Registered places: 44
Guide weekly rate: £303–£600
Specialist care: Nursing
Medical services: Podiatry, optician
Qualified staff: Exceeds standard: 60% at NVQ Level 2

Home details
Location: Residential area, 1 mile from New Romney
Communal areas: Lounge, dining room, library, garden
Accessibility: *Floors:* 3 • *Access:* Lift • *Wheelchair access:* Good
Smoking: In designated area
Pets: ✗
Routines: Flexible

Room details
Single: 44
Shared: 0
En suite: 10
Facilities: TV point

Door lock: ✗
Lockable place: ✓

Services provided
Beauty services: Hairdressing
Mobile library: ✗
Religious services: Monthly church services
Transport: ✓
Activities: *Coordinator:* ✓ • *Examples:* Arts and craft, gardening, walks • *Outings:* ✓
Meetings: ✓

Registered places: 32
Guide weekly rate: £330–£425
Specialist care: None
Medical services: Podiatry, optician
Qualified staff: Meets standard

Home details

Location: Residential area, 1.5 miles from Folkstone
Communal areas: 3 lounges, dining room, patio and garden
Accessibility: *Floors:* Undisclosed • *Access:* Lift
    Wheelchair access: Good
Smoking: ×
Pets: ×
Routines: Flexible

Room details

Single: 25
Shared: 4
En suite: 6
Facilities: TV point

Door lock: ×
Lockable place: ✓

Services provided

Beauty services: Hairdressing
Mobile library: ×
Religious services: Monthly
Transport: ×
Activities: *Coordinator:* ✓ • *Examples:* Bingo, knitting, gardening
    Outings: ×
Meetings: ✓

Cumbria House

Manager: Julia Carter
Owner: Cumbria House
Contact: 84–86 Shorncliffe Road,
Folkestone, Kent CT20 2PG
☎ 01303 254019

Cumbria House is a detached property in Folkestone, within walking distance of shops and transport links, approximately one and a half miles from the town centre. There is a large patio area with seating for residents to sit outside and socialise in better weather that looks out onto a well-maintained garden. There are activities organised for residents on a frequent basis by the activities coordinator. Activities include gardening knitting, bingo and bowls. There is a residents meeting every quarter.

Registered places: 13
Guide weekly rate: £350–£375
Specialist care: Day care, respite
Medical services: Podiatry
Qualified staff: Exceeds standard: 90% at NVQ Level 2

Home details

Location: Residential area, 4 miles from Gillingham
Communal areas: 2 lounges, dining room, patio and garden
Accessibility: *Floors:* 3 • *Access:* 2 stair lifts
    Wheelchair access: Good
Smoking: ×
Pets: ×
Routines: Flexible

Room details

Single: 5
Shared: 4
En suite: 8
Facilities: TV point, telephone point

Door lock: ×
Lockable place: ✓

Services provided

Beauty services: Hairdressing
Mobile library: ×
Religious services: ×
Transport: Car
Activities: *Coordinator:* × • *Examples:* Bingo, games, quizzes
    Outings: ×
Meetings: ×

Durland House

Manager: Royston Hartley
Owner: Margaret Hartley
Contact: 160 High Street,
Rainham, Gillingham, Kent ME8 8AT
☎ 01634 364305

Durland House is a Georgian Grade II listed building in Rainham town centre, four miles from Gillingham. The property retains many of the Georgian features with high-beamed ceilings, yet is also well suited for the residents needs. The home has its own transport and offers residents a variety of activities such as bingo and quizzes.

Eastfield

Manager: David Titherington
Owner: Bureaucom Ltd
Contact: 76 Sittingbourne Road,
Maidstone, Kent ME14 5HY
☎ 01622 755153

Eastfield is a large, detached property, approximately one and a half miles from Maidstone. The home has ties with the community with local schools coming in to do pantomimes. There are also one-to-one activities such as trips to the shops or the theatre. Entertainers also come regularly. The home arranges an Anglican and Catholic service every six weeks.

Registered places: 43
Guide weekly rate: £400–£475
Specialist care: Respite
Medical services: Podiatry, dentist, optician, physiotherapy
Qualified staff: Fails standard: 40% at NVQ Level 2

Home details

Location: Residential area, 1.5 miles from Maidstone
Communal areas: Lounge, dining room, patio and garden
Accessibility: *Floors:* 2 • *Access:* Lift • *Wheelchair access:* Good
Smoking: ×
Pets: ×
Routines: Flexible

Room details

Single: 29
Shared: 7
En suite: 30
Facilities: TV point, telephone point

Door lock: ✓
Lockable place: ✓

Services provided

Beauty services: Hairdressing
Mobile library: ✓
Religious services: Anglican and Catholic service every 6 weeks
Transport: ×
Activities: *Coordinator:* ✓ • *Examples:* Arts and crafts, bingo, music and movement • *Outings:* ✓
Meetings: ✓

Eaton Lodge Nursing Home

Manager: Maria Kallis
Owner: Mukesh Patel
Contact: 62 Westgate Bay Avenue,
Westgate-on-Sea, Kent CT8 8SN
☎ 01843 832184
@ Maria.eatonlodge@btconnect.com

Eaton Lodge is near the town centre and five minutes from the seafront. Residents are regularly taken out to the local shops, cafés and for walks along the seafront. Though no pets are allowed to stay at the home they can visit and there is a resident cat. The garden has seating areas for those who wish to enjoy the good weather or some fresh air. The home arranges a weekly Anglican Communion service but all denominations visit as and when required. There are also weekly residents meetings.

Registered places: 24
Guide weekly rate: From £575
Specialist care: Nursing
Medical services: Podiatry, dentist, optician
Qualified staff: Exceeds standard: 70% at NVQ Level 2

Home details

Location: Residential area, 0.5 miles from Westgate-on-Sea
Communal areas: Lounge, dining room, patio and garden
Accessibility: *Floors:* 3 • *Access:* Lift • *Wheelchair access:* Good
Smoking: ×
Pets: ×
Routines: Flexible

Room details

Single: 13
Shared: 5
En suite: 1
Facilities: TV point

Door lock: ✓
Lockable place: ✓

Services provided

Beauty services: Hairdressing, aromatherapy, massage
Mobile library: ✓
Religious services: Weekly Anglican Communion service
Transport: ×
Activities: *Coordinator:* ✓ • *Examples:* Exercise to music, current affairs talks • *Outings:* ✓
Meetings: ✓

Registered places: 71
Guide weekly rate: £303.25–£550
Specialist care: Physical disability
Medical services: Podiatry, dentist, optician, physiotherapy
Qualified staff: Fails standard: 46% at NVQ Level 2

Home details

Location: Residential area, 9 miles from Canterbury
Communal areas: 3 lounges, quiet lounge, library, garden
Accessibility: *Floors:* 3 • *Access:* 2 lifts • *Wheelchair access:* Good
Smoking: ✓
Pets: ✓
Routines: Flexible

Room details

Single: 65
Shared: 3
En suite: 68
Facilities: None

Door lock: ✗
Lockable place: ✓

Services provided

Beauty services: None
Mobile library: Library facilities
Religious services: Catholic and Anglican visits
Transport: ✗
Activities: *Coordinator:* ✓ • *Examples:* Arts and crafts, gardening, seasonal events • *Outings:* ✓
Meetings: ✓

Elliott House

Manager: Linda Elks
Owner: Ian Nicoll
Contact: 22 Reculver Road, Beltinge, Herne Bay, Kent CT6 6NA
☎ 01227 374084
@ elliothouse@btconnect.com

Elliot House is an impressive listed building, set in its own extensive grounds. It has undergone extensive renovation, but still retains many original features including a rotunda room. The home is approximately nine miles from Canterbury. The activities coordinator organises a range of activities, including visiting entertainers, specialist talks (eg from the air ambulance service, local historians) and seasonal events to mark Valentines Day, Christmas and the like. There are also small group outings to the seaside.

Registered places: 44
Guide weekly rate: Undisclosed
Specialist care: Day care, dementia, learning disability, respite
Medical services: Podiatry, dentist, occupational therapy, optician, physiotherapy
Qualified staff: Undisclosed

Home details

Location: Residential area, 1.5 miles from Chislehurst centre
Communal areas: 6 lounges, 3 dining rooms, kitchenette, library, hairdressing salon, garden
Accessibility: *Floors:* 3 • *Access:* Lift • *Wheelchair access:* Good
Smoking: In designated area
Pets: ✓
Routines: Flexible

Room details

Single: 23
Shared: 9
En suite: 9
Facilities: TV point, telephone point

Door lock: ✓
Lockable place: ✗

Services provided

Beauty services: Hairdressing, aromatherapy
Mobile library: Library facilities
Religious services: ✓
Transport: ✓
Activities: *Coordinator:* ✓ • *Examples:* Bingo, exercise • *Outings:* ✓
Meetings: ✗

Elmstead

Manager: Caroline Cheeseman
Owner: BUPA Care Homes Ltd
Contact: 104 Elmstead Lane, Chislehurst, Kent BR7 5EL
☎ 020 8467 0007
@ ElmsteadALL@BUPA.com
🖰 www.bupacarehomes.co.uk

Elmstead is situated in the suburb of Chislehurst, and is close to local shops and on a local bus route. It offers a choice of six spacious lounge and dining areas for residents to meet and relax or entertain guests. There is also a small garden and patio area with a pond, which is safe for all residents to enjoy. Regular entertainment and activities are arranged, and personal interests are encouraged. Elmstead also offers residential dementia care, and maintains links with the community by offering day care to a number of local older people.

Elvy Court Nursing Home

Manager: Keith Bartlett
Owner: Southern Cross Healthcare Ltd
Contact: 204 London Road,
Sittingbourne, Kent ME10 1QA
) 01795 437449
@ elvycourt@schealthcare.co.uk
⌂ www.schealthcare.co.uk

Elvy Court is a modern, purpose-built care home. The home is situated a five-minute drive from the centre of Sittingbourne. It has the facilities for 57 residents, including dementia patients. The home has lounges which open out onto the garden as well as a separate dining room. The residents' meals are freshly cooked on the premises. The home has a communal safe in the office to keep residents' valuables. Smoking is permitted in a designated area and pets would be allowed to visit. There is a regular newspaper delivery.

Registered places: 57
Guide weekly rate: Undisclosed
Specialist care: Nursing, dementia
Medical services: Podiatry, dentist, optician, physiotherapy
Qualified staff: Meets standard

Home details
Location: Residential area, 1 mile from Sittingbourne
Communal areas: Lounge, dining room, garden
Accessibility: *Floors:* 2 • *Access:* Lift • *Wheelchair access:* Good
Smoking: In designated area
Pets: ✗
Routines: Flexible

Room details
Single: 57	**Door lock:** ✗
Shared: 0	**Lockable place:** ✗
En suite: Undisclosed	
Facilities: None	

Services provided
Beauty services: Hairdressing
Mobile library: ✗
Religious services: ✓
Transport: ✓
Activities: *Coordinator:* ✓ • *Examples:* Bingo • *Outings:* ✗
Meetings: Undisclosed

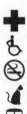

Emily Jackson Care Home

Manager: Vacant
Owner: Barchester Healthcare Ltd
Contact: 34 Eardley Road,
Sevenoaks, Kent TN13 1XT
) 01732 743 824
⌂ www.barchester.com

Emily Jackson Care Home is located in the pleasant market town of Sevenoaks in the county of Kent. The building has a purpose-built interior, whilst retaining the integrity of the original external Dutch design. Within the garden, there are landscaped areas, as well as areas where there are raised beds for the residents to grow there own plants. There are also seating areas and all pathways are suitable for wheelchair users. The home has residents meetings once a month and also arranges for visiting entertainers to come to the home.

Registered places: 60
Guide weekly rate: £945–£1,000
Specialist care: Nursing, respite
Medical services: Podiatry, dentist, optician, physiotherapy
Qualified staff: Exceeds standard: 80% at NVQ Level 2

Home details
Location: Residential area, 0.5 miles from Sevenoaks
Communal areas: 2 lounges, dining room, conservatory, garden
Accessibility: *Floors:* 3 • *Access:* Lift • *Wheelchair access:* Good
Smoking: ✗
Pets: At manager's discretion
Routines: Flexible

Room details
Single: 53	**Door lock:** ✗
Shared: 3	**Lockable place:** ✓
En suite: 53	
Facilities: TV point, telephone point	

Services provided
Beauty services: Hairdressing
Mobile library: ✓
Religious services: ✓
Transport: Minibus
Activities: *Coordinator:* ✓ • *Examples:* Barbecues, gardening, games, singing • *Outings:* ✓
Meetings: ✓

Registered places: 24
Guide weekly rate: £520–£730
Specialist care: None
Medical services: Podiatry, dentist, optician, physiotherapy
Qualified staff: Exceeds standard: 75% at NVQ Level 2

Home details
Location: Residential area, 1 mile from Bromley
Communal areas: 2 Lounge, dining room, garden
Accessibility: *Floors:* 2 • *Access:* Lift and stair lift
    Wheelchair access: Good
Smoking: In designated area
Pets: At manager's discretion
Routines: Flexible

Room details
Single: 24
Shared: 0
En suite: 15
Facilities: TV point

Door lock: ✓
Lockable place: ✓

Services provided
Beauty services: Hairdressing
Mobile library: ✓
Religious services: Fortnightly Baptist service
Transport: ✗
Activities: *Coordinator:* ✓ • *Examples:* Bingo, craft, reminiscence
    Outings: ✓
Meetings: ✓

Eversleigh

Manager: Mrs Offin
Owner: CNV Ltd
Contact: 13 Sundridge Avenue,
Bromley, Kent BR1 2PU
☎ 020 8464 2998

Eversleigh is a converted, three-storey Victorian house set off the road with pleasant, well-maintained gardens. There is a range of activities including art, flower arranging and music to choose from as well as frequent outings. The home has residents meetings twice a month as well as a Baptist service. The home also has visits from a mobile library.

Registered places: 30
Guide weekly rate: Undisclosed
Specialist care: Mental disorder
Medical services: Podiatry, dentist, optician, physiotherapy
Qualified staff: Meets standard

Home details
Location: Village location, 2 miles from Hartley
Communal areas: 3 lounges, dining room, patio and garden
Accessibility: *Floors:* 2 • *Access:* Stair lift
    Wheelchair access: Good
Smoking: In designated are
Pets: ✓
Routines: Flexible

Room details
Single: 30
Shared: 0
En suite: 8
Facilities: TV, telephone

Door lock. ✓
Lockable place: ✓

Services provided
Beauty services: Hairdressing, aromatherapy, manicures
Mobile library: ✗
Religious services: ✓
Transport: Car
Activities: *Coordinator:* ✓ • *Examples:* Bingo, cards, quizzes,
    reminiscence • *Outings :* ✓
Meetings: ✓

Fairby Grange Rest Home

Manager: Christine Brent
Owner: Gregory Reeve
Contact: Ash Road, Hartley,
Dartford, Kent DA3 8QD
☎ 01474 702223
@ enquiries@fairbygrange.co.uk
🌐 www.fairbygrange.co.uk

A listed Grade II property with purpose-built extension, Fairby Grange is situated in the centre of Hartley village, one mile from Longfield train station. With ample communal space which includes an oak-panelled lounge, a further room is allocated 'the quiet sitting room'. The home also has a dining room and a garden and a patio. The home also has its own activities coordinator and daily activities include bingo, cards, motivation sessions and reminiscence sessions. The home also arranges outings to local garden centre and to the theatre.

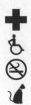

Fairlight and Fallowfield

Manager: Patrick Sena
Owner: The Mills Family Ltd
Contact: Ashfield Lane,
Chislehurst, Kent BR7 6LQ
☎ 020 8467 2781

Fairlight and Fallowfield was originally two facilities that are now joined by a walkway. Located in a residential area, the home is situated in the village of Chislehurst in Kent, where it is half mile to the next nearest village. The home has extensive well-maintained grounds, and from the lounge you can look out at the views across the garden. Visiting entertainment is brought in on a weekly basis to perform music and shows to keep the residents stimulated. There are also regular outings organised by the home.

Registered places: 68
Guide weekly rate: £540–£900
Specialist care: Nursing, respite
Medical services: Podiatry, dentist, optician, physiotherapy
Qualified staff: Meets standard

Home details
Location: Residential area, 2 miles from Bromley
Communal areas: Lounge, dining room, conservatory, patio and garden
Accessibility: *Floors:* 2 • *Access:* Lift and stair lift *Wheelchair access:* Good
Smoking: ✗
Pets: At manager's discretion
Routines: Flexible

Room details
Single: 60
Shared: 4
En suite: 64
Facilities: Telephone point

Door lock: ✗
Lockable place: ✓

Services provided
Beauty services: Hairdressing
Mobile library: ✗
Religious services: Weekly services
Transport: ✗
Activities: *Coordinator:* ✓ • *Examples:* Games, gentle exercise *Outings:* ✓
Meetings: ✗

Fairways Retirement Home

Manager: Alison Yarnley
Owner: David James
Contact: Madeira Road, Littlestone,
New Romney, Kent TN28 8QX
☎ 01797 362336

Fairways Retirement Home is a large Victorian house in its own grounds, one and a half miles from New Romney. There are a range of activities with crosswords and movement to music chiefly chosen by the residents. Outings are also regularly organised with trips to garden centres and the Rare Breeds Centre where residents can enjoy a day with animals and nature. Though no pets are allowed to stay in the home, they can visit with friends and family. There are also meetings every two months for residents to voice any concerns or issues they might have.

Registered places: 28
Guide weekly rate: £398–£430
Specialist care: Physical disability, respite
Medical services: Podiatry, dentist, optician, physiotherapy
Qualified staff: Meets standard

Home details
Location: Residential area, 1.5 miles from New Romney
Communal areas: Lounge, quiet lounge, dining room, garden
Accessibility: *Floors:* 3 • *Access:* Lift • *Wheelchair access:* Good
Smoking: ✗
Pets: ✗
Routines: Flexible

Room details
Single: 22
Shared: 3
En suite: 7
Facilities: TV point, telephone point

Door lock: ✓
Lockable place: ✓

Services provided
Beauty services: Hairdressing
Mobile library: ✓
Religious services: ✗
Transport: ✗
Activities: *Coordinator:* ✓ • *Examples:* Bingo, crosswords, movement to music • *Outings:* ✓
Meetings: ✓

Registered places: 28
Guide weekly rate: £377–£600
Specialist care: Dementia, respite
Medical services: Podiatry, dentist, optician
Qualified staff: Meets standard

Home details

Location: Residential area, 1.2 miles from Deal
Communal areas: Lounge, dining room, conservatory, garden
Accessibility: *Floors:* 2 • *Access:* Lift and stair lift
   Wheelchair access: Good
Smoking: ✕
Pets: ✓
Routines: Flexible

Room details

Single: 28   Door lock: ✓
Shared: 0   Lockable place: ✓
En suite: Undisclosed
Facilities: TV, telephone

Services provided

Beauty services: Hairdressing
Mobile library: ✓
Religious services: ✓
Transport: ✕
Activities: *Coordinator:* ✓ • *Examples:* Dominoes, visiting
   entertainers • *Outings:* ✕
Meetings: ✓

Fassaroe

Manager: Vacant
Owner: Fassaroe Ltd
Contact: 5–7 Warwick Road, Walmer,
Deal, Kent CT14 7JF
☏ 01304 361894
@ fassaroe.ch@gmail.com
🖱 www.fassaroehouse.co.uk

Fassaroe is situated in a residential area of the seaside town of Deal, close to the seafront. The home has a lounge and a dining room as well as a conservatory and a garden. There is a good range of activities including games and visiting entertainers as well as one-to-one sessions. There is a relatives meeting held once a month to discuss any issues that may arise. Religious services are available on request and the home arranges for a mobile library to visit.

Registered places: 16
Guide weekly rate: £303–£450
Specialist care: Learning disability
Medical services: Undisclosed
Qualified staff: Exceeds standard: 70% at NVQ Level 2

Home details

Location: Residential area, 7 miles from Canterbury
Communal areas: 2 lounges, dining room, conservatory
Accessibility: *Floors:* 2 • *Access:* Stair lift • *Wheelchair access:* Good
Smoking: In designated area
Pets: Undisclosed
Routines: Flexible

Room details

Single: 12   Door lock: ✕
Shared: 2   Lockable place: ✕
En suite: Undisclosed
Facilities: None

Services provided

Beauty services: Undisclosed
Mobile library: ✕
Religious services: ✕
Transport: ✕
Activities: *Coordinator:* ✕ • *Examples:* Bingo, skittles, games,
   music • *Outings:* ✕
Meetings: ✕

Favorita House

Manager: Pauline Gough
Owner: Kevin Post
Contact: 28 Canterbury Road,
Herne Bay, Kent CT6 5DJ
☏ 01227 374166

Favorita House is located on the main road into Herne Bay, seven miles from Canterbury. Activities offered in the home include bingo, skittles and music. Smoking is allowed in the home in designated areas. There are two lounges, a dining room and a conservatory as communal areas for the residents. The home also has the facilities for one resident with learning disabilities.

Firtree House Nursing Home

Manager: Catherine Brewster
Owner: Firtree Care Ltd
Contact: 30 St James' Road,
Tunbridge Wells, Kent TN1 2JZ
☏ 01892 523954

Firtree House Nursing Home resides in a residential area approximately half a mile from Tunbridge Wells. The home has a large rear garden with seating for residents. Daily activities include gardening, singalongs, carpet bowls and charades. Organised outings are frequent and give residents the chance to suggest ideas about where they would like to go in the local area. Pets are welcome to visit the home.

Registered places: 50
Guide weekly rate: £350–£450
Specialist care: Nursing
Medical services: Podiatry, optician
Qualified staff: Meets standard

Home details
Location: Residential area, 0.5 miles from Tunbridge Wells
Communal areas: 3 lounges, dining room, garden
Accessibility: *Floors:* 3 • *Access:* 2 lifts • *Wheelchair access:* Good
Smoking: In designated area
Pets: ✗
Routines: Flexible

Room details
Single: 29
Shared: 0
En suite: 28
Facilities: TV point

Door lock: ✗
Lockable place: ✗

Services provided
Beauty services: Hairdressing
Mobile library: ✓
Religious services: Monthly
Transport: ✗
Activities: *Coordinator:* ✓ • *Examples:* Gardening, singalongs
  Outings: ✓
Meetings: ✗

Fontenay Nursing Home

Manager: Florence Hussin
Owner: Thomas Kelly
Contact: 39 Watts Avenue,
Rochester, Kent ME1 1RX
☏ 01634 843753

The home is a detached Victorian house on a main bus route and within half a mile of Rochester. During the summer the home sets out benches and tables in the garden for residents to enjoy the weather. There is also a delivery of large print books and films every six months. The home allows for animals to visit but not to stay. Budgies are allowed to stay. There are residents meetings every three months.

Registered places: 27
Guide weekly rate: £496–£700
Specialist care: Nursing, dementia, respite
Medical services: Podiatry, hygienist, optician, physiotherapy
Qualified staff: Meets standard

Home details
Location: Residential area, 0.5 miles from Rochester
Communal areas: Lounge, dining room, garden
Accessibility: *Floors:* 3 • *Access:* Lift • *Wheelchair access:* Good
Smoking: In designated area
Pets: ✗
Routines: Flexible

Room details
Single: 8
Shared: 9
En suite: 2
Facilities: TV point

Door lock: ✓
Lockable place: ✓

Services provided
Beauty services: Hairdressing
Mobile library: ✓
Religious services: ✗
Transport: ✗
Activities: *Coordinator:* ✓ • *Examples:* Jigsaw puzzles,
  singalongs, films • *Outings:* ✗
Meetings: ✓

Registered places: 30
Guide weekly rate: £496–£575
Specialist care: Nursing, respite, terminal care
Medical services: Podiatry, dietician, dentist,
    occupational therapy, optician
Qualified staff: Meets standard

Home details

Location: Residential area, 2 miles from Chatham
Communal areas: Lounge, dining room, garden, conservatory
Accessibility: *Floors:* 1 • *Wheelchair access:* Good
Smoking: ✗
Pets: ✗
Routines: Flexible

Room details

Single: 24   Door lock: ✓
Shared: 3   Lockable place: ✓
En suite: 4
Facilities: TV point, telephone point

Services provided

Beauty services: Hairdressing
Mobile library: ✓
Religious services: Visits from local churches
Transport: ✗
Activities: *Coordinator:* ✓ • *Examples:* Arts and crafts, bingo,
    cake making • *Outings:* ✓
Meetings: ✓

Fort Horstead Nursing Home

Manager: Linda Edwards
Owner: Dr and Mrs Jana
Contact: Primrose Close, Chatham,
Kent ME4 6HZ
☎ 01634 406119

Fort Horstead is a purpose-built nursing home housed in a single-storey bungalow. This means that wheelchair access and movement around the home is excellent. The home offers meetings three times a year and relatives are invited to get involved or voice any concerns. The home offers a range of activities to help all residents stay active in body and mind as well as letting them continue any previous hobbies or interests. These include exercises, music and arts and crafts. The home also goes on outings. Pets can visit the home but are not allowed to stay.

Registered places: 25
Guide weekly rate: From £400
Specialist care: Physical disability, respite
Medical services: Podiatry, dentist, optician
Qualified staff: Fails standard

Home details

Location: Residential area, 2 miles from Dartford
Communal areas: 2 lounges, dining room, patio and garden
Accessibility: *Floors:* 3 • *Access:* Lift • *Wheelchair access:* Good
Smoking: ✗
Pets: At manager's discretion
Routines: Flexible

Room details

Single: 25   Door lock: ✓
Shared: 0   Lockable place: ✓
En suite: 25
Facilities: TV point, telephone point

Services provided

Beauty services: None
Mobile library: ✓
Religious services: ✓
Transport: Minibus
Activities: *Coordinator:* ✓ • *Examples:* Karaoke, bingo, games
    Outings: ✓
Meetings: ✓

Gardenia House

Manager: Wendy Clarke
Owner: Heritage Care Ltd
Contact: 19 Pilgrims Court, Farnol
Road, Dartford, Kent DA1 5LZ
☎ 01322 290837
@ gardenia.house@heritagecre.co.uk
🖥 www.heritagecare.co.uk

A modern, purpose-built home that lies next door to a church, Gardenia House is owned by Heritage Care. There is a small open garden to the rear and an enclosed garden area to the side of the property. For those more active residents, the activities programme includes trips to the local garden centre or pub for lunch. Some residents recently enjoyed a trip to Southend for the theatre. The home also organises daily activities such as karaoke and bingo.

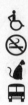

Garlinge Lodge

Manager: Heywantee Purmessur
Owner: Mr and Mrs Purmessur
Contact: 6 Garlinge Road,
Southborough, Tunbridge Wells,
Kent TN4 0NR
☎ 01892 528465

Garlinge Lodge is a large, detached property surrounded on three sides by gardens. The home organises an active schedule for those residents who wish to take part, including board games and exercise sessions. The home is located close to local shops and public transport, two miles from Tunbridge Wells. The home also arranges a weekly Anglican service.

Registered places: 14
Guide weekly rate: £340–£495
Specialist care: Respite
Medical services: Podiatry, dentist, optician, physiotherapy
Qualified staff: Exceeds standard: 60% at NVQ Level 2

Home details
Location: Residential area, 2 miles from Tunbridge Wells
Communal areas: Lounge, dining room, conservatory, garden
Accessibility: *Floors:* 3 • *Access:* Lift • *Wheelchair access:* Good
Smoking: ✗
Pets: At manager's discretion
Routines: Flexible

Room details
Single: 14
Shared: 0
En suite: 1
Facilities: TV point, telephone point

Door lock: ✓
Lockable place: ✓

Services provided
Beauty services: Hairdressing
Mobile library: ✓
Religious services: Weekly Anglican service
Transport: People carrier
Activities: *Coordinator:* ✓ • *Examples:* Board games, exercise sessions, quizzes • *Outings:* ✗
Meetings: ✓

Glebe Court Nursing Home

Manager: Gillian Payne
Owner: Glebe Housing Association
Contact: Glebe Way, West Wickham,
Kent BR4 0RZ
☎ 020 8462 6609

Glebe Court is part of the Glebe Housing Association and is set in its own grounds in Bencurtis Park. The home is half a mile from West Wickham. The activities coordinator arranges weekly activities, such as walks and drawing classes or history talks. The conservatory on the ground floor has under-floor heating, enabling its use all year round, and this opens out onto a large garden with seating for residents to sit outside and enjoy in the summer months. This includes activities such as barbecues.

Registered places: 51
Guide weekly rate: £525–£740
Specialist care: Nursing
Medical services: Podiatry, hygienist, optician, physiotherapy
Qualified staff: Exceeds standard

Home details
Location: Residential area, 0.5 miles from West Wickham
Communal areas: 2 lounges, dining room, conservatory, garden
Accessibility: *Floors:* 2 • *Access:* Lift • *Wheelchair access:* Good
Smoking: ✗
Pets: ✗
Routines: Flexible

Room details
Single: 47
Shared: 4
En suite: 51
Facilities: TV point, telephone point

Door lock: ✗
Lockable place: ✓

Services provided
Beauty services: Hairdressing
Mobile library: ✓
Religious services: Monthly
Transport: ✗
Activities: *Coordinator:* ✓ • *Examples:* Bowls, darts, drawing *Outings:* ✓
Meetings: ✓

Registered places: 20
Guide weekly rate: Undisclosed
Specialist care: Respite
Medical services: Podiatry, dentist, optician
Qualified staff: Fails standard

Home details
Location: Residential area, 0.5 miles from Tunbridge Wells
Communal areas: 2 lounges, dining room, garden
Accessibility: *Floors:* 3 • *Access:* Lift • *Wheelchair access:* Good
Smoking: ×
Pets: ×
Routines: Flexible

Room details
Single: 16
Shared: 2
En suite: 4
Facilities: TV

Door lock: ✓
Lockable place: ✓

Services provided
Beauty services: Hairdressing
Mobile library: Library facilities
Religious services: ✓
Transport: ×
Activities: *Coordinator:* ✓ • *Examples:* Musical entertainment, music and movement • *Outings:* ✓
Meetings: ✓

Glendale House

Manager: Judy Connor
Owner: Chistlehurst Care Ltd
Contact: 32 Boyne Park, Tunbridge Wells, Kent TN4 8ET
☏ 01892 524222

Glendale House is situated in a residential area, approximately half a mile from the town centre of Tunbridge Wells. The home has two lounges and a dining room, as well as a garden. The home has its own library facilities and residents are often taken out on walks and to the pantomime at Christmas. There are also daily activities in the home, which include games and musical performances.

Registered places: 25
Guide weekly rate: £410–£435
Specialist care: Respite
Medical services: Podiatry, dentist, optician, physiotherapy
Qualified staff: Meets standard

Home details
Location: Village location, 0.5 miles from Kingsdown
Communal areas: Lounge, 2 dining rooms, conservatory, garden
Accessibility: *Floors:* 2 • *Access:* Stair lift • *Wheelchair access:* Good
Smoking: ×
Pets: At manager's discretion
Routines: Flexible

Room details
Single: 23
Shared: 1
En suite: 15
Facilities: TV point, telephone point

Door lock: ✓
Lockable place: ✓

Services provided
Beauty services: Hairdressing, aromatherapy
Mobile library: ✓
Religious services: Monthly Anglican Communion service
Transport: ×
Activities: *Coordinator:* × • *Examples:* Arts and crafts, board games, singers • *Outings:* ✓
Meetings: ✓

Glendale Lodge Residential Care Home

Manager: Carole McNamara
Owner: Extrafriend Ltd
Contact: Glen Road, Kingsdown, Deal, Kent CT14 8BS
☏ 01304 363449

Glendale Lodge is a purpose-built care home in a village with impressive rural views. The home employs a chef which means that all dietary requirements can be catered for, and meals are served with a choice of beer, wine, juice or water. Entertainment visits including two different singers and they also go on outings. The home has most of its rooms on the ground floor and only two rooms on the first floor, therefore the home is wheelchair accessible. A mobile library visits with large print books and videos. The home has its own cat.

Gordon Lodge Rest Home

Manager: Diane Fleming
Owner: Fleming Care Homes Ltd
Contact: 43 Westgate Bay Avenue, Westgate-on-Sea, Kent CT8 8AH
☎ 01843 831491
@ lodgegordon@yahoo.co.uk

Gordon Lodge Rest Home is located in a residential area, half a mile from the town centre of Westgate-on-Sea. The home is within walking distance of the beach and local amenities. There is a Communion service held in the home on a monthly basis and there are regular outings organised. The home also arranges daily activities such as exercises and games. There is a garden with a patio area in the home as well as a lounge and a dining room.

Registered places: 33
Guide weekly rate: £309–£600
Specialist care: Respite
Medical services: Podiatry, dentist, optician
Qualified staff: Meets standard

Home details
Location: Residential area, 0.5 miles from Westgate-on-Sea
Communal areas: Lounge, dining room, patio and garden
Accessibility: *Floors:* 3 • *Access:* Stair lift • *Wheelchair access:* Good
Smoking: ✗
Pets: ✗
Routines: Flexible

Room details
Single: 29
Shared: 2
En suite: Undisclosed
Facilities: TV point, telephone point

Door lock: ✓
Lockable place: ✓

Services provided
Beauty services: Hairdressing
Mobile library: ✓
Religious services: Monthly Communion
Transport: ✓
Activities: *Coordinator:* ✗ • *Examples:* Games, visiting entertainers *Outings:* ✓
Meetings: ✓

Grafton Lodge

Manager: Anne Perkins
Owner: Lavinia, Lee, Rickie, Lesley and Sharon Boyson and Jo Weston
Contact: 40 Goddington Road, Strood, Rochester, Kent ME2 3DE
☎ 01634 722621
@ graftonlodge@havencarehomes.co.uk
🖰 www.havencarehomes.co.uk

Grafton Lodge is a detached property situated about 10 minutes' walk from Strood town centre in Rocester. The home arranges a variety of outings for the residents. Shopping trips are always popular, as are trips down to the river for a stroll along the prom followed by tea and cakes. Pub lunches are frequent, and a trip to see the Christmas lights is always well attended. The home also organises celebrations or seasonal events: summer barbecues, Pancake Day, a resident's birthday, bingo sessions, Easter, Christmas and New Year. There are also residents meetings once a month.

Registered places: 20
Guide weekly rate: £330–£340
Specialist care: None
Medical services: Podiatry, optician
Qualified staff: Meets standard

Home details
Location: Residential area, 0.5 miles from Strood
Communal areas: Lounge, dining room
Accessibility: *Floors:* 2 • *Access:* Lift and stair lift *Wheelchair access:* Good
Smoking: In designated area
Pets: At manager's discretion
Routines: Flexible

Room details
Single: 10
Shared: 5
En suite: 5
Facilities: TV point

Door lock: ✗
Lockable place: ✓

Services provided
Beauty services: Hairdressing
Mobile library: ✗
Religious services: Monthly church services
Transport: ✓
Activities: *Coordinator:* ✗ • *Examples:* Barbecues, bingo sessions, exercise sessions • *Outings:* ✓
Meetings: ✓

Registered places: 10
Guide weekly rate: £301–£350
Specialist care: Day care, respite
Medical services: Podiatry, optician
Qualified staff: Meets standard

Home details
Location: Residential area, 7.5 miles from Canterbury
Communal areas: 2 lounges, dining room, patio and garden
Accessibility: *Floors:* 2 • *Access:* Stair lift
    Wheelchair access: Limited
Smoking: ✗
Pets: ✓
Routines: Flexible

Room details
Single: 6   Door lock: ✓
Shared: 2   Lockable place: ✓
En suite: 0
Facilities: TV

Services provided
Beauty services: Hairdressing
Mobile library: ✗
Religious services: Monthly Catholic Communion service
Transport: ✗
Activities: *Coordinator:* ✗ • *Examples:* Bingo, games, karaoke
    Outings: ✓
Meetings: ✗

Grafton Villa

Manager: Lorraine Tyler
Owner: Mr and Mrs Rajaratnan
Contact: 31 Blackburn Road,
Greenhill, Herne Bay, Kent CT6 7RQ
☎ 01227 372937

Grafton Villa is a semi-detached house situated in Greenhill, a residential area near Herne Bay. It is approximately seven and a half miles from Canterbury. The home has a lounge and a sun lounge as well as a dining room. The manager organises activities in the home and residents play various games such as bingo; there are also karaoke sessions. Pets are allowed in the home and smoking is not permitted.

Registered places: 29
Guide weekly rate: £313–£361
Specialist care: Respite
Medical services: Podiatry, dentist, optician, physiotherapy
Qualified staff: Fails standards

Home details
Location: Residential area, 2.5 miles from Ashford
Communal areas: 2 lounges, dining room, conservatory, garden
Accessibility: *Floors:* 2 • *Access:* Lift • *Wheelchair access:* Limited
Smoking: ✗
Pets: At manager's discretion
Routines: Flexible

Room details
Single: 21   Door lock: ✓
Shared: 4   Lockable place: ✓
En suite: 7
Facilities: TV point, telephone point

Services provided
Beauty services: Hairdressing
Mobile library: ✓
Religious services: Monthly Anglican service
Transport: Car
Activities: *Coordinator:* ✗ • *Examples:* Exercise, bingo, music
    Outings: ✓
Meetings: ✓

The Grange

Manager: Karen Whiting
Owner: Mr and Mrs Friend
Contact: 2 The Street, Kennington,
Ashford, Kent TN24 9EX
☎ 01233 621824
@ thegrange1989@aol.com

The Grange is a detached property on the outskirts of Ashford. The home has a large enclosed garden with a fenced-in fishpond. There are many different activities for residents to get involved in, such as exercises and board games. Though not all denominations offer religious services at the home, the churches pick up residents for weekly services at local churches. There is an Anglican service once a month in the home. The home also has its own transport for outings.

The Grange Care Home

Manager: Carol Weeks
Owner: Ashwood Court Healthcare Ltd
Contact: 22 Cornwallis Avenue, Folkestone, Kent CT19 5JB
☏ 01303 252394

The Grange Care Home is situated in a residential area, approximately one mile from Folkestone town centre. The home is set in its own grounds with large, well-maintained gardens at the front and back. A spacious porch provides a relaxing sitting area. The home tries to cater for the individuals needs and offers a wide range of activities and religious services. These include visiting entertainers and outings for lunch. The home also arranges for Anglican and Catholic clergy to visit the home once a month.

Registered places: 28
Guide weekly rate: £312–£450
Specialist care: None
Medical services: Podiatry, optician, physiotherapy
Qualified staff: Meets standard

Home details
Location: Residential area, 1 mile from Folkestone
Communal areas: 2 lounge/dining rooms, library, patio and garden
Accessibility: *Floors:* 2 • *Access:* Lift • *Wheelchair access:* Good
Smoking: ✗
Pets: ✗
Routines: Flexible

Room details
Single: 28
Shared: 0
En suite: 20
Facilities: TV point, telephone point

Door lock: ✓
Lockable place: ✓

Services provided
Beauty services: Hairdressing
Mobile library: ✓
Religious services: Monthly Anglican and Catholic visits
Transport: ✗
Activities: *Coordinator:* ✗ • *Examples:* Entertainers, bingo
  Outings: ✓
Meetings: ✓

Green Gables

Manager: Annette Smith
Owner: Annette Smith and Carol Lewis
Contact: 6 Northdown Avenue, Cliftonville, Margate, Kent CT9 2NL
☏ 01843 227770

Green Gables is a detached property located in a residential part of Cliftonville about half a mile from the town centre. There is ample communal space, with three lounges, a dining room and a conservatory, where smoking is allowed. An activities coordinator works in the home two days a week and consults residents as to which activities they would like to participate in. There are day trips using the home's minibus, themed evenings, games and quizzes. There is a medium sized garden at the rear of the property with seating for the residents to enjoy in better weather.

Registered places: 18
Guide weekly rate: £294–£340
Specialist care: None
Medical services: Podiatry, hygienist, optician, physiotherapy
Qualified staff: Exceeds standard: 75% at NVQ Level 2

Home details
Location: Residential area, 0.5 miles from Cliftonville
Communal areas: 3 lounges, dining room, conservatory, garden
Accessibility: *Floors:* 3 • *Access:* Stair lifts
  Wheelchair access: Good
Smoking: In designated area
Pets: At manager's discretion
Routines: Flexible

Room details
Single: 14
Shared: 2
En suite: 5
Facilities: TV point

Door lock: ✗
Lockable place: ✓

Services provided
Beauty services: Hairdressing
Mobile library: ✓
Religious services: ✗
Transport: ✓
Activities: *Coordinator:* ✓ • *Examples:* Quizzes, games
  Outings: ✓
Meetings: ✓

Registered places: 32
Guide weekly rate: £312–£455
Specialist care: Day care, respite
Medical services: Podiatry, hygienist, optician, physiotherapy
Qualified staff: Meets standard

Home details

Location: Residential area, 0.7 miles from Birchington
Communal areas: 3 lounges, dining room, garden
Accessibility: *Floors:* 2 • *Access:* Lift • *Wheelchair access:* Good
Smoking: ✗
Pets: At manager's discretion
Routines: Flexible

Room details

Single: 32   Door lock: ✓
Shared: 0   Lockable place: ✗
En suite: Undisclosed
Facilities: TV point, telephone point

Services provided

Beauty services: Hairdressing
Mobile library: ✗
Religious services: Monthly Communion service
Transport: Minibus
Activities: *Coordinator:* ✓ • *Examples:* Sewing, quizzes,
      reminiscence • *Outings:* ✓
Meetings: ✓

Grenham Bay Court

Manager: Jacqueline Cross
Owner: Grenham Bay Care Ltd
Contact: Cliff Road, Birchington,
Kent CT7 9JX
☏ 01843 841008
@ juliemills@highmeadow.co.uk

Grenham Bay Court faces the sea in the residential area of Birchington, near Margate. Activities include fortnightly visits from entertainers, in addition to reminiscence sessions and quizzes. Residents regularly enjoy outings in the home's minibus to nearby villages and attractions, which include trips to the circus, picnic and local fish and chip shops. There is a residents meeting twice a month.

Registered places: 31
Guide weekly rate: £304–£344
Specialist care: Residential, respite
Medical services: Podiatry, hygienist, optician, physiotherapy
Qualified staff: Exceeds standard: 70% at NVQ Level 2

Home details

Location: Residential area, 1.5 miles from Margate
Communal areas: Lounge/dining room, conservatory, garden
Accessibility: *Floors:* 3 • *Access:* Lift • *Wheelchair access:* Good
Smoking: In designated area
Pets: ✗
Routines: Flexible

Room details

Single: 26   Door lock: ✓
Shared: 5   Lockable place: ✓
En suite: 31
Facilities: TV point, telephone point

Services provided

Beauty services: Hairdressing, manicures
Mobile library: ✓
Religious services: ✓
Transport: Minibus
Activities: *Coordinator:* ✗ • *Examples:* Exercise, film shows,
      reminiscence • *Outings:* ✓
Meetings: ✓

Gresham Residential Care Home

Manager: Jonathan Smith
Owner: Mr and Mrs Smith
Contact: 47–49 Norfolk Road,
Cliftonville, Margate, Kent CT9 2HU
☏ 01843 220178

Gresham Residential Care Home is a detached building located within one and a half miles of Margate. The home is near local shops and all public amenities and the seafront can be accessed via a short walk. The home boasts a small, enclosed back garden with fishpond, flowerbeds and seating area. Residents are allowed to maintain the flowerbeds if they choose. There are regular residents meetings and the home also arranges outings in its minibus.

Grimston House

Manager: Eileen Godden
Owner: MNP Complete Care Group
Contact: 16 Grimston Gardens,
Folkestone, Kent CT20 2PU
) 01303 244958

Grimston House is located in a residential area, approximately one and a half miles from Folkstone. The home has a good-sized, enclosed garden where residents like to spend time in summer. The home prides itself on giving the residents lots of activities and outings during the week. There is an Anglican and Catholic service once every three weeks and there are residents meetings three times a year.

Registered places: 21
Guide weekly rate: £312–£450
Specialist care: None
Medical services: Podiatry, hygienist, optician, physiotherapy
Qualified staff: Meets standard

Home details
Location: Residential area, 1.5 miles from Folkstone
Communal areas: Lounge, dining room, library, conservatory, patio and garden
Accessibility: *Floors:* 3 • *Access:* Lift • *Wheelchair access:* Good
Smoking: ✗
Pets: ✗
Routines: Flexible

Room details
Single: 17
Shared: 2
En suite: 18
Facilities: TV point, telephone point

Door lock: ✓
Lockable place: ✓

Services provided
Beauty services: Hairdressing, massage
Mobile library: Library facilities
Religious services: Anglican, Catholic and Communion service every 3 weeks
Transport: ✗
Activities: *Coordinator:* ✓ • *Examples:* Arts and crafts, bingo, quizzes • *Outings:* ✓
Meetings: ✓

The Grove

Manager: Rosemary Lee
Owner: Smartblade Ltd
Contact: Bower Mount Road,
Maidstone, Kent ME16 8AU
) 01622 755292

The Grove is set in its own grounds with a level pathway around it and the gardens are well used in summer. The home is next to Oakwood Park, with two railway stations less than a mile away. Activities are arranged regularly with arts and crafts and music and movement for residents to get involved in. Outings also take place with trips to local points of interest. There is also a Communion service performed once a month in the home.

Registered places: 32
Guide weekly rate: £400–£490
Specialist care: None
Medical services: Podiatry, dentist, optician
Qualified staff: Meets standard

Home details
Location: Residential area, 1.2 miles from Maidstone
Communal areas: 3 lounges, dining rom, garden
Accessibility: *Floors:* 2 • *Access:* Lift • *Wheelchair access:* Good
Smoking: ✗
Pets: ✗
Routines: Flexible

Room details
Single: 28
Shared: 2
En suite: 23
Facilities: TV point, telephone point

Door lock: ✓
Lockable place: ✓

Services provided
Beauty services: Hairdressing
Mobile library: ✓
Religious services: Monthly Communion service
Transport: ✗
Activities: *Coordinator:* ✗ • *Examples:* Arts and crafts, bingo, music and movement • *Outings:* ✓
Meetings: ✗

Registered places: 17
Guide weekly rate: £360–£400
Specialist care: Dementia
Medical services: Podiatry, dentist, optician
Qualified staff: Exceeds standard: 70% at NVQ Level 2

Home details

Location: Village location, 2 miles from Canterbury
Communal areas: Lounge, dining room, patio and garden
Accessibility: *Floors:* 2 • *Access:* None • *Wheelchair access:* Limited
Smoking: In designated area
Pets: ✗
Routines: Flexible

Room details

Single: 14
Shared: 1
En suite: 7
Facilities: TV, telephone

Door lock: ✓
Lockable place: ✓

Services provided

Beauty services: Hairdressing, manicures, aromatherapy massage
Mobile library: ✗
Religious services: ✓
Transport: ✗
Activities: *Coordinator:* ✗ • *Examples:* Bingo, exercises, games
Outings: ✓
Meetings: ✗

Hamiltons Residential Home

Manager: Vacant
Owner: MGL Healthcare Ltd
Contact: 26 Island Road, Upstreet, Canterbury, Kent CT3 4DA
✆ 01227 860128
@ michaellisis@btconnect.com

Hamiltons is a listed building, a large detached property situated on a main road in the village of Upstreet. The home is approximately two miles from Canterbury and the seaside towns of Whitstable and Hearne Bay are a 30-minute drive away.

The home does not have an activities coordinator, but staff engage residents in games, gentle exercises, singing sessions and the occasional outing. There are religious services available. The landscaped garden has seating areas and focal points throughout including a water feature.

Registered places: 46
Guide weekly rate: £401–£540
Specialist care: Dementia
Medical services: Podiatry, dentist
Qualified staff: Exceeds standard: 60% at NVQ Level 2

Home details

Location: Residential area, 1 mile from Greenhithe
Communal areas: 5 lounges, 3 dining rooms, garden
Accessibility: *Floors:* 3 • *Access:* Lift • *Wheelchair access:* Good
Smoking: In designated area
Pets: ✗
Routines: Flexible

Room details

Single: 46
Shared: 0
En suite: 44
Facilities: TV point, telephone point

Door lock: ✓
Lockable place: ✗

Services provided

Beauty services: Hairdressing
Mobile library: ✓
Religious services: Fortnightly visit from motivation leader, monthly visits from vicar
Transport: ✗
Activities: *Coordinator:* ✓ • *Examples:* Celebratory teas
Outings: ✗
Meetings: ✗

Haslington Residential Home

Manager: Frances Maynard
Owner: Carol and Edward Jansz
Contact: Cobham Terrace, Bean Road, Greenhithe, Kent DA9 9JB
✆ 01322 383229
@ haslingtonhome@aol.com

Haslington Residential Home is located on a quiet residential street close to rail and bus links. The home is approximately one mile from Greenhithe. There are many lounges and quiet areas for residents to enjoy and the residents also have many areas to walk in including a circular walkway for continuous movement and a sensory garden. There is an activities coordinator, visits from a mobile library and a motivational leader once a fortnight. There is also a hairdressing service and a vicar visits once a month. Smoking is allowed in a designated area and pets are not permitted.

Hatfield Lodge Residential Home

Manager: Yvonne Copleston
Owner: First Choice Homes
Contact: 1–3 Trinity Gardens,
Folkestone, Kent CT20 2RP
☎ 01303 253253
@ hatfieldlodge@1stchoice.com

Hatfield Lodge Residential Home is situated in the seaside town of Folkestone, less than half a mile from the town centre. Several bedrooms in the home are styled as semi-self-contained apartments and there is also a large lounge for residents to relax in. There is a garden with a patio area and smoking is permitted outside or in residents' rooms. The home arranges outings for the residents as well as activities such as games and a wine and cheese evening.

Registered places: 28
Guide weekly rate: £400–£600
Specialist care: None
Medical services: Podiatry, dentist, optician
Qualified staff: Exceeds standard: 71% at NVQ Level 2

Home details
Location: Urban area, 0.3 miles from Folkestone
Communal areas: Lounge, dining room, patio and garden
Accessibility: *Floors:* 4 • *Access:* Lift and stair lift
 Wheelchair access: Good
Smoking: In designated area
Pets: At manager's discretion
Routines: Flexible

Room details
Single: 28
Shared: 0
En suite: 11
Facilities: Telephone

Door lock: Undisclosed
Lockable place: Undisclosed

Services provided
Beauty services: Hairdressing
Mobile library: ✓
Religious services: Monthly Communion service
Transport: ✗
Activities: *Coordinator:* ✓ • *Examples:* Wine and cheese evenings, games • *Outings:* ✓
Meetings: ✓

Hazelwood Nursing Home

Manager: Valerie Setrem
Owner: Smartmove Homes Ltd
Contact: Brickfield Farm, Main Road,
Longfield, Kent DA3 7PW
☎ 01474 573800
🖰 www.hazelwoodnursing.com

Hazelwood Nursing Home is a purpose-built, detached home, located in the village of Longfield, which is accessible by public transport. The home includes a reminiscence room which is decorated with pictures and items relevant to different decades. A sensory room is also available. Musicians visit the home on a monthly basis to play live music for the residents. There are also regular visits from local schools and church and a good range of daily activities.

Registered places: 50
Guide weekly rate: Undisclosed
Specialist care: Nursing, Dementia
Medical services: Podiatry, dentist, optician, physiotherapy
Qualified staff: Meets standard

Home details
Location: Residential area, 1 mile from Longfield
Communal areas: 7 lounges, dining room, patio and garden
Accessibility: *Floors:* 2 • *Access:* Lift • *Wheelchair access:* Good
Smoking: ✗
Pets: At manager's discretion
Routines: Flexible

Room details
Single: 50
Shared: 0
En suite: 50
Facilities: TV point, telephone point

Door lock: ✓
Lockable place: ✓

Services provided
Beauty services: Hairdressing
Mobile library: Library facilities
Religious services: Monthly Anglican visits
Transport: ✗
Activities: *Coordinator:* ✗ • *Examples:* Bingo, flower arranging, quizzes • *Outings:* ✗
Meetings: ✓

Registered places: 12
Guide weekly rate: £500–£520
Specialist care: Respite
Medical services: None
Qualified staff: Exceeds standard: 80% at NVQ Level 2

Home details
Location: Residential area, 0.5 miles from Bromley
Communal areas: 2 lounges, 2 dining rooms, patio and garden
Accessibility: *Floors:* 3 • *Access:* Lift • *Wheelchair access:* Good
Smoking: ✗
Pets: ✓
Routines: Flexible

Room details
Single: 10
Shared: 1
En suite: 4
Facilities: TV, telephone

Door lock: ✓
Lockable place: ✓

Services provided
Beauty services: Hairdressing
Mobile library: ✓
Religious services: Monthly nondenominational church service
Transport: ✗
Activities: *Coordinator:* ✗ • *Examples:* Art class, exercise class, musical evenings • *Outings:* ✗
Meetings: ✗

The Heathers

Manager: Gillian Watkins
Owner: The Heathers Residential Care Home Ltd
Contact: 35 Farnaby Road, Shortlands, Bromley, Kent BR1 4BL
☏ 020 8460 6555

The Heathers consists of two adjoining semi-detached houses. It is situated in a quiet residential area, within walking distance of local shops and public transport. The residents have a flexible daily routine alongside structured meal times. There are scheduled weekly activities such as art and exercise classes and musical evenings – the home has a piano in its lounge. Services such as hairdressing, visits from a mobile library and a nondenominational church service once a month are arranged by the home. The home is currently undergoing a complete renovation and refurbishment. Parking is available for visitors.

Registered places: 8
Guide weekly rate: £515
Specialist care: Respite
Medical services: Podiatry, dentist, optician, physiotherapy
Qualified staff: Fails standard: 25% at NVQ level 2

Home details
Location: Urban area, 0.5 miles from Orpington
Communal areas: Lounge, dining room, patio and garden
Accessibility: *Floors:* 2 • *Access:* Stair lift
Wheelchair access: Limited
Smoking: ✗
Pets: At manager's discretion
Routines: Structured

Room details
Single: 4
Shared: 2
En suite: 0
Facilities: TV point

Door lock: ✗
Lockable place: ✓

Services provided
Beauty services: Hairdressing
Mobile library: ✓
Religious services: Fortnightly church group
Transport: ✗
Activities: *Coordinator:* ✗ • *Examples:* Bingo, movement to music, theatre group • *Outings:* ✗
Meetings: ✓

Heatherwood

Manager: Sally Perry
Owner: Chislehurst Care Ltd
Contact: 33 Station Road, Orpington, Kent BR6 0RZ
☏ 01689 813041
@ Alsh@tiscali.co.uk

Heatherwood is a small care home for eight people in a period property. The home is located in the town centre of Orpington. There is a veranda at the rear of the home which overlooks the home's enclosed gardens. The size of the home allows it to offer a personalised service and a homely atmosphere. Activities include bingo, movement to music, a theatre group and therapy dogs pets are allowed at the manager's discretion. There is a residents meeting every quarter.

Heathfield

Manager: Shelagh Lewis
Owner: Jason Prior and
Bonita Davis-Prior
Contact: Canterbury Road, Ashford,
Kent TN24 8QG
☎ 01233 610010
@ heathfield.prior@virgin.net

Heathfield is a detached property situated in a residential area of Ashford, one and a half miles from the town centre. There are a wide range of activities on offer with musical movement, coffee mornings, tea afternoons and trips out for lunches.

Though pets are not allowed to stay at Heathfield they can visit with family and friends. There are also residents meetings which occur every three months.

Registered places: 30
Guide weekly rate: £405–£431
Specialist care: Day care, physical disability, respite
Medical services: Podiatry, dentist, optician, physiotherapy
Qualified staff: Meets standard

Home details
Location: Residential area, 1.5 miles from Ashford
Communal areas: Lounge, 2 dining rooms, garden
Accessibility: *Floors:* 2 • *Access:* Lift • *Wheelchair access:* Good
Smoking: ✗
Pets: ✗
Routines: Flexible

Room details
Single: 22
Shared: 4
En suite: 11
Facilities: TV point

Door lock: ✓
Lockable place: ✓

Services provided
Beauty services: Hairdressing
Mobile library: ✓
Religious services: Weekly catholic and Anglican service
Transport: ✗
Activities: *Coordinator:* ✗ • *Examples:* Coffee mornings, musical movement, visiting entertainers • *Outings:* ✓
Meetings: ✓

High Hilden

Manager: Carol Tincombe
Owner: High Hilden Ltd
Contact: High Hilden Close, Tonbridge,
Kent TN10 3DD
☎ 01732 353070
@ highhilden@btconnect.com
🖰 www.highhilden.co.uk

High Hilden has been a residential care home for 60 years, located in a rural area, one mile from Tonbridge. There are extensive and attractive gardens with seating and views of the surrounding countryside. The home offers a vast array of activities for residents to take part in, including arts and crafts, visiting entertainers and classic board games. The home also goes on day trips to local points of interest.

Registered places: 40
Guide weekly rate: £435–£530
Specialist care: Respite
Medical services: Podiatry, dentist, optician, physiotherapy
Qualified staff: Exceeds standard: 80% at NVQ Level 2

Home details
Location: Rural area, 1 mile from Tonbridge
Communal areas: Lounge, dining room, activities room, library, hairdressing salon, garden
Accessibility: *Floors:* 2 • *Access:* Lift • *Wheelchair access:* Good
Smoking: In designated area
Pets: At manager's discretion
Routines: Flexible

Room details
Single: 40
Shared: 0
En suite: 9
Facilities: TV point, telephone point

Door lock: ✓
Lockable place: ✓

Services provided
Beauty services: Hairdressing
Mobile library: Library facilities
Religious services: Weekly service
Activities: *Coordinator:* ✓ • *Examples:* Craft, visiting shows, board games • *Outings:* ✓
Meetings: ✓

Registered places: 21
Guide weekly rate: £312–£397
Specialist care: None
Medical services: Podiatry, optician
Qualified staff: Exceeds standard: 75% at NVQ Level 2

Home details
Location: Village location, 2 miles from Hearne Bay
Communal areas: 2 lounges, dining room, garden
Accessibility: *Floors:* 2 • *Access:* Stair lift • *Wheelchair access:* Good
Smoking: In designated area
Pets: ✗
Routines: Flexible

Room details
Single: 18
Shared: 2
En suite: 12
Facilities: TV point

Door lock: ✓
Lockable place: ✗

Services provided
Beauty services: Hairdressing
Mobile library: ✗
Religious services: Monthly Anglican church service
Transport: Minibus
Activities: *Coordinator:* ✓ • *Examples:* Bingo, musical events
    Outings: ✗
Meetings: ✗

High Pines

Manager: Ann Huggins
Owner: High Pines Ltd
Contact: 47 Pigeon Lane, Herne Bay, Kent CT6 7ES
☏ 01227 368454
@ highpines47@aol.com

High Pines, a large detached property, is set in a quarter acre of land just outside of Herne. There is a bus stop just outside the home with buses to Hearne Bay, which is two miles away, and to Canterbury and Margate, both six miles away. Garden areas at the front and back of the property provide seating areas for residents in addition to the lounge. There is an activities coordinator who arranges games such as bingo and skittles and musical events and arts classes. Pets are not allowed and smoking is permitted only in the designated smoking room.

Registered places: 33
Guide weekly rate: £480–£800
Specialist care: Nursing, physical disability, terminal care
Medical services: None
Qualified staff: Meets standard

Home details
Location: Village location, 10 miles from Canterbury
Communal areas: 2 lounges, quiet lounge, dining room
Accessibility: *Floors:* 2 • *Access:* Lift • *Wheelchair access:* Good
Smoking: ✗
Pets: ✗
Routines: Flexible

Room details
Single: 13
Shared: 10
En suite: 7
Facilities: TV point, telephone point

Door lock: ✗
Lockable place: ✓

Services provided
Beauty services: Hairdressing
Mobile library: ✗
Religious services: Monthly church services
Transport: ✗
Activities: *Coordinator:* ✓ • *Examples:* Knitting, games, bowls
    Outings: ✗
Meetings: ✓

High View Oast Nursing Home

Manager: Sheelagah Sanford
Owner: New Century Care Ltd
Contact: Poulton Lane, Ash, Canterbury, Kent CT3 2HN
☏ 01304 813333

High View is a converted oast house, which retains many of its original features. The home is on a hill and has panoramic views of the Kent countryside. There is a local bus service into the village going to Canterbury, Sandwich and Deal. There are two interconnecting lounges and a quiet lounge which cater for the needs of all residents. If there is a daily activity going on in one room, there will still be a quiet lounge where residents can retreat to if they wish.

Highfield Private Rest Home

Manager: Simon Proctor
Owner: Mr and Mrs Wadmore
Contact: 77 Seabrook Road, Hythe, Kent CT21 5QW
☎ 01303 267036
🖰 www.highfieldresthome.com

The home is situated a few minutes' walk from the sea and within easy walking distance of the high street. In the garden there is a fishpond and aviary. The home creates traditional meals and varied menus using local produce so everything is fresh and wholesome. There is a variety of activities and outings for residents to take part in. These include handicraft sessions, quizzes and outings take place in the home's minibus.

Registered places: 31
Guide weekly rate: £445–£580
Specialist care: Day care, respite
Medical services: Podiatry, dentist, optician, physiotherapy
Qualified staff: Exceeds standard: 60% at NVQ level 2

Home details
Location: Residential area, 1 mile from Hythe
Communal areas: 3 lounges, dining room, 2 conservatories, patio and garden
Accessibility: *Floors:* 3 • *Access:* Lift • *Wheelchair access:* Good
Smoking: ✗
Pets: At manager's discretion
Routines: Flexible

Room details
Single: 30
Shared: 1
En suite: Undisclosed
Facilities: TV point, telephone point

Door lock: ✓
Lockable place: ✓

Services provided
Beauty services: Hairdressing
Mobile library: ✓
Religious services: Monthly Catholic, Anglican and Methodist services
Transport: Minibus
Activities: *Coordinator:* ✓ • *Examples:* Handicrafts, board and card games, quizzes • *Outings:* ✓
Meetings: ✓

Highfield

Manager: Melanie Baker
Owner: Egerton and Anne Eckersley
Contact: 51 Alpha Road, Birchington, Kent CT7 9EG
☎ 01843 842116
@ melanie4baker@hotmail.com

Highfield residential home is a detached three-storey building with an extension. It is located half a mile from the centre of Birchington. The home has two lounges and a dining room. At the rear of the property, there is a large garden. Activities include games and a weekly exercise session and the home arranges outings to the local fish shop. The home has two dogs and other pets would be allowed at the owners' discretion. Smoking is not permitted. There are residents meetings every month.

Registered places: 21
Guide weekly rate: £330–£460
Specialist care: None
Medical services: Podiatry, dentist, optician, physiotherapy
Qualified staff: Meets standard

Home details
Location: Residential area, 0.5 miles from Birchington
Communal areas: 2 lounges, dining room, garden
Accessibility: *Floors:* 3 • *Access:* Lift • *Wheelchair access:* Good
Smoking: ✗
Pets: At manager's discretion
Routines: Flexible

Room details
Single: 19
Shared: 2
En suite: 8
Facilities: TV, telephone

Door lock: ✓
Lockable place: ✓

Services provided
Beauty services: Hairdressing, aromatherapy
Mobile library: ✗
Religious services: Monthly church service
Transport: ✗
Activities: *Coordinator:* ✗ • *Examples:* Exercise, reminiscence sessions, visiting entertainers • *Outings:* ✓
Meetings: ✓

Registered places: 28
Guide weekly rate: Undisclosed
Specialist care: None
Medical services: Podiatry, dentist, optician
Qualified staff: Meets standard

Home details

Location: Residential area, 2 mile from Canterbury
Communal areas: 2 lounges, dining room, conservatory, garden
Accessibility: *Floors:* 2 • *Access:* Stair lift • *Wheelchair access:* Good
Smoking: x
Pets: At manager's discretion
Routines: Flexible

Room details

Single: 22
Shared: 3
En suite: 28
Facilities: TV, telephone point

Door lock: ✓
Lockable place: ✓

Services provided

Beauty services: Hairdressing, reflexology
Mobile library: x
Religious services: x
Transport: x
Activities: *Coordinator:* x • *Examples:* Bingo, music sessions, exercise sessions • *Outings:* ✓
Meetings: ✓

Highland House Retirement Home

Manager: Sue Page
Owner: Marian Walsh
Contact: Littlebourne Road, Canterbury, Kent CT3 4AE
☎ 01227 462921
@ highlandhousehc@aol.com

Highland House is situated two miles from Canterbury. Each of the rooms on the ground floor opens up onto the patio area and the home also has a conservatory. There is a wide range of activities that caters for all recreational and amusement needs such as exercise sessions and visiting entertainers. The home arranges outings for the residents, for example a ride in a limousine to see the Christmas lights. The home has its own pair of lovebirds and other pets are allowed at the manager's discretion. Each room in the home has en suite facilities, and four have en suite showers.

Registered places: 40
Guide weekly rate: £375–£450
Specialist care: Day care, respite
Medical services: Podiatry, dentist, optician
Qualified staff: Exceeds standard: 95% at NVQ Level 2

Home details

Location: Residential area, 0.5 miles from Gravesend
Communal areas: 2 lounges, dining room, 2 conservatories, hairdressing salon, garden
Accessibility: *Floors:* 2 • *Access:* Lift • *Wheelchair access:* Good
Smoking: In designated area
Pets: At manager's discretion
Routines: Flexible

Room details

Single: 37
Shared: 2
En suite: 39
Facilities: TV point

Door lock: ✓
Lockable place: ✓

Services provided

Beauty services: Hairdressing
Mobile library: x
Religious services: Weekly Anglican and Catholic service
Transport: Minibus
Activities: *Coordinator:* x • *Examples:* Exercise, bingo, visiting entertainers • *Outings:* ✓
Meetings: ✓

The Hollies

Manager: Peter Rogers
Owner: Mr and Mrs Rogers
Contact: 86–90 Darnley Road, Gravesend, Kent DA11 0SE
☎ 01474 568998
🖥 www.theholliesresidentialhome.co.uk

The Hollies was formerly two semi-detached houses that have been made into one house and extended. The home is half a mile from the town centre. The home offers a wealth of outings including pub lunches, mystery trips, seaside trips and blossom tours. These activities take place once a month and entertainers also visit once a month including singing and musical evenings. There are also frequently arranged parties such as tea dances and bingo evenings.

Holywell Park Residential Home

Manager: Sharon Apps
Owner: Holywell Park Ltd
Contact: Hodsoll Street, Ash-cum-Ridley, Wrotham, Kent TN15 7LE
) 01732 822215
@ holywellpark@aol.com
ᐯᕼ www.holywellpark.com

The home is a large, spacious, listed building set in its five acres of grounds with extensive countryside views. It comprises 48 bedrooms in the main house and two apartments in an adjoining stable block. The home has a dedicated hairdressing salon, which is very popular and lots of activities are available on a weekly basis. The home is located 11 and a half miles from Sevenoaks and arranges regular outings for the residents.

Registered places: 58
Guide weekly rate: £385–£650
Specialist care: Respite
Medical services: Podiatry, hygienist, optician, physiotherapy
Qualified staff: Exceeds standard: 60% at NVQ Level 2

Home details

Location: Residential area, 11.5 miles from Sevenoaks
Communal areas: 4 Lounges, dining room, library, conservatory, hairdressing salon, patio and garden
Accessibility: *Floors:* 3 • *Access:* 3 lifts • *Wheelchair access:* Good
Smoking: In designated area
Pets: ✗
Routines: Flexible

Room details

Single: 38
Shared: 10
En suite: Undisclosed
Facilities: TV point, telephone point

Door lock: ✓
Lockable place: ✓

Services provided

Beauty services: Hairdressing, aromatherapy
Mobile library: Library facilities
Religious services: Monthly Anglican service, Catholic visits
Transport: ✗
Activities: *Coordinator:* ✓ • *Examples:* Art classes, motivation class, jewellery making • *Outings:* ✓
Meetings: ✓

Hythe Nursing Home

Manager: Linda Hazrati
Owner: Premium Healthcare Ltd
Contact: 91 North Road, Hythe, Kent CT21 5ET
) 01303 265441
@ premiumhythe@btconnect.com

Hythe Nursing Home is located one mile from Hythe and provides care for 27 residents. The rooms at the rear of the home have panoramic views of the town and the English Channel. There is a large patio area which overlooks the sloping garden, although access is limited. The home arranges a lot of activities for residents with visiting singers and board games. There is also a regular Anglican communion service.

Registered places: 27
Guide weekly rate: £600–£650
Specialist care: Nursing, respite
Medical services: Podiatry, dentist, optician
Qualified staff: Fails standard

Home details

Location: Residential area, 1 mile from Hythe
Communal areas: Lounge, dining room, patio and garden
Accessibility: *Floors:* 2 • *Access:* Lift • *Wheelchair access:* Good
Smoking: In designated area
Pets: At manager's discretion
Routines: Flexible

Room details

Single: 19
Shared: 3
En suite: 5
Facilities: TV point, telephone point

Door lock: ✓
Lockable place: ✓

Services provided

Beauty services: Hairdressing
Mobile library: ✗
Religious services: Anglican Communion service
Transport: ✗
Activities: *Coordinator:* ✓ • *Examples:* Bingo, board games, flower arranging • *Outings:* ✓
Meetings: ✗

Registered places: 51
Guide weekly rate: £728–£894
Specialist care: Nursing, dementia, respite
Medical services: Podiatry, dentist, optician, physiotherapy
Qualified staff: Exceeds standard: 75% at NVQ Level 2

Home details

Location: Village location, 5 miles from Maidstone
Communal areas: Lounge/dining room, lounge, garden
Accessibility: *Floors:* 4 • *Access:* Lift and stair lift
     Wheelchair access: Good
Smoking: In designated area
Pets: ✗
Routines: Flexible

Room details

Single: 42
Shared: 4
En suite: 35
Facilities: TV point, telephone point

Door lock: ✗
Lockable place: ✓

Services provided

Beauty services: Hairdressing, aromatherapy, reflexology
Mobile library: ✗
Religious services: Monthly Anglican and Communion service
Transport: ✓
Activities: *Coordinator:* ✗ • *Examples:* Bingo, strawberry tea
     evenings, history talks • *Outings:* ✓
Meetings: ✓

Iden Manor Care Home

Manager: Sandra Gower
Owner: Whitepost Health Care Centre
Contact: Cranbrook Road, Staplehurst,
Tonbridge, Kent TN12 0ER
☎ 01580 891261
🖥 www.whiteposthealthcare.co.uk

Iden Manor Care Home is a Victorian manor house situated in 15 acres of land on the edge of Staplehurst. The grounds are extensive and well maintained offering views of the countryside. The staff at Iden Manor plan trips for the residents such as trips to Hastings and trips to London to the. There is also entertainment on a daily basis at the home such as history talks about the local area, classic film night and strawberry tea evenings.

Registered places: 44
Guide weekly rate: Undisclosed
Specialist care: Physical disability
Medical services: Podiatry, dentist, optician, physiotherapy
Qualified staff: Meets standard

Home details

Location: Residential area, 9 miles from Sheerness
Communal areas: 2 lounges, 2 dining rooms, balcony,
     patio and garden
Accessibility: *Floors:* 2 • *Access:* Lift • *Wheelchair access:* Good
Smoking: In designated area
Pets: ✓
Routines: Flexible

Room details

Single: 44
Shared: 0
En suite: 4
Facilities: TV, telephone

Door lock: ✓
Lockable place: ✓

Services provided

Beauty services: Hairdressing, manicures
Mobile library: Library facilities
Religious services: ✓
Transport: ✓
Activities: *Coordinator:* ✓ • *Examples:* Swimming • *Outings:* ✓
Meetings: ✓

The Island Home

Manager: Christine Strawbridge
Owner: Jagjit and Kuldish Pawar
Contact: Main Road, Leysdown-on-Sea,
Sheerness, Kent ME12 4LH
☎ 01795 510271

The Island Home is located in the village of Leysdown, which has local facilities such as shops and a library. There is a bus service to Sheerness which is nine miles away. The home has 44 single rooms for permanent residents but four have double capacity for respite patients. The home has an activities coordinator who visits four days a week and arranges a rota to take residents to the shops and swimming. There is also an outing to the local library once a month. The home allows budgies and cats. There are residents meetings every week.

Jeanette Lodge

Manager: Richard Raj
Owner: Golden Slumbers Ltd
Contact: 15–17 Park Avenue,
Gillingham, Kent ME7 4AS
☏ 01634 852894

Jeanette Lodge is a large detached property situated in a residential area and directly opposite a park. Chatham and Gillingham are approximately one mile away. There is a lounge, a dining room and a large garden. The home has three floors and although it has a lift wheelchair access is limited. Activities include quizzes, cooking, arts and crafts, exercises, bingo and flower arranging. Outings are also arranged by the home. Pets are not permitted and smoking is allowed outside. There a residents meeting every two months.

Registered places: 20
Guide weekly rate: £323–£408
Specialist care: Dementia
Medical services: Podiatry, dentist
Qualified staff: Meets standard

Home details

Location: Residential area, 1.2 miles from Gillingham
Communal areas: Lounge, dining room, garden
Accessibility: *Floors:* 3 • *Access:* Stair lift
  Wheelchair access: Limited
Smoking: In designated area
Pets: ✗
Routines: Flexible

Room details

Single: 10	Door lock: ✗
Shared: 5	Lockable place: ✓
En suite: 0	
Facilities: TV, telephone point	

Services provided

Beauty services: Hairdressing
Mobile library: ✓
Religious services: Monthly church service
Transport: ✗
Activities: *Coordinator:* ✗ • *Examples:* Arts and crafts, cooking, quizzes • *Outings:* ✓
Meetings: ✓

Kearsney Manor Nursing Home

Manager: Karen Wilczek
Owner: Sisters of the Christian Retreat
Contact: Alkham Road,
Kearsney, Dover, Kent CT16 3EQ
☏ 01304 822135
@ kmnh@btconnect.com

Kearsney Manor is a large detached stone building in 21 acres of land in Temple Ewell with views of the countryside. The complex also includes a convent for the nuns that work and volunteer at the home. A kitchen garden supplies the fresh vegetables used for the home's meals. There are daily activities such as cookery lessons as well as outings organised by the home. There is also mass three times a week.

Registered places: 44
Guide weekly rate: £400–£735
Specialist care: Nursing, respite
Medical services: Podiatry, optician, physiotherapy, speech therapy
Qualified staff: Exceeds standard: 67% at NVQ Level 2

Home details

Location: Rural area, 3 miles from Dover
Communal areas: 5 lounges, dining room, chapel/prayer room, garden
Accessibility: *Floors:* 3 • *Access:* Lift • *Wheelchair access:* Good
Smoking: ✗
Pets: At manager's discretion
Routines: Structured

Room details

Single: 38	Door lock: ✓
Shared: 3	Lockable place: ✓
En suite: 0	
Facilities: TV point	

Services provided

Beauty services: Hairdressing
Mobile library: ✓
Religious services: Mass 3 times a week
Transport: ✗
Activities: *Coordinator:* ✓ • *Examples:* Bingo, cookery, quizzes *Outings:* ✓
Meetings: ✗

Registered places: 31
Guide weekly rate: £303–£349
Specialist care: Respite
Medical services: Podiatry, dentist
Qualified staff: Exceeds standard: 60% at NVQ Level 2

Home details
Location: Urban area, 0.5 miles from Ramsgate
Communal areas: 3 lounges, dining room, patio and garden
Accessibility: *Floors:* 3 • *Access:* 2 lifts • *Wheelchair access:* Good
Smoking: ✗
Pets: ✗
Routines: Flexible

Room details
Single: 27
Shared: 2
En suite: 25
Facilities: TV point

Door lock: ✓
Lockable place: ✓

Services provided
Beauty services: Hairdressing, manicures
Mobile library: ✗
Religious services: Weekly Anglican visits,
    fortnightly Catholic services
Transport: ✗
Activities: *Coordinator:* ✗ • *Examples:* Bingo, exercise, quizzes
    Outings: ✗
Meetings: ✓

Keele House

Manager: Joan Smith
Owner: Soory and Co Ltd
Contact: 176 High Street, Ramsgate,
Kent CT11 9TS
☎ 01843 591735

Keele House is a detached building located approximately half a mile from Ramsgate town centre. The town offers a variety of shops, restaurants and pubs. The Edwardian Ellington Park with bandstand is 30 yards from the home. To the rear of the home, there is an enclosed garden with patio and seating area for residents' use. The home arranges weekly visits from Anglican ministers and there is a Catholic Mass performed every two weeks.

Registered places: 22
Guide weekly rate: From £313
Specialist care: None
Medical services: Podiatry, dentist, optician, physiotherapy
Qualified staff: Exceeds standard: 80% at NVQ Level 2

Home details
Location: Residential area, 1 mile from Broadstairs
Communal areas: 2 lounges, dining room, conservatory, garden
Accessibility: *Floors:* 4 • *Access:* Lift • *Wheelchair access:* Good
Smoking : ✗
Pets: ✓
Routines: Flexible

Room details
Single: 20
Shared: 1
En suite: 22
Facilities: TV, telephone

Door lock: ✓
Lockable place: ✓

Services provided
Beauty services: Hairdressing, beautician, massage
Mobile library: Library facilities
Religious services: ✓
Transport: ✗
Activities: *Coordinator:* ✗ • *Examples:* Bingo, craft, exercises
    Outings: ✗
Meetings: ✗

Kent House

Manager: Toni Selfridge
Owner: Choicecare 2000 Ltd
Contact: Fairfield Road, Broadstairs,
Kent CT10 2JY
☎ 01843 602720

Situated in a residential area, one mile from Broadstairs, Kent House is spread over four floors which are serviced by a lift, providing good wheelchair access throughout the home. There is a beauty salon in the home where residents can benefit from the home's services including hairdressing and holistic massage. The home also offers religious services and daily activities such as bingo and exercise sessions are arranged.

The Knoll Nursing Home

Manager: Amita Patel
Owner: Raj and Knoll Ltd
Contact: 196 Dover Road, Walmer, Deal, Kent CT14 7NB
☏ 01304 374679

The Knoll Nursing Home is a large, detached building, situated seven miles from Dover. Outdoor space is limited to a patio area. There is no garden attached to the premises, but there is a public park opposite the home, where residents are taken for walks. There are monthly visits from an Anglican minister and the home offers hairdressing, aromatherapy and manicures to its residents.

Registered places: 29
Guide weekly rate: £475–£675
Specialist care: Nursing, terminal care
Medical services: Podiatry, optician, physiotherapy
Qualified staff: Meets standard

Home details
Location: Residential area, 7 miles from Dover
Communal areas: Lounge, dining room, patio
Accessibility: *Floors:* 2 • *Access:* Lift • *Wheelchair access:* Good
Smoking: ✗
Pets: ✗
Routines: Flexible

Room details
Single: 29
Shared: 0
En suite: 8
Facilities: TV point

Door lock: ✓
Lockable place: ✓

Services provided
Beauty services: Hairdressing, aromatherapy, manicures
Mobile library: ✗
Religious services: Monthly Anglican visits
Transport: ✗
Activities: *Coordinator:* ✓ • *Examples:* Ball games, quizzes, singalongs • *Outings:* ✗
Meetings: ✓

The Laleham

Manager: Vacant
Owner: Kent County Ltd
Contact: 117–121 Central Parade, Herne Bay, Kent CT6 5JN
☏ 01227 363340

Situated close to the centre of Herne Bay The Laleham offers care to 75 residents, with one place for learning disability and one for dementia. The home consists of five older properties which have been converted into one building. To the front of the home there are views across the promenade and the sea. The home has 43 single rooms and 15 double rooms. The double rooms are used for single occupancy unless residents specifically request to share.

Registered places: 75
Guide weekly rate: £305–£380
Specialist care: Dementia, learning disability
Medical services: None
Qualified staff: Meets standard

Home details
Location: Residential area, 9 miles from Canterbury
Communal areas: Undisclosed
Accessibility: *Floors:* 3 • *Access:* Lift • *Wheelchair access:* Good
Smoking: Undisclosed
Pets: Undisclosed
Routines: Flexible

Room details
Single: 43
Shared: 15
En suite: Undisclosed
Facilities: None

Door lock: ✗
Lockable place: ✗

Services provided
Beauty services: Undisclosed
Mobile library: ✗
Religious services: ✗
Transport: ✗
Activities: *Coordinator:* ✗ • *Examples:* Undisclosed • *Outings:* ✗
Meetings: ✗

Registered places: 33
Guide weekly rate: £560–£730
Specialist care: Nursing
Medical services: Podiatry, optician
Qualified staff: Fails standard: 25% at NVQ Level 2

Home details

Location: Village location, 3 miles from Stapleton
Communal areas: Lounge, dining room, library,
    conservatory, garden
Accessibility: *Floors:* 2 • *Access:* Lift • *Wheelchair access:* Good
Smoking: In designated area
Pets: At manager's discretion
Routines: Flexible

Room details

Single: 23	Door lock: ✗
Shared: 5	Lockable place: ✓
En suite: 8	
Facilities: TV point	

Services provided

Beauty services: Hairdressing
Mobile library: Library facilities
Religious services: Monthly
Transport: ✗
Activities: *Coordinator:* ✓ • *Examples:* Flower arranging, games
    Outings: ✓
Meetings: ✓

Larchmere House

Manager: Daphne Brockman
Owner: Family Care UK Ltd
Contact: Biddenden Road, Frittenden,
Kent TN17 2EN
☎ 01580 852335
@ family.care@btconnect.com

Larchmere House is situated in the small village of Frittenden, only three miles from Staplehurst where there is a mainline railway station and bus station. The home has two activities coordinators, who offer residents activities including flower arranging, games, quizzes. There are also regular outings to Staplehurst where residents have the opportunity to shop or simply stop and have a pub lunch. The home has a resident cat and there is a large garden for residents to enjoy in nice weather.

Registered places: 21
Guide weekly rate: Undisclosed
Specialist care: Respite
Medical services: Podiatry, dentist, optician, physiotherapy
Qualified staff: Exceeds standard: 60% at NVQ Level 2

Home details

Location: Residential area, 0.5 miles from Dover
Communal areas: 2 lounges, dining room, patio and garden
Accessibility: *Floors:* 3 • *Access:* Lift • *Wheelchair access:* Good
Smoking: ✗
Pets: At manger's discretion
Routines: Flexible

Room details

Single: 13	Door lock: ✓
Shared: 4	Lockable place: ✓
En suite: 1	
Facilities: TV point	

Services provided

Beauty services: Hairdressing
Mobile library: ✗
Religious services: Monthly Communion service
Transport: ✗
Activities: *Coordinator:* ✗ • *Examples:* Crafts, bingo, shopping
    Outings: ✓
Meetings: ✓

Laureston House Residential Home

Manager: Ann Lott
Owner: Mr and Mrs Roberts
Contact: Laureston Place, Dover, Kent
CT16 1QU
☎ 01304 204283

Laureston House is located on a hill overlooking Dover and is five minutes' walk from public transport. Every Friday the home arranges activities including arts and crafts, bingo and shopping. Outings are arranged frequently and other events such as a summer tea party. All of these events are chosen by residents through the monthly residents meetings. The home also arranges for a priest to visit and there is a Communion service once a month.

Lauriston House Nursing Home

Manager: Silvia Rahaman
Owner: Southern Cross Healthcare Ltd
Contact: Bickley Park Road, Bickley,
Kent BR1 2AZ
) 020 8295 3000
@ Lauriston.house@
southerncrosshealthcare.co.uk
www.southerncrosshealthcare.co.uk

An exceptionally large, purpose-built home, Lauriston House is located two miles from Bromley town centre. The home has three lounges, three dining rooms and there are computer facilities. The home has its own transport and takes residents on outings. There is also an activities coordinator. Pets are not allowed in the home and smoking is permitted in designated area. All of the rooms have en suite facilities and there are regular residents meetings.

Registered places: 92
Guide weekly rate: Undisclosed
Specialist care: Nursing, physical disability, respite
Medical services: Podiatry, dentist, optician, physiotherapy
Qualified staff: Undisclosed

Home details
Location: Residential area, 2 miles from Bromley
Communal areas: 3 lounges, 3 dining rooms, computer facilities, patio and garden
Accessibility: *Floors:* 3 • *Access:* 2 lifts • *Wheelchair access:* Good
Smoking: In designated area
Pets: ✗
Routines: Flexible

Room details

Single: 28	**Door lock:** ✗
Shared: 32	**Lockable place:** ✗
En suite: 92	
Facilities: TV, telephone	

Services provided
Beauty services: Hairdressing, manicures
Mobile library: ✓
Religious services: ✗
Transport: ✓
Activities: *Coordinator:* ✓ • *Examples:* Bingo, visiting entertainers
Outings: ✓
Meetings: ✓

Lavenders

Manager: Candyce Brockwell
Owner: Mr and Mrs Webb
Contact: Lavenders Road,
West Malling, Kent ME19 6HP
) 01732 844744

Lavenders is made up of three wings and is suitable for the elderly with low care needs. It is a purpose-built care home with a garden, located half a mile from West Malling. There are extensive, well-kept grounds. The home organises weekly activities including musical entertainers and guest speakers. The home arranges for an outside group to take small groups of residents out for trips as the home does not have its own transport. There are evening songs and hymns performed in the home and a vicar visits regularly.

Registered places: 61
Guide weekly rate: £410–£495
Specialist care: Respite
Medical services: Podiatry, dentist, optician, physiotherapy
Qualified staff: Meets standard

Home details
Location: Rural area, 0.5 miles from West Malling
Communal areas: 5 lounges, 4 dining rooms, garden
Accessibility: *Floors:* 2 • *Access:* Stair lift • *Wheelchair access:* Good
Smoking: In designated area
Pets: ✗
Routines: Flexible

Room details

Single: 61	**Door lock:** ✓
Shared: 0	**Lockable place:** ✓
En suite: 60	
Facilities: TV point, telephone point	

Services provided
Beauty services: Hairdressing
Mobile library: ✓
Religious services: Evening songs and hymns, Communion service
Transport: ✗
Activities: *Coordinator:* ✓ • *Examples:* Motivation exercise, speakers, musical entertainers • *Outings:* ✓
Meetings: ✗

Registered places: 26
Guide weekly rate: £313–£430
Specialist care: Day care, respite
Medical services: Podiatry, dentist, optician
Qualified staff: Meets standard

Home details

Location: Rural area, 0.5 miles from Little Romney
Communal areas: Lounge/dining room, quiet room, garden
Accessibility: *Floors:* 2 • *Access:* Lift and stair lift
    Wheelchair access: Good
Smoking: ✗
Pets: ✓
Routines: Flexible

Room details

Single: 26
Shared: 0
En suite: 12
Facilities: TV point, telephone point

Door lock: ✓
Lockable place: ✓

Services provided

Beauty services: Hairdressing
Mobile library: Library facilities
Religious services: Communion and church group visits
Transport: ✗
Activities: *Coordinator:* ✗ • *Examples:* Games, visiting entertainers
    Outings: ✓
Meetings: ✓

Lindau Retirement Home

Manager: Stephen Cooper
Owner: Care Excellence Ltd
Contact: 104 Littlestone Road, Littlestone, New Romney, Kent TN28 8NH
☏ 01797 364371
@ landau.newromney@uwclub.net

Lindau Retirement Home is situated in a rural area close to the seafront, approximately half a mile from the town of Little Romney. The home has a lounge and a dining room and a quiet room with library facilities. There is also a garden for residents to enjoy in the warmer weather. The home arranges a Communion service and a church group visits regularly. The home provides daily activities for the residents such as games and performances by visiting entertainers. There are also outings in the local area, for example for cream tea.

Registered places: 28
Guide weekly rate: Undisclosed
Specialist care: Nursing
Medical services: Podiatry, occupational therapy, optician, physiotherapy
Qualified staff: Undisclosed

Home details

Location: Village location, 4 miles from Royal Tunbridge Wells
Communal areas: Lounge, conservatory
Accessibility: *Floors:* 2 • *Access:* Lift • *Wheelchair access:* Good
Smoking: ✗
Pets: At manager's discretion
Routines: Flexible

Room details

Single: 20
Shared: 4
En suite: 10
Facilities: TV point, telephone point

Door lock: ✗
Lockable place: ✓

Services provided

Beauty services: Hairdressing
Mobile library: ✓
Religious services: ✓
Transport: ✗
Activities: *Coordinator:* ✓ • *Examples:* Bingo, quizzes
    Outings: ✗
Meetings: ✓

Little Court Nursing Home

Manager: Peter Hart
Owner: Neatbell Ltd
Contact: Roopers, Speldhurst, Tunbridge Wells, Kent TN3 0NY
☏ 01892 863414
@ manager@thelittlecourt.co.uk
🖱 www.thelittlecourt.co.uk

Little Court Nursing Home is located in the picturesque village of Speldhurst, only four miles away from the spa town of Royal Tunbridge Wells. It is a large building that stands in its own grounds with a lounge and a conservatory for residents to enjoy. There is a voluntary service run by a lady of St Marys Church, who visits the home once a week. They talk with residents, partake in activities, or take them for strolls around the village.

Littlebourne House

Manager: Luciana Jarmaine
Owner: Maralyn Hussein and Michael Moreland
Contact: 2 High Street, Littlebourne, Canterbury, Kent CT3 1UN
☏ 01227 721527
@ care@littlebournecarehome.co.uk
🖱 www.littlebournecarehome.co.uk

Littlebourne House is situated in Littlebourne village, approximately five miles from Canterbury. The home is an older property which has been modernised and extended. The home boasts a large all-weather conservatory that looks out onto the garden. A range of activities are provided for residents, such as bingo, quizzes, video afternoons, ball games and walks during the warmer months.

Registered places: 41
Guide weekly rate: £300–£550
Specialist care: Day care, residential
Medical services: Podiatry, optician, physiotherapy
Qualified staff: Exceeds standard: 100% at NVQ Level 2

Home details
Location: Village location, 5 miles from Canterbury
Communal areas: Conservatory, garden
Accessibility: *Floors:* 2 • *Access:* Stair lift • *Wheelchair access:* Good
Smoking: In designated area
Pets: ✗
Routines: Flexible

Room details
Single: 37
Shared: 2
En suite: 39
Facilities: TV point, telephone point

Door lock: ✓
Lockable place: ✓

Services provided
Beauty services: Hairdressing
Mobile library: ✓
Religious services: Fortnightly
Transport: ✓
Activities: *Coordinator:* ✓ • *Examples:* Bingo, video afternoons
   Outings: ✓
Meetings: ✓

Loose Valley Nursing Home

Manager: Janet Poole
Owner: Nellsar Ltd
Contact: 15 Linton Road, Loose, Maidstone, Kent ME15 0AG
☏ 01622 745959
@ loosevalley@nellsar.com

Loose Valley Nursing Home is set in a rural location and is situated approximately two miles from Maidstone. There is a garden at the rear of the property which offers seating for the residents, with views over the Loose Valley. Residents take part in daily activities such as bingo, skittles, cards and backgammon. There are also a variety of outings arranged for small groups, for example to the theatre or to a wine tasting. The residents enjoy a flexible daily schedule with lunch being the only meal with a set time.

Registered places: 39
Guide weekly rate: £600–£800
Specialist care: None
Medical services: Podiatry, optician, physiotherapy
Qualified staff: Meets standard

Home details
Location: Rural area, 2 miles from Maidstone
Communal areas: Lounge, dining room, conservatory, patio and garden
Accessibility: *Floors:* 2 • *Access:* Lift and stair lift
   Wheelchair access: Good
Smoking: ✗
Pets: ✓
Routines: Flexible

Room details
Single: 22
Shared: 7
En suite: Undisclosed
Facilities: TV point

Door lock: ✓
Lockable place: ✓

Services provided
Beauty services: Hairdressing, aromatherapy
Mobile library: ✗
Religious services: ✓
Transport: ✗
Activities: *Coordinator:* ✗ • *Examples:* Bingo, reading, music
   Outings: ✓
Meetings: ✓

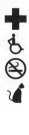

Registered places: 15
Guide weekly rate: £597–£680
Specialist care: Nursing
Medical services: Podiatry, optician, physiotherapy
Qualified staff: Meets standard

Home details

Location: Residential area, 1 mile from Westgate-on-Sea
Communal areas: Lounge, dining room, chapel, garden
Accessibility: *Floors:* 2 • *Access:* Lift • *Wheelchair access:* Good
Smoking: ✗
Pets: At manager's discretion
Routines: Flexible

Room details

Single: 15
Shared: 0
En suite: 15
Facilities: TV point

Door lock: ✗
Lockable place: ✓

Services provided

Beauty services: Hairdressing
Mobile library: ✓
Religious services: Daily Bible readings
Transport: ✗
Activities: *Coordinator:* ✓ • *Examples:* Gardening, knitting
    Outings: ✓
Meetings: ✓

Lourdes Nursing Home

Manager: Josephine Cutting
Owner: The Trustees for the Roman Union
Contact: Ursuline Convent, 225 Canterbury Road, Westgate-on-Sea, Kent CT8 8LX
☎ 01843 833242

Situated within the grounds of Ursuline Convent, Lourdes Community is a purpose-built home which is located within extensive grounds, one mile from Westgate-on-Sea. The grounds have level access for wheelchair users, and those that are mobile are welcome to walk round the grounds and even help with gardening. There is a chapel at the home where there a daily prayers and Bible readings for those that want to join in. Being located near the seafront, there are regular walks along the seafront for fish and chips.

Registered places: 40
Guide weekly rate: £313–£350
Specialist care: Respite
Medical services: Podiatry, dentist, optician
Qualified staff: Exceeds standard: 70% at NVQ Level 2

Home details

Location: Residential area, 1 mile from Folkstone
Communal areas: Lounge, dining room, hairdressing salon, sluice room, patio and garden
Accessibility: *Floors:* 3 • *Access:* 2 lifts • *Wheelchair access:* Good
Smoking: ✗
Pets: ✓
Routines: Flexible

Room details

Single: 40
Shared: 0
En suite: 40
Facilities: TV point

Door lock: ✓
Lockable place: ✓

Services provided

Beauty services: Hairdressing
Mobile library: ✓
Religious services: Monthly
Transport: ✗
Activities: *Coordinator:* ✓ • *Examples:* Arts and crafts, bingo, chair aerobics • *Outings:* ✓
Meetings: ✓

Mandalay Residential Home

Manager: Shirley Brook
Owner: Stargate Partnership Ltd
Contact: 10 Julian Road, Folkstone, Kent CT19 5HB
☎ 01303 258095

Mandalay Residential Home is around a mile from Folkestone town centre. There are local shops near the home and the main bus route into town runs close to the home. As well as daily activities such as bingo and aerobics, the home puts on fêtes and birthday parties for residents in its grounds. Residents also have the opportunity to go on outings, for example to the local pantomime. The home has a lounge and a dining room as communal areas and there is also a hairdressing salon. Pets are allowed in the home and smoking is not permitted.

MaryCare Homes

Manager: Vacant
Owner: Mary Smith
Contact: 8 Marine Road, Deal,
Kent CT14 7DN
☏ 01304 366447
@ careletonmead@tesco.net

MaryCare Homes are two separate facilities, Carleton Mead and Carleton Lodge, which are adjacent buildings with a driveway between them. They specialise in care for Parkinson's and Huntington's disease sufferers. The home also caters for special dietary requirements such as vegans and food intolerances. The home is situated on the seafront in Deal and there is access to local shops and public transport close by. Residents can also enjoy a garden at the rear of the property.

Registered places: 37
Guide weekly rate: £365–£385
Specialist care: Nursing
Medical services: Podiatry, hygienist, optician, physiotherapy
Qualified staff: Exceeds standard: 70% at NVQ Level 2

Home details
Location: Residential area, 8 miles from Dover
Communal areas: 2 dining rooms, garden
Accessibility: *Floors:* 2 • *Access:* Lift and stair lift
   Wheelchair access: Good
Smoking: ✓
Pets: ✓
Routines: Flexible

Room details
Single: 29
Shared: 5
En suite: 1
Facilities: TV point

Door lock: ✗
Lockable place: ✓

Services provided
Beauty services: None
Mobile library: ✓
Religious services: Monthly Communion service
Transport: ✗
Activities: *Coordinator:* ✗ • *Examples:* Bingo, exercises, organised activities • *Outings:* ✗
Meetings: ✓

Mill House

Manager: Heather Karslake
Owner: Renuha and Niranjan Francis
Contact: Salters Lane, Faversham,
Kent ME13 8ND
☏ 01795 533276

Mill House is a large, detached property which is a listed building. Mill House is located two miles from Faversham town centre. The home has a large garden to the rear of the property with an ornamental fishpond, bird aviary and seating for residents. The home arranges daily activities such as bingo and takes the residents on walks in the local area. There is an Anglican service once a month and a Catholic service every two weeks.

Registered places: 24
Guide weekly rate: £370–£400
Specialist care: Day care, dementia, respite
Medical services: Podiatry, dentist, optician, physiotherapy
Qualified staff: Exceeds standard: 70% at NVQ Level 2

Home details
Location: Residential area, 2 miles from Faversham
Communal areas: Lounge, dining room, patio and garden
Accessibility: *Floors:* 2 • *Access:* Lift • *Wheelchair access:* Good
Smoking: In designated area
Pets: At manger's discretion
Routines: Flexible

Room details
Single: 19
Shared: 3
En suite: 11
Facilities: TV point, telephone point

Door lock: ✓
Lockable place: ✓

Services provided
Beauty services: Hairdressing
Mobile library: ✗
Religious services: Monthly Anglican service, fortnightly Catholic service
Transport: ✗
Activities: *Coordinator:* ✗ • *Examples:* Bingo, keep fit
   Outings: ✓
Meetings: ✓

Registered places: 30
Guide weekly rate: £295–£365
Specialist care: Day care, respite
Medical services: Podiatry, optician
Qualified staff: Fails standard

Home details

Location: Residential area, 1 mile from Cliftonville
Communal areas: 2 lounges, dining room, hairdressing salon, patio and garden
Accessibility: *Floors:* 3 • *Access:* Lift and stair lift
  Wheelchair access: Good
Smoking: In designated area
Pets: At manager's discretion
Routines: Flexible

Room details

Single: 24
Shared: 3
En suite: 27
Facilities: TV point, telephone point

Door lock: ✓
Lockable place: ✓

Services provided

Beauty services: Aromatherapy, manicures
Mobile library: ✗
Religious services: ✗
Transport: ✗
Activities: *Coordinator:* ✓ • *Examples:* Arts and crafts, games, exercise • *Outings:* ✓
Meetings: ✓

Montagu Court Residential Home

Manager: Margaret Woods
Owner: Alan Morris
Contact: 49–51 Edgar Road,
Cliftonville, Margate, Kent CT9 2EQ
☏ 01843 223648

Montagu Court Residential Home is a large, family-run property, approximately one mile from Cliftonville. It is within a short walking distance from the local shopping centre, the seafront and public transport. The residents partake in various excursions and activities including watching films on the home's own cinema screen. There are also arts and crafts and exercise sessions. The home has a garden for residents to enjoy as well as its own hairdressing salon.

Registered places: 22
Guide weekly rate: £432–£550
Specialist care: None
Medical services: Podiatry, hygienist, optician, physiotherapy
Qualified staff: Meets standard

Home details

Location: Residential area, 1 mile from Bromley
Communal areas: Lounge, dining room, conservatory, garden
Accessibility: *Floors:* 3 • *Access:* Lift • *Wheelchair access:* Good
Smoking: ✗
Pets: ✓
Routines: Flexible

Room details

Single: 14
Shared: 4
En suite: 0
Facilities: TV point, telephone point

Door lock: ✓
Lockable place: ✓

Services provided

Beauty services: Hairdressing, manicures
Mobile library: ✓
Religious services: Weekly church service
Transport: ✗
Activities: *Coordinator:* ✓ • *Examples:* Quizzes, bingo, exercise
  Outings: ✓
Meetings: ✓

Nettlestead

Manager: Kim Thomas
Owner: Nightingale Retirement Care Ltd
Contact: 19 Sundridge Avenue,
Bromley, Kent BR1 2PU
☏ 020 8460 2279
🖰 www.nightingale.co.uk

Nettlestead is a detached three-storey Victorian house situated in a quiet residential area within one mile of Bromley. The house is set within its own grounds, with a secluded rear garden. An activities coordinator arranges pub lunches, visits to art centres, and exercise sessions. There is a wide menu range and residents have the option to dine where they like. There is a residents meeting arranged once a month.

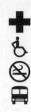

Newington Court Nursing Home

Manager: Alison Butler
Owner: Barchester Healthcare Ltd
Contact: Keycol Hill, Newington, Sittingbourne, Kent ME9 7LG
) 01795 843033
www.barchester.com

Newington Court is a purpose-built home on the main road between Newington and Sittingbourne. The home is approximately two miles from Sittingbourne. The home has a Pets As Therapy scheme that residents can enjoy. The home also arranges outings for residents using its minibus as transportation. A monthly newsletter is issued to residents. Families and friends are able to visit at any time.

Registered places: 50
Guide weekly rate: £750–£875
Specialist care: Nursing, dementia, respite
Medical services: Podiatry, optician
Qualified staff: Exceeds standard: 68% at NVQ Level 2

Home details
Location: Rural area, 2 miles from Sittingbourne
Communal areas: 3 lounges, 3 dining rooms, garden
Accessibility: *Floors:* 3 • *Access:* Lift • *Wheelchair access:* Good
Smoking: ✗
Pets: ✗
Routines: Flexible

Room details
Single: 46	**Door lock:** ✓
Shared: 2	**Lockable place:** ✓
En suite: 48	
Facilities: TV point, telephone point	

Services provided
Beauty services: Hairdressing, massages, manicures
Mobile library: ✗
Religious services: Weekly
Transport: Minibus
Activities: *Coordinator:* ✓ • *Examples:* Hanging baskets, painting, Pets As Therapy • *Outings:* ✓
Meetings: ✓

Newlyn Residential Home

Manager: Linda Goldsmith
Owner: Linda Goldsmith
Contact: 2 Cliftonville Avenue, Newington, Ramsgate, Kent CT12 6DS
) 01843 589191
@ cherylgoldsmith@fsmail.net

Newlyn Residential Home is a family-run home, located approximately one and a half miles from Ramsgate. The home is close both train and bus routes. There is a garden with a patio area for residents to enjoy in warmer months, as well as a lounge. The home arranges daily activities such as exercise sessions and visiting entertainment and also takes the residents on outings. The home has its own car for this purpose. There are also regular residents meetings.

Registered places: 13
Guide weekly rate: £303–£390
Specialist care: Respite
Medical services: Podiatry, hygienist, optician, physiotherapy
Qualified staff: Meets standard

Home details
Location: Residential area, 1.5 miles from Ramsgate
Communal areas: Lounge, dining room, patio and garden
Accessibility: *Floors:* 2 • *Access:* Stair lift • *Wheelchair access:* Good
Smoking: ✗
Pets: At manager's discretion
Routines: Flexible

Room details
Single: 7	**Door lock:** ✓
Shared: 3	**Lockable place:** ✓
En suite: 6	
Facilities: TV point	

Services provided
Beauty services: Hairdressing
Mobile library: ✓
Religious services: ✗
Transport: Car
Activities: *Coordinator:* ✓ • *Examples:* Exercises, painting and entertainment • *Outings:* ✓
Meetings: ✓

Registered places: 30
Guide weekly rate: £303–£448
Specialist care: Respite
Medical services: Podiatry, dentist, optician
Qualified staff: Exceeds standard: 70% at NVQ Level 2

Home details

Location: Residential area, 0.5 miles from Westgate-on-Sea
Communal areas: 4 lounges, 1 dining, hairdressing salon,
   patio and garden
Accessibility: *Floors:* 3 • *Access:* Lift • *Wheelchair access:* good
Smoking: ×
Pets: ×
Routines: Flexible

Room details

Single: 30
Shared: 0
En suite: 7
Facilities: TV point, telephone point

Door lock: ✓
Lockable place: ✓

Services provided

Beauty services: Hairdressing, aromatherapy, manicures
Mobile library: ×
Religious services: Weekly Catholic visits
Transport: ×
Activities: *Coordinator:* × • *Examples:* Arts and crafts, games,
   keep fit • *Outings:* ✓
Meetings: ✓

Norfolk House

Manager: Vacant
Owner: Choicecare 2000 Ltd
Contact: 39–41 Sea Road,
Westgate-on-Sea, Kent CT8 8QW
☎ 01843 831667

Norfolk House is situated close to the seafront, giving uninterrupted sea views from the home. The seafront itself can be accessed easily via ramps and walkways and trips to the promenade are often arranged. The home is approximately half a mile from Westgate-on-Sea. The home has an attractive rear garden with a patio area and decorative pergola. The staff occasionally arrange garden parties during the summer months.

Registered places: 26
Guide weekly rate: £326–£420
Specialist care: Respite
Medical services: Podiatry, dentist, optician
Qualified staff: Exceeds standard: 70% at NVQ Level 2

Home details

Location: Residential area, 2 miles from Sheerness
Communal areas: 2 dining rooms, 2 lounge, conservatory, garden
Accessibility: *Floors:* 2 • *Access:* Lift • *Wheelchair access:* Good
Smoking: In designated area
Pets: At manager's discretion
Routines: Flexible

Room details

Single: 16
Shared: 5
En suite: 0
Facilities: TV point

Door lock: ✓
Lockable place: ✓

Services provided

Beauty services: Hairdressing
Mobile library: ✓
Religious services: Monthly Communion service
Transport: ×
Activities: *Coordinator:* × • *Examples:* Arts and crafts,
   floor basketball, paintings • *Outings:* ✓
Meetings: ×

Oakdene Rest Home

Manager: Tracey Gobbi
Owner: Tracey Gobbi
Contact: 165 Minster Road,
Minster-on-Sea, Sheerness, Kent
ME12 3LH
☎ 01795 874985

Oakdene Rest Home is located in Minister-on-Sea, approximately two miles from Sheerness. Activities are organised regularly including arts and crafts, painting and floor basketball. Outings take place frequently such as trips to the beach and concerts. The home also arranges for an Anglican vicar to visit and a Communion service occurs once a month.

Oakfield House

Manager: Robin Field
Owner: Roger, Robin and Gloria Field
Contact: High Street, Wingham, Canterbury, Kent CT3 1BU
☎ 01227 721107
@ robin.field@btinternet.com

Originally a village schoolhouse, Oakfield House is found in the quiet village of Wingham, between Canterbury and Sandwich. It is a family-run home approximately seven miles from Canterbury. There are a wide variety of books and DVDs at the home for residents to access, as well as a varied activities programme. Smoking is permitted in a designated area in the home and there is a residents meeting annually. The home has its own transport and takes residents on outings.

Registered places: 30
Guide weekly rate: £377–£495
Specialist care: Day care, respite
Medical services: Podiatry, physiotherapy dentist, optician
Qualified staff: Exceeds standard: 80% at NVQ Level 2

Home details
Location: Village location, 7 miles from Canterbury
Communal areas: Lounge, dining room, conservatory, patio and garden
Accessibility: *Floors:* 2 • *Access:* Stair lift
   Wheelchair access: Limited
Smoking: In designated area
Pets: ✓
Routines: Structured

Room details
Single: 24	Door lock: ✓
Shared: 3	Lockable place: ✓
En suite: 27	

Facilities: TV point, telephone point

Services provided
Beauty services: Hairdressing
Mobile library: ✗
Religious services: Weekly and monthly services
Transport: People carrier
Activities: *Coordinator:* ✓ • *Examples:* Bingo, reminiscence, quizzes • *Outings:* ✓
Meetings: ✓

The Old Farm House Residential Home

Manager: Vivien Fuller
Owner: Paul Straker
Contact: 48 Hollow Lane, Canterbury, Kent CT1 3SA
☎ 01227 453685

The Old Farm House Residential Home is located approximately one and a half miles from Canterbury town centre, which offers shops and other amenities. The home is set in a residential area, which affords views of Canterbury cathedral. The home was originally a farmhouse and is a detached building with a purpose-built extension. It is set within an enclosed, attractive garden which includes a seating area. The home also arranges for an Anglican minister to visit the residents once a month.

Registered places: 23
Guide weekly rate: £395–£440
Specialist care: None
Medical services: Podiatry, dentist, optician, physiotherapy
Qualified staff: Exceeds standard: 90% at NVQ Level 2

Home details
Location: Residential area, 1.5 miles from Canterbury
Communal areas: 2 lounges 1 dining room, library, conservatory, garden
Accessibility: *Floors:* 2 • *Access:* Lift • *Wheelchair access:* good
Smoking: ✗
Pets: ✗
Routines: Flexible

Room details
Single: 19	Door lock: ✓
Shared: 2	Lockable place: ✓
En suite: 21	

Facilities: TV point, telephone point

Services provided
Beauty services: Hairdressing
Mobile library: Library facilities
Religious services: Monthly Anglican visits
Transport: ✗
Activities: *Coordinator:* ✓ • *Examples:* Bingo, exercise, flower craft *Outings:* ✓
Meetings: ✓

Registered places: 26
Guide weekly rate: £329–£450
Specialist care: Respite
Medical services: Podiatry, dentist, optician physiotherapy
Qualified staff: Exceeds standard: 80% at NVQ Level 2

Home details

Location: Village location, 4.5 miles from Romney Marsh
Communal areas: Lounge, dining room, library, 2 conservatories, patio and garden
Accessibility: *Floors:* 3 • *Access:* Lift and stair lift
    Wheelchair access: Good
Smoking: ✗
Pets: At manager's discretion
Routines: Flexible

Room details

Single: 19
Shared: 3
En suite: 15
Facilities: TV point, telephone point

Door lock: ✓
Lockable place: ✓

Services provided

Beauty services: Hairdressing, aromatherapy
Mobile library: ✓
Religious services: Monthly Anglican service, Catholic visits
Transport: Minibus and car
Activities: *Coordinator:* ✓ • *Examples:* Puzzles, reminiscence, visiting entertainers • *Outings:* ✓
Meetings: ✓

The Old Rectory

Manager: Janet Blundred
Owner: Mr and Mrs Blundred
Contact: New Hall Close, Dymchurch, Kent TN29 0LE
) 01303 874470
@ oldrec@btconnect.com

The Old Rectory is a detached, three-storey Victorian house. A post office, church, shops, public transport and a pub are all within easy walking distance. The home is situated on the beach and arranges a range of activities for the residents, such as visiting entertainers and shows, as well as bingo and puzzles. Pets are welcome at the agreement of other residents. The home has both a covered and an uncovered patio area.

Registered places: 26
Guide weekly rate: £430–£516
Specialist care: None
Medical services: Podiatry, dentist, optician
Qualified staff: Meets standard

Home details

Location: Residential area, 1.5 miles from Canterbury
Communal areas: Lounge, dining room, patio and garden
Accessibility: *Floors:* 2 • *Access:* Lift • *Wheelchair access:* Good
Smoking: In designated area
Pets: ✗
Routines: Flexible

Room details

Single: 20
Shared: 3
En suite: 23
Facilities: TV point, telephone point

Door lock: ✓
Lockable place: ✓

Services provided

Beauty services: Hairdressing
Mobile library: ✓
Religious services: Monthly visiting ministers
Transport: ✗
Activities: *Coordinator:* ✓ • *Examples:* Garden parties, visiting choirs, quizzes • *Outings:* ✓
Meetings: ✓

Oldroyd House

Manager: Alison Haley
Owner: RBS Care Homes Foundation
Contact: 55 London Road, Canterbury, Kent CT2 8HQ
) 01227 454315
@ oldroydhouse@
    rbscarehomesfoundation.co.uk

Oldroyd home only accepts ex-employees of the Westminster Bank or Royal Bank of Scotland. The home is situated in a residential area of Canterbury, close to local amenities and one and a half miles from the town centre. The home has a planned activity programme each month, including garden parties, rides in the countryside and celebrations. The home also arranges for ministers to visit the residents once a month.

Orchard Cottage

Manager: Richy Khaira
Owner: Tersaim Khaira
Contact: 78 Old Road East,
Gravesend, Kent DA12 1PE

☎ 01474 321127
@ info@orchardcarehome.co.uk
🖰 www.orchardcarehome.co.uk

Orchard Cottage is a detached house set in attractive gardens. It is a small home situated in a residential area one and a half miles from Gravesend. The home focuses on creating a comfortable atmosphere for residents to enjoy, while also arranging activities to keep them active and entertained. There are monthly visits from the Anglican minister and residents are welcome to attend local services.

Registered places: 10
Guide weekly rate: £385–£600
Specialist care: Respite
Medical services: Podiatry, dentist, optician
Qualified staff: Exceeds standard: 90% at NVQ Level 2

Home details
Location: Residential area, 1.5 miles from Gravesend
Communal areas: Lounge, dining room, conservatory, garden
Accessibility: *Floors:* 2 • *Access:* Stair lift
　　Wheelchair access: Limited
Smoking: In designated area
Pets: ✗
Routines: Flexible

Room details
Single: 6	**Door lock:** ✓
Shared: 2	**Lockable place:** ✓
En suite: 1	

Facilities: TV point, telephone point

Services provided
Beauty services: Hairdressing
Mobile library: ✓
Religious services: Monthly Anglican minister visits
Transport: ✗
Activities: *Coordinator:* ✗ • *Examples:* Bingo, bowles,
　　exercises • *Outings:* ✓
Meetings: ✗

Park Avenue Care Centre

Manager: Arlette Beebeejaun
Owner: Park Avenue Healthcare Ltd
Contact: 69 Park Avenue,
Bromley, Kent BR1 4HJ

☎ 020 8466 5027

Situated in a residential area of Bromley, one mile from the town centre, Park Avenue Care Centre cares for older individuals. The home has regular visits from visiting entertainers, singing or playing musical instruments as well as daily exercises such as movement to music. There is a church service arranged once a month and the home has its own hairdressing salon.

Registered places: 51
Guide weekly rate: £575–£670
Specialist care: Nursing, dementia
Medical services: Podiatry, dentist, optician
Qualified staff: Meets standard

Home details
Location: Residential area, 1 mile from Bromley
Communal areas: 2 lounges, dining room, garden
Accessibility: *Floors:* 4 • *Access:* Lift • *Wheelchair access:* Good
Smoking: In designated area
Pets: At manager's discretion
Routines: Flexible

Room details
Single: 51	**Door lock:** ✗
Shared: 0	**Lockable place:** ✓
En suite: 51	

Facilities: TV point

Services provided
Beauty services: Hairdressing salon
Mobile library: ✓
Religious services: Monthly church service
Transport: ✗
Activities: *Coordinator:* ✓ • *Examples:* Exercise to music, visiting
　　entertainers • *Outings:* ✓
Meetings: ✓

Registered places: 88
Guide weekly rate: £433–£850
Specialist care: Nursing, dementia, respite
Medical services: Podiatry, dentist, optician
Qualified staff: Undisclosed

Home details

Location: Residential area, 2.5 miles from Ashford
Communal areas: 2 lounges, 2 lounge/dining rooms,
    patio and garden
Accessibility: *Floors:* 2 • *Access:* Lift • *Wheelchair access:* Good
Smoking: In designated area
Pets: ✗
Routines: Flexible

Room details

Single: 88
Shared: 0
En suite: 88
Facilities: TV, telephone point

Door lock: ✓
Lockable place: ✗

Services provided

Beauty services: Hairdressing
Mobile library: ✗
Religious services: Weekly church service
Transport: ✗
Activities: *Coordinator:* ✓ • *Examples:* Baking, knitting, visiting
    entertainers • *Outings:* ✓
Meetings: ✗

Park View Care Centre

Manager: Sarah Erasmus
Owner: Ranc Care Homes Ltd
Contact: Field View, Park Farm, Ashford,
Kent TN23 3NZ
☎ 01233 501748
@ Parkview-1@btconnect.com

Park View Care Centre is a purpose-built two-storey home located on the outskirts of Ashford. It is set in its own grounds, surrounded by gardens with seating areas, bird feeders and raised flowerbeds. There are two fenced-off garden areas for those with dementia to wander freely in. The home arranges daily activities such as baking and there are visiting entertainers who come to the home on a weekly basis. There is also a church service once a week. Fund-raising events are also organised regularly.

Registered places: 22
Guide weekly rate: £320–£500
Specialist care: Respite
Medical services: Podiatry, dentist, optician, physiotherapy
Qualified staff: Meets standard

Home details

Location: Residential area, 0.5 miles from Folkestone
Communal areas: 3 lounges, 2 dining rooms, conservatory, garden
Accessibility: *Floors:* 2 • *Access:* None • *Wheelchair access:* Limited
Smoking: ✗
Pets: ✗
Routines: Structured

Room details

Single: 22
Shared: 0
En suite: 2
Facilities: TV, telephone point

Door lock: ✓
Lockable place: ✓

Services provided

Beauty services: Hairdressing
Mobile library: ✗
Religious services: Monthly church service,
    weekly Communion service
Transport: ✗
Activities: *Coordinator:* ✓ • *Examples:* Bingo, cards, skittles
    Outings: ✗
Meetings: ✓

Pelham House Residential Home

Manager: George Thomas
Owner: Margaret and George Thomas
Contact: 5–6 Pelham Gardens,
Folkestone, Kent CT20 2LF
☎ 01303 252145

Pelham House is a residential home located approximately half a mile from Folkestone town centre. The home has a number of small lounges, enabling residents to sit peacefully if they wish. As the home is set in a conservation area, there is no lift or stair lift; therefore those with rooms on the second floor must be mobile. There is a well-maintained garden with two garden houses in providing pleasant seating areas. While the home does not allow pets, there is a resident cat.

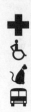

Pembroke House

Manager: Carole Davis
Owner: The Royal Naval Benevolent Trust
Contact: 11 Oxford Road, Gillingham, Kent ME7 4BS

☎ 01634 852431

Pembroke House provides residential and nursing care for former sailors, Royal Marines, their wives and widows. The home was originally built in the 1920s and extended and modernised in 2000. The home is spread across three floors each with its own dining room and day room. Wheelchair access is very good at the home as even the garden was purpose-built for wheelchairs. The home has its own minibus and takes residents on regular outings.

Registered places: 50
Guide weekly rate:
Specialist care: Nursing, day care, respite
Medical services: Podiatry, hygienist, optician, physiotherapy
Qualified staff: Meets standard

Home details

Location: Residential area, 1 mile from Gillingham
Communal areas: 3 lounges, 3 dining rooms, library, 2 conservatories, garden
Accessibility: *Floors:* 3 • *Access:* 2 lifts *Wheelchair access:* Good
Smoking: In designated area
Pets: At manager's discretion
Routines: Flexible

Room details

Single: 47
Shared: 2
En suite: 49
Facilities: TV point, telephone point

Door lock: ✓
Lockable place: ✓

Services provided

Beauty services: Hairdressing
Mobile library: ✗
Religious services: ✗
Transport: Minibus and car
Activities: *Coordinator:* ✓ • *Examples:* Arts and crafts, bingo, exercise • *Outings:* ✓
Meetings: ✓

Philbeach Nursing Home

Manager: Lorna Smith
Owner: Philbeach Care Centre Ltd
Contact: Tanners Hill, Hythe, Kent CT21 5UE

☎ 01303 262421
🖥 www.highmeadow.co.uk

Philbeach Nursing Home is situated in on the outskirts of Hythe, approximately half a mile from the town centre. The home is set in well-kept grounds which consist of nine acres. There is also a patio which is south facing, so often the residents sit out to enjoy the sun. Those who enjoy gardening as a hobby are encouraged to have some input into the gardening and help the gardener with his daily activities. The home also has a large lounge which is the good place for entertaining visitors or reading.

Registered places: 61
Guide weekly rate: £425–£625
Specialist care: Nursing, respite
Medical services: Podiatry, dentist, optician
Qualified staff: Exceeds standard: 70% at NVQ Level 2

Home details

Location: Residential area, 0.5 miles from Hythe
Communal areas: 2 lounges, dining room, library, conservatory, patio and garden
Accessibility: *Floors:* 3 • *Access:* Lift • *Wheelchair access:* Good
Smoking: ✗
Pets: At manager's discretion
Routines: Flexible

Room details

Single: 61
Shared: 0
En suite: Undisclosed
Facilities: TV, telephone point

Door lock: Undisclosed
Lockable place: ✓

Services provided

Beauty services: Hairdressing
Mobile library: ✓
Religious services: Monthly church services
Transport: ✗
Activities: *Coordinator:* ✓ • *Examples:* Exercise classes, magic shows, musical entertainment • *Outings:* ✗
Meetings: ✓

Registered places: 26
Guide weekly rate: £378–£450
Specialist care: Dementia, learning disability
Medical services: Undisclosed
Qualified staff: Meets standard

Home details

Location: Residential area, 1 mile from Canterbury
Communal areas: Garden
Accessibility: *Floors:* 2 • *Access:* None • *Wheelchair access:* None
Smoking: ✗
Pets: ✗
Routines: Flexible

Room details

Single: 18
Shared: 4
En suite: 0
Facilities: None

Door lock: ✗
Lockable place: ✗

Services provided

Beauty services: Hairdressing
Mobile library: ✗
Religious services: ✗
Transport: ✗
Activities: *Coordinator:* Undisclosed • *Examples:* Undisclosed
   Outings: Undisclosed
Meetings: ✗

Pilgrims Lodge Residential Home for the Elderly

Manager: Margery Martin
Owner: David Barzotelli
Contact: 10–12 Pilgrims Way,
Canterbury, Kent CT1 1XT
☏ 01227 760199

Situated in a residential area and comprising of two houses, Pilgrims Lodge cares for 26 residents. The home is located in a residential part of Canterbury, approximately one mile from the city centre. The home has no lift or stair lift so residents on the first floor are required to have a fair degree of mobility. The home has a garden for the residents to enjoy and offers a hairdressing service.

Registered places: 30
Guide weekly rate: Undisclosed
Specialist care: Nursing, palliative care, respite, terminal care
Medical services: Podiatry, physiotherapy
Qualified staff: Exceeds standard: 90% at NVQ Level 2

Home details

Location: Residential area, 2 miles from Sevenoaks centre
Communal areas: 2 lounges, dining room, library,
   hairdressing salon, garden
Accessibility: *Floors:* 1 • *Wheelchair access:* Good
Smoking: ✗
Pets: ✗
Routines: Flexible

Room details

Single: 30
Shared: 0
En suite: 0
Facilities: TV, telephone point

Door lock: ✓
Lockable place: ✓

Services provided

Beauty services: Hairdressing, manicures
Mobile library: ✓
Religious services: ✓
Transport: ✓
Activities: *Coordinator:* ✓ • *Examples:* Flower arranging,
   exercises, quizzes, speakers • *Outings:* ✓
Meetings: ✓

Pinehurst House Nursing Home

Manager: Helena Coetzee
Owner: BUPA Care Homes Ltd
Contact: Pinehurst, off Filmer Lane,
Sevenoaks, Kent TN14 5AQ
☏ 01732 762871
@ PinehurstHouseALL@BUPA.com
🖰 www.bupacarehomes.co.uk

Pinehurst House is a purpose-built home set in a quiet cul-de-sac near Sevenoaks, with easy access to the Kent countryside. The landscaped gardens and sensory courtyard provide seating areas, and are accessible for the disabled. All bedrooms have doors to the attractive landscaped gardens. Daily activities are offered, including flower arranging, exercises, quizzes and speakers. Pinehurst House offers care to a small number of physically disabled residents, residents who have had a stroke or require terminal care. It is also able to offer long-term and respite care to people with Parkinson's disease and Progressive Supranuclear Palsy.

The Poplars Nursing Home

Manager: Sandra Wilmshurst
Owner: Tamehaven Ltd
Contact: 158 Tonbridge Road,
Maidstone, Kent ME16 8SU
☎ 01622 752872
@ poplarnursinghome@btconnect.com

The Poplars Nursing Home is divided into two wings with a unit manager for each wing. The home is one mile from Maidstone town centre. The home regularly organises outings in and around the centre of town such as museum visits. There is a large garden at the home where there are regular barbecues in the summer months. In the winter, bingo and quiz night are more popular for a get together with other residents. Residents are welcome to bring their pets if they are capable of caring for them, and pets are always welcome to visit.

Registered places: 71
Guide weekly rate: £519–£780
Specialist care: Nursing, physical disability, respite, terminal care
Medical services: Podiatry, hygienist, optician, physiotherapy
Qualified staff: Meets standard

Home details
Location: Residential area, 1 mile from Maidstone
Communal areas: 4 lounges, dining room, garden
Accessibility: *Floors:* Undisclosed • *Access:* Lift
Wheelchair access: Good
Smoking: In designated area
Pets: At manager's discretion
Routines: Flexible

Room details
Single: 41
Shared: 15
En suite: 33
Facilities: TV point, telephone point
Door lock: ✗
Lockable place: ✓

Services provided
Beauty services: Hairdressing
Mobile library: ✓
Religious services: Monthly
Transport: ✗
Activities: *Coordinator:* ✓ • *Examples:* Bingo, pottery, quiz night
Outings: ✓
Meetings: ✓

Ramsgate Care Centre

Manager: Julie Cuthbert
Owner: Choicecare 2000 Ltd
Contact: 66–68 Boundary Road,
Ramsgate, Kent CT11 7NP
☎ 01843 585444
@ ramsgatecare@msn.com

Ramsgate Care Centre is a purpose-built, detached property located in a residential area of Ramsgate, half a mile from the town centre. There is easy access to public transport, shops and amenities. The home is spacious, offering wide corridors throughout the building for good wheelchair access. The home arranges a variety of activities, for example an arts and crafts teacher visits twice a week and a music man visits. The home has its own hairdressing salon and arranges monthly religious services.

Registered places: 41
Guide weekly rate: £303–£520
Specialist care: None
Medical services: Podiatry, dentist, hygienist, optician, physiotherapy
Qualified staff: Exceeds standard: 100% at NVQ Level 2

Home details
Location: Urban area, 0.5 miles from Ramsgate
Communal areas: 3 lounges, dining room, quiet area, garden
Accessibility: *Floors:* 2 • *Access:* Lift • *Wheelchair access:* Good
Smoking: ✗
Pets: ✗
Routines: Flexible

Room details
Single: 41
Shared: 0
En suite: 41
Facilities: TV point, telephone point
Door lock: ✓
Lockable place: ✓

Services provided
Beauty services: Hairdressing salon, aromatherapy, manicures, massages
Mobile library: ✗
Religious services: Monthly
Transport: ✗
Activities: *Coordinator:* ✗ • *Examples:* Arts and crafts, music, exercise • *Outings:* ✓
Meetings: ✓

Registered places: 31
Guide weekly rate: £600–£665
Specialist care: Nursing, dementia
Medical services: Podiatry, dentist, optician, physiotherapy
Qualified staff: Fails standard

Home details
Location: Residential area, 1.5 miles from Canterbury
Communal areas: Lounge, quiet lounge, dining room, patio and garden
Accessibility: *Floors:* 2 • *Access:* Lift • *Wheelchair access:* Good
Smoking: In designated area
Pets: ✗
Routines: Flexible

Room details
Single: 21
Shared: 5
En suite: 26
Facilities: TV, telephone point

Door lock: ✓
Lockable place: ✓

Services provided
Beauty services: Hairdressing
Mobile library: Library facilities
Religious services: ✓
Transport: ✗
Activities: *Coordinator:* ✓ • *Examples:* Crafts, flower arranging, visiting entertainers • *Outings:* ✓
Meetings: ✗

The Red House Nursing Home

Manager: Susanne Williams
Owner: The Red House Nursing Home Ltd
Contact: London Road, Canterbury, Kent CT2 8NB
☏ 01227 464171

The Red House Nursing Home is a large detached property which used to be a Victorian vicarage. It is set in its own grounds with large attractive gardens and a patio area. It is situated one and a half miles from Canterbury. The home has its own activities coordinator who organises activities such as reminiscing, as well as visiting entertainers, such as bell ringers. There are also outings to the seaside. Pets are allowed to visit the home. The home has its own library facilities, receiving large print books, which are changed every three months.

Registered places: 18
Guide weekly rate: £300–£376
Specialist care: Respite
Medical services: Podiatry, dentist, optician
Qualified staff: Exceeds standard: 80% at NVQ Level 2

Home details
Location: Residential area, 1 mile from Margate
Communal areas: 2 lounges, dining room, garden
Accessibility: *Floors:* 2 • *Access:* Lift • *Wheelchair access:* Good
Smoking: ✗
Pets: At manager's discretion
Routines: Flexible

Room details
Single: 14
Shared: 2
En suite: 5
Facilities: TV point, telephone point

Door lock: ✓
Lockable place: ✓

Services provided
Beauty services: Hairdressing, manicure, pedicure
Mobile library: ✗
Religious services: Regular Anglican and Catholic visits
Transport: ✗
Activities: *Coordinator:* ✓ • *Examples:* Bingo, board games *Outings:* ✓
Meetings: ✓

Redcot Lodge

Manager: Emma Sambrook
Owner: Redcot Care Ltd
Contact: 1 Lower Northdown Avenue, Cliftonville, Margate, Kent CT9 2NJ
☏ 01843 220131
@ redcotcare@btinternet.com

Redcot Lodge is a large, detached house with a garden at the rear of the building. Accommodation for residents is provided on two floors. The home accepts some animals including budgies and cockatoos (which they already have) but not cats or dogs. The home arranges regular visits from both Anglican and Catholic clergy. There are regular outings as well as daily activities such as bingo and board games.

Redlynch House Residential Home

Manager: Susan Hambelton
Owner: Redlynch Residential Home Ltd
Contact: 19 Hillcrest Road,
Hythe, Kent CT21 5EX
☎ 01303 264252

The home is situated on the outskirts of Hythe, approximately one mile from the town centre. The home is not suitable for wheelchair users as there are no lifts. The activities organised can include gentle exercises and cookery. The home also arranges visiting entertainers to come to the home. The home will offer religious services on request.

Registered places: 13
Guide weekly rate: £295–£450
Specialist care: Respite
Medical services: Podiatry, dentist, optician
Qualified staff: Meets standard

Home details
Location: Residential area, 1 mile from Hythe
Communal areas: Lounge, dining room, garden
Accessibility: *Floors:* 2 • *Access:* None • *Wheelchair access:* None
Smoking: ✗
Pets: At manager's discretion
Routines: Flexible

Room details
Single: 13	**Door lock:** ✓
Shared: 0	**Lockable place:** ✓
En suite: 5	

Facilities: TV point, Telephone point

Services provided
Beauty services: Hairdressing
Mobile library: ✗
Religious services: ✓
Transport: ✗
Activities: *Coordinator:* ✓ • *Examples:* Arts and crafts, cookery, entertainers • *Outings:* ✗
Meetings: ✗

Resthaven Residential Retirement Home

Manager: Adrian Clarke
Owner: Fairlawn Investments Ltd
Contact: 123 Grand Drive, Herne Bay,
Kent CT6 8HS
☎ 01227 369607
@ pidoux@aol.com

Resthaven Residential Retirement Home is a three-storey detached building which has been adapted for its present use. The property is located within a quiet residential area, approximately eight miles from Canterbury. The rooms on the top floor have a panoramic view over Herne Bay. Residents are provided with a varied, nutritious meal to suit their preferences, with flexibility as to where they can dine. The home arranges regular outings and daily activities which include bingo and exercise sessions.

Registered places: 16
Guide weekly rate: £318–£360
Specialist care: Respite
Medical services: Podiatry, optician
Qualified staff: Exceeds standard: 100% at NVQ Level 2

Home details
Location: Residential area, 8 miles from Canterbury
Communal areas: Lounge, dining room, garden
Accessibility: *Floors:* 3 • *Access:* Lift • *Wheelchair access:* Good
Smoking: In designated area
Pets: ✓
Routines: Flexible

Room details
Single: 16	**Door lock:** ✓
Shared: 0	**Lockable place:** ✓
En suite: 9	

Facilities: TV point, telephone point

Services provided
Beauty services: Hairdressing, aromatherapy, manicures
Mobile library: ✗
Religious services: Anglican
Transport: ✗
Activities: *Coordinator:* ✓ • *Examples:* Bingo, bowls, exercises *Outings:* ✓
Meetings: ✓

Registered places: 17
Guide weekly rate: £310–£350
Specialist care: Day care, respite
Medical services: Podiatry, dentist, optician, physiotherapy
Qualified staff: Meets standard

Home details

Location: Village location, 7 miles from Canterbury
Communal areas: 3 lounges, dining room, conservatory,
    patio and garden
Accessibility: *Floors:* 2 • *Access:* Stair lift • *Wheelchair access:* Good
Smoking: In designated area
Pets: At manager's discretion
Routines: Flexible

Room details

Single: 13
Shared: 2
En suite: 0
Facilities: TV point, telephone point

Door lock: ✓
Lockable place: ✓

Services provided

Beauty services: Hairdressing, aromatherapy
Mobile library: ✗
Religious services: Monthly Catholic and Methodist visits
Transport: Minibus
Activities: *Coordinator:* ✗ • *Examples:* Arts and craft, bingo,
    cooking • *Outings:* ✓
Meetings: ✓

Roberta House

Manager: Mrs Tarry
Owner: Mr and Mrs Tarry
Contact: 99–103 Island Road,
Upstreet, Canterbury, Kent CT3 4DE
☏ 01227 860704

Roberta House is situated in the village of Upstreet, approximately seven miles from Canterbury. The premises consist of three terrace houses that have been converted into one dwelling. The home organises outings and recent trips have included the circus. The home has its own minibus for this purpose. There are visits from Catholic and Methodist clergy once a month. The home has a garden with a patio area for residents to enjoy.

Registered places: 21
Guide weekly rate: £320–£400
Specialist care: Day care
Medical services: Podiatry, dentist, optician, physiotherapy
Qualified staff: Exceeds standard: 82% at NVQ Level 2

Home details

Location: Residential area, 1.5 miles from Margate
Communal areas: 2 lounges, dining room, conservatory, garden
Accessibility: *Floors:* 2 • *Access:* Lift • *Wheelchair access:* Good
Smoking: In designated area
Pets: At manager's discretion
Routines: Flexible

Room details

Single: 21
Shared: 0
En suite: 2
Facilities: TV point, telephone point

Door lock: ✓
Lockable place: ✓

Services provided

Beauty services: Hairdressing
Mobile library: ✗
Religious services: Weekly Catholic service
Transport: ✗
Activities: *Coordinator:* ✓ • *Examples:* Art club, bingo, exercise
    Outings: ✓
Meetings: ✓

Rosedene Residential Home

Manager: Vivienne Conway
Owner: Richard Raj
Contact: 29–31 Westonville Avenue,
Westbrook, Margate, Kent CT9 5DY
☏ 01843 220087
@ richardraj@
    rosedenerch.freeserve.co.uk

Rosedene Residential Home is situated in a residential area, one and a half miles from Margate. The home caters for all hobbies with card and games mornings and an art club. There are regular outings as well as exercise classes to help keep residents active. In the home there is a resident cat and other pets would be allowed at the manager's discretion. There are three lounges including a conservatory to enjoy in fine weather.

Roselawn Residential Home

Manager: Christopher Zacharia

Owner: Mr and Mrs Zacharia

Contact: 2 Eaton Road, Margate, Kent CT9 1XE

☎ 01843 223240

@ c.zacharia@btconnect.com

Roselawn is situated a short distance from the seafront and half a mile from the town of Margate. The home has its own library facilities and the books are replaced every three months. There is also a hairdressing service as well as regular religious services. The home arranges activities such as music and bingo and in the summer months arranges a picnic for the residents. There is no resident tenants association but the manager does hand out questionnaires to the residents.

Registered places: 13
Guide weekly rate: Undisclosed
Specialist care: Respite
Medical services: Podiatry, dentist, optician, physiotherapy
Qualified staff: Meets standard

Home details

Location: Residential area, 0.5 miles from Margate
Communal areas: 2 lounges, dining room, patio, conservatory
Accessibility: *Floors:* 3 • *Access:* Lift • *Wheelchair access:* Limited
Smoking: ✗
Pets: At manager's discretion
Routines: Flexible

Room details

Single: 9
Shared: 2
En suite: 11
Facilities: TV point, telephone point

Door lock: ✓
Lockable place: ✓

Services provided

Beauty services: Hairdressing, aromatherapy, manicures
Mobile library: Library facilities
Religious services: ✓
Transport: People carrier
Activities: *Coordinator:* ✗ • *Examples:* Bingo, games, music
 Outings: ✓
Meetings: ✗

Roxburgh House

Manager: Vacant

Owner: Discovery Care Ltd

Contact: 29 Roxburgh Road, Westgate-on-Sea, Kent CT8 8RX

☎ 01843 832022

Roxburgh House is a large property that is located in a residential area, within walking distance of the seafront. The home has a garden with patio area to the rear, where residents can enjoy the good weather in the seating area. There is a mobile library which visits the home and every six to eight weeks there is an Anglican service. The home also arranges regular outings for the residents.

Registered places: 22
Guide weekly rate: £300–£500
Specialist care: Physical disability, respite
Medical services: Podiatry, optician
Qualified staff: Exceeds standard: 70% at NVQ Level 2

Home details

Location: Residential area, 0.5 miles from Westgate-on-Sea
Communal areas: Lounge, dining room, conservatory, patio and garden
Accessibility: *Floors:* 3 • *Access:* Lift • *Wheelchair access:* Good
Smoking: ✗
Pets: At manager's discretion
Routines: Flexible

Room details

Single: 14
Shared: 4
En suite: 17
Facilities: TV point, telephone point

Door lock: ✓
Lockable place: ✓

Services provided

Beauty services: Hairdressing
Mobile library: ✓
Religious services: Anglican service every 6–8 weeks
Transport: ✗
Activities: *Coordinator:* ✗ • *Examples:* Arts and craft, bingo, games
 Outings: ✓
Meetings: ✓

Registered places: 23
Guide weekly rate: £390.22–£550
Specialist care: Day care, respite
Medical services: Podiatry, dentist, optician, physiotherapy
Qualified staff: Exceeds standard: 80% at NVQ Level 2

Home details
Location: Village location, 3.5 miles from Canterbury
Communal areas: Lounge, dining room, patio and garden
Accessibility: *Floors:* 2 • *Access:* Lift • *Wheelchair access:* Good
Smoking: ✗
Pets: At manager's discretion
Routines: Flexible

Room details
Single: 23
Shared: 0
En suite: 12
Facilities: TV point, telephone point

Door lock: ✓
Lockable place: ✓

Services provided
Beauty services: Hairdressing
Mobile library: ✓
Religious services: Monthly Communion service
Transport: People carrier
Activities: *Coordinator:* ✓ • *Examples:* Arts and crafts, bingo,
    quizzes • *Outings:* ✓
Meetings: ✓

Saxon Lodge

Manager: Wendy Richards
Owner: Saxon Lodge Residential Home Ltd
Contact: 30 Western Avenue, Bridge,
Canterbury, Kent CT4 5LT
☏ 01227 831737

Saxon Lodge is situated in the village of Bridge, approximately three and a half miles from Canterbury. The home takes residents on many outings including bus tours of places of interest and afternoon teas. In the home there is a resident cat and an abundance of activities for residents to partake in. These include bingo and arts and crafts sessions. There is also a residents meeting every quarter.

Registered places: 50
Guide weekly rate: £303–£397
Specialist care: Residential
Medical services: Podiatry, hygienist, optician, physiotherapy
Qualified staff: Exceeds standard: 65% at NVQ Level 2

Home details
Location: Residential area, 2 miles from Ashford
Communal areas: 2 dining rooms, conservatory, garden
Accessibility: *Floors:* 2 • *Access:* Lift • *Wheelchair access:* Good
Smoking: In designated area
Pets: ✗
Routines: flexible

Room details
Single: 40
Shared: 5
En suite: 10
Facilities: TV point

Door lock: ✗
Lockable place: ✓

Services provided
Beauty services: Hairdressing
Mobile library: ✓
Religious services: Weekly Catholic and Anglican visits
Transport: ✗
Activities: *Coordinator:* ✗ • *Examples:* Arts and crafts, keep fit
    Outings: ✓
Meetings: ✓

Sevington Mill Residential Home

Manager: Anne Hooper
Owner: Kent County Ltd
Contact: Sevington Lane, Willesborough,
Ashford, Kent TN24 0LB
☏ 01233 639800

Sevingdon Mill is situated on the outskirts of Ashford, around two miles from the town centre. Residents have access to a garden, and outings are often arranged. Activities such as bingo, jigsaw puzzles and carpet bowls occur on a nightly basis to keep residents stimulated. There are also weekly visits from Anglican and Catholic clergy. The residents have regular meetings to discuss any issues they may have.

Shakti Lodge

Manager: Chan Teeluck
Owner: Shakti Lodge Ltd
Contact: 208–212 Princes Road, Dartford, Kent DA1 3HR
☎ 01322 288070

Shakti Lodge is located one and a half miles from the town of Dartford and there are good travel links provided by a bus service. The home has two lounges, a dining room and a conservatory. There is a garden to the rear of the property. An activities coordinator comes in five days a week to run games such as monopoly, cards and hangman and reminiscence sessions. Trips are also organised to musicals and the theatre. The home also offers services such as a mobile library and religious services.

Registered places: 26
Guide weekly rate: From £410
Specialist care: Dementia
Medical services: Podiatry, dentist, optician, physiotherapy
Qualified staff: Exceeds standard: 75% at NVQ Level 2

Home details
Location: Residential area, 1.5 miles from Dartford
Communal areas: 2 lounges, dining room, conservatory, patio and garden
Accessibility: *Floors:* 2 • *Access:* Lift • *Wheelchair access:* Good
Smoking: In designated area
Pets: ✓
Routines: Flexible

Room details
Single: 14
Shared: 6
En suite: 1
Facilities: TV, telephone

Door lock: ✓
Lockable place: ✓

Services provided
Beauty services: Hairdressing
Mobile library: ✓
Religious services: ✓
Transport: ✗
Activities: *Coordinator:* ✓ • *Examples:* Arts and crafts, games, reminiscence sessions • *Outings:* ✓
Meetings: ✓

Sheila Stead House

Manager: Philomena Winterboer
Owner: Shaw Healthcare Ltd
Contact: Bushell Way, Chislehurst, Kent BR7 6SF
☎ 020 8468 7021

Sheila Stead House is a large, purpose-built residential home located one mile from Chislehurst. The home has a safe enclosed garden with a patio area, and attractive well-maintained garden with seating to the front. There is also a garden area to the back of the property, especially created for the residents. The home has its own activities coordinator who arranges activities suited to the individual needs of the residents.

Registered places: 48
Guide weekly rate: Undisclosed
Specialist care: Dementia
Medical services: Undisclosed
Qualified staff: Meets standard

Home details
Location: Residential area, 1 mile from Chislehurst
Communal areas: Lounges, patio and garden
Accessibility: *Floors:* 2 • *Access:* Lift • *Wheelchair access:* Good
Smoking: ✗
Pets: ✗
Routines: Structured

Room details
Single: 48
Shared: 0
En suite: Undisclosed
Facilities: None

Door lock: ✗
Lockable place: ✗

Services provided
Beauty services: Undisclosed
Mobile library: ✗
Religious services: ✗
Transport: ✗
Activities: *Coordinator:* ✓ • *Examples:* Bingo, games • *Outings:* ✗
Meetings: Undisclosed

Registered places: 27
Guide weekly rate: £350–£400
Specialist care: Day care, respite
Medical services: Podiatry, optician, physiotherapy
Qualified staff: Exceeds standard: 83% at NVQ Level 2

Home details

Location: Village location, 1.5 miles from Deal
Communal areas: Lounge, dining room, conservatory, garden
Accessibility: *Floors:* 2 • *Access:* Lift and stair lift
    Wheelchair access: Good
Smoking: In designated area
Pets: At manager's discretion
Routines: Flexible

Room details

Single: 18
Shared: 4
En suite: 15
Facilities: TV point, telephone point

Door lock: ✓
Lockable place: ✓

Services provided

Beauty services: Hairdressing, reflexology, head massage
Mobile library: ✗
Religious services: Monthly Communion service
Transport: ✗
Activities: *Coordinator:* ✗ • *Examples:* Bingo, crafts, gardening
    Outings: ✗
Meetings: ✓

Sholden Hall

Manager: Clare Stephens
Owner: Dean Williams and
Maria Eagland
Contact: London Road,
Sholden, Deal, Kent CT14 0AB
☎ 01304 375445
🖰 www.sholdenhall.co.uk

Sholden Hall is a listed building that has been extended and adapted for use as a care home. Situated in the village of Sholden, the home is one and a half miles from the town of Deal. The home is surrounded by its own grounds where residents enjoy the gardens and conservatory. Residents benefit from the flexible approach to daily routines and are free to carry out their own activities. Children from the nearby Sholden Primary School occasionally visit to re-enact performances they have done at school.

Registered places: 38
Guide weekly rate:
Specialist care: Nursing, respite
Medical services: Podiatry, optician, physiotherapy
Qualified staff: Exceeds standard: 60% at NVQ Level 2

Home details

Location: Residential area, 1 mile from Margate
Communal areas: 2 lounges, dining room, garden
Accessibility: *Floors:* 3 • *Access:* Lift • *Wheelchair access:* Good
Smoking: ✗
Pets: ✗
Routines: Flexible

Room details

Single: 30
Shared: 4
En suite: 25
Facilities: TV point

Door lock: ✗
Lockable place: ✓

Services provided

Beauty services: Hairdressing
Mobile library: ✓
Religious services: Monthly
Transport: ✓
Activities: *Coordinator:* ✓ • *Examples:* Singalong, games, puzzles
    Outings: ✗
Meetings: ✓

Shottendane Nursing Home

Manager: Tracey Fullagar
Owner: Norman Temple, Laurence Waitt
and Nigel Cripps
Contact: Shottendane Road, Margate,
Kent CT9 4BS
☎ 01843 291888

A converted property, Shottendane Nursing Home is situated in secluded grounds, one mile from Margate. In and around the grounds there are seating areas for residents to enjoy the garden if they wish. Activities are planned for the residents on a daily basis and include singalongs, puzzles and carpet bowls. The local library also loans books to the home on a three monthly basis so residents can order books that they wish to read. The home offers a small, quiet room on the first floor which can be used as overnight accommodation for relatives if needed.

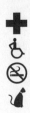

The Sidcup Nursing and Residential Centre

Manager: Jane Brock
Owner: BUPA Care Home Ltd
Contact: 2–8 Hatherley Road,
Sidcup, Kent DA14 4BG
☎ 020 8300 7711
🖰 www.bupacarehomes.co.uk

The Sidcup Nursing and Residential Centre is situated in a residential area of a small town in Kent near to the town centre and local shops. The home has its own hairdressing salon and library facilities. The home has weekly religious visits and a flexible daily routine for its residents. There are two activities coordinators who organise a range of activities such as bingo, chair exercises, quizzes and outings. There are residents meetings every quarter and pets are allowed at the manager's discretion.

Registered places: 100
Guide weekly rate: £695–£895
Specialist care: Nursing, emergency admissions, physical disability, respite
Medical services: Podiatry, dentist, optician, physiotherapy
Qualified staff: Meets standard

Home details
Location: Residential area, 0.5 miles from Sidcup
Communal areas: 8 lounges, 3 dining rooms, quiet room, hairdressing salon, library, garden
Accessibility: *Floors:* 3 • *Access:* Lift • *Wheelchair access:* Good
Smoking: ✗
Pets: At manager's discretion
Routines: Flexible

Room details
Single: 100
Shared: 0
En suite: 100
Facilities: TV point, telephone point
Door lock: ✓
Lockable place: ✓

Services provided
Beauty services: Hairdressing
Mobile library: Library facilities
Religious services: Weekly church visits
Transport: ✗
Activities: *Coordinators:* ✓ • *Examples:* Bingo, chair exercise, flower arranging • *Outings:* ✓
Meetings: ✓

Singleton Nursing and Residential Home

Manager: Elizabeth Obousy
Owner: Singleton Nursing and Residential Home Ltd
Contact: Hoxton Close, Singleton, Ashford, Kent TN23 5LB
☎ 01233 666768
@ Singleton.nursinghome@ totalserve.co.uk

Singleton Nursing and Residential Home is situated four miles from Ashford town centre, close to a GP and primary school. It is also near a shopping centre, which is convenient for small shopping trips. The home's close proximity to the school means that residents not only watch the activities but are also involved in them. The home is also near to Singleton Park which features a lake with wildlife. Often residents go on walks round the park. There are also regular activities organised in the home such as singalongs and games, and there is also visiting entertainment including singers and magicians.

Registered places: 36
Guide weekly rate: Undisclosed
Specialist care: Nursing
Medical services: None
Qualified staff: Meets standard

Home details
Location: Residential area, 4 miles from Ashford
Communal areas: 3 lounges, 2 dining rooms, patio
Accessibility: *Floors:* 2 • *Access:* Lift • *Wheelchair access:* Good
Smoking: ✗
Pets: ✓
Routines: Flexible

Room details
Single: 30
Shared: 3
En suite: 30
Facilities: TV point, telephone point
Door lock: ✗
Lockable place: ✓

Services provided
Beauty services: Hairdressing
Mobile library: ✓
Religious services: ✓
Transport: ✗
Activities: *Coordinator:* ✓ • *Examples:* Games, magician, singalongs • *Outings:* ✓
Meetings: ✓

Registered places: 13
Guide weekly rate: £410–£465
Specialist care: Dementia
Medical services: Podiatry, optician
Qualified staff: Meets standard

Home details
Location: Village location, 0.5 miles from Sandhurst
Communal areas: Lounge, dining room, garden
Accessibility: *Floors:* 3 • *Access:* Stair lift • *Wheelchair access:* Good
Smoking: In designated area
Pets: ✗
Routines: Flexible

Room details
Single: 7
Shared: 3
En suite: 1
Facilities: TV point, telephone point

Door lock: ✗
Lockable place: ✓

Services provided
Beauty services: Hairdressing
Mobile library: ✓
Religious service: Fortnightly
Transport: ✓
Activities: *Coordinator:* ✓ • *Examples:* Bingo, ball games,
    reminiscence • *Outings:* ✗
Meetings: ✓

Slate House

Manager: Liza Khan
Owner: Ahmad and Anne-Marie Beeharry and Nasar and Liza Khan
Contact: 26 Wellington Road, Sandhurst, Kent GU47 9AN
☏ 01344 773358
@ Nasar_g_khan@hotmail.com

Slate House is a privately run care home close to the centre of Sandhurst. A specialist activities coordinator comes in on Saturdays to give one-to-one time to all residents. The coordinator also organises group activity such as ball games, bingo and reminiscence. There is also a garden at the rear of the property which is enjoyed in summer months, and pets are welcome. There is a residents meeting once a fortnight.

Registered places: 29
Guide weekly rate: £800–£850
Specialist care: Nursing, respite
Medical services: Podiatry, hygienist, optician, physiotherapy
Qualified staff: Exceeds standard: at NVQ Level 2

Home details
Location: Residential area, 1 mile from Beckenham
Communal areas: Lounge, dining room, conservatory, garden
Accessibility: *Floors:* Undisclosed • *Access:* Undisclosed
    Wheelchair access: Undisclosed
Smoking: ✗
Pets: At manager's discretion
Routines: Flexible

Room details
Single: 26
Shared: 4
En suite: 30
Facilities: TV point, telephone point

Door lock: ✓
Lockable place: ✓

Services provided
Beauty services: Hairdressing
Mobile library: ✓
religious services: Fortnightly
Transport: ✗
Activities: *Coordinator:* ✓ • *Examples:* Arts and crafts, bingo,
    entertainers • *Outings:* ✓
Meetings: ✓

Sloane House Nursing Home

Manager: Traute Gladstone
Owner: The Mills Family Ltd
Contact: 28 Southend Road, Beckenham, Kent BR3 5AA
☏ 020 8650 3410
@ sloanenursinghome@dsl.pipex.com

Sloane House Nursing Home is a large, detached building in a residential area of Beckenham. The home provides a team of qualified nurses, supported by care and ancillary staff. An activities coordinator also provides residents with arts and crafts sessions, bingo and visiting entertainers. The home also organises religious services for the residents and arranges for a mobile library to come to the home.

Sonya Lodge

Manager: Jean Wright
Owner: Nellsar Ltd
Contact: 10 High Road, Wilmington,
Nr Dartford, Kent DA2 7EG

) 01322 289768
@ Sonya.lodge@nellsar.com
⌨ www.nellsar.com

Sonya Lodge resides in a residential area four miles from the centre of Dartford. The home has a garden with a patio area for residents to relax in. The home employs an activities coordinator who arranges a wide range of activities and events for the residents. These include visiting entertainers, outings to coffee mornings and craft sessions. There are residents meetings held in the home on a quarterly basis and there is an Anglican service held once a month.

Registered places: 37
Guide weekly rate: £410–£575
Specialist care: Dementia, respite
Medical services: Podiatry
Qualified staff: Meets standard

Home details
Location: Residential area, 4 miles from Dartford
Communal areas: Lounge, patio and garden
Accessibility: *Floors:* 2 • *Access:* Lift • *Wheelchair access:* Good
Smoking: ✗
Pets: ✗
Routines: Flexible

Room details
Single: 37
Shared: 0
En suite: 27
Facilities: TV

Door lock: ✓
Lockable place: ✓

Services provided
Beauty services: Hairdressing
Mobile library: Library facilities
Religious services: Monthly Anglican service
Transport: ✗
Activities: *Coordinator:* ✓ • *Examples:* Coffee mornings, crafts, visiting entertainers • *Outings:* ✓
Meetings: ✓

Sovereign House

Manager: Louise Ibrahim
Owner: Hassan Ibrahim
Contact: 30 Canterbury Road,
Herne Bay, Kent CT6 5DJ

) 01227 368796

Sovereign House is a detached property, located eight and a half miles from Canterbury. It has a grassed front garden and is concreted at the rear. The home is close to local amenities in the town centre and to the beach. Pets and smoking are not permitted. The residents have a flexible daily routine and the home arranges a hairdressing service.

Registered places: 10
Guide weekly rate: Undisclosed
Specialist care: None
Medical services: Podiatry, dentist, optician, physiotherapy
Qualified staff: Undisclosed

Home details
Location: Residential area, 8.5 miles from Canterbury
Communal areas: Lounge, dining room, garden
Accessibility: *Floors:* 3 • *Access:* Lift • *Wheelchair access:* Good
Smoking: ✗
Pets: ✗
Routines: Flexible

Room details
Single: 10
Shared: 0
En suite: 8
Facilities: TV point

Door lock: ✗
Lockable place: ✓

Services provided
Beauty services: Hairdressing
Mobile library: ✗
Religious services: ✗
Transport: ✗
Activities: *Coordinator:* ✗ • *Examples:* Undisclosed • *Outings:* ✗
Meetings: ✗

Registered places: 25
Guide weekly rate: £312–£420
Specialist care: None
Medical services: Podiatry, dentist, optician, physiotherapy
Qualified staff: Exceeds standard: 90% at NVQ Level 2

Home details

Location: Residential area, 0.7 miles from Birchington
Communal areas: 2 lounges, 2 dining rooms, garden
Accessibility: *Floors:* 3 • *Access:* Stair lifts
    Wheelchair access: Limited
Smoking: In designated area
Pets: At manager's discretion
Routines: Flexible

Room details

Single: 19
Shared: 3
En suite: 8
Facilities: TV, telephone point

Door lock: ✓
Lockable place: ✓

Services provided

Beauty services: Hairdressing
Mobile library: ✗
Religious services: Fortnightly Communion service
Transport: ✗
Activities: *Coordinator:* ✗ • *Examples:* Singing, reminiscence,
    quizzes • *Outings:* ✓
Meetings: ✗

Spencer House

Manager: Simee Cooppen
Owner: Vinaigum Cooppen
Contact: Spencer Road,
Birchington, Kent CT7 9EZ
☎ 01843 841460

Spencer House is located in a residential area on the outskirts of Birchington. The home organises some outings but the residents are mostly taken out by their families to pubs, theatres and cinemas. Age Concern also comes to take a group of residents to visit garden centres and on other trips. The home has an assortment of activities including board games and card games, singing and quizzes. There is a resident cat and other animals are allowed so long as they are approved by the manager.

Registered places: 37
Guide weekly rate: £450–£500
Specialist care: Day care, dementia, learning disability, respite
Medical services: Podiatry, hygienist, optician, physiotherapy
Qualified staff: Exceeds standard: 80% at NVQ Level 2

Home details

Location: Residential area, 9 miles from Canterbury
Communal areas: 4 Lounges, 2 dining rooms, conservatory,
    patio and garden
Accessibility: *Floors:* 3 • *Access:* Stair lift
    Wheelchair access: Good
Smoking: ✗
Pets: ✗
Routines: Flexible

Room details

Single: 21
Shared: 8
En suite: 23
Facilities: TV point

Door lock: ✗
Lockable place: ✓

Services provided

Beauty services: Hairdressing, massages
Mobile library: ✗
Religious services: Monthly Anglican visits, fortnightly Catholic visits
Transport: ✗
Activities: *Coordinator:* ✗ • *Examples:* Art and pottery, puzzles,
    musical exercises • *Outings:* ✓
Meetings: ✗

St Brelades

Manager: Catherine Chuck
Owner: St Brelades Retirement
Homes Ltd
Contact: 5–6 Beacon Hill, Herne Bay,
Kent CT6 6AU
☎ 01227 375301

Located on the seafront and close to Hearn Bay town centre, St Brelades is a home providing care for women only. Residents enjoy the seasonal garden fête the home offers, and can participate in games, musical exercises and art sessions. The locality of the seafront makes coastal trips easily accessible for residents who are able enjoy the beautiful views. The home arranges for Anglican clergy to visit once a month and Catholic clergy to visit twice a month.

The St John Home

Manager: Joyce Mitchell
Owner: The Priory of England and the Islands of the Order of St John
Contact: 1 Gloucester Road, Whitstable, Kent CT5 2DS
☎ 01227 273043

The home is a Royal Charter Home and has charitable status. The St John Home is located in a residential area, one and a half miles from Whitstable. They offer a nondenominational service as well as an Anglican service. There is a trolley shop for residents' convenience. The home arranges outings for the residents and has its own library facilities.

Registered places: 18
Guide weekly rate: From £484
Specialist care: Nursing, respite
Medical services: Podiatry, hygienist, optician, physiotherapy
Qualified staff: Exceeds standard: 77% at NVQ Level 2

Home details
Location: Residential area, 1.5 miles from Whitstable
Communal areas: Lounge, dining room, library, patio and garden
Accessibility: *Floors:* 2 • *Access:* Stair lift • *Wheelchair access:* Good
Smoking: ✗
Pets: ✗
Routines: Flexible

Room details
Single: 16
Shared: 1
En suite: 0
Facilities: TV point, telephone point

Door lock: ✓
Lockable place: ✓

Services provided
Beauty services: Hairdressing
Mobile library: Library facilities
Religious services: Monthly Free Church and Anglican service
Transport: ✗
Activities: *Coordinator:* ✓ • *Examples:* Bingo, exercise, quizzes
　　　Outings: ✓
Meetings: ✓

St Margarets Nursing Home

Manager: Amanda Atkins
Owner: Charmdale Healthcare Ltd
Contact: 20 Twiss Avenue, Hythe, Kent CT21 5NU
☎ 01303 267557
@ asastmargarets@aol.com
🖰 www.stmargaretshythe.com

St Margarets Nursing Home is situated in Hythe alongside the Royal Military Canal, within easy walking distance of the seafront and town centre. The home has disabled access to the front door and there is a shop next door to the home. The home arranges for visiting entertainment to come to the home and the residents are taken on walks through the surrounding area. Residents enjoy a walk along the canal with a carer. Staff also encourage residents to speak with the activities coordinators and have direct input into the activities that are being planned for the month.

Registered places: 24
Guide weekly rate: £386–£739
Specialist care: Nursing
Medical services: Podiatry, dentist, optician, physiotherapy
Qualified staff: Exceeds standard: 75% at NVQ Level 2

Home details
Location: Residential area, 0.5 miles from Hythe
Communal areas: Lounge, dining room, garden
Accessibility: *Floors:* 2 • *Access:* Lift • *Wheelchair access:* Good
Smoking: ✗
Pets: At manager's discretion
Routines: Flexible

Room details
Single: 20
Shared: 2
En suite: 0
Facilities: TV point

Door lock: ✗
Lockable place: ✓

Services provided
Beauty services: Hairdressing
Mobile library: ✓
Religious services: Monthly Communion service
Transport: ✗
Activities: *Coordinator:* ✗ • *Examples:* Games, visiting entertainers
　　　Outings: ✓
Meetings: ✓

Registered places: 23
Guide weekly rate: £367–£580
Specialist care: Dementia, respite
Medical services: Podiatry, dentist, optician
Qualified staff: Meets standard

Home details

Location: Residential area, 0.5 miles from Whitstable
Communal areas: 2 lounges, 2 dining rooms, garden
Accessibility: *Floors:* 2 • *Access:* 2 stair lifts
    Wheelchair access: Good
Smoking: In designated area
Pets: At manager's discretion
Routines: Flexible

Room details

Single: 17 | Door lock: ✓
Shared: 3 | Lockable place: ✓
En suite: 11
Facilities: TV, telephone point

Services provided

Beauty services: Hairdressing
Mobile library: ✗
Religious services: ✓
Transport: ✗
Activities: *Coordinator:* ✗ • *Examples:* Visiting entertainers,
    wine and film night • *Outings:* ✓
Meetings: ✓

St Martins

Manager: Joanne Thomas
Owner: HU Investments Ltd
Contact: 3 Joy Lane, Whitstable,
Kent CT5 4LS
☏ 01227 261340
@ saintmartin@btconnect.com

St Martins is located in a residential area, approximately half a mile from Whitstable. There is a garden for residents to enjoy in the warmer weather and the home is within walking distance of the seafront. The home has ample communal space and there is a varied activities programme including visiting entertainers, bingo and bowling. There are also regular residents meetings.

Registered places: 30
Guide weekly rate: £303–£364
Specialist care: None
Medical services: None
Qualified staff: Exceeds standard: 55% at NVQ Level 2

Home details

Location: Residential area, 0.5 miles from Dover
Communal areas: 4 lounges, dining room, activities room, chapel,
    hairdressing salon, patio and garden
Accessibility: *Floors:* 4 • *Access:* Lift • *Wheelchair access:* Good
Smoking: ✓
Pets: ✗
Routines: Flexible

Room details

Single: 30 | Door lock: ✗
Shared: 0 | Lockable place: ✓
En suite: 30
Facilities: TV point, telephone point

Services provided

Beauty services: Hairdressing, aromatherapy
Mobile library: ✗
Religious services: ✗
Transport: ✗
Activities: *Coordinator:* ✓ • *Examples:* Armchair aerobics,
    cooking, embroidery • *Outings:* ✓
Meetings: ✓

St Mary's Home

Manager: M Smith
Owner: A Kupendrarajah
Contact: 8 Eastbrook Place, Dover,
Kent CT16 1RP
☏ 01304 204232
@ Maureensmith1204@aol.com

St Mary's is located in Dover, approximately 10 minutes' walk from the seafront and close to shops and the train station. Bedrooms are spread on four floors, and each floor has a lounge area and kitchenette. There is also a dedicated activities room. The home has a book club and musicians regularly visit. The home has a vast range of activities to keep the residents stimulated such as cookery, embroidery, poetry writing, exercise classes and outings. Outings are often down to the seafront or into the town centre to shop.

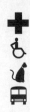

Staplehurst Manor Nursing Home

Manager: Louise Foster
Owner: BUPA Care Homes Ltd
Contact: Frittenden Road, Staplehurst, Tonbridge, Kent TN12 0DG

📞 0113 3816100
@ StaplehurstManorALL@BUPA.com
🖥 www.bupacarehomes.co.uk

Situated in the village of Staplehurst and surrounded by extensive wooded grounds, Staplehurst Manor is a fine example of a Georgian country house. A particular feature is the marble-pillared hallway, leading to the main staircase with its balustrades, stained-glass window and galleried landings. Beautifully furnished reception rooms include a drawing room with floor-to-ceiling Georgian windows overlooking the garden. Daily activities are offered, including painting, music appreciation, quizzes and gardening, while the home has its own library and quiet lounge. Leeds Castle and Sissinghurst gardens are nearby, and residents also enjoy the home's extensive grounds.

Registered places: 31
Guide weekly rate: Undisclosed
Specialist care: Nursing, palliative care, respite, terminal care
Medical services: Podiatry, physiotherapy
Qualified staff: Meets standard

Home details
Location: Village location, 9 miles from Maidstone
Communal areas: 2 lounges, 2 dining rooms, hairdressing salon, library, garden
Accessibility: *Floors:* 3 • *Access:* Lift and stair lift *Wheelchair access:* Good
Smoking: In designated area
Pets: At manager's discretion
Routines: Flexible

Room details
Single: 31
Shared: 0
En suite: 19
Facilities: TV, telephone point

Door lock: ✓
Lockable place: ✓

Services provided
Beauty services: Hairdressing, aromatherapy
Mobile library: ✓
Religious services: ✓
Transport: ✓
Activities: *Coordinator:* ✓ • *Examples:* Painting, music appreciation, visiting musicians • *Outings:* ✓
Meetings: ✓

Sundridge Court Nursing Home

Manager: Vacant
Owner: Harley Healthcare Nursing Homes Ltd
Contact: 19 Edward Road, Bromley, Kent BR1 3NG

📞 020 8466 6553
@ office@sundridgecourt.fslife.co.uk
🖥 www.sundridgecourt.fslife.co.uk

Sundridge Court is situated in a quiet residential area, one mile from the centre of Bromley. It is a purpose-built home providing nursing care for up to 30 people. Communal space includes a lounge, large conservatory and a dining room.

The home has a large back garden with patio seating and a gazebo to sit in. An activities coordinator devises a programme of activities, arranges occasional trips out from the home, and organises various entertainers to visit the home.

Registered places: 30
Guide weekly rate: £750–£1,100
Specialist care: Nursing, physical disability
Medical services: Podiatry
Qualified staff: Meets standard

Home details
Location: Residential area, 1 mile from Bromley
Communal areas: Lounge, dining room, conservatory, patio and garden
Accessibility: *Floors:* 3 • *Access:* Lift • *Wheelchair access:* Good
Smoking: ✗
Pets: ✗
Routines: Flexible

Room details
Single: 24
Shared: 3
En suite: 30
Facilities: None

Door lock: ✗
Lockable place: ✗

Services provided
Beauty services: Hairdressing
Mobile library: ✗
Religious services: ✗
Transport: ✗
Activities: *Coordinator:* ✓ • *Examples:* Arts and crafts, baking, musical afternoons • *Outings:* ✓
Meetings: Undisclosed

Registered places: 44
Guide weekly rate: £550–£660
Specialist care: Nursing, terminal care
Medical services: Dietician, occupational therapy, physiotherapy
Qualified staff: Exceeds standard: 70% at NVQ Level 2

Home details

Location: Village location, 3 miles from Dover
Communal areas: Lounge, dining room, sensory room,
conservatory, patio and garden
Accessibility: *Floors:* 3 • *Access:* Lift • *Wheelchair access:* Good
Smoking: ✗
Pets: ✗
Routines: Flexible

Room details

Single: 38
Shared: 3
En suite: 10
Facilities: TV, telephone

Door lock: ✓
Lockable place: ✓

Services provided

Beauty services: Hairdressing, aromatherapy, massage, reflexology
Mobile library: ✗
Religious services: Monthly Anglican services
Transport: ✗
Activities: *Coordinator:* ✓ • *Examples:* Arts and crafts, bingo,
exercises • *Outings:* ✗
Meetings: ✓

Temple Ewell Nursing Home

Manager: Yvonne Mhlanga-Kayoni
Owner: Charing Cross Investments Ltd
Contact: Wellington Road, Temple Ewell,
Dover, Kent CT16 3DB
☎ 01304 822206

Temple Ewell is a detached, purpose-built home situated in the village of Temple Ewell, three miles from Dover. The home is set on a slight hill which gives residents views over Alkham Valley and the neighbouring village. Facilities at the home include a conservatory and sensory room. The sensory garden is an enclosed section of the spacious main garden. The home has an extensive activities programme which includes Pets as Therapy, as well as bingo and exercise sessions.

Registered places: 44
Guide weekly rate: £303–£395
Specialist care: Day care, respite
Medical services: Podiatry, dentist, optician, physiotherapy
Qualified staff: Undisclosed

Home details

Location: Residential area, 1 mile from Folkestone
Communal areas: 2 lounges, 2 dining room, library, garden
Accessibility: *Floors:* 4 • *Access:* Lift and stair lifts
Wheelchair access: Good
Smoking: In designated area
Pets: ✗
Routines: Flexible

Room details

Single: 38
Shared: 3
En suite: 35
Facilities: TV point, telephone point

Door lock: ✓
Lockable place: ✓

Services provided

Beauty services: Hairdressing
Mobile library: Library facilities
Religious services: ✓
Transport: Minibus
Activities: *Coordinator:* ✓ • *Examples:* Bingo, reminiscence,
quizzes • *Outings:* ✓
Meetings: ✗

Tudor Lodge

Manager: Julie Williams
Owner: Kanagaratnam Rajaseelan and
Kanagaratnam Rajamenon
Contact: 18–20 Manor Road,
Folkestone, Kent CT20 2SA
☎ 01303 251195
@ info@1stchoicecarehomes.com
🖱 www.1stchoicecarehomes.com

Tudor Lodge is situated near local amenities and one mile Folkestone town centre. It has a large car park and garden at the rear of the home. There are a range of activities and outings for residents to get involved in, such as bingo and reminiscence classes. The home provides a choice of menus offering nutritional home-cooked meals. Individual preferences and suggestions to broaden the current selection, special dietary requirements can be catered for. The home also has its own library facilities.

Valley View Residential Nursing Home

Manager: Hazel Beattie-Burrows
Owner: Prathap and Jyothi Jana
Contact: Maidstone Road, Rochester,
Kent ME1 3LT
☎ 01634 409797

Valley View is a purpose-built home, located in a square with an attractive courtyard garden in the centre. It is in a residential area of Rochester, close to local amenities and a bus route. The home organises a range of activities for residents to take part in, either enhancing their own hobbies or discovering new ones. These include arts and crafts, board and card games and film showings. Outings are also arranged to local points of interest.

Registered places: 33
Guide weekly rate: £525–£590
Specialist care: Nursing, physical disability, respite, terminal care
Medical services: Podiatry, dentist, optician
Qualified staff: Exceeds standard: 80% at NVQ Level 2

Home details
Location: Residential area, 2 miles from Rochester
Communal areas: Lounge/dining room, visitor's room, conservatory, garden
Accessibility: *Floors:* 3 • *Access:* Lift • *Wheelchair access:* Good
Smoking: In designated area
Pets: ✗
Routines: Flexible

Room details
Single: 27	**Door lock:** ✓
Shared: 3	**Lockable place:** ✓
En suite: 30	
Facilities: TV point, telephone point	

Services provided
Beauty services: Hairdressing
Mobile library: ✓
Religious services: Monthly Anglican service
Transport: ✗
Activities: *Coordinator:* ✓ • *Examples:* Arts and crafts, bingo, films
Outings: ✓
Meetings: ✓

Wantsum Lodge

Manager: Vacant
Owner: Choicecare 2000 Ltd
Contact: 32 St Mildreds Road,
Ramsgate, Kent CT11 0EF
☎ 01843 582666

Wantsum House is situated in a residential area in the costal town of Ramsgate. The home is located one mile from the town centre which offers community facilities such as health centres, library, railway station and a shopping centre. The home arranges activities such as beauty sessions and exercise sessions, as well as outings. There are regular residents meetings and a weekly religious service. The home caters for a great a deal of flexibility for both residents' daily routines, and for meals. Staff encourage residents to participate in activities, such a bingo, exercise and quizzes.

Registered places: 32
Guide weekly rate: £303–£570
Specialist care: None
Medical services: Podiatry, hygienist, optician, physiotherapy
Qualified staff: Exceeds standard: 80% at NVQ Level 2

Home details
Location: Residential area, 1 mile from Ramsgate
Communal areas: 3 lounges, 2 dining rooms, garden
Accessibility: *Floors:* 4 • *Access:* Lift • *Wheelchair access:* Good
Smoking: In designated area
Pets: ✓
Routines: Flexible

Room details
Single: 26	**Door lock:** ✓
Shared: 3	**Lockable place:** ✓
En suite: 29	
Facilities: TV point, telephone point	

Services provided
Beauty services: Hairdressing
Mobile library: ✗
Religious services: Weekly
Transport: ✗
Activities: *Coordinator:* ✗ • *Examples:* Beauty sessions, exercises, quizzes • *Outings:* ✓
Meetings: ✓

Registered places: 25
Guide weekly rate: £575–£700
Specialist care: Nursing, respite
Medical services: Podiatry, dentist, optician
Qualified staff: Exceeds standard: 59% at NVQ Level 2

Home details

Location: Residential area, 1 mile from Tunbridge Wells
Communal areas: Lounge, dining room, library, quiet room/
 conservatory, patio and garden
Accessibility: *Floors:* 3 • *Access:* Lift and stair lift
 Wheelchair access: Good
Smoking: In designated area
Pets: At manager's discretion
Routines: Flexible

Room details

Single: 15
Shared: 6
En suite: 0
Facilities: TV point, telephone point

Door lock: ✓
Lockable place: ✓

Services provided

Beauty services: Hairdressing
Mobile library: Library facilities
Religious services: Monthly Anglican service,
 visiting ministers and rabbis
Transport: ✗
Activities: *Coordinator:* ✓ • *Examples:* Arts and crafts, croquet,
 quizzes • *Outings:* ✓
Meetings: ✓

Warwick Park Nursing Home

Manager: Karen Pratt
Owner: Up-Beat Enterprises Ltd
Contact: 55 Warwick Park,
Tunbridge Wells, Kent TN2 5EJ
☎ 01892 541434

Warwick Park is a large detached house set in extensive grounds close to Tunbridge Wells town centre. The home is also close to The Pantiles, an 18th-century colonnaded shopping street, with shops and cafés lining the pedestrian area. There are regular outings, taking residents for cream teas, to the theatre and a local garden centre. In the summer there is the annual fête for residents to enjoy. There is a large, well-maintained and attractive garden for sitting in during the warmer weather. There is also a resident cat.

Registered places: 22
Guide weekly rate: £580
Specialist care: Nursing
Medical services: Podiatry, dentist, optician
Qualified staff: Exceeds standard: 55% at NVQ Level 2

Home details

Location: Residential area, 2 miles from Folkstone
Communal areas: Lounge, dining room, patio and garden
Accessibility: *Floors:* 3 • *Access:* Lift • *Wheelchair access:* Good
Smoking: In designated area
Pets: ✗
Routines: Flexible

Room details

Single: 22
Shared: 0
En suite: 18
Facilities: TV, telephone

Door lock: ✗
Lockable place: ✓

Services provided

Beauty services: Hairdressing
Mobile library: ✗
Religious services: ✗
Transport: ✗
Activities: *Coordinator:* ✓ • *Examples:* Exercises, occupational
 therapy, visiting entertainers • *Outings:* ✗
Meetings: ✗

Wells House Nursing Home

Manager: Chak Ng
Owner: Wells Care Ltd
Contact: Radnor Cliff Crescent,
Folkestone, Kent CT20 2JQ
☎ 01303 850727
🖰 www.wellscare.com

Wells House Nursing Home is a listed building situated in an elevated position, overlooking the sea on the outskirts of Sandgate. Wells House Nursing Home is the former residence of the author HG Wells. Several of the rooms at the home have excellent sea views. The rear garden also overlooks the sea and has a seating area for residents to observe the views of the channel. The home has an activities coordinator who arranges occupational therapy three times a week and visiting entertainers throughout the year. Pets are allowed to visit the home and smoking is permitted outside.

Wells Lodge Nursing Home

Manager: Vacant
Owner: Wells Care Ltd
Contact: 60 Earls Avenue,
Folkestone, Kent CT20 2HA
✆ 01303 850898

Wells Lodge Nursing Home is an adapted property that lies close to local amenities including shops and a train station. The home has two lounges, a dining room and a garden with a patio. The home offers a hairdressing service and there are visits from the local vicar. Pets are allowed to visit the home. There is a call system in each room as well as a TV.

Registered places: 22
Guide weekly rate: Undisclosed
Specialist care: Nursing
Medical services: Podiatry, dentist, optician, physiotherapy
Qualified staff: Undisclosed

Home details
Location: Residential area, 1 mile from Folkestone
Communal areas: 2 lounges, dining room, patio and garden
Accessibility: *Floors:* 3 • *Access:* Lift • *Wheelchair access:* Good
Smoking: ✗
Pets: ✗
Routines: Flexible

Room details
Single: 22
Shared: 0
En suite: 22
Facilities: TV

Door lock: ✓
Lockable place: ✓

Services provided
Beauty services: Hairdressing
Mobile library: ✗
Religious services: ✓
Transport: ✗
Activities: *Coordinator:* ✗ • *Examples:* Undisclosed • *Outings:* ✗
Meetings: ✗

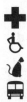

Westbank Nursing Home

Manager: Ruth Varley
Owner: New Century Care Ltd
Contact: 64 Sevenoaks Road,
Borough Green, Kent TN15 8AP
✆ 01732 780066

Westbank is located in a village, around seven miles from Sevenoaks. The home is a detached purpose-built property set in beautiful grounds with views extending across the countryside. The grounds have different decking and seating areas with level access for wheelchair users. There are daily activities planned for the residents to keep them stimulated and proactive, such as games, quizzes and visiting dogs. There are also visiting entertainers that come in monthly and put on shows or sing to the residents.

Registered places: 40
Guide weekly rate: £700–£1,000
Specialist care: Nursing, physical disability
Medical services: Podiatry
Qualified staff: Exceeds standard: 70% at NVQ Level 2

Home details
Location: Rural area, 7 miles from Sevenoaks
Communal areas: Lounge/dining room, visiting room, garden
Accessibility: *Floors:* 1 • *Wheelchair access:* Good
Smoking: In designated area
Pets: ✓
Routines: Flexible

Room details
Single: 40
Shared: 0
En suite: 3
Facilities: TV point, telephone point

Door lock: ✗
Lockable place: ✓

Services provided
Beauty services: Hairdressing, manicures
Mobile library: ✓
Religious services: Monthly church services
Transport: ✓
Activities: *Coordinator:* ✓ • *Examples:* Exercise to music, games, visiting entertainers • *Outings:* ✗
Meetings: ✓

Registered places: 20
Guide weekly rate: £304–£500
Specialist care: Respite
Medical services: Podiatry, dentist, optician
Qualified staff: Exceeds standard: 60% at NVQ Level 2

Home details

Location: Residential area, 1 mile from Folkestone
Communal areas: Lounge, dining room, patio and garden
Accessibility: *Floors:* 3 • *Access:* Lift • *Wheelchair access:* Limited
Smoking: ✗
Pets: ✗
Routines: Flexible

Room details

Single: 20
Shared: 0
En suite: 4
Facilities: TV point

Door lock: ✓
Lockable place: ✓

Services provided

Beauty services: Hairdressing
Mobile library: ✗
Religious services: Monthly Anglican and Life Church services
Transport: ✗
Activities: *Coordinator:* ✓ • *Examples:* Bingo, gentle exercise, table games • *Outings:* ✓
Meetings: ✓

Westleas

Manager: Sita Bhadye
Owner: Kestrel Care Ltd
Contact: 47 Earls Avenue, Folkestone, Kent CT20 2HB
) 01303 242784
@ info@westleascarehome.com
🖰 www.westleascarehome.com

Westleas is a Victorian building built in the 1900s which was converted over 25 years ago. The home does not allow pets to stay but there are visiting dogs. There are also lots of activities and musical afternoons with visiting entertainers. There are also barbecues in the summer and more restful activities such as quizzes and puzzles. The home also arranges religious services once a month.

Registered places: 36
Guide weekly rate: £606–£731
Specialist care: Nursing
Medical services: Podiatry, dentist, optician, physiotherapy
Qualified staff: Meets standard

Home details

Location: Residential area, 1.2 miles from Bromley
Communal areas: Lounge, dining room, activities area, patio and garden
Accessibility: *Floors:* 4 • *Access:* Lift • *Wheelchair access:* Good
Smoking: ✗
Pets: At manager's discretion
Routines: Flexible

Room details

Single: 13
Shared: 2
En suite: 2
Facilities: TV, telephone

Door lock: ✗
Lockable place: ✓

Services provided

Beauty services: Hairdressing
Mobile library: ✓
Religious services: ✓
Transport: ✗
Activities: *Coordinator:* ✓ • *Examples:* Arts and crafts, quizzes, visiting entertainers • *Outings:* ✗
Meetings: ✗

Westmeria Nursing Home

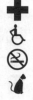

Manager: Susan Clarke
Owner: Westmeria Nursing Home Ltd
Contact: 47 Park Avenue, Bromley, Kent BR1 4EG
) 020 8460 5695
@ westmerian@btconnect.com
🖰 www.westmerianursingcentre.co.uk

Westmeria Nursing Home is located over a mile from Bromley and has a good bus service linking it to the town centre. The home has 13 single rooms and two double rooms. One single room and one double room have en suite facilities. A lockable facility for the room is available on request. The home is expecting a refurbishment so there may be locks on the doors. The home has its own activities coordinator and the programme includes games, quizzes, arts and crafts and visiting entertainers. Pets are allowed at the manager's discretion.

Westonville Lodge

Manager: Susan Neal
Owner: Susan Neal
Contact: 24 Royal Esplanade,
Westbrook, Kent CT9 5DX
☎ 01843 220669

Westonville Lodge is a small home located in a residential area of Margate, in close proximity to the seafront and local amenities. Residents' views are sought at the meetings held twice a month and they involved in decisions such as menu planning and what activities are organised by the home. The home has regular coffee mornings for residents, friends, families and local people. The home also arranges regular religious services for the residents.

Registered places: 10
Guide weekly rate: £320–£360
Specialist care: Day care
Medical services: Podiatry, optician
Qualified staff: Meets standard

Home details

Location: Residential area, 1.5 miles from Margate
Communal areas: Lounge, dining room, garden
Accessibility: *Floors:* 1 • *Wheelchair access:* Good
Smoking: ✗
Pets: At manager's discretion
Routines: Flexible

Room details

Single: 9
Shared: 1
En suite: 0
Facilities: TV point, telephone point

Door lock: ✓
Lockable place: ✓

Services provided

Beauty services: Hairdressing, aromatherapy, manicures
Mobile library: ✓
Religious services: ✓
Transport: ✗
Activities: *Coordinator:* ✓ • *Examples:* Shows, magicians, barbecues • *Outings:* ✓
Meetings: ✓

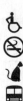

White Lodge

Manager: Christine Almichael
Owner: Michael and Christine Topping
Contact: 44–46 Madeira Road,
Cliftonville, Margate, Kent CT9 2QQ
☎ 01843 225956
@ michaeljtopping@aol.com

White Lodge is located in a residential area close to local shops and amenities and is five minutes from the seafront. The home has a homely atmosphere with three lounges and a large garden. The home has its own activities coordinator and arranges daily activities such as bingo and card games. There are also organised outings to the theatre. The home has its own budgies and other pets are allowed at the manager's discretion.

Registered places: 23
Guide weekly rate: From £375
Specialist care: None
Medical services: Podiatry, dentist, optician
Qualified staff: Fails standard

Home details

Location: Residential area, 0.7 miles from Margate
Communal areas: 3 lounges, dining room, garden
Accessibility: *Floors:* 3 • *Access:* Lift • *Wheelchair access:* Good
Smoking: ✗
Pets: At manager's discretion
Routines: Flexible

Room details

Single: 19
Shared: 2
En suite: 18
Facilities: TV

Door lock: ✓
Lockable place: ✓

Services provided

Beauty services: Hairdressing
Mobile library: ✗
Religious services: ✗
Transport: Car
Activities: *Coordinator:* ✓ • *Examples:* Bingo, cards, scrabble *Outings:* ✗
Meetings: ✗

Registered places: 19
Guide weekly rate: £297–£400
Specialist care: Respite, day care
Medical services: Podiatry, dentist, optician, physiotherapy
Qualified staff: Meets standard

Home details
Location: Residential area, 0.5 miles from Herne Bay
Communal areas: 2 lounges, dining room, garden
Accessibility: *Floors:* 2 • *Access:* Stair lift • *Wheelchair access:* Good
Smoking: In designated area
Pets: At manager's discretion
Routines: Flexible

Room details
Single: 19
Shared: 0
En suite: 19
Facilities: TV point, telephone point

Door lock: ✓
Lockable place: ✓

Services provided
Beauty services: Hairdressing
Mobile library: ✗
Religious services: ✗
Transport: 7-seater vehicle
Activities: *Coordinator:* ✓ • *Examples:* Cards, visiting entertainers
    Outings: ✓
Meetings: ✗

Whitebirch Lodge

Manager: Marilyn Squire
Owner: Krystlegate Ltd
Contact: 104 Canterbury Road,
Herne Bay, Kent CT6 5SE
☎ 01227 374633
@ Hernebay@home-service.uk.com

Whitebirch Lodge is a detached three-storey building that has been extended to include ground floor accommodation in the building next door. The family-run home is located approximately 100 yards from the seafront and half a mile from local shops. Excursions that are organised by the staff include visits to the local theatre and trips around the local coastal areas using the home's own transport.

Registered places: 27
Guide weekly rate: Undisclosed
Specialist care: Nursing, respite
Medical services: Podiatry, dentist, optician, physiotherapy
Qualified staff: Exceeds standard: 100% at NVQ Level 2

Home details
Location: Residential area, 1 mile from Chislehurst
Communal areas: Lounge, dining room, garden
Accessibility: *Floors:* 2 • *Access:* Lift • *Wheelchair access:* Good
Smoking: ✗
Pets: ✗
Routines: Flexible

Room details
Single: 23
Shared: 2
En suite: 6
Facilities: TV point, telephone point

Door lock: ✓
Lockable place: ✓

Services provided
Beauty services: Hairdressing
Mobile library: ✓
Religious services: ✗
Transport: ✗
Activities: *Coordinator:* ✓ • *Examples:* Exercise, music,
    reminiscence • *Outings:* ✗
Meetings: ✗

Whiteoak Court Nursing Home

Manager: Mary Lyons
Owner: I and R Tappin and S Schluep
Contact: 15 Selby Close,
Chislehurst, Kent BR7 5RU
☎ 020 8467 0954
@ matron@whiteoakcourt.co.uk
🖰 www.whiteoakcourt.co.uk

Whiteoak Court Nursing Home has been caring for the elderly for 25 years. The food is home cooked and they use as much local produce as possible. This means that special diets can be catered for. There is also a laundry service, library facilities and newspapers and magazines can be ordered. At present no religious services are arranged but if requested the home will organise a service or Communion. Pets are also allowed to visit but not to stay.

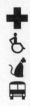

Wilmington Manor Nursing Home

Manager: Mary Bazeley

Owner: BUPA Care Homes Ltd

Contact: Common Lane, Wilmington, Dartford, Kent DA2 7BA

☎ 01322 288746

@ WilmingtonManorALL@BUPA.com

🖰 www.bupacarehomes.co.uk

Originally a 19th-century private house, Wilmington Manor has been converted and extended. It is situated in a semi-rural location with shops and amenities close at hand, and only three miles from Dartford which can be reached using the local bus service. There is a choice of well-furnished lounges which provide meeting places for residents and guests. The dining room overlooks the patio and well-kept garden, which also contains a summerhouse. Daily activities include games, musical entertainment, gardening and trips to local places of interest. Wilmington Manor is also able to offer specialist care to older people with physical disabilities.

Registered places: 50

Guide weekly rate: Undisclosed

Specialist care: Nursing, respite, physical disability

Medical services: Podiatry, physiotherapy

Qualified staff: Undisclosed

Home details

Location: Rural area, 3 miles from Dartford centre

Communal areas: 2 lounges, 2 dining rooms, library, hairdressing salon, garden

Accessibility: *Floors:* 2 • *Access:* Lift • *Wheelchair access:* Good

Smoking: In designated area

Pets: ✓

Routines: Flexible

Room details

Single: 50

Shared: 0

En suite: 50

Facilities: TV point, telephone point

Door lock: ✓

Lockable place: ✓

Services provided

Beauty services: Hairdressing, aromatherapy

Mobile library: ✗

Religious services: ✓

Transport: ✓

Activities: *Coordinator:* ✓ • *Examples:* Games, musical entertainment, gardening • *Outings:* ✓

Meetings: ✓

Winchester House

Manager: Susan Watson

Owner: Barchester Healthcare Ltd

Contact: 180 Wouldham Road, Rochester, Kent ME1 3TR

☎ 01634 685001

@ Winchester@barchester.com

🖰 www.barchester.com

Winchester House is run by Barchester Healthcare and has a dementia unit attached. The home is a former rectory and was recently refurbished. The home is surrounded by two acres of land. It is situated in a rural area, two miles from the city of Rochester. The home provides transport for residents and taxis are available. A dedicated activities coordinator organises stimulating activities for residents to participate in if they wish. These activities include baking and games. There are also organised outings to the seaside. The home has on-site hairdressing and aromatherapy and manicures are available.

Registered places: 123

Guide weekly rate: From £950

Specialist care: Dementia, physical disability, respite

Medical services: Podiatry, dentist, optician, physiotherapy

Qualified staff: Meets standard

Home details

Location: Rural area, 1 mile from Wouldham

Communal areas: Lounges, dining rooms, patio and garden

Accessibility: *Floors:* 2 • *Access:* Lift • *Wheelchair access:* Good

Smoking: ✗

Pets: ✗

Routines: Flexible

Room details

Single: 123

Shared: 0

En suite: Undisclosed

Facilities: TV

Door lock: ✗

Lockable place: ✓

Services provided

Beauty services: Hairdressing, aromatherapy, manicures

Mobile library: ✓

Religious services: ✓

Transport: ✓

Activities: *Coordinator:* ✓ • *Examples:* Baking, Elvis day, games *Outings:* ✓

Meetings: ✗

Registered places: 33
Guide weekly rate: Up to £750
Specialist care: Nursing
Medical services: Podiatry, dentist, optician, physiotherapy
Qualified staff: Meets standard

Home details
Location: Rural area, 4 miles from Gravesend
Communal areas: Lounge, dining room, conservatory, garden
Accessibility: *Floors:* 2 • *Access:* Lift • *Wheelchair access:* Good
Smoking: ✗
Pets: ✗
Routines: Flexible

Room details
Single: 23
Shared: 5
En suite: 7
Facilities: Telephone point

Door lock: ✓
Lockable place: ✓

Services provided
Beauty services: Hairdressing
Mobile library: ✗
Religious services: ✓
Transport: ✗
Activities: *Coordinator:* ✓ • *Examples:* Arts and crafts, reading
    Outings: ✗
Meetings: ✓

The Withens Nursing Home

Manager: Mrs Chandler
Owner: Ranc Care Homes Ltd
Contact: Hook Green Road, Southfleet, Kent DA13 9NQ
  ✆ 01474 834109

The Withens is situated in a rural location with an acre of land surrounding it. The home is not purpose built so retains an individual atmosphere with each room having its own character. The home offers a hairdressing service and could offer other services such as aromatherapy. The local library is nearby and there are books brought for the residents. The home has an activities coordinator who structures the activities programme around the residents' individual needs and wishes. Pets are allowed to visit the home but smoking is not permitted. The home has regular residents meetings.

Registered places: 120
Guide weekly rate: Undisclosed
Specialist care: Nursing, respite
Medical services: Podiatry, occupational therapy, physiotherapy
Qualified staff: Meets standard

Home details
Location: Residential area, 1.5 miles from Gravesend centre
Communal areas: 4 lounges, 4 dining rooms, hairdressing salon, garden
Accessibility: *Floors:* 1 • *Wheelchair access:* Good
Smoking: In designated area
Pets: ✗
Routines: Flexible

Room details
Single: 120
Shared: 0
En suite: 0
Facilities: TV point, telephone point

Door lock: ✓
Lockable place: ✗

Services provided
Beauty services: Hairdressing
Mobile library: ✓
Religious services: ✓
Transport: ✓
Activities: *Coordinator:* ✓ • *Examples:* Bingo, entertainers, games
    Outings: ✓
Meetings: ✓

Wombwell Hall Nursing Home

Manager: Elaine Rosenthal
Owner: BUPA Care Homes Ltd
Contact: Wombwell Gardens, Northfleet, Gravesend, Kent DA11 8BL
  ✆ 01474 569699
  @ WombwellALL@BUPA.com
  🖳 www.bupacarehomes.co.uk

Set in a residential area of Gravesend, Wombwell Hall is close to local shops and on a local bus route. Built in the grounds of Wombwell Hall Girls Grammar School, this purpose-built home has been designed to meet the needs of elderly residents. It comprises four separate houses, all providing nursing care. Each house has a lounge, conservatory and dining area, and all houses have access to the landscaped gardens. Daily activities include games, bingo, entertainers and trips to local shops. Wombwell Hall is also able to care for those who have had strokes, and who require palliative or terminal care.

Woodlands Care Home

Manager: Andrea Callow
Owner: Ashbourne Ltd
Contact: Fairfield Road,
Broadstairs, Kent CT10 2JU

✆ 01843 860998
@ woodlandsnh@schealthcare.co.uk
🖳 www.southerncrosshealthcare.co.uk

A purpose-built home situated next to Fairfield Manor Care Centre, Woodlands Care Home is situated in a residential area, one mile from Broadstairs. The home is set in well-kept, scenic gardens surrounded by trees and local wildlife. The home has two resident cats and birds, and residents pets are welcome to visit. The home's activities coordinator arranges events for the residents such as afternoon tea and there is a mobile library which visits.

Registered places: 33
Guide weekly rate: £396–£698
Specialist care: Nursing
Medical services: Podiatry, dentist, optician, physiotherapy
Qualified staff: Fails standard: 44% at NVQ Level 2

Home details
Location: Residential area, 1 mile from Broadstairs
Communal areas: 2 lounges, dining room, garden
Accessibility: *Floors:* 2 • *Access:* Lift • *Wheelchair access:* Good
Smoking: ✗
Pets: ✗
Routines: Flexible

Room details
Single: 28
Shared: 1
En suite: 29
Facilities: TV point, telephone point

Door lock: ✗
Lockable place: ✓

Services provided
Beauty services: Hairdressing
Mobile library: ✓
Religious services: ✗
Transport: ✗
Activities: *Coordinator:* ✓ • *Examples:* Afternoon teas, cooking, gardening • *Outings:* ✗
Meetings: ✓

Woodstock Residential Home

Manager: Gail Edey
Owner: Nellsar Ltd
Contact: 80 Woodstock Road,
Sittingbourne, Kent ME10 4HN

✆ 01795 420202
🖳 www.woodstock@nelsar.com

Woodstock Residential Home is located in a residential area on the outskirts of Sittingbourne, approximately two miles from the town centre and a main line railway station. The home organise a number of social events such as barbecues, 'strawberries and champagne' parties, and gin and tonic afternoons. The garden and patio at the rear of the home is very well maintained and includes a pleasant seating area for residents to enjoy. The home arranges for local clergy to visit the home twice a month and there is also a mobile library which come to the home.

Registered places: 60
Guide weekly rate: £338–£550
Specialist care: Dementia, respite
Medical services: Podiatry, Optician
Qualified staff: Exceeds standard: 100% at NVQ Level 2

Home details
Location: Residential area, 2 miles from Sittingbourne
Communal areas: 4 lounges, 2 dining rooms, hairdressing salon, activities room, 2 conservatories, patio and garden
Accessibility: *Floors:* 2 • *Access:* 2 lifts • *Wheelchair access:* Good
Smoking: ✗
Pets: ✗
Routines: Flexible

Room details
Single: 40
Shared: 7
En suite: 9
Facilities: None

Door lock: ✗
Lockable place: ✗

Services provided
Beauty services: Hairdressing
Mobile library: ✓
Religious services: Fortnightly church visits
Transport: ✗
Activities: *Coordinator:* ✓ • *Examples:* Arts and crafts, exercise, films • *Outings:* ✓
Meetings: ✗

Registered places: 20
Guide weekly rate: £375–£575
Specialist care: Respite
Medical services: Podiatry, dentist, optician
Qualified staff: Exceeds standard: 100% at NVQ Level 2

Home details
Location: Residential area, 1.5 miles from Folkestone
Communal areas: Lounge, dining room, patio
Accessibility: *Floors:* 4 • *Access:* Lift • *Wheelchair access:* Good
Smoking: ✗
Pets: At manager's discretion
Routines: Flexible

Room details
Single: 10
Shared: 10
En suite: 17
Facilities: TV point, telephone point

Door lock: ✓
Lockable place: ✓

Services provided
Beauty services: Hairdressing
Mobile library: ✗
Religious services: Weekly church visits
Transport: Car
Activities: *Coordinator:* ✓ • *Examples:* Bingo, musical sessions,
   quizzes • *Outings:* ✗
Meetings: ✓

Mont Calm

Manager: Vacant
Owner: Comforts of Home Ltd
Contact: 3 Clifton Crescent,
Folkestone, Kent CT20 2EL
✆ 01303 242940
@ m.davies@wyncare.co.uk

Mont Calm is a Grade II listed, detached Victorian building, overlooking the cliffs with spectacular sea views. The grassed area allows resident's to freely enjoy the scenic coast, particularly in the warmer months. The home offers good wheelchair access throughout, and residents are provided with an activities coordinator who offers social quizzes, bingo and musical sessions. There is a residents meetings every six to eight weeks.

Registered places: 13
Guide weekly rate: £390–£500
Specialist care: Dementia
Medical services: Podiatry, optician
Qualified staff: Meets standard

Home details
Location: Village location, 14 miles from Ashford
Communal areas: Lounge, dining room, garden
Accessibility: *Floors:* 2 • *Access:* None • *Wheelchair access:* None
Smoking: ✗
Pets: ✗
Routines: flexible

Room details
Single: 11
Shared: 1
En suite: 3
Facilities: TV point, telephone point

Door lock: ✗
Lockable place: ✓

Services provided
Beauty services: Hairdressing
Mobile library: ✗
Religious services: ✗
Transport: ✗
Activities: *Coordinator:* ✗ • *Examples:* Games, quizzes
   Outings: ✗
Meetings: ✓

Yew Tree House Residential Care Home for the Elderly

Manager: Michael Discombe
Owner: Michael Discombe
Contact: 9 Station Road, Headcorn,
Ashford, Kent TN27 9SA
✆ 01622 890112

Situated a 15-minute walk from local facilities in Headcorn village, Yew Tree House is in a quite residential area near Ashford. The home does not have a lift or stair lift and therefore upstairs bedrooms are limited to residents with some mobility. Aside from the main house, a separate building at the front of the premises provides two en suite studio bedrooms. The staff organise daily activities for residents such as quizzes and games, and the residents' pets are always welcome to visit the home.

Yew Tree Lodge

Manager: Sharon Edmunds
Owner: Abida and Syed Ali
Contact: Stoke Road, Hoo, Rochester, Kent ME3 9BJ

☎ 01634 251312
@ info@yewtreelodge.com
🖰 www.yewtreelodge.com

Yew Tree Lodge is situated in Hoo St Werburgh, six miles from Rochester. It is an old village surrounded by a picturesque and peaceful countryside. The home has landscaped gardens and there is a fishpond which is overlooked from the front of the house. There are three extensive lounges, including one on the first floor with panoramic views over the Medway Estuary. Outings are arranged on request by individuals, couples or groups, and there is also daily activities planned such as cards as well as visiting entertainment. The home also arranges one-to-one activities session with the residents.

Registered places: 29
Guide weekly rate: £416–£450
Specialist care: Dementia
Medical services: Podiatry, dentist, optician
Qualified staff: Exceeds standard: 60% at NVQ Level 2

Home details

Location: Rural area, 6 miles from Rochester
Communal areas: Lounge, dining room, garden
Accessibility: *Floors:* 2 • *Access:* Lift • *Wheelchair access:* Good
Smoking: ✗
Pets: At manager's discretion
Routines: Flexible

Room details

Single: 17
Shared: 6
En suite: 0
Facilities: TV point

Door lock: ✗
Lockable place: ✓

Services provided

Beauty services: Hairdressing
Mobile library: ✓
Religious services: Monthly church services
Transport: ✗
Activities: *Coordinator:* ✗ • *Examples:* Arts and crafts, games, tea afternoons • *Outings:* ✓
Meetings: ✓

Registered places: 66
Guide weekly rate: £765–£845
Specialist care: Nursing, dementia, mental disorder, respite
Medical services: Podiatry, physiotherapy
Qualified staff: Fails standard: 20% at NVQ Level 2

Home details

Location: Village location, 4 miles from Oxford
Communal areas: 8 lounges, 4 dining rooms, patio and garden
Accessibility: *Floors:* 3 • *Access:* Lift • *Wheelchair access:* Good
Smoking: x
Pets: At manager's discretion
Routines: Flexible

Room details

Single: 66
Shared: 0
En suite: 66
Facilities: TV point, telephone point

Door lock: ✓
Lockable place: ✓

Services provided

Beauty services: Hairdressing
Mobile library: x
Religious services: Fortnightly Communion service
Transport: Minibus
Activities: *Coordinator:* ✓ • *Examples:* Bingo, games, painting, quizzes • *Outings:* ✓
Meetings: x

Brookfield Christian Care Home

Manager: Susan Chapman
Owner: Trinity Care Ltd
Contact: Little Bury, Greater Leyes, Oxford OX4 7UY
☎ 01865 779888
@ Brookfield@schousecare.co.uk
🖰 www.schousecare.co.uk

Brookfield Christian Care Home is a purpose-built home situated on the outskirts of the Greater Leys area of Oxford, overlooking open countryside. The home currently has two of its own cats and several fish which residents enjoy caring for. The home organises various outings using its minibus. In the past, trips have included a visit to Monkey World in Poole.

Registered places: 24
Guide weekly rate: Undisclosed
Specialist care: Nursing, respite
Medical services: Audiologist, podiatry
Qualified staff: Meets standard

Home details

Location: Residential area, in Banbury
Communal areas: Lounge/dining room, 4 patio areas and garden
Accessibility: *Floors:* 3 • *Access:* Lift • *Wheelchair access:* Good
Smoking: x
Pets: At manager's discretion
Routines: Flexible

Room details

Single: 9
Shared: 7
En suite: 0
Facilities: None

Door lock: x
Lockable place: ✓

Services provided

Beauty services: Hairdressing
Mobile library: x
Religious services: ✓
Transport: x
Activities: *Coordinator:* x • *Examples:* Crafts, entertainment, gardening • *Outings:* ✓
Meetings: ✓

Brooklands 1 Nursing Home

Manager: Julie Richardson
Owner: Brooklands 1 Ltd
Contact: 14 Dashwood Road, Banbury, Oxfordshire OX16 5HD
☎ 01295 268522

Brooklands 1 Home is conveniently located five minutes' walk from Banbury's shops and public transport. It is situated in a residential area and has a front lawn and several small patio areas as outside space. An occupational therapist runs activities for residents, including bulb planting, crafts and outings. There are also visits from outside performers. The owners have two dogs who regularly visit the home and two pet birds reside in the communal area.

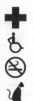

Chervil Cottage

Manager: Wendy Drewett
Owner: Mr and Mrs Drewett
Contact: Brighthampton, Standlake, Oxfordshire OX29 7QW
) 01865 300820
@ Wendy.drewett@virgin.net

Chervil Cottage is located near the village of Standlake, around six miles from Witney. The village nearby has shops and pubs, with a local bus service providing easy access. The home provides ground-floor accommodation opening on to attractive gardens. All rooms exit onto the gardens for residents to enjoy. A daily routine of activities is provided, such as arts and crafts, keep fit and quizzes.

Registered places: 17
Guide weekly rate: £580–£650
Specialist care: None
Medical services: Podiatry, dentist
Qualified staff: Fails standard: 40% at NVQ Level 2

Home details
Location: Rural area, 6 miles from Witney
Communal areas: Lounge, dining room, 2 conservatories, garden
Accessibility: *Floors:* 1 • *Wheelchair access:* Good
Smoking: ✗
Pets: ✗
Routines: Flexible

Room details
Single: 17
Shared: 0
En suite: 17
Facilities: TV point, telephone point

Door lock: ✓
Lockable place: ✓

Services provided
Beauty services: Hairdressing
Mobile library: ✓
Religious services: Monthly Communion service
Transport: ✗
Security:
Activities: *Coordinator:* ✓ • *Examples:* Arts and crafts, keep fit, quizzes • *Outings:* ✓
Meetings: ✓

Cherwood House Care Centre

Manager: Yvonne Bazylkiewicz
Owner: Ellenbern Holdings Ltd
Contact: Buckingham Road, Caversfield, Bicester, Oxfordshire OX27 8RA
) 01869 245005
@ yvonne.cherwood@ cherwoodhouse.co.uk
🖰 www.cherwoodhouse.co.uk

Cherwood House is located in Caversfield in Bicester and is very near shops, facilites and public transport links. The home was originally a Royal Airforce Officers Mess and retains many of its original furnishings. Cherwood House is set in extensive grounds which have raised flowerbeds and a greenhouse as well as a 'safe area' for those vulnerable residents. Residents are very welcome to help maintain the garden or grow vegetables in the greenhouse if they enjoy gardening. Activities are planned for the residents on a daily basis including gardening, walks, bingo and quizzes.

Registered places: 103
Guide weekly rate: £409–£817
Specialist care: Nursing, dementia, learning disability, mental disorder, physical disability, sensory impairment
Medical services: Physiotherapy
Qualified staff: Meets standard

Home details
Location: Village location, 1.5 miles from Bicester
Communal areas: 5 lounges, dining room, conservatory, garden
Accessibility: *Floors:* 2 • *Access:* Lift • *Wheelchair access:* Good
Smoking: In designated area
Pets: ✓
Routines: Flexible

Room details
Single: 61
Shared: 21
En suite: 50
Facilities: TV point, telephone point

Door lock: ✗
Lockable place: ✓

Services provided
Beauty services: Hairdressing
Mobile library: ✓
Religious services: Anglican and Catholic Communion services
Transport: ✓
Activities: *Coordinator:* ✓ • *Examples:* Bingo, gardening, walks *Outings:* ✗
Meetings: ✗

Registered places: 97
Guide weekly rate: £409–£850
Specialist care: Nursing, respite
Medical services: Podiatry, dentist, optician
Qualified staff: Exceeds standard: 62% at NVQ Level 2

Home details

Location: Rural area, 6 miles from Oxford
Communal areas: 4 lounges, dining room, conservatory, garden
Accessibility: *Floors:* 2 • *Access:* Lift • *Wheelchair access:* Good
Smoking: In designated area
Pets: ✗
Routines: Flexible

Room details

Single: 87
Shared: 10
En suite: 97
Facilities: TV point, telephone point

Door lock: ✓
Lockable place: ✓

Services provided

Beauty services: Hairdressing
Mobile library: ✗
Religious services: Monthly Anglican and Catholic visits
Transport: Minibus
Activities: *Coordinator:* ✓ • *Examples:* Games, music, quizzes
   Outings: ✓
Meetings: ✓

The Close Nursing and Residential Home

Manager: Nyembezi Chipara
Owner: Cavendish Close Ltd
Contact: Burcot, Abingdon, Oxfordshire OX14 3DP
☏ 01865 407343

The Close was originally a Tudor-style Victorian country house set in four acres of ground. A recent refurbishment of the home has modernised, while leaving many of the attractive Victorian features intact. The home is situated close to the market town of Abingdon and approximately six miles south of the city of Oxford. The local pub is within walking distance from the home. The River Thames is at the end of the garden, providing a peaceful retreat for residents who wish to go on walks. There is also a pond and a seating area with spectacular views due to the homes slightly raised position.

Registered places: 51
Guide weekly rate: Undisclosed
Specialist care: Nursing, convalescent, palliative,
   physical disability, respite
Support services available: Podiatry, optician, physiotherapy
Qualified staff: Exceeds standard: 75% at NVQ Level 2

Home details

Location: Rural area, 2 miles from Burford
Communal areas: Lounge, dining room, garden
Accessibility: *Floors:* 2 • *Access:* Lift • *Wheelchair access:* Good
Smoking: ✗
Pets: ✗
Routines: Flexible

Room details

Single: 51
Shared: 0
En suite: 51
Facilities: TV point, telephone point

Door lock: ✗
Lockable place: ✓

Services provided

Beauty services: Hairdressing, aromatherapy
Mobile library: ✓
Religious services: Fortnightly Anglican service
Transport: Minibus
Activities: *Coordinator:* ✓ • *Examples:* Exercise classes, quizzes
   Outings: ✓
Meetings: ✗

Cotswold Home

Manager: Pat Hamilton
Owner: Elizabeth Finn Homes Ltd
Contact: Woodside Drive,
Bradwell Village, Burford,
Oxfordshire OX18 4XA
☏ 01993 824225
@ thecotswoldhome@efhl.co.uk
🖰 www.efhl.co.uk

Built in the traditional Cotswold style, this nursing and residential home is situated in open countryside two miles from Burford. Cotswold Home runs an events programme aided by a committee of local volunteers who work with the activities coordinator to take residents on outings and to their houses for tea. Twice weekly, physiotherapists run a gentle exercise class and residents can also take part in yoga and art sessions. The home's minibus transports residents to the local shops, pubs and gardens as well as nearby attractions. Budding gardeners also benefit from the raised flowerbeds in the home itself.

Culworth House

Manager: Martha Cromhout
Owner: Blanchworth Care
Contact: Queens Street, Culworth,
Banbury, Oxfordshire OX17 2AT

⟩ 08453 455 744
⌐Ь www.blanchworth.co.uk

This classical Georgian-style mansion is set in four acres of land in a rural village north of Oxford. This home provides a support group for relatives of residents and emphasises the importance of involving them in their relative's care plan. With three reception rooms and a conservatory, residents enjoy ample communal space. The part-time activities coordinator organises a good variety of activities. This home has a smoking lounge.

Registered places: 35
Guide weekly rate: £300–£680
Specialist care: Nursing, physical disability, respite
Medical services: Chiropody
Qualified staff: Undisclosed

Home details
Location: Village location, 7 miles from Banbury
Communal areas: 3 lounges, dining room, smoking room,
   hairdressing salon, conservatory, garden
Accessibility: *Floors:* 3 • *Access:* Lift • *Wheelchair access:* Good
Smoking: In designated area
Pets: ✗
Routines: Flexible

Room details
Single: 27
Shared: 4
En suite: 5
Facilities: TV, telephone

Door lock: ✓
Lockable place: ✗

Services provided
Beauty services: Hairdressing
Mobile library: ✗
Religious services: ✗
Transport: ✗
Activities: *Coordinator:* ✓ • *Examples:* Craftwork, flower arranging,
   parties • *Outings:* ✗
Meetings: ✗

Eden House

Manager: Deborah del Rosario
Owner: Marjorie Chungtuyco
Contact: 50 Horspath Road, Cowley,
Oxfordshire OX4 2QT

⟩ 01865 776012
@ eden.house@ntlworld.com

Eden House is a private family-run business situated in a residential area on the outskirts of Oxford. The majority of the staff are family members living in the vicinity of the home and as a consequence of this the residents form part of an extended family. Activities are on offer and residents are encouraged to go on visits to the pub or to get more involved with the local community. Residents' rooms are personalised by the residents' own possessions and photographs.

Registered places: 8
Guide weekly rate: £491–£500
Specialist care: Dementia, physical disability
Medical services: Podiatry, dentist, optician
Qualified staff: Undisclosed

Home details
Location: Residential area, 3 miles from Oxford centre
Communal areas: Lounge, dining room, garden
Accessibility: *Floors:* 2 • *Access:* Undisclosed
   Wheelchair access: Good
Smoking: ✗
Pets: ✗
Routines: Structured

Room details
Single: 4
Shared: 2
En suite: 0
Facilities: None

Door lock: ✓
Lockable place: ✗

Services provided
Beauty services: Hairdressing
Mobile library: ✓
Religious services: ✗
Transport: ✗
Activities: *Coordinator:* ✗ • *Examples:* One-to-one sessions
   Outings: ✓
Meetings: ✗

Registered places: 28
Guide weekly rate: £490–£550
Specialist care: Dementia, physical disability
Medical services: Podiatry, dentist, optician, physiotherapy
Qualified staff: Fails standard: 20% at NVQ Level 2

Home details
Location: Village location, 5 miles from Chipping Norton
Communal areas: Lounge, dining room, garden
Accessibility: *Floors:* 3 • *Access:* Lift • *Wheelchair access:* Good
Smoking: x
Pets: ✓
Routines: Flexible

Room details
Single: 14
Shared: 7
En suite: Undisclosed
Facilities: TV point, telephone point

Door lock: ✓
Lockable place: x

Services provided
Beauty services: Hairdressing
Mobile library: x
Religious services: Monthly church service
Transport: x
Activities: *Coordinator:* ✓ • *Examples:* Games • *Outings:* x
Meetings: x

Enstone House

Manager: Caroline Dyett
Owner: Dilrukshan Wijayaratnam, Selvan Kularatnam and Thevaratnam Selvaratnam
Contact: Cox's Lane, Enstone, Oxfordshire OX7 4LF
☏ 01608 677375
@ enstonehouse01@btconnect.com

Enstone House was originally an 18th-century coaching inn and is situated in the village of Enstone. Local buses stop outside the home and the village post office and shop are within easy walking distance. The home has three floors with a lift and good wheelchair access. There is an activities coordinator in the home and services such as hairdressing and a monthly church service are available. The residents have a flexible daily routine and meal times are flexible.

Registered places: 30
Guide weekly rate: £450–£500
Specialist care: None
Medical services: Podiatry, optician
Qualified staff: Meets standard

Home details
Location: Residential area, 2 miles from Oxford centre
Communal areas: Lounge, dining room, garden
Accessibility: *Floors:* 2 • *Access:* Lift • *Wheelchair access:* Good
Smoking: x
Pets: x
Routines: Flexible

Room details
Single: 30
Shared: 0
En suite: 22
Facilities: TV point

Door lock: x
Lockable place: ✓

Services provided
Beauty services: Hairdressing
Mobile Library: ✓
Religious services: Fortnightly Communion service
Transport: x
Activities: *Coordinator:* x • *Examples:* Arts and crafts, exercise, quizzes • *Outings:* x
Meetings: ✓

Fairfield Residential Home

Manager: Alison Parry
Owner: The Management Committee of Fairfield
Contact: 115 Banbury Road, Oxford OX2 6LA
☏ 01865 558413

Fairfield Residential Home is situated on the edge of Oxford city centre, which is easily accessed by bus or on foot. The home is also within walking distance of Summertown, a suburban shopping area. The property is a large town house with extensive well-maintained grounds and gardens that residents can walk around any time. The home provides a thorough range of daily activities as well as theatrical shows, fashion and shoe sales which are held quarterly.

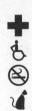

Freeland House Nursing Home

Manager: Frances Payne
Owner: Dove Care Homes Ltd
Contact: Wroslyn Road, Freeland, Witney, Oxfordshire OX29 8AH
☎ 01993 881258
@ frhouse@rock.com

Freeland House is a nursing home set in a 19th-century building, with six acres of woodland and landscaped gardens at the southern edge of Freeland village. It is approximately five miles from the market town of Witney, with good amenities. The home consists of two buildings and extensive views over the gardens and fields at the rear of the home provide pleasant scenery for residents.

Registered places: 76
Guide weekly rate: £567–£850
Specialist care: Nursing, physical disability, respite.
Medical services: Podiatry, dentist, optician, physiotherapy
Qualified staff: Undisclosed

Home details

Location: Rural area, 5 miles from Witney
Communal areas: 3 lounges, 2 dining rooms, garden
Accessibility: *Floors:* 3 • *Access:* Lift • *Wheelchair access:* Good
Smoking: ✗
Pets: At manager's discretion
Routines: Flexible

Room details

Single: 56
Shared: 10
En suite: 50
Facilities: TV point, telephone point

Door lock: ✓
Lockable place: ✓

Services provided

Beauty services: Hairdressing, beauty treatments, manicures,
Mobile library: ✗
Religious services: Fortnightly Communion service
Transport: ✗
Activities: *Coordinator:* ✓ • *Examples:* Games, visiting entertainers
     Outings: ✓
Meetings: ✓

The Grange Nursing Home

Manager: Kenneth Mead
Owner: Bonneycourt Ltd
Contact: 25 Church Green, Stanford-in-the-Vale, Faringdon, Oxfordshire SN7 8HU
☎ 01367 718836
@ thegrange@bonneycourt.co.uk
🖰 www.grangenursing.co.uk

The Grange Nursing Home is a mature country house set in the centre of Stanford in the Vale with beautiful country surroundings. It is next to St Deny's Church and was once the vicarage. The market towns of Wantage and Faringdon can be reached by car or public transport. The home has strong links with the local village, which contains a post office, public house and shops. Many rooms have pleasant views and a few are accessed by a short flight of stairs. The home has its own activities coordinator and organises weekly entertainment and exercise sessions twice a week.

Registered places: 49
Guide weekly rate: £626–£799
Specialist care: Nursing, physical disability
Medical services: Podiatry, dentist, optician.
Qualified staff: Exceeds standard: 85% at NVQ Level 2

Home details

Location: Village location, 4 miles from Farringdon
Communal areas: 2 lounges, dining room, patio and garden
Accessibility: *Floors:* 2 • *Access:* Lift and stair lift
     Wheelchair access: Good
Smoking: ✗
Pets: At manager's discretion
Routines: Flexible

Room details

Single: 39
Shared: 5
En suite: 30
Facilities: TV

Door lock: ✓
Lockable place: ✓

Services provided

Beauty services: Hairdressing
Mobile library: ✓
Religious services: Monthly church service
Transport: ✗
Activities: *Coordinator:* ✓ • *Examples:* Entertainment,
     exercise sessions • *Outings:* ✗
Meetings: ✓

Registered places: 40
Guide weekly rate: Undisclosed
Specialist care: Nursing, respite, palliative care, terminal care
Medical services: Podiatry, occupational therapy, physiotherapy
Qualified staff: Undisclosed

Home details

Location: Residential area, 3 miles from Oxford centre
Communal areas: 4 lounges, dining room, garden,
     hairdressing salon, kitchenette, garden
Accessibility: *Floors:* 2 • *Access:* Lift • *Wheelchair access:* Good
Smoking: In designated area
Pets: At manager's discretion
Routines: Flexible

Room details

Single: 24
Shared: 15
En suite: 26
Facilities: TV, telephone point

Door lock: ✓
Lockable place: ✓

Services provided

Beauty services: Hairdressing, aromatherapy
Mobile library: ✓
Religious services: Monthly church service
Transport: ✓
Activities: *Coordinator:* ✓ • *Examples:* Arts and crafts, films,
     visiting entertainers • *Outings:* ✓
Meetings: ✗

Green Gates Nursing Home

Manager: Margo Wilcock
Owner: BUPA Care Homes Ltd
Contact: 2 Hernes Road, Summertown,
Oxford OX2 7PT
☏ 01865 558815
@ GreenGatesALL@BUPA.com
🖰 www.bupacarehomes.co.uk

Originally a private house, Green Gates has been tastefully converted into a welcoming nursing home set in the residential area of Summertown. It is close to local shops and on a local bus route. The entrance hall retains three stained-glass windows depicting the streets and colleges of Oxford. Each bedroom is individually decorated, and all offer en suite facilities. Regular activities include musical entertainment, gardening, games and even French conversation, as well as trips to local places of interest. Green Gates is also able to offer palliative and terminal care.

Registered places: 30
Guide weekly rate: £604–£654
Specialist care: Nursing
Medical services: Podiatry, physiotherapy
Qualified staff: Exceeds standard: 60% at NVQ Level 2

Home details

Location: Residential area, 1 mile from Banbury centre
Communal areas: Lounge, dining room, conservatory, garden
Accessibility: *Floors:* 2 • *Access:* Lift • *Wheelchair access:* Good
Smoking: ✗
Pets: ✗
Routines: Structured

Room details

Single: 26
Shared: 2
En suite: 8
Facilities: TV point, telephone point

Door lock: ✗
Lockable place: ✗

Services provided

Beauty services: Hairdressing
Mobile library: ✗
Religious services: Weekly church service,
     monthly Communion service
Transport: ✗
Activities: *Coordinator:* ✓ • *Examples:* Games • *Outings:* ✗
Meetings: ✗

Green Pastures Christian Care Home

Manager: Belinda Woodward
Owner: Green Pastures Ltd
Contact: The Hawthorns, Banbury,
Oxfordshire OX16 9FA
☏ 01295 279963

Green Pastures Christian Nursing Home is a purpose-built care home located on the outskirts of Banbury. The home is operated as a not-for-profit Christian organisation through Green Pastures Ltd, and is a registered charity. The home has a strong Christian ethos, but this does not preclude those people who belong to other denominations and have different religious beliefs. There is a lounge, dining room and garden and a conservatory. There is an activities coordinator and both a structured daily routine and set meal times.

Hempton Field

Manager: Elizabeth Norris

Owner: Hamilton House Medical Ltd

Contact: 36 Lower Icknield Way, Chinnor, Oxfordshire OX39 4EB

☏ 01844 351766

@ Admin1@hamiltoncare.com

🖰 www.hamiltoncare.com

Hempton Field is one of the oldest established nursing homes in the county. The home aims to give quality of life to their residents and prides itself on the homely atmosphere created by its staff. This is further helped by the layout of the home, avoiding long, clinical corridors. There is a large courtyard garden with raised flowerbeds and a lily pond leading to an orchard that overlooks the Chiltern Hills. As well as attending to resident's needs, the home feels it is very important to provide support to relatives also.

Registered places: 29

Guide weekly rate: £575–£925

Specialist care: Podiatry, dentist, optician, physiotherapy

Medical services: Nursing, respite, palliative

Qualified staff: Meets standard

Home details

Location: Village location, 0.5 miles from Chinnor

Communal areas: 2 lounges, dining room, garden

Accessibility: *Floors:* 2 • *Access:* Lift • *Wheelchair access:* Good

Smoking: ✗

Pets: ✓

Routines: Structured

Room details

Single: 28

Shared: 1

En suite: 17

Facilities: TV point, telephone point

Door lock: ✗

Lockable place: ✓

Services provided

Beauty services: Hairdressing, manicures

Mobile library: ✗

Religious services: Weekly Anglican Communion, monthly nondenominational service

Transport: ✗

Activities: *Coordinator:* ✓ • *Examples:* Art classes, exercise classes, knitting • *Outings:* ✓

Meetings: ✓

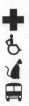

Huntercombe Hall Care Home

Manager: Lisa Archer

Owner: Caring Homes Ltd

Contact: Huntercombe Place, Nuffield Henley-on-Thames, Oxfordshire RG9 5SE

☏ 01491 641792

Set in extensive grounds in a rural location, Huntercombe Hall is located in well-kept, landscaped gardens, however, due to its rural location, access to public transport is limited. The home is isolated from local shops and transport, however the home does have its own transport, so transporting residents around is not a problem. There are extensive grounds for residents to socialise in or walk around. There are daily activities organise for the residents by the activities coordinator, and visiting entertainers who come in on a monthly basis and do historical talks, sing live or act a play.

Registered places: 48

Guide weekly rate: £650–£950

Specialist care: Nursing

Medical services: Podiatry, optician

Qualified staff: Meets standard

Home details

Location: Rural area, 8 miles to Henley-on-Thames

Communal areas: 3 lounges, dining room, garden

Accessibility: *Floors:* 2 • *Access:* Lift • *Wheelchair access:* Good

Smoking: In designated area

Pets: ✓

Routines: Flexible

Room details

Single: 40

Shared: 4

En suite: 44

Facilities: TV point, telephone point

Door lock: ✗

Lockable place: ✓

Services provided

Beauty services: Hairdressing

Mobile library: ✓

Religious services: ✓

Transport: ✓

Activities: *Coordinator:* ✓ • *Examples:* Visiting entertainers *Outings:* ✓

Meetings: ✗

Registered places: 12
Guide weekly rate: £464–£555
Specialist care: Dementia, physical disability
Medical services: Podiatry, optician
Qualified staff: Meets standard

Home details
Location: Village location, 2 miles from Oxford centre
Communal areas: Lounge, dining room, patio and garden
Accessibility: *Floors: 2* • *Access:* Lift • *Wheelchair access:* Good
Smoking: ✗
Pets: At manager's discretion
Routines: Flexible

Room details
Single: 10
Shared: 1
En suite: 10
Facilities: TV point, telephone point

Door lock: ✓
Lockable place: ✓

Services provided
Beauty services: Hairdressing
Mobile library: Library facilities
Religious services: Monthly Communion service,
    prayer meetings every 3 weeks
Transport: ✗
Activities: *Coordinator:* ✗ • *Examples:* Board games, summer
    bazaars, video sessions • *Outings:* ✓
Meetings: ✓

Kirlena House

Manager: Vedenath Audit
Owner: Vedenath and Ellen Audit
Contact: 18 Kennington Road,
Oxford OX1 5NZ
✆ 01865 730510
@ enquiries@auditcare.com
🖥 www.auditcare.com

Kirlena House is located near Oxford in the village of Kennington, close to shops and transport facilities. The house itself is detached, with a patio area and large attractive garden at the rear. The home has a lounge, a dining room and a garden with a large patio and is spread over two floors with a shaft lift. The residents have a flexible daily routine but have structured mealtimes with a provision for changes. There are outings arranged to the local village library and an over 60s club in the village. Daily activities include video sessions and visits from professional entertainers. There is a resident tenants association which meets every quarter.

Registered places: 36
Guide weekly rate: £515–£730
Specialist care: Nursing, respite
Medical services: Podiatry, optician
Qualified staff: Fails standard

Home details
Location: Village location, 5 miles from Chipping Norton
Communal areas: Lounge, dining room, patio and garden
Accessibility: *Floors: 4* • *Access:* Lift • *Wheelchair access:* Good
Smoking: ✗
Pets: At manager's discretion
Routines: Flexible

Room details
Single: 28
Shared: 4
En suite: 18
Facilities: Telephone

Door lock: ✓
Lockable place: ✓

Services provided
Beauty services: Hairdressing
Mobile library: ✗
Religious services: Monthly Anglican service
Transport: ✗
Activities: *Coordinator:* ✓ • *Examples:* Quizzes, visiting entertainers
    Outings: ✓
Meetings: ✓

The Langston

Manager: Vacant
Owner: J Sai Country Home Ltd
Contact: Station Road, Kingham,
Oxfordshire OX7 6UP
✆ 01608 658233

The Langston is a Grade II listed building situated in the village of Kingham, five miles from Chipping Norton. The home has a courtyard area for residents to enjoy in warmer weather as well as a lounge and a dining room inside the home. There is a dedicated activities coordinator who arranges reminiscence sessions, quizzes and performances by visiting entertainers. There are also outings in the local area and an Anglican service is held at the home on a monthly basis.

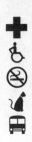

Lashbrook House

Manager: Suresh Gogna
Owner: Majestic Number One Ltd
Contact: Mill Road, Shiplake,
Henley-on-Thames, Oxfordshire
RG9 3LP
☏ 01189 401770

Lashbrook House is situated in an attractive part of Oxfordshire near the River Thames. There is a railway station in the nearby village of Shiplake, as well as a post office and shop. The home is set in extensive grounds with views across open countryside. There is level access in most parts of the grounds, and various seating and decking areas for residents to sit outside. Weekly activities include a variation of arts and crafts, bingo, board games and visiting entertainers. Visiting entertainers include live singing and magic.

Registered places: 46
Guide weekly rate: £700–£900
Specialist care: Nursing, dementia
Medical services: Podiatry, dentist, optician, physiotherapy
Qualified staff: Exceeds standard: 60% at NVQ Level 2

Home details
Location: Village location, 2.5 miles from Henley-on-Thames
Communal areas: 2 lounges, lounge/dining room, dining room
Accessibility: *Floors:* 2 • *Access:* Lift • *Wheelchair access:* Good
Smoking: ✗
Pets: ✓
Routines: Flexible

Room details
Single: 42
Shared: 2
En suite: 39
Facilities: TV point, telephone point

Door lock: ✗
Lockable place: ✓

Services provided
Beauty services: Hairdressing
Mobile library: ✓
Religious services: Monthly church services
Transport: ✓
Activities: *Coordinator:* ✓ • *Examples:* Arts and crafts, games, visiting entertainers • *Outings:* ✗
Meetings: ✓

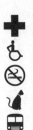

Longlands Nursing Home

Manager: Susan Jones
Owner: Chiltern Care Homes Ltd
Contact: Pound Lane, Cassington,
Oxfordshire OX28 1DL
☏ 01865 881440
@ longlands@schealthcare.co.uk

Longlands Nursing Home is located in an attractive situation close to the church and village centre of Witney. The grounds are extensive and provide a pleasant outlook from every room. It has a well-maintained interior and offers homely accommodation for the residents. There is a range of activities available, and the notice boards in the entrance corridor display village events, such as a coffee morning or a flower festival.

Registered places: 35
Guide weekly rate: £653–£900
Specialist care: Nursing, terminal care
Medical services: Podiatry, dentist, optician
Qualified staff: Meets standard

Home details
Location: Village location
Communal areas: 2 dining rooms, garden
Accessibility: *Floors:* 2 • *Access:* Lift • *Wheelchair access:* Good
Smoking: ✗
Pets: At manager's discretion
Routines: Flexible

Room details
Single: 31
Shared: 2
En suite: 33
Facilities: TV point

Door lock: ✓
Lockable place: ✓

Services provided
Beauty services: Hairdressing
Mobile library: ✗
Religious services: Communion services
Transport: ✓
Activities: *Coordinator:* ✓ • *Examples:* Exercises, Pets As Therapy *Outings:* ✓
Meetings: ✓

Registered places: 23
Guide weekly rate: Undisclosed
Specialist care: Dementia, mental disorder
Medical services: Undisclosed
Qualified staff: Meets standard

Home details
Location: Village location, 10 miles from Reading
Communal areas: 3 lounges, dining room, garden
Accessibility: *Floors:* 3 • *Access:* Lift • *Wheelchair access:* Good
Smoking: In designated area
Pets: At manager's discretion
Routines: Flexible

Room details
Single: 17
Shared: 3
En suite: 15
Facilities: TV point, telephone

Door lock: ✓
Lockable place: ✗

Services provided
Beauty services: Hairdressing, beautician
Mobile library: Library facilities
Religious services: Monthly Anglican visits,
fortnightly Catholic visits
Transport: ✗
Activities: *Coordinator:* ✗ • *Examples:* Cooking, exercise, t'ai chi
Outings: ✓
Meetings: ✓

Lyndhurst Residential Home

Manager: Julia Collyer
Owner: Lyndhurst Ltd
Contact: Lyndhurst Road,
Goring-on-Thames, Oxfordshire
RG8 9BL
☎ 01491 871325

Lyndhurst Residential Home is a Victorian-style house that has been altered and adapted for its purpose. Many rooms have attractive views of the countryside and the village green. The village offers shops, pubs and cafés with transport links to Reading and Oxford. The home strives to engage with its residents and to keep them as mobile as possible. Outings are arranged to the local library and shops as well as to Reading. Afternoon activities include t'ai chi as well as games such as scrabble and bingo and arts and crafts. There are monthly meetings for the residents which their families are welcome to attend.

Registered places: 42
Guide weekly rate: £589–£740
Specialist care: Nursing, day care, dementia, respite
Medical services: Podiatry, optician, physiotherapy
Qualified staff: Exceeds standard: 85% at NVQ Level 2

Home details
Location: Village location, 6 miles from Witney
Communal areas: 3 lounges, 2 dining rooms,
conservatory, garden
Accessibility: *Floors:* 2 • *Access:* Lift • *Wheelchair access:* Good
Smoking: ✗
Pets: ✗
Routines: Flexible

Room details
Single: 37
Shared: 5
En suite: 20
Facilities: TV point, telephone point

Door lock: ✓
Lockable place: ✓

Services provided
Beauty services: Hairdressing, aromatherapy, manicures, massages
Mobile library: ✗
Religious services: ✗
Transport: ✓
Activities: *Coordinator:* ✓ • *Examples:* Bingo, knitting, painting
Outings: ✓
Meetings: ✓

Meadowview Nursing Home

Manager: Caroline Campbell Schofield
Owner: Farhad Pardhan
Contact: 48 Rack End, Standlake,
Witney, Oxfordshire OX29 7SB
☎ 01865 300205
@ farhadpardhan@aol.com
🖰 www.meadowviewnh.com

Meadowview is a privately owned home situated in a residential area of Standlake village. A local bus service provides easy access to shops and pubs, and the minibus service provides its own outings to farms, garden centres and most recently, Blenheim Palace. Residents enjoy the enclosed, secure garden during the warmer seasons that provides a calm and relaxing environment. The home has recently begun a monthly newsletter that informs residents of current affairs, activities and staff profiles.

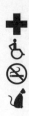

Merryfield House

Manager: Jill Timms
Owner: Kuldip Dhanani
Contact: 33 New Yatt Road, Witney,
Oxfordshire OX28 1NX
☏ 01993 775776
@ jill@merryfieldcare.co.uk
℥ www.merryfieldhouse.co.uk

Merryfield House is a beautiful Cotswold stone small manor house near the village of Witney, within 10 minutes' walk to local amenities. Some original features remain, such as a large stone fireplace in the main lounge where activities take place. There is also space to relax in peace and quiet in the smaller lounge, which also has a piano. An extension was built to accommodate more bedrooms and is linked to the central house by a glass walkway. Planning permission is being requested to build a conservatory and create a separate dining area for residents.

Registered places: 24
Guide weekly rate: £589–£660
Specialist care: Nursing, respite
Medical services: Podiatry, optician
Qualified staff: Meets standard

Home details
Location: Village location, 0.5 miles from Witney centre
Communal areas: 2 lounges, garden
Accessibility: *Floors:* 2 • *Access:* Lift • *Wheelchair access:* Good
Smoking: ✗
Pets: At manager's discretion
Routines: Flexible

Room details
Single: 14	**Door lock:** ✓
Shared: 5	**Lockable place:** ✓
En suite: 14	
Facilities: TV, telephone point	

Services provided
Beauty services: Hairdressing, aromatherapy, massage
Mobile library: ✗
Religious services: Monthly nondenominational service
Transport: ✗
Activities: *Coordinator:* ✓ • *Examples:* Music and exercise, painting, quizzes • *Outings:* ✗
Meetings: ✓

Mon Choisy

Manager: Ellen Audit
Owner: Mr and Mrs Audit
Contact: 128 Kennington Road,
Kennington, Oxford OX1 5PE
☏ 01865 739223
@ enquiries@auditcare.com
℥ www.auditcare.com

Mon Choisy resides in the village of Kennington three minutes' walk from shops and local facilities. The home is situated close to its sister home, Kirlena House, which is also owned by Mr and Mrs Audit. The home offers day care and is in contact with a podiatrist and an optician. The home arranges a variety of outings and daily activities such as board games and summer bazaars. The residents have a structured daily routine and although there are set meal times these are open to change to accommodate the residents' needs.

Registered places: 28
Guide weekly rate: £491–£562
Specialist care: Day care, dementia
Medical services: Podiatry, optician
Qualified staff: Meets standard

Home details
Location: Village location, 2.5 miles from Oxford centre
Communal areas: 3 lounges, dining room, conservatory, patio and garden
Accessibility: *Floors:* 2 • *Access:* Lift • *Wheelchair access:* Good
Routines: Flexible
Pets: At manager's discretion
Smoking: ✗

Room details
Single: 21	**Door lock:** ✓
Shared: 3	**Lockable place:** ✓
En suite: 0	
Facilities: TV point, telephone point	

Services provided
Beauty services: Hairdressing
Mobile library: Library facilities
Religious services: Monthly Communion service, prayer meetings every 3 weeks
Transport: ✗
Activities: *Coordinator:* ✗ • *Examples:* Bingo, board games, entertainers • *Outings:* ✓
Meetings: ✓

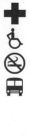

Registered places: 80
Guide weekly rate: £518–£1,108
Specialist care: Nursing, dementia, physical disability, respite
Medical services: Podiatry, dentist, physiotherapy, optician
Qualified staff: Fails standards

Home details

Location: Rural area, 4 miles from Oxford centre
Communal areas: 4 lounges, 4 dining rooms, conservatory,
    library, garden
Accessibility: *Floors:* 2 • *Access:* Lift • *Wheelchair access:* Good
Smoking: ✗
Pets: ✗
Routines: Flexible

Room details

Single: 0   Door lock: ✓
Shared: 55   Lockable place: ✗
En suite: 55
Facilities: TV, telephone point

Services provided

Beauty services: Hairdressing, aromatherapy, manicures, massage
Mobile library: ✓
Religious services: Anglican and Catholic services
Transport: Minibus
Activities: *Coordinator:* ✓ • *Examples:* Games, visiting entertainers
    Outings: ✓
Meetings: ✗

Oaken Holt House Nursing and Residential Home

Manager: Mandy Vettraino
Owner: Oaken Holt Care Ltd
Contact: Eynsham Road, Farmoor, Oxfordshire OX2 9NL
☏ 01865 863710
🖳 www.oakenholt.co.uk

Oaken Holt House Nursing and Residential Home is a Victorian building set in 22 acres of landscaped grounds in a secluded elevated position four miles from the city of Oxford. The gardens have numerous seating areas, a fishpond and flowerbeds.

All rooms can either be used for single or double occupancy, so the home can accommodate couples. A range of outings are organised – from theatre trips to a drink at a pub, and there are two activities coordinators to ensure residents have a varied activity programme.

Registered places: 49
Guide weekly rate: £788–£1,674
Specialist care: Nursing, day care, physically disabled, respite,
    terminal care
Medical services: Podiatry, dentist, optician, physiotherapy
Qualified staff: Fails standard

Home details

Location: Residential area, 3.5 miles from Oxford
Communal areas: Lounge, garden
Accessibility: *Floors:* 2 • *Access:* Lift • *Wheelchair access:* Good
Smoking: ✗
Pets: Undisclosed
Routines: Flexible

Room details

Single: 42   Door lock: Undisclosed
Shared: 3   Lockable place: ✗
En suite: 41
Facilities: TV point, telephone

Services provided

Beauty services: Undisclosed
Mobile library: Undisclosed
Religious services: Catholic and Anglican services
Transport: Minibus
Activities: *Coordinator:* Undisclosed • *Examples:* Knitting group
    Outings: ✓
Meetings: ✓

Oxford Beaumont

Manager: Lesley Widdicombe
Owner: Barchester Healthcare Ltd
Contact: Bayworth Corner, Bayworth Lane, Boars Hill, Oxford OX1 5DE
☏ 01865 730990
@ oxford@barchester.com
🖳 www.barchester.com

Oxford Beaumont is located in a residential area, three and a half miles from Oxford. The home is set in five and a half acres of ground and there is ample communal space inside the home. The home produces a regular newsletter outlining changes in the home and there are also quarterly residents meetings. The home arranges both Catholic and Anglican services and there are daily activities such as knitting groups.

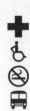

Rush Court

Manager: Dina Rodriguez
Owner: Elizabeth Finn Homes Ltd
Contact: Shillingford Road, Wallingford, Oxfordshire OX10 8LL
) 01491 837223
@ rushcourt@efhl.co.uk
ᵹ www.efhl.co.uk

Rush Court is approximately two and a half miles from the market town of Wallingford's town centre. Outings to the local pub are a regular occurrence and residents make regular trips out in the home's minibus. Additionally, a monthly tea party is organised by staff and relatives are invited to an annual garden party at the home, held in its well-maintained gardens. The home has three lounges and a separate dining room for residents to enjoy. There is also a hairdressing salon, a library and a dedicated activities room. The residents have a structured daily routine and there are residents meetings every quarter. The home has its own minibus and there is a Communion service every two weeks.

Registered places: 50
Guide weekly rate: £550–£965
Specialist care: Nursing, respite, physical disability
Medical services: Podiatry, physiotherapy
Qualified staff: Undisclosed

Home details
Location: Rural area, 2.5 miles from Wallingford
Communal areas: 3 lounges, dining room, physiotherapy room, activities room, hairdressing salon, library, garden
Accessibility: *Floors:* 2 • *Access:* Lift • *Wheelchair access:* Good
Smoking: ✗
Pets: ✗
Routines: Structured

Room details
Single: 50   **Door lock:** ✗
Shared: 0   **Lockable place:** ✓
En suite: 50
Facilities: TV point, telephone point

Services provided
Beauty services: Hairdressing
Mobile library: ✓
Religious services: Fortnightly Communion service, Catholic visits
Transport: Minibus
Activities: *Coordinator:* ✓ • *Examples:* Arts and crafts, cinema club, music appreciation • *Outings:* ✓
Meetings: ✓

Sotwell Hill House

Manager: Joy Butterfield
Owner: Joy Butterfield
Contact: Brightwell Cum Sotwell, Wallingford, Oxfordshire OX10 0PS
) 01491 836685
ᵹ www.sotwellhillhouse.co.uk

Set in nearly 20 acres of landscaped parklands, this late-Victorian converted country house is only half a mile away from the town of Wallingford. The large garden is well maintained and residents are able to take exercise in safety. The dining room, conservatory and main lounges have views over the lawns and Chiltern Hills. The home is family owned and run, aiming to therefore maintain personal relationships with the residents. On the second floor there is a fully equipped hairdressing salon and a hairdresser comes in regularly.

Registered places: 36
Guide weekly rate: £550–£690
Specialist care: None
Medical services: Podiatry, dentist, optician, physiotherapy
Qualified staff: Meets standard

Home details
Location: Village location, 0.5 miles from Wallingford
Communal areas: 3 lounges, dining room, conservatory, hairdressing salon, garden
Accessibility: *Floors:* 2 • *Access:* Lift • *Wheelchair access:* Good
Smoking: ✗
Pets: ✗
Routines: Flexible

Room details
Single: 35   **Door lock:** ✗
Shared: 1   **Lockable place:** ✗
En suite: 36
Facilities: TV, telephone

Services provided
Beauty services: Hairdressing
Mobile library: ✗
Religious services: Fortnightly Communion service
Transport: Car
Activities: *Coordinator:* ✓ • *Examples:* Crosswords, music and movement, quizzes • *Outings:* ✓
Meetings: ✓

Registered places: 87
Guide weekly rate: £750–£1,000
Specialist care: Nursing, dementia, mental disorder, physical disability, respite
Medical services: Podiatry, optician, physiotherapy
Qualified staff: Exceeds standard: 65% at NVQ Level 2

Home details

Location: Residential area, 1 mile from Chipping Norton
Communal areas: Lounge, dining room, garden
Accessibility: *Floors:* 2 • *Access:* Lift • *Wheelchair access:* Good
Smoking: ✗
Pets: ✓
Routines: Flexible

Room details

Single: 79
Shared: 4
En suite: 56
Facilities: TV point, telephone point

Door lock: ✗
Lockable place: ✓

Services provided

Beauty services: Hairdressing
Mobile library: ✓
Religious services: Monthly church services
Transport: Minibus
Activities: *Coordinator:* ✓ • *Examples:* Games, reminiscence
    Outings: ✓
Meetings: ✓

Southdown Nursing Home

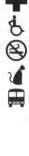

Manager: Shirley Archer
Owner: Barchester Healthcare Ltd
Contact: Worcester Road,
Chipping Norton, Oxfordshire OX7 5YF
☎ 01608 644129
🖥 www.barchester.com

Southdown Nursing Home is a purpose-built property consisting of two units that are linked by a covered walkway. The original house caters for residents who are physically frail. The second unit, the Memory Lane building, was constructed in 2002 and provides for residents with mental health needs. On the outskirts of the market town of Chipping Norton, the home enjoys panoramic views across an unspoilt valley and the Cotswolds. To the rear of the main house is a secure garden with fencing, shrubbery and garden furniture for the residents' use.

Registered places: 51
Guide weekly rate: Undisclosed
Specialist care: Nursing, dementia, physically disabled, respite, terminal care
Medical services: Podiatry, hygienist, optician, physiotherapy
Qualified staff: Meets standard

Home details

Location: Residential area, 2 miles from Oxford centre
Communal areas: 3 lounges, dining room, garden
Accessibility: *Floors:* 2 • *Access:* Lift • *Wheelchair access:* Good
Smoking: ✗
Pets: ✗
Routines: Flexible

Room details

Single: 48
Shared: 0
En suite: 48
Facilities: TV, telephone

Door lock: ✓
Lockable place: ✓

Services provided

Beauty services: Hairdressing, aromatherapy, manicures
Mobile library: ✓
Religious services: Weekly Anglican service,
    monthly Catholic service
Transport: ✗
Activities: *Coordinator:* ✓ • *Examples:* Music, Pets As Therapy
    Outings: ✗
Meetings: ✗

St Luke's Hospital

Manager: Zannifer Mason
Owner: The Council of St Luke's Hospital
Contact: 4 Latimer Road, Headington,
Oxford OX3 7PF
☎ 01865 228800
@ admin@stlukeshosp.co.uk
🖥 www.stlukeshosp.co.uk

St Luke's Hospital is a care home with nursing and is managed by a non-profit-making Christian charitable trust, The Council of St Luke's Hospital. Situated close to Headington town centre, the home provides a warm and friendly environment for residents and is near local shops. Care is provided on a medical basis and residents are referred to as 'patients'. St Luke's admits patients on a long-term basis and also as respite patients. There is a tropical fish tank on the first floor, installed at the request of a resident.

The Triangle Nursing Home

Manager: Amanda Longford
Owner: Southern Cross Healthcare Ltd
Contact: London Road, Wheatley, Oxfordshire OX33 1YW

☎ 01865 875596
🖱 www.schealthcare.co.uk

The Triangle Nursing Home is located in the village of Wheatley on the old A40, east of Oxford. Regular bus services stop near to the home. There are regular visits from locals in the community giving different types of talk such as historical talks about the area. The home also has its own minibus which makes outings easier, and residents can go shopping on a weekly basis. Outings are monthly to points of interest in and around Oxfordshire, and on a daily basis there are activities in the home such as chair exercises to music and gardening.

Registered places: 28
Guide weekly rate: £518–£714
Specialist care: Nursing, terminal care
Medical services: Podiatry, optician
Qualified staff: Meets standard

Home details
Location: Village location, 3 miles from Oxford
Communal areas: Lounge, dining room, garden
Accessibility: *Floors:* 2 • *Access:* Lift • *Wheelchair access:* Good
Smoking: In designated area
Pets: ✗
Routines: Flexible

Room details
Single: 26
Shared: 1
En suite: 27
Facilities: TV point

Door lock: ✗
Lockable place: ✓

Services provided
Beauty services: Hairdressing
Mobile library: ✗
Religious services: Monthly church service
Transport: Minibus
Activities: *Coordinator:* ✓ • *Examples:* Chair exercises, gardening, quizzes • *Outings:* ✗
Meetings: ✗

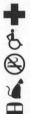

Wardington House Nursing Home

Manager: George Tuthill
Owner: Wardington House Partnership
Contact: Wardington, Banbury, Oxfordshire OX17 1SD

☎ 01295 750622

Wardington House Nursing Home has been providing care for individuals with dementia and other mental disorders since 1965. The home lies on the edge of Wardington village, close to the town of Banbury. The home has its own minibus, so it can take residents shopping and to local attractions. There are extensive grounds which are accessible to residents and three areas which double as a lounge and a dining room. The home's chef sources foods locally as much as possible.

Registered places: 60
Guide weekly rate: £750–£900
Specialist care: Nursing, dementia, learning disability, mental disorder, physical disability
Medical services: Podiatry, dentist, optician, physiotherapy
Qualified staff: Fails standard: 13% at NVQ Level 2

Home details
Location: Village location, 5 miles from Banbury
Communal areas: 3 lounge/dining rooms, garden
Accessibility: *Floors:* 3 • *Access:* Lift • *Wheelchair access:* Good
Smoking: ✗
Pets: ✓
Routines: Flexible

Room details
Single: 19
Shared: 20
En suite: Undisclosed
Facilities: TV point, telephone point

Door lock: ✓
Lockable place: ✓

Services provided
Beauty services: Hairdressing
Mobile library: ✗
Religious services: ✓
Transport: Minibus
Activities: *Coordinator:* ✓ • *Examples:* Entertainers • *Outings:* ✓
Meetings: ✗

Registered places: 63

Guide weekly rate: £565–£850

Specialist care: Nursing, dementia, physical disabled, respite, terminal care

Medical services: Audiologist, podiatry, physiotherapy

Qualified staff: Meets standard

Home details

Location: Village location, 3 miles from Weybridge

Communal areas: 2 lounges, 3 dining rooms, reading room, garden

Accessibility: *Floors:* 2 • *Access:* Lift
Wheelchair access: Limited

Smoking: ✗

Pets: ✗

Routines: Structured

Room details

Single: 53

Shared: 5

En suite: Undisclosed

Facilities: TV point, telephone point

Door lock: ✗

Lockable place: ✗

Services provided

Beauty services: Hairdressing

Mobile library: ✗

Religious services: Monthly church service

Transport: ✗

Activities: *Coordinator:* ✓ • *Examples:* Visits from school children, Salvation Army • *Outings:* ✗

Meetings: ✗

Abbey Chase Residential and Nursing Home

Manager: Jean Short

Owner: Abbey Chase Residential and Nursing Homes Ltd

Contact: Bridge Road, Chertsey, Surrey KT16 8JW

☏ 01932 569768

@ admin@abbeychase.co.uk

🖱 www.abbeychase.co.uk

Abbey Chase lies in 10 acres of abbey grounds in the ancient Thameside town of Chertsey near Weybridge. The garden looks out onto the river and there are ramps and pathways to ensure wheelchair access. There is also a central courtyard with seating for residents to enjoy and many riverside walks. The home offers outdoor pursuits such as private angling and gardening. The activities coordinator ensures there is something available for less able residents and organises performances from local schools and the Salvation Army.

Registered places: 25

Guide weekly rate: £600–£675

Specialist care: Nursing, day care, respite

Medical services: Podiatry, dentist, optician, physiotherapy

Qualified staff: Fails standards

Home details

Location: Residential area, in Addlestone

Communal areas: Lounge, dining room, patio and garden

Accessibility: *Floors:* 3 • *Access:* Lift • *Wheelchair access:* Good

Smoking: ✗

Pets: ✗

Routines: Flexible

Room details

Single: 24

Shared: 1

En suite: 9

Facilities: TV point, telephone point

Door lock: ✓

Lockable place: ✗

Services provided

Beauty services: Hairdressing

Mobile library: ✓

Religious services: Anglican visits

Transport: ✗

Activities: *Coordinator:* ✓ • *Examples:* Exercises, reminiscence, quizzes • *Outings:* ✗

Meetings: ✓

Addlestone Lodge

Manager: Mrs Tharani

Owner: Addlestone Care Home Ltd

Contact: Ongar Hill, Addlestone, Surrey KT15 1BS

☏ 01932 846268

Addlestone Lodge is located in Addlestone and accommodation is set over three floors accessed by stairs or a lift and comprises of a lounge, dining area, kitchen, laundry, office, bathrooms, toilets and shared and single bedrooms. The home has built an extension to increase the number of places available at the home. There is a part-time activities coordinator who organises exercises, reminiscence, quizzes and more. Outside, there is a patio and landscaped garden for residents to enjoy.

Albury House

Manager: Deborah Parratt
Owner: Eric Goozee
Contact: 6 Albury Road, Guildford,
Surrey GU1 2BT
☎ 01483 573847
@ alburyhouse@btconnect.com
🖰 www.alburyhouse.co.uk

Situated in a residential area of Guilford, Albury House is a detached home close to local shops, bus routes and a train station. Guildford town centre is a five-minute drive away. Some suites have kitchenette facilities which include a kettle and fridge. An activities coordinator provides a range of sessions, including exercise classes, flower arranging and visiting entertainers. The home has recently added a new conservatory.

Registered places: 33
Guide weekly rate: £450–£640
Specialist care: Respite
Medical services: Podiatry, optician, physiotherapy
Qualified staff: Exceeds standard: 75% for NVQ level 2

Home details
Location: Residential area, 1 mile from Guildford centre
Communal areas: Lounge, dining room, conservatory, garden
Accessibility: *Floors:* 3 • *Access:* Lift • *Wheelchair access:* Good
Smoking: ✗
Pets: ✗
Routines: Flexible

Room details
Single: 31
Shared: 2
En suite: 33
Facilities: TV point, telephone point

Door lock: ✓
Lockable place: ✓

Services provided
Beauty services: Hairdressing
Mobile library: ✓
Religious service: ✓
Transport: ✗
Activities: *Coordinator:* ✓ • *Examples:* Exercise classes, flower arranging, visiting entertainers • *Outings:* ✓
Meetings: ✓

Alvington House

Manager: S Ludlow
Owner: Mr and Mrs Ludlow and
Mrs Stephenson
Contact: 59 Wray Park Road, Reigate,
Surrey RH2 0EQ
☎ 01737 222042

Alvington House is situated in a residential area of Reigate. Shops, post office, chemist, pub, train station, library and bank are all under a mile away. There is a varied activity plan at the home with knitting circles and reminiscence sessions. Outings are planned to local points of interest and garden centres. The home has two budgies and other pets may stay at the home at the discretion of the manager. There are meetings every two months for residents to raise any issues or concerns.

Registered places: 25
Guide weekly rate: £420–£520
Specialist care: Mental disorder, respite
Medical services: Podiatry, dentist, optician, physiotherapy
Qualified staff: Meets standard

Home details
Location: Residential area, 1 mile from Reigate centre
Communal areas: Lounge, dining room, conservatory, garden
Accessibility: *Floors:* 3 • *Access:* Stair lifts
Wheelchair access: Good
Smoking: ✗
Pets: At manager's discretion
Routines: Flexible

Room details
Single: 25
Shared: 0
En suite: 22
Facilities: TV point, telephone point

Door lock: ✓
Lockable place: ✓

Services provided
Beauty services: Hairdressing
Mobile library: ✓
Religious services: Monthly Anglican service
Transport: ✗
Activities: *Coordinator:* ✓ • *Examples:* Bingo, knitting circle, reminiscence • *Outings:* ✓
Meetings: ✓

Registered places: 60
Guide weekly rate: £515–£750
Specialist care: Nursing, dementia, respite
Medical services: Podiatry, dentist, optician, physiotherapy
Qualified staff: Exceeds standard: 65% at NVQ Level 2

Home details

Location: Residential area, 0.5 miles from Purley Junction
Communal areas: 3 lounges, 3 dining rooms, library, garden
Accessibility: *Floors:* 3 • *Access:* Lift • *Wheelchair access:* Good
Smoking: In designated area
Pets: ✓
Routines: Flexible

Room details

Single: 59
Shared: 1
En suite: 60
Facilities: TV point, telephone point

Door lock: ✗
Lockable place: ✓

Services provided

Beauty services: Hairdressing
Mobile library: Library facilities
Religious services: ✓
Transport: ✗
Activities: *Coordinator:* ✓ • *Examples:* Bingo, dominoes, live music • *Outings:* ✓
Meetings: ✓

Amberley Lodge Nursing Home

Manager: Osborne Acquaye
Owner: Care UK Community Partnerships Ltd
Contact: 86–94 Downlands Road, Purley, Surrey CR8 4JF
✆ 020 8668 0999
@ manager.burroughs@careuk.com
🖰 www.careuk.com

Amberly Lodge is a purpose-built care home, on three floors. The first two floors provide nursing care and the top floor residential care. It is located in Purley, close to its shops and facilities. There are lounge and dining areas on each floor. The unit is managed by Care UK, a private healthcare provider, contracted directly to Croydon Health Authority. The home boasts a large landscaped garden which the residents enjoy in summer months, and pets are welcome which brings a lively and homely atmosphere to the home.

Registered places: 40
Guide weekly rate: £650–£700
Specialist care: Nursing care, day care, dementia, respite
Medical services: Podiatry, hygienist, optician, physiotherapy
Qualified staff: Exceeds standard: 75% at NVQ Level 2

Home details

Location: Urban area, 250 yards from Farnham centre
Communal areas: 2 lounges, dining room, conservatory, library, garden
Accessibility: *Floors:* 2 • *Access:* Lift • *Wheelchair access:* Good
Smoking: In designated area
Pets: ✓
Routines: Structured

Room details

Single: 34
Shared: 2
En suite: 36
Facilities: TV point, telephone point

Door lock: ✓
Lockable place: ✓

Services provided

Beauty services: Hairdressing, aromatherapy, manicures
Mobile library: Library facilities
Religious services: ✗
Transport: ✗
Activities: *Coordinator:* ✗ • *Examples:* Knitting, films, music and movement, quizzes, bingo • *Outings:* ✓
Meetings: ✓

Anchorstone Services Ltd

Manager: Esperanza Bevan
Owner: Anchorstone Services Ltd
Contact: 8–10a Searle Road, Farnham, Surrey GU9 8LJ
✆ 01252 727378
🖰 www.careatanchorstone.co.uk

Situated 250 yards from the town centre of Farnham, Anchorstone Services Ltd is a well-established care home that provides residents with an array of activities and services. The home boasts a 60ft dining room providing residents an ample communal area for socialising. Although the home provides a structured daily routine, those more physically able are allowed to follow a more flexible schedule to suit their needs. Anchorstone provides residents with a range of yearly activities, which include reminiscence, hairdressing, outings, and a visiting clothes shop. The home also provides an in-house library for residents to enjoy.

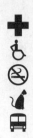

Arbrook House

Manager: Keena Millar
Owner: BUPA Care Homes Ltd
Contact: 36 Copsem Lane,
Esher, Surrey KT10 9HE
☎ 01372 468246
@ millark@bupa.com
🖱 www.bupacarehomes.co.uk

Arbrook House is located near Esher town centre and Claremont Landscaped Gardens. The home itself is situated in its own landscaped grounds with its own lake. The home prides itself on its comfortable and relaxed atmosphere. Much effort has been put into providing residents with areas representing the past including collections of objects and pictures; there is also much opportunity for reminiscence. Several of the residents take part in a 'super supper' which takes place every Wednesday and gives residents the chance to make a request for their wants and wishes. The home has recently undergone major refurbishment to improve all rooms and facilities.

Registered places: 44
Guide weekly rate: Undisclosed
Specialist care: Nursing, respite
Medical services: Podiatry, hygienist, optician, physiotherapy
Qualified staff: Meets standard

Home details
Location: Residential area, 1 mile from Esher centre
Communal areas: Lounge, dining room, conservatory, hairdressing salon, patio and garden
Accessibility: *Floors:* 2 • *Access:* Lift • *Wheelchair access:* Good
Smoking: ✗
Pets: ✓
Routines: Structured

Room details
Single: 44
Shared: 0
En suite: 44
Facilities: TV point, telephone point

Door lock: ✓
Lockable place: ✓

Services provided
Beauty services: Hairdressing, manicures
Mobile library: ✓
Religious services: Church visits
Transport: ✓
Activities: *Coordinator:* ✓ • *Examples:* Board games, exercise, Pets As Therapy • *Outings:* ✓
Meetings: ✓

Ashley House

Manager: Christine Back
Owner: Penelope McKenna
Contact: Christmas Hill, Kings Road,
Shalford Nr Guildford, Surrey GU4 8HN
☎ 01483 561406

Ashley House is a large detached property on the outskirts of Guildford. The home is set in spacious grounds, accessible to residents. The grounds contain various wildlife, including foxes, badgers and ducks. The residents are mostly over 85 years old and therefore outings and activities cannot be too taxing, so trips to the village and activities such as quizzes and bingo are organised. The home also has visiting entertainers come in regularly. Pets are not allowed to stay but can visit with family and friends.

Registered places: 29
Guide weekly rate: £450–£800
Specialist care: Dementia, physical disability
Medical services: Podiatry, dentist, optician
Qualified staff: Fails standards

Home details
Location: Village location, 3 miles from Guildford centre
Communal areas: 2 lounges, dining room, conservatory, garden
Accessibility: *Floors:* 3 • *Access:* Lift and stair lift *Wheelchair access:* Limited
Smoking: ✗
Pets: ✗
Routines: Flexible

Room details
Single: 17
Shared: 6
En suite: 16
Facilities: TV point

Door lock: ✓
Lockable place: ✓

Services provided
Beauty services: Hairdressing
Mobile library: ✓
Religious services: Communion every 6 weeks, monthly church service
Transport: ✗
Activities: *Coordinator:* ✗ • *Examples:* Bingo, games, quizzes *Outings:* ✓
Meetings: ✗

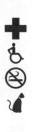

Registered places: 47
Guide weekly rate: Undisclosed
Specialist care: Nursing, dementia, physical disability, respite
Medical services: Podiatry, dentist, optician, physiotherapy
Qualified staff: Meets standard

Home details

Location: Rural area, 4 miles from Guildford
Communal areas: 2 lounges, dining room, hairdressing salon,
physiotherapy room, garden
Accessibility: *Floors:* 3 • *Access:* Lift • *Wheelchair access:* Good
Smoking: ✗
Pets: ✓
Routines: Flexible

Room details

Single: 43
Shared: 2
En suite: Undisclosed
Facilities: TV point, telephone point

Door lock: ✗
Lockable place: ✓

Services provided

Beauty services: Hairdressing
Mobile library: ✓
Religious services: ✓
Transport: ✗
Activities: *Coordinator:* ✓ • *Examples:* Art classes, bingo,
exercise • *Outings:* ✓
Meetings: ✓

Ashley Park Nursing Home

Manager: Ladan French
Owner: BUPA Care Homes Ltd
Contact: The Street, West Clandon,
Guildford, Surrey GU4 7SU
☏ 01483 222296
@ Frenchla@bupa.com
🖰 www.bupacarehomes.co.uk

Set in its own large grounds that run to the nearby golf course, Ashley Park Nursing Home is a detached property set in the village of West Clandon. The home consists of a sun lounge, drawing room, and a large dining room that is the centre of activities. The home offers a hairdressing salon and physiotherapy room for residents. There is a sun gazebo in the grounds for residents to enjoy, particularly in the warmer months. An activities coordinator organises art classes, bingo and exercise sessions for residents.

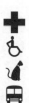

Registered places: 30
Guide weekly rate: £350–£500
Specialist care: Nursing, day care, dementia,
mental disorder, respite
Medical services: Podiatry, dentist, optician, physiotherapy
Qualified staff: Exceeds standard: 100% at NVQ Level 2

Home details

Location: Village location, 2 miles from Redhill
Communal areas: 3 lounges, dining room, conservatory, garden
Accessibility: *Floors:* 3 • *Access:* Lift • *Wheelchair access:* Good
Smoking: In designated area
Pets: ✓
Routines: Flexible

Room details

Single: 20
Shared: 5
En suite: 23
Facilities: TV point, telephone point

Door lock: ✓
Lockable place: ✓

Services provided

Beauty services: Hairdressing, aromatherapy
Mobile library: ✗
Religious services: Monthly Anglican visits
Transport: Minibus
Activities: *Coordinator:* ✗ • *Examples:* Gardening, exercise, cards
Outings: ✓
Meetings: ✓

The Barn House

Manager: Permal Gungaloo
Owner: Permal Gungaloo
Contact: Quality Street,
Merstham, Surrey RH1 3BB
☏ 01737 643273

The Barn House is a detached property in a quiet cul-de-sac in the village of Merstham. It provides care for those with mental health needs or assistance with nursing. The staff organise several social activities throughout the year including summer parties for residents and relatives. With its own minibus, outings are regular occurrences.

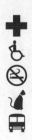

Barrington Lodge Nursing Home

Manager: Veronica Raynor
Owner: London Residential Healthcare Ltd
Contact: 9–15 Morland Road, Croydon, Surrey CR0 6HA
) 020 8654 9136
@ info@lrh-homes.com
⌐ᵇ www.lrh-homes.com

Barrington Lodge Nursing Home is situated in a residential area near to Croydon centre. The home has two lounges, a dining room and a garden with a patio. The home provides services such as hairdressing, a mobile library and a twice-weekly church service. The home has its own activities coordinator who arranges activities such as arts and crafts, board games and exercise sessions. The residents enjoy a flexible daily routine alongside structured meal times. Pets are allowed at the manager's discretion and there is a resident tenant's association.

Registered places: 44
Guide weekly rate: £525–£700
Specialist care: Nursing, physical disability
Medical services: Podiatry, dentist, hygienist, optician, physiotherapy
Qualified staff: Undisclosed

Home details
Location: Urban area, 1.5 miles from Croydon centre
Communal areas: 2 lounges, dining room, patio and garden
Accessibility: *Floors:* 3 • *Access:* Lift • *Wheelchair access:* Good
Smoking: ✗
Pets: At manager's discretion
Routines: Flexible

Room details
Single: 22
Shared: 11
En suite: 0
Facilities: TV

Door lock: ✗
Lockable place: ✗

Services provided
Beauty services: Hairdressing
Mobile library: ✓
Religious services: Fortnightly church service
Transport: ✓
Activities: *Coordinator:* ✓ • *Examples:* Arts and crafts, board games, keep fit • *Outings*
Meetings: ✓

Beaufort Lodge

Manager: Vacant
Owner: CHD Care Homes Ltd
Contact: 38 Beaufort Road, Kingston-upon-Thames, Surrey KT1 2TQ
) 020 8546 2073
@ info@carehomesofdistinction.co.uk
⌐ᵇ www.carehomesofdistinction.co.uk

Beaufort Lodge is situated in a quiet residential street in Surbiton with good access to public transport. As well as holding a church service, the home offers outings to the local church. The home's activities coordinator also arranges exercise sessions, games and visiting entertainers. The residents enjoy a flexible daily routine as well as flexible mealtimes. The home prides itself on its sense of choice and independence. There are visits from a mobile library and the services of a hairdresser are provided.

Registered places: 20
Guide weekly rate: £500–£600
Specialist care: Dementia
Medical services: Podiatry, dentist, hygienist, optician, physiotherapy
Qualified staff: Exceeds standard: 90% at NVQ Level 2

Home details
Location: Residential area, 1 mile from Kingston centre
Communal areas: 2 lounges, dining room, conservatory, garden
Accessibility: *Floors:* 2 • *Access:* Lift • *Wheelchair access:* Good
Smoking: ✗
Pets: At manager's discretion
Routines: Flexible

Room details
Single: 18
Shared: 1
En suite: 3
Facilities: TV, telephone point

Door lock: ✓
Lockable place: ✗

Services provided
Beauty services: Hairdressing, aromatherapy
Mobile library: ✓
Religious services: Church service
Transport: ✗
Activities: *Coordinator:* ✓ • *Examples:* Exercise, games, visiting entertainers • *Outings:* ✓
Meetings: ✓

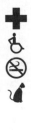

Registered places: 43
Guide weekly rate: £565–£725
Specialist care: Nursing, dementia, respite
Medical services: Podiatry, dentist, optician.
Qualified staff: Fails standard

Home details

Location: Residential are, 0.5 miles from Camberley centre
Communal areas: 2 lounges, dining room, garden
Accessibility: *Floors:* 3 • *Access:* Lift • *Wheelchair access:* Good
Smoking: ✗
Pets: At manager's discretion
Routines: Flexible

Room details

Single: 35
Shared: 4
En suite: 30
Facilities: TV point

Door lock: ✓
Lockable place: ✓

Services provided

Beauty services: Hairdressing, manicures, massage
Mobile library: ✓
Religious services: ✗
Transport: ✗
Activities: *Coordinator:* ✓ • *Examples:* Arts and crafts, outings,
visiting musicians • *Outings:* ✓
Meetings: ✓

Beaumont Lodge Nursing and Residential Home

Manager: Robeen and Indira Roopun
Owner: Indira Roopun
Contact: 19–21 Heatherley Road,
Camberley, Surrey GU15 3LX
☏ 01276 23758
@ rdroopen@hotmail.com
🖥 www.beautmontlodge.com

Situated in a quiet residential area of Camberley, near the local park, amenities and public transport links, Beaumont Lodge is designed to help residents maintain their independence and provide them with a friendly, non-institutional homely atmosphere. The home has well-maintained garden at the front and rear and runs an activities programme with current affairs discussions, a mini casino and cooking as just some examples. Every month, a musician, comedian or visiting entertainer comes to perform for the residents. Included in the weekly fee are manicures and hand massages. On residents' birthdays, relatives are invited for a mini-party.

Registered places: 18
Guide weekly rate: £535
Specialist care: Dementia
Medical services: None
Qualified staff: Exceeds standard: 65% at NVQ Level 2

Home details

Location: Residential area, 1.5 miles from Purley
Communal areas: Lounge/dining room, garden
Accessibility: *Floors:* 2 • *Access:* Lift • *Wheelchair access:* Good
Smoking: ✗
Pets: ✓
Routines: Flexible

Room details

Single: 16
Shared: 0
En suite: 16
Facilities: TV point

Door lock: ✗
Lockable place: ✓

Services provided

Beauty services: Hairdressing
Mobile library: ✓
Religious services: ✓
Transport: ✗
Activities: *Coordinator:* ✗ • *Examples:* Exercise, quizzes,
readings • *Outings:* ✓
Meetings: ✓

Beth Ezra Home

Manager: Janet Brooks
Owner: Beth Ezra Trust
Contact: 52 Smitham Bottom Lane,
Purley, Surrey CR8 3DB
☏ 020 8668 7116

Beth Ezra Home is owned and managed by Beth Ezra Trust, a Christadelphian Community charity. An activities programme is displayed in the lounge and outings are organised every three weeks. There are also regular lunchtime concerts, as well as visits to local National Trust sites. There is a spacious, well-maintained garden with a large summerhouse at the rear of the property with seating areas and ramps for wheelchair users. There is a local village shop opposite the home on the village green and it is only a short distance from the major town of Purley. The home is positioned on the main bus route.

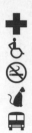

Birtley House Nursing Home

Manager: Jacqueline Sadler
Owner: Eyhurst Court Ltd
Contact: Birtley Road, Bramley, Guildford, Surrey GU5 0LB
) 01483 892055
@ info@birtleyhouse.co.uk
⌂ www.birtleyhouse.co.uk

Birtley House is a family-run nursing home that has been providing care for over 70 years, throughout which the home has stayed within the same family. Lying at the foot of the Surrey Hills, in a designated area of 'outstanding natural beauty', the estate is set in 48 acres of woodland and parkland with country gardens and its own lake. The woods are full of wildlife and birds and are carpeted in bluebells in May. A continuing programme of enhancements to the gardens has resulted in the development of a rose garden and a secret garden with a pergola walk and a new summerhouse.

Registered places: 47
Guide weekly rate: £735–£1,085
Specialist care: Nursing, physical disability
Medical services: Aromatherapy, podiatry, dentist, optician, physiotherapy
Qualified staff: Exceeds standard: 55% at NVQ Level 2

Home details
Location: Rural area, 5 miles from Guildford
Communal areas: Lounge, dining room, garden
Accessibility: *Floors:* 2 • *Access:* Lift • *Wheelchair access:* Good
Smoking: ✗
Pets: ✓
Routines: Flexible

Room details
Single: 41
Shared: 3
En suite: 35
Facilities: TV point, telephone point

Door lock: ✗
Lockable place: ✓

Services provided
Beauty services: Hairdressing
Mobile library: ✗
Religious services: Monthly Communion service
Transport: ✓
Activities: *Coordinator:* ✗ • *Examples:* Arts and crafts, beauty sessions, exercise • *Outings:* ✓
Meetings: ✓

Bourne House Nursing Home

Manager: Paula Gratton
Owner: London Residential Healthcare Ltd
Contact: 45 Langley Avenue, Surbiton, Surrey KT6 6QR
) 020 8399 6022
@ bourne@lrh-homes.com
⌂ www.lrh-homes.com

Situated at the heart of prestigious Southborough conservation area of Royal Borough of Kingston-upon-Thames, the home is near local amenities, pubs, leisure facilities and religious buildings. There are views from all rooms of the conservation area and the residents go on regular outings. The staff aim to create a flexible and pleasant atmosphere for their residents, striving for the best form of care for those suffering from dementia.

Registered places: 40
Guide weekly rate: £619–£800
Specialist care: Nursing, dementia, physically disabled
Medical services: Podiatry, hygienist, occupational therapy, optician, physiotherapy
Qualified staff: Exceeds standard: 95% at NVQ level 2

Home details
Location: Residential area, 1 mile from Surbiton centre
Communal areas: Lounge, dining room, conservatory, garden
Accessibility: *Floors:* 3 • *Access:* Lift • *Wheelchair access:* Good
Smoking: In designated area
Pets: At manager's discretion
Routines: Flexible

Room details
Single: 36
Shared: 2
En suite: 38
Facilities: TV point, telephone

Door lock: ✓
Lockable place: ✓

Services provided
Beauty services: Hairdressing, aromatherapy, manicures
Mobile library: ✗
Religious services: Weekly Catholic clergy visit, regular Anglican Communion service
Transport: ✗
Activities: *Coordinator:* ✓ • *Examples:* Arts and crafts, bingo, karaoke • *Outings:* ✓
Meetings: ✓

Registered places: 23
Guide weekly rate: £500–£550
Specialist care: Day care, dementia, respite
Medical services: Podiatry, dentist, optician, physiotherapy
Qualified staff: Exceeds standard: 75% at NVQ Level 2

Home details

Location: Residential area, close to Guildford centre
Communal areas: Lounge, dining room, conservatory, garden
Accessibility: *Floors:* 3 • *Access:* Stair lifts
    Wheelchair access: None
Smoking: ×
Pets: At manager's discretion
Routines: Flexible

Room details

Single: 15
Shared: 4
En suite: 19
Facilities: TV point, telephone point

Door lock: ✓
Lockable place: ✓

Services provided

Beauty services: Hairdressing
Mobile library: ×
Religious services: Monthly Anglican Service
Transport: ×
Activities: *Coordinator:* × • *Examples:* Board games, poetry,
    exercises • *Outings:* ✓
Meetings: ×

Braemar Court

Manager: Hazel Al-Nakeeb
Owner: Dr and Mrs Al-Nakeeb and
Mr and Mrs Al-Nasrawi
Contact: 16 Sydney Road, Guildford,
Surrey GU1 3LJ
❫ 01483 502828

Braemar House is situated in a residential area close to Guildford town centre. Part of the house has been extended to provide a conservatory at the rear. The home offers a range of activities for all hobbies and tastes. There are poetry clubs and current events discussions. The home also offers outings for those residents who wish to go on shopping trips or to local points of interest. There is a resident cat.

Registered places: 35
Guide weekly rate: £550–£725
Specialist care: Nursing, dementia, physical disability,
    terminal care
Medical services: Podiatry, dentist, optician, physiotherapy
Qualified staff: Exceeds standard: 100% at NVQ Level 2

Home details

Location: Residential area, 1 mile from Wallington centre
Communal areas: Lounge, dining room, conservatory, garden
Accessibility: *Floors:* 3 • *Access:* Lift • *Wheelchair access:* Good
Smoking: ×
Pets: ✓
Routines: Flexible

Room details

Single: 29
Shared: 3
En suite: 17
Facilities: TV point

Door lock: ✓
Lockable place: ×

Services provided

Beauty services: Hairdressing
Mobile library: ×
Religious services: ✓
Transport: ×
Activities: *Coordinator:* ✓ • *Examples:* Cards, scrabble, quizzes
    Outings: ✓
Meetings: ✓

Bridge House Nursing Home

Manager: Patricia Reid
Owner: Ryedowns Ltd
Contact: 280–282 London Road,
Wallington, Surrey SM6 7DJ
❫ 020 8647 8419

Bridge House is located in a quiet residential road in Wallington, about a mile from the centre of town. There is a bus stop on both sides of the road directly outside the home, which goes into Wallington town centre. Beddington Park is opposite the home, where residents go on regular walks, and at the back of the home, the conservatory overlooks a river. There is a small garden with seating. Activities are organised for the residents on a regular basis such as scrabble, cards, bingo and quiz night. This keeps the residents stimulated and socialising with one another.

Brownscombe House Nursing and Residential Home

Manager: Elizabeth McAllister
Owner: Mr Hasham
Contact: Hindhead Road, Haslemere, Surrey GU27 3PL
☎ 01428 643528

Brownscombe House is located outside the village of Haslemere near Guildford. The house boasts a well-maintained garden which slopes up the back of the property so that there is a garden on each level of the home. The garden is frequently used for barbecues and garden parties in the summer. The home is a half-mile walk from Haslemere where there are local shops and amenities, and a 15-minute drive from the centre of Guildford. The home welcome pets and has 'pat-a-pet' once a week, when visitors bring in their animals for the residents to see.

Registered places: 36
Guide weekly rate: £442–£725
Specialist care: Nursing, dementia, sensory impairment
Medical services: Podiatry, optician
Qualified staff: Exceeds standard: 60% at NVQ level 2

Home details
Location: Village location, 0.5 miles from Haslemere
Communal areas: 2 lounges, conservatory/dining room, garden
Accessibility: *Floors:* 3 • *Access:* Lift • *Wheelchair access:* Good
Smoking: ✓
Pets: ✓
Routines: Flexible

Room details
Single: 28
Shared: 4
En suite: 32
Facilities: TV point, telephone point

Door lock: ✗
Lockable place: ✓

Services provided
Beauty services: Hairdressing
Mobile library: ✗
Religious services: Monthly Communion service
Transport: ✗
Activities: *Coordinator:* ✗ • *Examples:* Exercise, garden parties, musical entertainment • *Outings:* ✗
Meetings: ✓

Cambridge House

Manager: Naushad Heeroo
Owner: Naushad and Christine Heeroo
Contact: 141 Gordon Avenue, Camberley, Surrey GU15 2NR
☎ 01276 691035

Cambridge House is situated in a residential area of Camberley, within walking distance from the town centre and the train station. The M3 motorway is close by for commuting visitors from London. Care staff provide an activities programme which includes indoor games and board games as well as beauty therapy. The garden is accessed down a ramp and has seating areas for residents. At the home fluent French is spoken adding to the multi-cultural feel of the home.

Registered places: 16
Guide weekly rate: Undisclosed
Specialist care: Dementia, mental disorder, respite
Medical services: Podiatry, optician
Qualified staff: Exceeds standard: 60% at NVQ Level 2

Home details
Location: Residential area, in Camberley
Communal areas: Lounge, dining room, garden
Accessibility: *Floors:* 2 • *Access:* Lift • *Wheelchair access:* Good
Smoking: In designated area
Pets: At manager's discretion
Routines: Flexible

Room details
Single: 12
Shared: 2
En suite: 0
Facilities: TV point

Door lock: ✗
Lockable place: ✓

Services provided
Beauty services: Hairdressing, manicures
Mobile library: ✗
Religious services: ✗
Transport: ✗
Activities: *Coordinator:* ✗ • *Examples:* Indoor bowling, quizzes, trivial pursuit • *Outings:* ✗
Meetings: ✗

Registered places: 63
Guide weekly rate: £650–£750
Specialist care: Nursing, dementia
Medical services: Podiatry, optician
Qualified staff: Meets standard

Home details

Location: Residential area, 2 miles from Farnborough
Communal areas: Lounge, dining room, garden
Accessibility: *Floors:* 2 • *Access:* Lift • *Wheelchair access:* Good
Smoking: In designated area
Pets: At manager's discretion
Routines: Flexible

Room details

Single: 62
Shared: 1
En suite: 63
Facilities: TV point, telephone point

Door lock: ✗
Lockable place: ✓

Services provided

Beauty services: Hairdressing
Mobile library: ✓
Religious services: ✓
Transport: ✗
Activities: *Coordinator:* ✓ • *Examples:* Bingo, games, gardening
    Outings: ✗
Meetings: ✓

Cedar Lodge Nursing and Residential Home

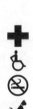

Manager: Jane McAuley
Owner: Forest Care Ltd
Contact: St Catherine's Road, Frimley Green, Camberley, Surrey GU16 6PY
☏ 01420 487732

Cedar Lodge is a purpose-built home, set in its own landscaped gardens and overlooking Frimley Green. Beyond the gardens, the home is surrounded by woodland. The home has a GP surgery within a quarter of a mile. Shop, post office, chemist, library, bank and bus stop all within half a mile's walk. The main shopping centre at Camberley is one mile away. There are facilities for family or friends to stay overnight if they wish which is a great convenience if there is something planned for the next day. There are regular activities planned for the residents by the activities coordinator which includes bingo, boards games, cards and gardening.

Registered places: 37
Guide weekly rate: £550–£850
Specialist care: Nursing, day care, respite
Medical services: Podiatry, dentist, optician, physiotherapy
Qualified staff: Exceeds standard: 97% at NVQ level 2

Home details

Location: Residential area, 2 miles from Sutton centre
Communal areas: 2 lounges, conservatory and garden
Accessibility: *Floors:* 2 • *Access:* Lift • *Wheelchair access:* Good
Smoking: ✗
Pets: At manager's discretion
Routines: Flexible

Room details

Single: 29
Shared: 4
En suite: 7
Facilities: TV point, telephone point

Door lock: ✗
Lockable place: ✗

Services provided

Beauty services: Hairdressing, aromatherapy
Mobile library: ✓
Religious services: Monthly Communion service
Transport: ✗
Activities: *Coordinator:* ✗ • *Examples:* Chairobics, karaoke,
    visiting entertainers • *Outings:* ✓
Meetings: ✓

Chegworth Nursing Home

Manager: Puspavani Barkakaty
Owner: Bayswift Ltd
Contact: 23 Downs Side, Sutton, Surrey SM2 7EH
☏ 020 8642 9453

Situated on a quiet road with access to a bus stop and close to Banstead Downs, Chegworth Nursing Home is a domestic-style property with an extensive activities programme. Although there is currently no designated dining room, tables can be set in the lounge or conservatory. Residents are able to use the garden for their own purposes and one resident has grown herbs and plants there. Activities include chairobics, karaoke and visiting entertainers are arranged. Pets are allowed at the manager's discretion. The home has visits from a mobile library and monthly Communion.

Cherry Lodge Rest Home

Manager: Cherie Callender
Owner: Cherie Callender
Contact: 75 Whyteleafe Road,
Caterham, Surrey CR3 5EJ
) 01883 341471

Cherry Lodge Rest Home is a large detached property located in a quiet residential area of Caterham, located opposite a school, and park called Caterham-on-the-Hill. It is near to public transport links into Caterham town centre. The residents have regular outings arranged for them, including walks, shopping trip and visits to historical sites in the area. Activities in the home include movement to music, singalongs and board games. The staff like to allow residents as much independence as they possibly can, to help them enjoy their freedom.

Registered places: 14
Guide weekly rate: £525–£600
Specialist care: Dementia, physical disability, respite
Medical services: Podiatry, hygienist, optician, physiotherapy
Qualified staff: Fails standard: 40% at NVQ Level 2

Home details
Location: Residential area, in Caterham
Communal areas: Lounge, dining room, garden
Accessibility: *Floors:* 2 • *Access:* Stair lift
   Wheelchair access: Good
Smoking: ✗
Pets: ✗
Routines: Flexible

Room details
Single: 10
Shared: 2
En suite: 6
Facilities: TV point, telephone point

Door lock: ✗
Lockable place: ✓

Services provided
Beauty services: Hairdressing
Mobile library: ✓
Religious services: Monthly church services
Transport: ✗
Activities: *Coordinator:* ✗ • *Examples:* Games, movement to
   music, singalongs • *Outings:* ✓
Meetings: ✓

Cherrydale

Manager: Jean Joyce
Owner: Nightingale Residential Care Home
Contact: Springfield Road,
Camberley, Surrey GU15 1AE
) 01276 682585
@ cherrydale@hotmail.co.uk

Cherrydale Home is set in spacious grounds and gardens, in a residential area close to Camberley. Local amenities are a distance away, but the home has its own car in which to transport residents to shops. Activities and outings are organised, such as a trip on a canal boat. All denomination of religion is welcome; the home aims to accommodate residents needs as much as possible. Pets are welcome and the home currently has a fish tank.

Registered places: 22
Guide weekly rate: £403–£565
Specialist care: Dementia
Medical services: Podiatry, hygienist, optician, physiotherapy
Qualified staff: Meets standard

Home details
Location: Residential area, 1.5 miles from Camberley
Communal areas: 2 lounges, dining room, patio and garden
Accessibility: *Floors:* 3 • *Access:* Lift • *Wheelchair access:* Good
Smoking: ✗
Pets: ✓
Routines: Flexible

Room details
Single: 18
Shared: 2
En suite: 3
Facilities: TV point, telephone point

Door lock: ✗
Lockable place: ✓

Services provided
Beauty services: Hairdressing
Mobile library: ✓
Religious services: Anglican visits
Transport: Car
Activities: *Coordinator:* ✓ • *Examples:* Music and movement,
   board games, visiting entertainers • *Outings:* ✓
Meetings: ✗

Registered places: 60
Guide weekly rate: £565–£720
Specialist care: Nursing, dementia, respite
Medical services: Podiatry, dentist, optician, physiotherapy
Qualified staff: Meets standard

Home details
Location: Village location, in Haslemere
Communal areas: 3 lounges, 3 dining rooms, 2 gardens
Accessibility: *Floors:* 3 • *Access:* Lift • *Wheelchair access:* Good
Smoking: ✗
Pets: ✗
Routines: Flexible

Room details
Single: 60
Shared: 0
En suite: 60
Facilities: TV point

Door lock: ✓
Lockable place: ✓

Services provided
Beauty services: Hairdressing, manicure
Mobile library: ✓
Religious services: ✓
Transport: ✗
Activities: *Coordinator:* ✓ • *Examples:* Bingo, painting, quizzes
   Outings: ✓
Meetings: ✓

Chestnut View Care Home

Manager: Susannah Stanesby
Owner: St Cloud Care Plc
Contact: Lion Green, Haslemere, Surrey GU27 1LD
☎ 01428 652622
@ admin@chestnutview.plus.com
🖰 www.chestnutview.plus.com

Set in private gardens overlooking Lion Green, Chestnut View Care Home is located opposite a leisure centre with many shops and local amenities like a chemist. The home has two gardens and a lounge and dining room on each of the three floors. The home has an activities programme which each resident receives a copy of and includes games and painting. There is a separate one-to-one programme for the dementia patients. The home offers services such as weekly hairdressing and manicures. The residents enjoy a flexible routine with set meal times and the option to have their meals in their room.

Registered places: 32
Guide weekly rate: Undisclosed
Specialist care: Nursing, physical disability, respite
Medical services: Podiatry, dentist, optician, physiotherapy,
   occupational therapy, speech therapy
Qualified staff: Undisclosed

Home details
Location: Urban area, in Walton-on-Thames
Communal areas: 3 lounges, dining room, conservatory, activities
   room, kitchenette, hairdressing salon, patio and garden
Accessibility: *Floors:* 3 • *Access:* Lift • *Wheelchair access:* Good
Smoking: ✗
Pets: ✓
Routines: Flexible

Room details
Single: 29
Shared: 1
En suite: 26
Facilities: TV point

Door lock: ✗
Lockable place: ✓

Services provided
Beauty services: Hairdressing, aromatherapy, manicures
Mobile library: ✓
Religious services: ✓
Transport: Minibus
Activities: *Coordinator:* ✓ • *Examples:* Arts and crafts, exercise,
   reading • *Outings:* ✓
Meetings: ✓

Clare House Nursing Home

Manager: Gilly Podd
Owner: BUPA Care Homes Ltd
Contact: 36 Hersham Road, Walton-on-Thames, Surrey KT12 1JJ
☎ 01932 224881
@ ClareHSEWalton@Bupa.com
🖰 www.bupacarehomes.co.uk

Clare House is a Tudor-style home situated in a residential area of Walton-on-Thames. Formerly a private residence, it retains a homely atmosphere while meeting the needs of elderly residents requiring nursing care. There is also a secluded garden and a new conservatory. Local amenities are within walking distance, and attractions such as Hampton Court and the River Thames are near by. There is a dedicated activities room; Panting, trips to local places of interest and cheese and wine evenings for relatives are among the activities offered.

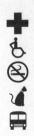

Coppice Lea Care Home

Manager: Norah Davey
Owner: Coppice Lea Ltd
Contact: 151 Bletchingley Road, Merstham, Surrey RH1 3QN
☎ 01737 645117
@ coppicelea@caringhomes.org
🖥 www.caringhomes.org

Set in five acres of wooded grounds this detached Victorian home is in a semi-rural area, on the outskirts of Merstham and Bletchingly, three miles from Redhill. The home prides itself on a high standard of care giving residents the opportunity to get involved in group and individual activities. Residents are taken on frequent outings in shared transportation with another home, such as garden centres. There is a full-time maintenance person and in 2007 the home was refurbished to make room for a conservatory and a further nine rooms. From all of the rooms there is a view of the surrounding wooded and landscaped grounds.

Registered places: 44
Guide weekly rate: £770–£875
Specialist care: Nursing (29), dementia, physically disabled, respite
Medical services: Physiotherapy
Qualified staff: Meets standard

Home details
Location: Village location, 3 miles from Redhill
Communal areas: 2 lounges, dining room, conservatory, garden
Accessibility: *Floors:* 3 • *Access:* 3 lifts
Wheelchair access: Good
Smoking: ✗
Pets: At manager's discretion
Routines: Flexible

Room details
Single: 42   **Door lock:** ✗
Shared: 1   **Lockable place:** ✓
En suite: All
Facilities: TV, telephone

Services provided
Beauty services: Hairdressing, manicures, aromatherapy
Mobile library: ✓
Religious services: Fortnightly Anglican service
Transport: ✓
Activities: *Coordinator:* ✓ • *Examples:* Bingo, carpet bowls, quizzes • *Outings:* ✓
Meetings: ✓

Cossins House Care Home

Manager: Carol Kirby
Owner: Four Seasons Healthcare Ltd
Contact: 1 Downside Road, Downside, Cobham, Surrey KT11 3LZ
☎ 01932 862038
🖥 www.fshc.co.uk

Cossins House is situated in a semi-rural location, around a mile from Cobham centre. Many of the residents of Cossins House are able to care for themselves with minimal assistance. The most independent of the residents live in bungalows in the grounds where pets are allowed to live at manager's discretion. There is a regular monthly inspection carried out by the providers. Residents are taken on outings every other week when a minibus comes for trips to garden centres, local points of interest and for afternoon teas.

Registered places: 24
Guide weekly rate: £690–£780
Specialist care: Respite
Medical services: Podiatry, dentist, optician
Qualified staff: Fails standard: 40% at NVQ Level 2

Home details
Location: Village location, 1 mile from Cobham centre
Communal areas: Lounge, dining room, garden
Accessibility: *Floors:* 2 • *Access:* Lift
Wheelchair access: Limited
Smoking: ✗
Pets: ✗
Routines: Flexible

Room details
Single: 18   **Door lock:** ✓
Shared: 3   **Lockable place:** ✓
En suite: 21
Facilities: TV point, telephone point

Services provided
Beauty services: Hairdressing
Mobile library: ✓
Religious services: Fortnightly Anglican, weekly Catholic services
Transport: ✗
Activities: *Coordinator:* ✓ • *Examples:* Games, keep fit, manicures • *Outings:* ✓
Meetings: ✗

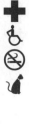

Registered places: 72
Guide weekly rate: £580–£1,165
Specialist care: Nursing, dementia, respite
Medical services: Podiatry, optician, physiotherapy
Qualified staff: Meets standard

Home details

Location: Village location, 3 miles from Woking
Communal areas: 3 lounges, 4 dining rooms,
    conservatory, garden
Accessibility: *Floors:* 3 • *Access:* 2 lifts
    Wheelchair access: Good
Smoking: ✗
Pets: At manager's discretion
Routines: Flexible

Room details

Single: 40   Door lock: ✓
Shared: 18   Lockable place: ✓
En suite: 58
Facilities: TV point, telephone point

Services provided

Beauty services: Hairdressing, massage
Mobile library: ✓
Religious services: Fortnightly Anglican services
Transport: ✗
Activities: *Coordinator:* ✓ • *Examples:* Arts and crafts, crossword,
    musical recitals, poetry club
Meetings: ✓

Coxhill Manor Nursing and Residential Home

Manager: Janet Varndell
Owner: Caring Homes
Contact: Station Road, Chobham,
Woking, Surrey GU24 8AU
☎ 01276 858926
@ matron@coxhillmanor.com
🖰 www.coxhillmanor.com

This Elizabethan Manor House is set in four acres of ground with good views from all the rooms. Coxhill Manor is a quarter of a mile from the nearest local amenities. There is a fishpond in the garden and the home holds annual garden parties as well as buffets throughout the year. The home aims to accommodate residents as much as possible while also keeping them active, a physiotherapist comes into the home twice a week to lead exercise programmes. Meals can be requested at different times and if residents need to visit a dentist or any other local amenities the home will arrange travel. There are also two full time maintenance personnel.

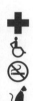

Registered places: 56
Guide weekly rate: £750–£900
Specialist care: Nursing, dementia respite, palliative, physical
    disability, terminal care
Medical services: Podiatry, physiotherapy
Qualified staff: Meets standard

Home details

Location: Village location, 1.5 miles from Warlingham
Communal areas: 2 lounges, 2 dining rooms,
    activities room, garden
Accessibility: *Floors:* 2 • *Access:* Lift • *Wheelchair access:* Good
Smoking: ✗
Pets: ✓
Routines: Structured

Room details

Single: 56   Door lock: ✓
Shared: 0   Lockable place: ✓
En suite: 56
Facilities: TV, telephone point

Services provided

Beauty services: Hairdressing, aromatherapy, manicures
Mobile library: ✗
Religious services: ✗
Transport: Bus
Activities: *Coordinator:* ✓ • *Examples:* Drama, keep fit, painting,
    reading • *Outings:* ✓
Meetings: ✓

Cranmer Court

Manager: Margaret Faulkner-Shotter
Owner: Cranmer Court Ltd
Contact: Farleigh Road, Farleigh
Common, Warlingham,
Surrey CR6 9PE
☎ 01883 627713
🖰 www.caringhomes.org

Cranmer Court is a purpose-built home completed in 2006 and is for those with moderate, severe or complex nursing needs on a short-term or long-term basis. It is located within a conservation area, on the edge of the village of Farleigh, close to Warlingham. The home is constructed from a mellow brick, and there are Romeo and Juliet-inspired balconies on the first floor and patio doors leading out onto terraces with patio gardens on the ground floor. All rooms have a TV with a DVD player so residents can watch a film from the home's DVD library in their room. There is a large garden, with plenty of places for residents to sit. There are a few churches near the home where residents can attend if they wish.

Crann Mor Nursing Home

Manager: Vacant
Owner: Mr and Mrs Emambux
Contact: 151 Old Woking Road, Pyrford, Woking, Surrey GU22 8PD
☏ 01932 344090
@ crannmor@hotmail.com

With ample parking for visitors and gardens to the front and rear of the property, Crann Mor Nursing Home is a detached property situated in a residential area close to Woking town. The home is decorated in a homely style, equipped and maintained to meet the needs of residents. Activities such as games, music entertainment and exercise are also arranged. Although residents are encouraged to participate in activities, they are not obliged to and are free to carry out their own programmes.

Registered places: 24
Guide weekly rate: £650–£750
Specialist care: Nursing, dementia
Medical services: Podiatry, dentist, optician, psychiatrist
Qualified staff: Meets standard

Home details
Location: Residential area, 2 miles from Woking centre
Communal areas: 2 lounges, dining room, garden
Accessibility: *Floors:* 2 • *Access:* Lift • *Wheelchair access:* Good
Smoking: In designated area
Pets: ✗
Routines: Flexible

Room details
Single: 20
Shared: 2
En suite: 0
Facilities: TV point, telephone point

Door lock: ✗
Lockable place: ✓

Services provided
Beauty services: Hairdressing
Mobile library: ✗
Religious services: ✓
Transport: ✗
Activities: *Coordinator:* ✗ • *Examples:* Games, exercise, visiting entertainers • *Outings:* ✗
Meetings: ✓

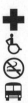

Crispins and Loadhams Nursing Homes

Manager: Angela Ashby
Owner: BUPA Care Homes Ltd
Contact: 43 Waverley Lane, Farnham, Surrey GU9 8BH
☏ 01252 710574
@ CrispinsandLoadhamsEveryone@ BUPA.com
🖰 www.bupacarehomes.co.uk

Crispins and Loadhams Nursing Homes are situated in a quiet residential area. Built as residential properties in the 1920s, the buildings retain many original features and have been sympathetically converted to provide nursing care for older people. The homes' spacious lounge and dining areas overlook two acres of gardens and a small orchard. The home has a varied activities programme; the social calendar includes trips to local places of interest such as Bird World and Kings Pond. Personal interests and hobbies are also encouraged at Crispins and Loadhams.

Registered places: 37
Guide weekly rate: Undisclosed
Specialist care: Nursing, respite
Medical services: Podiatry
Qualified staff: Meets standard

Home details
Location: Residential area, 1 mile from Farnham centre
Communal areas: 2 lounges, dining room, garden
Accessibility: *Floors:* 2 • *Access:* Lift • *Wheelchair access:* Good
Smoking: ✗
Pets: ✗
Routines: Flexible

Room details
Single: 32
Shared: 1
En suite: 26
Facilities: TV point, telephone point

Door lock: ✓
Lockable place: ✗

Services provided
Beauty services: Hairdressing, aromatherapy
Mobile library: ✓
Religious services: Monthly Communion service
Transport: Minibus
Activities: *Coordinator:* ✓ • *Examples:* Arts and crafts, bingo *Outings:* ✓
Meetings: ✗

Registered places: 40
Guide weekly rate: £600–£800
Specialist care: Nursing, dementia
Medical services: Podiatry, hygienist, optician, physiotherapy
Qualified staff: Exceeds standard: 90% at NVQ Level 2

Home details

Location: Residential area, in Sutton
Communal areas: 3 lounges, dining room, patio and garden
Accessibility: *Floors:* 3 • *Access:* 2 lifts
Wheelchair access: Good
Smoking: ✗
Pets: ✗
Routines: Flexible

Room details

Single: 36
Shared: 2
En suite: 19
Facilities: TV point, telephone point

Door lock: ✓
Lockable place: ✓

Services provided

Beauty services: Hairdressing
Mobile library: ✓
Religious services: Monthly Catholic and Anglican service
Transport: ✗
Activities: *Coordinator:* ✓ • *Examples:* Exercises, music,
reminiscence, shows
Meetings: ✓

Crossways Care Nursing Home

Manager: Alison Churchill
Owner: Crossway Nursing Home
Contact: 17 Overton Road, Sutton,
Surrey SM2 6RH
☏ 020 8642 0955
@ crosswaysnursinghome@
hotmail.co.uk

The Crossways is a large Edwardian property on a residential road near Sutton high street. The home has its own surrounding gardens for residents to enjoy, particularly in the summer months. Residents have the option of a birthday celebration where friends and family can attend. Residents are also able to bring personal items including furniture into the home if they wish, which helps form a settled and relaxed environment for the resident. An activities coordinator organises daily programmes for residents that includes exercises, reminiscence and occasional shows.

Registered places: 12
Guide weekly rate: £374–£430
Specialist care: Dementia
Medical services: Podiatry, dentist, optician
Qualified staff: Exceeds standards

Home details

Location: Residential area, in Coulsdon
Communal areas: Lounge, dining room, garden
Accessibility: *Floors:* 2 • *Access:* Lift • *Wheelchair access:* Good
Smoking: In designated area
Pets: At manager's discretion
Routines: Flexible

Room details

Single: 8
Shared: 2
En suite: 1
Facilities: TV point, telephone point

Door lock: ✓
Lockable place: ✓

Services provided

Beauty services: Hairdressing
Mobile library: ✗
Religious service: ✓
Transport: ✗
Activities: *Coordinator:* ✗ • *Examples:* Bingo, quizzes
Outings: ✗
Meetings: ✗

Crystal Residential Home

Manager: Jaisree Nemchand
Owner: Jaisree Nemchand
Contact: 97 Woodcote Grove Road,
Coulsdon, Surrey CR5 2AN
☏ 020 8660 8643

Crystal Residential Home is located in the attractive suburb of Coulsdon, close to Purley. The home does not have an activities coordinator, but staff run various activities such as bingo and quizzes for residents. Communal facilities include a comfortable lounge, dining room and accessible garden.

Dalmuir Home

Manager: Mike Noorbaccus
Owner: Mike Noorbaccus
Contact: 25 Gresham Road,
Limpsfield, Oxted, Surrey RH8 0BU
) 01883 715630
@ mikenoorbaccus@btinternet.com
⌂ www.surreycarehome.co.uk

Dalmuir Home is located in a residential area close to public amenities and other facilities. The home is a three-minute walk from the town centre. The home has a garden which is private and secure with wheelchair access. The home also grows its own vegetables which are used in the residents' meals. There is also a patio area to be enjoyed in summer months. The home has an activities coordinator who arranges reminiscence sessions, exercise and karaoke for the residents. There are also outings for the residents to the theatre. Pets are not allowed in the home but smoking is permitted in a designated area.

Registered places: 16
Guide weekly rate: £575
Specialist care: Nursing, dementia
Medical services: Podiatry, dentist, optician, physiotherapy
Qualified staff: Meets standard

Home details
Location: Residential area, in Oxted
Communal areas: Lounge, dining room, patio and garden
Accessibility: *Floors:* 3 • *Access:* Lift • *Wheelchair access:* Good
Smoking: In designated area
Pets: ✗
Routines: Flexible

Room details
Single: 12
Shared: 2
En suite: Undisclosed
Facilities: TV

Door lock: ✗
Lockable place: ✓

Services provided
Beauty services: Hairdressing
Mobile library: ✗
Religious services: ✓
Transport: ✓
Activities: *Coordinator:* ✓ • *Examples:* arts and crafts, exercise, karaoke • *Outings:* ✓
Meetings: ✓

Deepdene Care Centre

Manager: William Jones
Owner: Life Style Care Plc
Contact: Hill View, Reigate Road,
Dorking, Surrey RH4 1SY
) 01306 732880
@ manager@lifestylecare.co.uk
⌂ www.lifestylecare.co.uk

Deepdene Care Centre is a purpose-built home, ideally located for the facilities of Dorking town. The home is set on three floors, with each floor having a dining room and two lounges. There is a courtyard garden at the back of the home, which is easily accessible to residents. The home is very close to a sports centre, next to a doctor's surgery and close to Dorking Hall. Its location makes it easy for residents to go to the theatre and cinema in the hall.

Registered places: 66
Guide weekly rate: From £795
Specialist care: Nursing, dementia, respite
Medical services: Audiologist, Podiatry, dentist, hygienist, optician
Qualified staff: Meets standard

Home details
Location: Residential area, 0.5 miles from Dorking centre
Communal areas: 6 lounges, 3 dining rooms, garden
Accessibility: *Floors:* 3 • *Access:* 2 lifts
Wheelchair access: Good
Smoking: ✗
Pets: At manager's discretion
Routines: Structured

Room details
Single: 66
Shared: 0
En suite: 66
Facilities: TV point, telephone point

Door lock: ✓
Lockable place: ✓

Services provided
Beauty services: Hairdressing
Mobile library: ✓
Religious services: Monthly church visits
Transport: ✓
Activities: *Coordinator:* ✓ • *Examples:* Arts and crafts, knitting, videos • *Outings:* ✓
Meetings: ✗

Registered places: 32
Guide weekly rate: Undisclosed
Specialist care: Nursing, dementia, palliative care, respite
Support services: Podiatry, occupational therapy, physiotherapy
Qualified staff: Undisclosed

Home details

Location: Rural area, 6.5 miles from Guildford
Communal areas: Lounge, dining room, hairdressing salon,
   activities room, garden
Accessibility: *Floors:* 3 • *Access:* Lift • *Wheelchair access:* Good
Smoking: ✗
Pets: ✗
Routines: Flexible

Room details

Single: 21
Shared: 6
En suite: 18
Facilities: TV, telephone point

Door lock: ✓
Lockable place: ✗

Services provided

Beauty services: Hairdressing, aromatherapy
Mobile library: ✓
Religious services: ✓
Transport: ✓
Activities: *Coordinator:* ✓ • *Examples:* Cooking, flower arranging,
   visiting entertainers • *Outings:* ✓
Meetings: ✗

Dene Place

Manager: Tracy Manzi
Owner: BUPA Care Homes Ltd
Contact: Ripley Lane, West Horsley,
Leatherhead, Surrey KT24 6JW
☎ 01483 282733
@ DenePlaceALL@BUPA.com
🖰 www.bupacarehomes.co.uk

This elegant stucco Queen Anne-style house is set in a nine-acre estate of National Trust countryside near the village of West Horsley, a few minutes' drive from the A3 and M25. Built in 1910, it forms part of the Hatchlands Estate, the family home of Admiral Boscawen. The home retains its original character, including hand-carved fireplaces and decorative friezes. The dining room features graceful columns and garden views. Daily activities are offered, and there is a separate activities room for residents' use. Guest speakers and piano recitals are other popular events. Residents are involved in the local community and enjoy regular visits from local musicians.

Registered places: 31
Guide weekly rate: From £475
Specialist care: Dementia, respite, physical disability
Medical services: Podiatry, dentist, dietician, optician,
   physiotherapy
Qualified staff: Meets standard

Home details

Location: Residential area, 0.5 miles from New Malden centre
Communal areas: 3 lounges, 2 dining rooms, library,
   patio and garden
Accessibility: *Floors:* 3 • *Access:* Lift • *Wheelchair access:* Good
Smoking: In designated area
Pets: ✗
Routines: Flexible

Room details

Single: 31
Shared: 0
En suite: Undisclosed
Facilities: TV point, telephone point

Door lock: ✓
Lockable place: ✓

Services provided

Beauty services: Hairdressing, manicures
Mobile library: Library facilities
Religious services: ✓
Transport: Minibus
Activities: *Coordinator:* ✓ • *Examples:* Arts and crafts, board
   games, exercise • *Outings:* ✓
Meetings: ✓

The Devonshire

Manager: Jean Loughran
Owner: Annar and Abdul Mangalji
Contact: 213 Malden Road,
New Malden, Surrey KT3 6AG
☎ 020 8949 0818
@ Thedevonshire213@aol.com
🖰 www.thedevonshirecarehome.com

The Devonshire is a large detached property situated in easy reach of the A3 and close to New Malden high street, with its shops and local amenities. There is a library at the top of the home, with a wide selection of books with large print. A monthly newsletter is put together by the home and made available to residents, detailing forthcoming events and news. The home offers a range of activities, such as exercise sessions, board games and arts and crafts.

Downs Cottage

Manager: Norma Thomas
Owner: Mr and Mrs Thomas
Contact: 183 Great Tattenhams, Epsom Downs, Epsom, Surrey KT18 5RA
☎ 01737 352632
@ n.thomas@downscottage.co.uk
🖰 www.downscottage.co.uk

Downs Cottage is a property that has been converted and extended over the years, retaining the domestic style and character of the building. Standing in its own extensive grounds, Downs Cottage is close to Epsom Downs racecourse. Tattenham Corner village is within walking distance from the home, which offers local shops, a pleasant pub and train station. A bus route operates through Tattenham Corner, which gives access to Epsom town centre.

Registered places: 23
Guide weekly rate: £500–£650
Specialist care: Nursing, dementia, mental disorder
Medical services: Podiatry, dentist, optician, physiotherapy
Qualified staff: Meets standard

Home details
Location: Residential area, 3 miles from Epsom
Communal areas: Lounge, lounge/dining room, patio and garden
Accessibility: *Floors:* 2 • *Access:* Stair lift
Wheelchair access: Limited
Smoking: ✗
Pets: ✗
Routines: Flexible

Room details
Single: 17
Shared: 3
En suite: 8
Facilities: TV point

Door lock: ✗
Lockable place: ✓

Services provided
Beauty services: Hairdressing
Mobile library: ✓
Religious services: Weekly Communion service
Transport: ✓
Activities: *Coordinator:* ✗ • *Examples:* Exercises, games, music, quizzes • *Outings:* ✗
Meetings: ✓

Dungate Manor Care Home

Manager: Vacant
Owner: Southern Cross Healthcare Ltd
Contact: Flanchford Road, Reigate Heath, Surrey RH2 8QT
☎ 01737 244149
🖰 www.schealthcare.co.uk

Dungate Manor is a large, Edwardian building set in its own five acres of grounds. The home looks out onto the local golf course. The building has been extended to provide additional accommodation. There are many activities for residents and also frequent trips to local garden centres and scenic drives around the countryside. Dietary requirements can be catered for such as vegetarian and low fat.

Registered places: 45
Guide weekly rate: £500–£750
Specialist care: Respite, dementia, mental disorder, physical disability
Medical services: Podiatry, dentist, optician, physiotherapy
Qualified staff: Meets standard

Home details
Location: Rural area, 1.5 miles from Reigate
Communal areas: 2 lounges, dining room, conservatory, patio and garden
Accessibility: *Floors:* 2 • *Access:* 2 lifts
Wheelchair access: Good
Smoking: In designated area
Pets: At manager's discretion
Routines: Flexible

Room details
Single: 38
Shared: 2
En suite: Undisclosed
Facilities: TV point, telephone point

Door lock: ✓
Lockable place: ✓

Services provided
Beauty services: Hairdressing
Mobile library: ✓
Religious services: Monthly Anglican service
Transport: ✗
Activities: *Coordinator:* ✓ • *Examples:* Entertainers, games, painting, music • *Outings:* ✓
Meetings: ✓

Registered places: 33
Guide weekly rate: Undisclosed
Specialist care: Nursing, respite
Medical services: Podiatry, physiotherapy, occupational therapy
Qualified staff: Meets standard

Home details

Location: Village location, 5 miles from Guildford
Communal areas: Lounge, quiet lounge, dining room, hairdressing salon, garden
Accessibility: *Floors:* 2 • *Access:* Lift • *Wheelchair access:* Good
Smoking: In designated area
Pets: ✓
Routines: Flexible

Room details

Single: 24
Shared: 2
En suite: 22
Facilities: TV point, telephone point

Door lock: ✓
Lockable place: ✗

Services provided

Beauty services: Hairdressing, aromatherapy
Mobile library: ✓
Religious services: ✓
Transport: ✓
Activities: *Coordinator:* ✓ • *Examples:* Flower arranging, cooking, arts and crafts, quizzes • *Outings:* ✓
Meetings: ✗

Eastbury Manor

Manager: Jane Marquis
Owner: BUPA Care Homes Ltd
Contact: The Street, Compton, Guildford, Surrey GU3 1EE
☎ 01483 810346
@ EastburyManorALL@BUPA.com
🖥 www.bupacarehomes.co.uk

Eastbury Manor is a country house in the heart of the village of Compton, near Guildford. It is surrounded by cedar trees, extensive lawns and a picturesque lake, and residents regularly attend the 14th-century church next door. This home retains many original features including an ornate oak staircase, wood panelled reception rooms and large stone mullioned windows. The home is very involved in the local community, and hosts annual events in its grounds for the whole village. Popular trips include garden centres and afternoon teas, while a quiet lounge and library are available for those who prefer to read or catch up on correspondence.

Registered places: 14
Guide weekly rate: £410–£450
Specialist care: Dementia
Medical services: Podiatry, dentist, hygienist, optician, physiotherapy
Qualified staff: Exceeds standard: 60% at NVQ Level 2

Home details

Location: Village location, 2 miles from Woking centre
Communal areas: Lounge, dining room, conservatory, garden
Accessibility: *Floors:* 2 • *Access:* Lift • *Wheelchair access:* None
Smoking: ✗
Pets: ✗
Routines: Flexible

Room details

Single: 12
Shared: 1
En suite: 0
Facilities: TV point, telephone point

Door lock: ✓
Lockable place: ✗

Services provided

Beauty services: Hairdressing
Mobile library: Library facilities
Religious services: Fortnightly church service
Transport: ✗
Activities: *Coordinator:* ✗ • *Examples:* Singing • *Outings:* ✓
Meetings: ✓

Elmbank Residential Care Home

Manager: Chinder Saggu
Owner: Elmbank Residential Care Home Ltd
Contact: Woodham Road, Woking, Surrey GU21 4EN
☎ 01483 765984
@ elmb4nk@hotmail.co.uk

Elmbank is a detached property in a residential area of Woking. Services such as hairdressing and a fortnightly church service are available and the home arranges outings for its residents. The home has two floors with a lift but is unable to accommodate wheelchairs. The home has a lounge, a dining room, a conservatory and a garden and its own library facilities. The residents have a flexible daily routine and can choose when they have their mealtimes. There is no activities coordinator, but staff arrange activities such as singing and organise outings.

Elmfield House

Manager: Linda Marsh
Owner: Alex Findlay and Linda Marsh
Contact: Church Lane, Bisley,
Surrey GU24 9ED
- 01483 489522
- @ elmfieldhouse@hotmail.com
- www.elmfieldhouse.com

Elmfield House is located on the village green in Bisley and is a large detached property, which has been modified to provide suitable accommodation for its residents. A selection of shops, the village post office and a public house are close to the home in the village. The home is situated between the towns of Woking and Camberley. Each of the rooms is single occupancy and has en suite facilities. Staff aim to create a 'home from home' feel and arrange daily activities such as bingo, movies, a crossword afternoon and exercise sessions.

Registered places: 10
Guide weekly rate: £520
Specialist care: Dementia, mental disorder
Medical services: Podiatry, dentist, optician
Qualified staff: Meets standard

Home details
Location: Village location of Bisley, 4 miles from Woking
Communal areas: Lounge, dining room, conservatory, garden
Accessibility: *Floors:* 2 • *Access:* Stair lift
    Wheelchair access: Limited
Smoking: ✗
Pets: ✗
Routines: Flexible

Room details
Single: 10
Shared: 0
En suite: 10
Facilities: TV, telephone

Door lock: ✓
Lockable place: ✓

Services provided
Beauty services: Hairdressing, manicures
Mobile library: ✗
Religious services: ✗
Transport: ✗
Activities: *Coordinator:* ✗ • *Examples:* Bingo, games, movies, pottery • *Outings:* ✗
Meetings: ✓

The Elms Nursing Home

Manager: Michael Faulkner
Owner: Dr and Mrs David
Contact: The Whitepost Health Care Centre, Ranelagh Road, Redhill, Surrey RH1 6YY
- 01737 764664

The Elms Nursing Home is situated in a residential road in Redhill and is in the same site as another home separated from The Elms by internal doors. The home overlooks Redhill Park, where mobile residents often go for walks accompanied by a carer. The activities coordinator organises flower arranging, arts and crafts and games evening for those residents who would like to take part. The home caters for a variety of residents including those suffering with Alzheimer's, dementia, EMI, Huntington's chorea, mental illness, physical disability, visual impairment and old age.

Registered places: 49
Guide weekly rate: £550–£750
Specialist care: Nursing, dementia, mental illness, physical disability, respite
Medical services: Podiatry, dentist, optician, physiotherapy
Qualified staff: Exceeds standard: 65% at NVQ Level 2

Home details
Location: Residential area, in Redhill
Communal areas: Lounge, dining room, garden, conservatory
Accessibility: *Floors:* 2 • *Access:* Lift • *Wheelchair access:* Good
Smoking: In designated area
Pets: ✗
Routines: Flexible

Room details
Single: 27
Shared: 11
En suite: 10
Facilities: TV point, telephone point

Door lock: ✗
Lockable place: ✓

Services provided
Beauty services: Hairdressing
Mobile library: ✓
Religious services: ✓
Transport: ✓
Activities: *Coordinator:* ✓ • *Examples:* Arts and crafts, flower arranging • *Outings:* ✓
Meetings: ✗

Registered places: 10
Guide weekly rate: £500–£550
Specialist care: Dementia, respite
Medical services: Podiatry, dentist, physiotherapy
Qualified staff: Meets standard

Home details
Location: Residential area, 0.5 miles to Epsom centre
Communal areas: Lounges, dining room, patio and garden
Accessibility: *Floors:* 2 • *Access:* Lift • *Wheelchair access:* Good
Smoking: ✗
Pets: At manager's discretion
Routines: Flexible

Room details
Single: 8
Shared: 1
En suite: 3
Facilities: TV point, telephone point

Door lock: ✓
Lockable place: ✓

Services provided
Beauty services: Hairdressing
Mobile library: ✗
Religious services: Monthly Communion service
Transport: ✗
Activities: *Coordinator:* ✓ • *Examples:* Flower arranging, model
    making, music • *Outings:* ✗
Meetings: ✓

Epsom Lodge

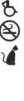

Manager: Helen Pugh
Owner: Kevin Middleton and
Ninawatie Seepaul
Contact: Burgh Heath Road, Epsom,
Surrey KT17 4LW
☏ 01372 724722

Epsom Lodge is a large, detached house with a landscaped garden at the rear for residents' use. The garden has an attractive seating area where residents can congregate and enjoy the warmer months. The home is approximately half a mile from Epsom town centre which offers a range of amenities such as a large shopping centre, restaurants, pubs and parks. Epsom also has extensive transport links with various bus routes and a train station.

Registered places: 32
Guide weekly rate: £665
Specialist care: Respite
Medical services: Podiatry, dentist, optician, physiotherapy
Qualified staff: Undisclosed

Home details
Location: Urban area, 1 mile from Reigate centre
Communal areas: 3 lounges, dining room, garden
Accessibility: *Floors:* 3 • *Access:* Lift • *Wheelchair access:* Good
Smoking: ✗
Pets: ✗
Routines: Flexible

Room details
Single: 32
Shared: 0
En suite: 32
Facilities: TV point, telephone point

Door lock: ✗
Lockable place: ✓

Services provided
Beauty services: Hairdressing
Mobile library: ✓
Religious services: ✓
Transport: Minibus
Activities: *Coordinator:* ✓ • *Examples:* Bingo, board games,
    music • *Outings:* ✓
Meetings: ✓

Eversfield Care Home

Manager: Ann Reid
Owner: Elizabeth Finn Homes Ltd
Contact: 56 Reigate Road, Reigate,
Surrey RH2 0QP
☏ 01737 229899
🖳 www.elizabethfinntrust.org.uk

Eversfield Care Home is situated close to Reigate town centre. Residents are encouraged to lead independent lives, and the home has good links with the local community. A group of local people work with the activities coordinator arranging events and outings for residents. There is a generous garden that is well kept. The home is close to local amenities such as shops, post office, library, pubs and local transport links. The staff aim to create a warm and welcoming environment for residents to enjoy. Visitors are welcomed at any time and may bring pets if they wish, though no animals are allowed to stay in the home.

Fermoyle House Nursing Home

Manager: Angela Partridge
Owner: Pinebird Ventures Ltd
Contact: 121–125 Church Road,
Addlestone, Surrey KT15 1SH
✆ 01932 849023
@ Graham.samuel@talk21.com

Situated in a residential area, Fermoyle House is within easy access to local bus services. The home provides hairdressing and manicures for residents on a regular basis, and a range of activities for them to enjoy. These include community visits, musical entertainment, hand massages and singalongs. Staff aim to create a warm, friendly and relaxed environment for residents to enjoy.

Registered places: 32
Guide weekly rate: £500–£650
Specialist care: Nursing
Medical services: Podiatry, hygienist, optician
Qualified staff: Meets standard

Home details
Location: Residential area, in Addlestone
Communal areas: 2 lounges, dining room, garden
Accessibility: *Floors:* 2 • *Access:* Lift • *Wheelchair access:* Good
Smoking: ✗
Pets: ✗
Routines: Flexible

Room details
Single: 21
Shared: 4
En suite: 0
Facilities: TV point, telephone point

Door lock: ✓
Lockable place: ✗

Services provided
Beauty services: Hairdressing, manicures
Mobile library: ✗
Religious services: ✓
Transport: ✗
Activities: *Coordinator:* ✗ • *Examples:* Community visits, musical entertainment, singalongs • *Outings:* ✓
Meetings: ✗

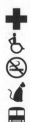

Fieldway Nursing and Residential Centre

Manager: Isabella Mackenzie
Owner: BUPA Care Homes Ltd
Contact: 40 Tramway Path, Mitcham,
Surrey CR4 4SJ
✆ 020 8648 3435
@ FieldwayEveryone@BUPA.com
🖳 www.bupacarehomes.co.uk

Fieldway is situated close to the town of Mitcham and is a purpose-built nursing and residential home providing care for elderly residents with a range of needs including dementia. All of the bedrooms are single occupancy and have en suite facilities and satellite TV; some have views out onto the home's landscaped gardens. Activities play an important part of life at Fieldway; the homes activities coordinator ensures a stimulating and enjoyable programme that includes afternoon reminiscence therapy sessions, singalongs with local entertainers and trips to nearby cafés for afternoon tea.

Registered places: 68
Guide weekly rate: Undisclosed
Specialist care: Nursing, dementia, palliative care, physical disability, terminal care, respite
Medical services: Podiatry, hygienist, optician, physiotherapy
Qualified staff: Meets standard

Home details
Location: Residential area, 1 mile from Mitcham centre
Communal areas: 4 lounges, 2 dining rooms, garden
Accessibility: *Floors:* 2 • *Access:* 2 lifts
Wheelchair access: Good
Smoking: ✗
Pets: ✓
Routines: Flexible

Room details
Single: 68
Shared: 0
En suite: 68
Facilities: TV, telephone point

Door lock: ✓
Lockable place: ✓

Services provided
Beauty services: Hairdressing, aromatherapy
Mobile library: ✓
Religious services: ✓
Transport: ✓
Activities: *Coordinator:* ✓ • *Examples:* Arts and crafts, exercise to music, skittles, reminiscence • *Outings:* ✓
Meetings: ✗

Registered places: 9
Guide weekly rate: £397–£440
Specialist care: Day care, respite
Medical services: Podiatry, hygienist, optician, physiotherapy
Qualified staff: Exceeds standard: 60% at NVQ Level 2

Home details

Location: Residential area, in Wallington
Communal areas: Lounge, dining room, patio and garden
Accessibility: *Floors:* 2 • *Access:* Stair lift
   Wheelchair access: Limited
Smoking: ✗
Pets: ✗
Routines: Flexible

Room details

Single: 1   Door lock: ✗
Shared: 4   Lockable place: ✓
En suite: 0
Facilities: TV point, telephone point

Services provided

Beauty services: Hairdressing
Mobile library: ✓
Religious services: Weekly church visits
Transport: Minibus
Activities: *Coordinator:* ✓ • *Examples:* Bingo, exercises, quizzes
   Outings: ✗
Meetings: ✓

Gable Lodge

Manager: June Wallace
Owner: June Wallace
Contact: 66 Beddington Gardens,
Carshalton, Surrey SM5 3HL
　☏ 020 8669 5513

Gable Lodge home is based in Carshalton, Surrey on a quiet residential road. It is a five-minute stroll for Wallington town centre, which has all needed amenities. The residents have their transport arranged by the carers in the home, and the owner's transport is used to drop and collect residents if they leave the home. The home has a large, rear, well-kept garden, with shrubs and a fishpond which is much enjoyed by residents in summer months.

Registered places: 15
Guide weekly rate: £500–£570
Specialist care: Day care, dementia, respite
Medical services: Podiatry, dentist, optician, physiotherapy
Qualified staff: Undisclosed

Home details

Location: Residential area, 2 miles from Esher centre
Communal areas: 2 lounges, dining room, conservatory, garden
Accessibility: *Floors:* 2 • *Access:* Lift • *Wheelchair access:* Good
Smoking: In designated area
Pets: ✗
Routines: Flexible

Room details

Single: 11   Door lock: ✗
Shared: 2   Lockable place: ✗
En suite: 9
Facilities: TV point

Services provided

Beauty services: Hairdressing, manicures
Mobile library: ✗
Religious services: Communion service
Transport: ✗
Activities: *Coordinator:* ✗ • *Examples:* Bingo, gardening, music
   for health • *Outings:* ✓
Meetings: ✓

Grace Lodge

Manager: Lopa Thakur
Owner: Grace Bridge Ltd
Contact: 4 Manor Road South, Hinchley Wood, Esher, Surrey KT10 0QL
　☏ 020 8398 0580
　@ thakur@gracelodge.freeserve.co.uk

Grace Lodge is a detached property located approximately two miles from Esher town centre. The property provides two sitting rooms, conservatory and dining room. The home has a mature garden, which surrounds the rear of the house. There is no designated activities coordinator, but staff ensure that residents keep active and take them shopping into Esher town. They also organise in-house activities such as games, gardening and exercises.

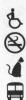

The Grange Chertsey

Manager: Diana McWilliam
Owner: The Grange Chertsey Ltd
Contact: Ruxbury Road, St Anne's Hill, Chertsey, Surrey KT16 9EP
) 01932 562361

The Grange Chertsey is a large detached property set in a spacious private garden. The home does not go on outings as the residents are too frail, but entertainers and small trips for shopping or afternoon teas are organised. The home can offer religious services if requested and there is a resident parrot.

Registered places: 61
Guide weekly rate: £545–£750
Specialist care: Day care, dementia, sensory impairment,
Medical services: Podiatry, dentist, optician
Qualified staff: Meets standard

Home details
Location: Residential area, in Chertsey
Communal areas: 2 lounges, 2 dining rooms, conservatory, garden
Accessibility: *Floors:* 2 • *Access:* Lift • *Wheelchair access:* Good
Smoking: ✗
Pets: At manager's discretion
Routines: Flexible

Room details
Single: 61	**Door lock:** ✓
Shared: 0	**Lockable place:** ✓
En suite: 61	

Facilities: TV point, telephone point

Services provided
Beauty services: Hairdressing
Mobile library: ✓
Religious services: ✗
Transport: Car
Activities: *Coordinator:* ✗ • *Examples:* Bingo, music, quizzes • *Outings:* ✗
Meetings: ✓

The Grange Nursing Home

Manager: Helena Grafton
Owner: Mr Baily
Contact: 22 Grange Road, New Haw, Addlestone, Surrey KT15 3RQ
) 01932 344940

The Grange Nursing Home is a family-run home close to Addlestone town centre in New Haw. There is a bus service to the town. The home cares for 24 residents and offers nursing care. There is a lounge, a dining room and a garden with a patio area. The home has a flexible daily routine and an activities coordinator organises chair-based activities for the residents. Each room in the home has a call system and a TV can be arranged. The home arranges for a mobile library to visit and religious services are available.

Registered places: 24
Guide weekly rate: £500
Specialist care: Nursing, dementia
Medical services: Podiatry, dentist, optician
Qualified staff: Fails standards

Home details
Location: Residential area, 2 miles from Addlestone centre
Communal areas: Lounge, dining room, patio and garden
Accessibility: *Floors:* 2 • *Access:* Lift • *Wheelchair access:* Good
Smoking: ✗
Pets: ✗
Routines: Flexible

Room details
Single: 14	**Door lock:** ✗
Shared: 5	**Lockable place:** ✗
En suite: 0	

Facilities: TV

Services provided
Beauty services: Hairdressing, manicures
Mobile library: ✓
Religious services: ✓
Transport: ✗
Activities: *Coordinator:* ✓ • *Examples:* Chair-based activities *Outings:* ✗
Meetings: ✗

Registered places: 25
Guide weekly rate: Up to £568
Specialist care: Respite
Medical services: Podiatry, dentist, optician, physiotherapy
Qualified staff: Meets standard

Home details

Location: Residential area, 0.5 miles from Sutton centre
Communal areas: 2 lounges, dining room, patio and garden
Accessibility: *Floors:* 4 • *Access:* Lift • *Wheelchair access:* Good
Smoking: In designated area
Pets: ✓
Routines: Structured

Room details

Single: 25
Shared: 0
En suite: Undisclosed
Facilities: TV point, telephone

Door lock: ✓
Lockable place: ✓

Services provided

Beauty services: Hairdressing, aromatherapy
Mobile library: ✗
Religious services: Church visits
Transport: ✗
Activities: *Coordinator:* ✗ • *Examples:* Exercises, singalongs,
  quizzes, skittles • *Outings:* ✓
Meetings: ✓

Grasmere

Manager: Sandra Sawyer
Owner: Mr and Mrs Nanji
Contact: 49 Grange Road, Sutton,
Surrey SM2 6SY
☎ 020 8642 8612

The original building for Grasmere has been extended over the years and some of the bedrooms open out directly into gardens. Good wheelchair access allows residents to access the garden in suitable weather. The home is within walking distance of shops and public transport. Residents have the opportunity to participate in activities or outings, an example being a trip to London to see the Christmas lights. A wide variety of well-balanced, nutritional food was available for residents, meeting all their dietary needs and preferences.

Registered places: 20
Guide weekly rate: £450–£575
Specialist care: Residential, respite
Medical services: Podiatry, hygienist, optician, physiotherapy
Qualified staff: Exceeds standard: 75% at NVQ Level 2

Home details

Location: Residential area, 1.5 miles from Woking centre
Communal areas: 2 lounges, 2 dining rooms, garden
Accessibility: *Floors:* 2 • *Access:* Lift
  Wheelchair access: Limited
Smoking: ✓
Pets: ✓
Routines: Flexible

Room details

Single: 19
Shared: 1
En suite: 20
Facilities: TV point, telephone point

Door lock: ✓
Lockable place: ✓

Services provided

Beauty services: Hairdressing, aromatherapy, manicures
Mobile library: ✗
Religious services: ✓
Transport: ✓
Activities: *Coordinator:* ✓ • *Examples:* Croquet, singers,
  exercises • *Outings:* ✗
Meetings: ✓

Greys Residential Home Ltd

Manager: Stephen Kennedy
Owner: Greys Residential Home Ltd
Contact: Hook Heath Road,
Woking, Surrey GU22 0JQ
☎ 01483 771523
🖰 www.greysresidential.co.uk

Greys Residential Home is a family-run home located on a quiet residential street in Woking, around one and a half miles from the town centre. There is a large lounge on the ground floor with a period fireplace and a large dining room, whilst on the second floor, there is a smaller lounge and dining area. There is a pleasant garden with a pond and rock garden and seating. All activities organised by the home are detailed in a newsletter, and there is a designated coordinator at the home.

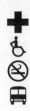

Haldane House Nursing Home

Manager: Margaret Ritchie
Owner: Atkinsons Care Homes
Contact: 127 Yorktown Road,
Sandhurst, Camberley, Surrey
GU47 9BW

☎ 01252 872218
@ diana@atkinsonshomes.com
🖰 www.atkinsonshomes.com

Haldane House is a large, converted, detached residence situated on a main road in Sandhurst. Staff often take residents out for a walk to the local shops, the coffee shop or to the park. Though pets are unable to stay at the home they can visit and religious service can be arranged on request. There is a wide variety of activities for residents such as football and dancing for the more active or board games for those wanting a restful time. Residents' meetings are held twice annually.

Registered places: 25
Guide weekly rate: From £850
Specialist care: Nursing, dementia, physical disability
Medical services: Podiatry, dentist, optician, physiotherapy
Qualified staff: Exceeds standard: 73% at NVQ Level 2

Home details
Location: Residential area, in Sandhurst
Communal areas: Lounge, dining room, patio and garden
Accessibility: *Floors:* 3 • *Access:* Stair lift
   Wheelchair access: Good
Smoking: ✗
Pets: ✗
Routines: Flexible

Room details
Single: 5
Shared: 10
En suite: 6
Facilities: TV point

Door lock: ✗
Lockable place: ✓

Services provided
Beauty services: Hairdressing
Mobile library: ✗
Religious services: ✗
Transport: Minibus
Activities: *Coordinator:* ✓ • *Examples:* Bingo, painting, singing
   Outings: ✓
Meetings: ✓

Hatch Mill

Manager: Tracey Scurr
Owner: Abbeyfield Society Ltd
Contact: Mike Hawthorn Drive,
Farnham, Surrey GU9 8AS

☎ 01252 899000
@ hatchmill@ukonline.co.uk

Completed in 2005, Hatch Mill incorporates the remains of an old mill which was built on the River Way. It is close to the town centre at Farnham where there is an abundance of amenities and shops. Residents are encouraged to participate in a range of outings, including trips to the local garden centre, to Southsea and out for picnics. The staff view these as important in keeping the residents motivated and busy, which helps maintain their independence. The home also offers aromatherapy to help keep the residents relaxed and comfortable, and in a positive state of mind.

Registered places: 36
Guide weekly rate: Undisclosed
Specialist care: Dementia, mental disorder, physical disability
Medical services: Undisclosed
Qualified staff: Meets standard

Home details
Location: Residential area, in Farnham
Communal areas: Lounge, dining room, sensory room, garden
Accessibility: *Floors:* 2 • *Access:* Lift
   Wheelchair access
Smoking: In designated area
Pets: At manager's discretion
Routines: Flexible

Room details
Single: 36
Shared: 0
En suite: 36
Facilities: TV point, telephone point

Door lock: ✗
Lockable place: ✓

Services provided
Beauty services: Hairdressing, aromatherapy
Mobile library: ✓
Religious services: ✓
Transport: ✗
Activities: *Coordinator:* ✓ • *Examples:* Cooking, gardening, walks
   Outings: ✓
Meetings: ✓

Registered places: 26
Guide weekly rate: £540–£570
Specialist care: Day care, dementia, respite
Medical services: Podiatry, dentist, optician, physiotherapy
Qualified staff: Exceeds standard: 60% at NVQ Level 2

Home details

Location: Residential area, 1 mile from Weybridge centre
Communal areas: 2 lounges, dining room, garden
Accessibility: *Floors:* 2 • *Access:* Stair lift
 Wheelchair access: Limited
Smoking: ✗
Pets: ✗
Routines: Flexible

Room details

Single: 22   Door lock: ✓
Shared: 2   Lockable place: ✓
En suite: 14
Facilities: TV point

Services provided

Beauty services: Hairdressing
Mobile library: ✓
Religious services: Fortnightly Anglican service
Transport: ✗
Activities: *Coordinator:* ✓ • *Examples:* Board games, card games, music and movement
Meetings: ✓

Heath Lodge

Manager: Marjorie Ladwig
Owner: Surrey Rest Homes Ltd
Contact: St Georges Avenue,
Weybridge, Surrey KT13 0DA
 ☏ 01932 854680
 @ enquiries@surreyresthomesltd.co.uk
 🖰 www.surreyresthomesltd.co.uk

Heath Lodge is a large detached property with a purpose-built extension. It is close to Weybridge station and town centre, on a residential road. It is easily accessed from both the M25 and the A3. The home borders on a large heathland, retaining its own character and is unspoiled. There are many activities organised including a summer barbecue and quiz sessions. Pets are allowed to visit the home, but cannot stay.

Registered places: 23
Guide weekly rate: £410–£500
Specialist care: Respite
Medical services: Podiatry, dentist, optician, physiotherapy
Qualified staff: Exceeds standard: 80% at NVQ Level 2

Home details

Location: Residential area, 0.5 miles from Sutton centre
Communal areas: Lounge, dining room, garden
Accessibility: *Floors:* 2 • *Access:* Stair lift
 Wheelchair access: Limited
Smoking: In designated area
Pets: At manager's discretion
Routines: Flexible

Room details

Single: 21   Door lock: ✓
Shared: 1   Lockable place: ✗
En suite: 3
Facilities: None

Services provided

Beauty services: Hairdressing
Mobile library: ✓
Religious services: ✓
Transport: ✗
Activities: *Coordinator:* ✗ • *Examples:* Exercise, quizzes, visiting entertainers
Meetings: ✓

Heatherbank

Manager: Hazel Hawkins
Owner: Adrian Hawkins
Contact: 7–9 Cavendish Road,
Sutton, Surrey SM2 5EY
 ☏ 020 8642 2930
 @ Hazel_hawkins@hotmail.com

Heatherbank is situated in a quiet residential area near Sutton town centre and has good travel links by both bus and train. Residents are encouraged to maintain good contact with friends and relatives, as well as the local community. The home has residents' meetings every three months and residents' opinions are top priority, for example with regards to pets the residents would be given the opportunity to vote on the matter. The home has some activities such as visiting entertainers and reminiscence sessions but the home allows residents to spend their day as they choose, allowing for a flexible daily routine.

Hill Brow

Manager: Elizabeth Butt
Owner: Woodlands and Hill Brow Ltd
Contact: Beacon Hill Road, Ewshot, Farnham, Surrey GU10 5DB

☎ 01252 851011
@ info@woodlands-hillbrow.co.uk
🖳 www.woodlands-hillbrow.co.uk

Hill Brow is set in well-kept grounds, where residents can enjoy the scenery and wildlife. The home is located two and a half miles from Farnham town centre, between Farnham and Fleet. The home is family run and aims to encourage independence for as long as possible. Residents regularly go on outings to the local garden centre and pub. There are a variety of activities that include armchair exercises and art classes. The home has 29 rooms but some of these can be used as a double for a married couple. All of the rooms have en suite facilities.

Registered places: 32
Guide weekly rate: £525–£650
Specialist care: Day care, dementia, respite
Medical services: Podiatry, dentist, optician, physiotherapy
Qualified staff: Exceeds standard: 80% at NVQ Level 2

Home details
Location: Village location, 2.5 miles from Farnham centre
Communal areas: Lounge, dining room, patio and garden
Accessibility: *Floors:* 2 • *Access:* Lift • *Wheelchair access:* Good
Smoking: In designated area
Pets: ✓
Routines: Flexible

Room details
Single: 29
Shared: 0
En suite: 29
Facilities: TV, telephone

Door lock: ✓
Lockable place: ✓

Services provided
Beauty services: Hairdressing, manicures
Mobile library: ✓
Religious services: Monthly Communion service
Transport: ✓
Activities: *Coordinator:* ✓ • *Examples:* Art classes, exercises, scrabble • *Outings:* ✓
Meetings: ✓

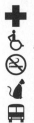

Hill House Nursing Home

Manager: Elana Follwell
Owner: Hill House Nursing Home Ltd
Contact: 48–50 Park Road, Kenley, Surrey CR8 5AR

☎ 020 8660 9336

Hill House Nursing Home is situated in a residential area, approximately one mile from Purley and its amenities. The home has a spacious front garden and enclosed courtyard to the rear of the property. The home also has its own library and hairdressing salon for the residents use. The activities coordinator ensures that the activities available are extensive and stimulating for the residents. Activities can include art therapy and visits from local entertainers.

Registered places: 65
Guide weekly rate: £600–£950
Specialist care: Nursing, day care, respite, terminal care
Medical services: Dentist, optician, Podiatry
Qualified staff: Exceeds standard: 80% at NVQ Level 2

Home details
Location: Residential area, 1 mile from Purley
Communal areas: 3 lounges, 2 dining room, conservatory, hairdressing salon, library, patio and garden
Accessibility: *Floors:* 3 • *Access:* 2 lifts *Wheelchair access:* Good
Smoking: ✗
Pets: At manager's discretion
Routines: Flexible

Room details
Single: 35
Shared: 15
En suite: 30
Facilities: TV point, telephone point

Door lock: ✓
Lockable place: ✓

Services provided
Beauty services: Hairdressing, alternative therapies, manicures
Mobile library: Library facilities
Religious services: Weekly Anglican and Catholic services
Transport: Minibus
Activities: *Coordinator:* ✓ • *Examples:* Arts and crafts, games, music, quizzes • *Outings:* ✓
Meetings: ✓

Registered places: 48
Guide weekly rate: £750–£850
Specialist care: Nursing, dementia, mental disorder
Medical services: Podiatry, dentist, optician, physiotherapy
Qualified staff: Exceeds standard: 90% at NVQ Level 2

Home details
Location: Residential area, in Tadworth
Communal areas: Lounge, dining room/conservatory,
    patio and garden
Accessibility: *Floors:* 2 • *Access:* Lift • *Wheelchair access:* Good
Smoking: In designated area
Pets: ✓
Routines: Flexible

Room details
Single: 37
Shared: 7
En suite: 44
Facilities: TV point, telephone point

Door lock: ✗
Lockable place: ✗

Services provided
Beauty services: Hairdressing
Mobile library: ✓
Religious services: ✓
Transport: ✓
Activities: *Coordinator:* ✓ • *Examples:* Arts and crafts,
    country walks, gardening • *Outings:* ✗
Meetings: ✗

Holmwood Nursing Home

Manager: Urmila Kumar
Owner: Robert Kibble
Contact: 53 The Avenue,
Tadworth, Surrey KT20 5DB
☏ 01737 217 000
@ info@homlwoodnursinghome.co.uk
🖰 www.holmwoodnursinghome.co.uk

Holmwood Nursing Home is situated in the heart of Tadworth, five minutes from the station and has very easy access from junction 8 of the M25. The home is set in an acre of land, which has picturesque landscaped gardens, decking areas, seating and a small fountain and fishpond. The home employs an occupational therapist who supervises a varied social calendar and library books, newspapers and magazines are all available every day. Activities include walks around the grounds, arts and crafts, gentle exercise to music classes and bingo. The conservatory boasts lovely views onto the grounds and is fully air-conditioned.

Registered places: 19
Guide weekly rate: Up to £475
Specialist care: Dementia, respite
Medical services: Podiatry
Qualified staff: Exceeds standard: 100% at NVQ level 2

Home details
Location: Residential area, 0.5 miles from Epsom centre
Communal areas: 2 lounges, dining room, garden
Accessibility: *Floors:* 2 • *Access:* Stair lift
    Wheelchair access: Limited
Smoking: ✗
Pets: At manager's discretion
Routines: Flexible

Room details
Single: 9
Shared: 5
En suite: 1
Facilities: TV point

Door lock: ✓
Lockable place: ✓

Services provided
Beauty services: Hairdressing
Mobile library: ✗
Religious services: ✗
Transport: ✗
Activities: *Coordinator:* ✗ • *Examples:* Bingo, cards • *Outings:* ✗
Meetings: ✗

Homelea

Manager: Mary Oozeerally
Owner: Kaltan Ltd
Contact: 68 Worple Road, Epsom,
Surrey KT18 7AG
☏ 01372 740730

Homelea is a large, detached property which has easy access to Epsom town centre. Contact with family and friends is encouraged and residents are able to have visitors in the privacy of their own room. The home exceeds government standards, with its entire staff trained at NVQ level two.

Horsell Lodge

Manager: Jane Manion
Owner: Caring Home Group Ltd
Contact: Kettlewell Hill, Horsell, Woking, Surrey GU21 4JA

- 01483 760706
- @ admin@caringhomegroup.org
- www.caringhomegroup.org

Horsell Lodge, a large, detached manor house, is found close to Horsell village, not far from Woking. Therapists are brought in from outside the home and the residents can book physiotherapy sessions. There is a garden terrace with summerhouse for use in warmer months. There is ample communal space, with tea lounges, a designated smoking room and a visitors lounge for residents to entertain guests. Trips into the village and many activities including 'seniorcise', skittles, and a reminiscence quiz are also available.

Registered places: 46
Guide weekly rate: From £365
Specialist care: Dementia, physically disabled, mental disorder, respite
Medical services: Podiatry, optician, physiotherapy
Qualified staff: Meets standard

Home details

Location: Residential area, 1 mile from Woking
Communal areas: 2 Lounges, dining room, smoking room, dining/visitors room, conservatory, garden
Accessibility: *Floors:* 3 • *Access:* Lift • *Wheelchair access:* Limited
Smoking: In designated area
Pets: At manager's discretion
Routines: Flexible

Room details

Single: 40
Shared: 5
En suite: 27
Facilities: TV point

Door lock: ✓
Lockable place: ✓

Services provided

Beauty services: Hairdressing
Mobile library: ✓
Religious services: Anglican and Catholic clergy visit
Transport: ✗
Activities: *Coordinator:* ✓ • *Examples:* Bingo, exercise classes • *Outings:* ✓
Meetings: ✓

Howards Care Home

Manager: Nicola Crossley
Owner: Greydales Ltd
Contact: 24 Rowtown, Addlestone, Surrey KT15 1EY

- 01932 856665

Howards Care Home is situated in a quiet residential area on the outskirts of Addlestone. The garden is well maintained and has two fishponds and ample garden furniture. The home has its own minibus and regularly goes on outings to Brighton Pier, Sea Life, Harry Ramsden's for lunch, river trips on the Thames, London tours and trips to see the Christmas lights. The home has two resident dogs.

Registered places: 21
Guide weekly rate: £350–£600
Specialist care: Day care, dementia, respite
Medical services: Podiatry, dentist, optician, physiotherapy
Qualified staff: Meets standard

Home details

Location: Residential area, 1 mile from Addlestone
Communal areas: 2 lounges, conservatory/dining room, garden
Accessibility: *Floors:* 2 • *Access:* Lift • *Wheelchair access:* Good
Smoking: ✗
Pets: At manager's discretion
Routines: Flexible

Room details

Single: 19
Shared: 1
En suite: 15
Facilities: TV point, telephone point

Door lock: ✓
Lockable place: ✓

Services provided

Beauty services: Hairdressing
Mobile library: ✓
Religious services: ✗
Transport: Minibus
Activities: *Coordinator:* ✗ • *Examples:* Board games, visiting entertainers • *Outings:* ✓
Meetings: ✗

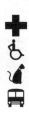

Registered places: 41
Guide weekly rate: From £875
Specialist care: Nursing
Medical services: Podiatry, dentist, optician, physiotherapy
Qualified staff: Exceeds standard: 75% at NVQ level 2

Home details

Location: Village location, 1 mile from Greyshot
Communal areas: 3 lounges, dining room, 2 conservatories, library, garden
Accessibility: *Floors:* 2 • *Access:* Lift • *Wheelchair access:* Good
Smoking: In designated area
Pets: ✓
Routines: Flexible

Room details

Single: 35
Shared: 3
En suite: 33
Facilities: TV, telephone point

Door lock: ✓
Lockable place: ✓

Services provided

Beauty services: Hairdressing
Mobile library: Library facilities
Religious services: Monthly Catholic service
Transport: Minibus
Activities: *Coordinator:* ✓ • *Examples:* Activity sessions, gardening, talks • *Outings:* ✓
Meetings: ✓

Huntington House

Manager: Kate Desmond
Owner: Marilyn Hoare
Contact: Huntington House Drive, Hindhead, Surrey GU26 6BG
☏ 01428 604600
@ kate@bmlhealthcare.co.uk
🖰 www.huntingtonhouse.co.uk

Huntington House is a family-run manor house offering comfortable surroundings with nursing care. Set in 30 acres of National Trust woodland, residents are invited to explore the home's formal gardens. Complimentary drinks and a meal are offered to visitors and an evening pre-dinner drinks trolley circulates daily. Huntington House has a well-advertised activities programme including weekly shopping trips, visiting musicians, knitting club and various outings to, for example, Bluebell Woods, or a nearby winery. Residents enjoy seasonal events, such as champagne with strawberries and cream on Wimbledon final day, a fireworks display for Bonfire night and a Christmas party.

Registered places: 33
Guide weekly rate: £485–£550
Specialist care: Dementia
Medical services: Podiatry, dentist, optician, physiotherapy
Qualified staff: Exceeds standard: 87% at NVQ Level 2

Home details

Location: Residential area, 1 mile from Purley
Communal areas: 3 lounges, dining room, 2 conservatories, 2 gardens
Accessibility: *Floors:* 3 • *Access:* Lift • *Wheelchair access:* Good
Smoking: ✗
Pets: At manager's discretion
Routines: Flexible

Room details

Single: 33
Shared: 0
En suite: 30
Facilities: TV, telephone

Door lock: ✓
Lockable place: ✗

Services provided

Beauty services: Hairdressing, aromatherapy, manicures
Mobile library: ✓
Religious services: ✓
Transport: ✗
Activities: *Coordinator:* ✓ • *Examples:* Chairobics, visiting entertainers • *Outings:* ✓
Meetings: ✓

Ingleside

Manager: Lynne Damaliti
Owner: Nightingale Premier
Contact: 20 Roke Road, Kenley, Surrey CR8 5DY
☏ 020 8660 1253
@ Ingleside.res@btconnect.com

Ingleside is a detached property situated in suburbs of Croydon and 15 minutes by bus from Purley town centre. The home has its own hairdresser and manicures are available every weekend as well as other beauty treatments. There is a mobile library that visits and there are religious services twice a month. The home holds a residents meeting every two months to discuss the activities programme and the upcoming outings. There is also a minimum of one visit a month from an external entertainer. Outings in the past have been to the local church, the pantomime and the garden centre.

James Terry Court

Manager: Diane Collins
Owner: Royal Masonic Benevolent Institution
Contact: 51 Warham Road, South Croydon, Surrey CR2 6LH
) 020 8688 1745
 @ jamesterry@rmbi.org.uk
 ⌂ www.rmbi.org.uk

James Terry Court is owned and run by the Royal Masonic Benevolent Institution and is for freemasons and female dependants of Masonic members. The home offers outings to parks, the theatre and brings in entertainers such as singers and dancers. There are also pantomimes during the winter months. Though pets are not allowed to stay they can visit. There is a bus stop right outside the home, and within a one mile radius there is a cinema, Croydon town centre, a museum and train station.

There are plans to redevelop the site in 2009.

Registered places: 58
Guide weekly rate: £450–£735
Specialist care: Nursing, respite
Medical services: Podiatry, dentist, optician
Qualified staff: Meets standard

Home details
Location: Residential area, 1 mile from Croydon centre
Communal areas: Lounge, dining room, conservatory, library, patio and garden
Accessibility: *Floors:* 4 • *Access:* Lift *Wheelchair access:* Limited
Smoking: In designated area
Pets: ✗
Routines: Flexible

Room details
Single: 58
Shared: 0
En suite: 0
Facilities: TV point, telephone point

Door lock: ✓
Lockable place: ✓

Services provided
Beauty services: Hairdressing
Mobile library: ✓
Religious services: Monthly Anglican service
Transport: Minibus
Activities: *Coordinator:* ✓ • *Examples:* Knitting, reminiscence, sewing • *Outings:* ✓
Meetings: ✗

Kettlewell House

Manager: Sarah Cook
Owner: Matthew and Jessica Liddle
Contact: Kettlewell Hill, Chobham Road, Woking, Surrey GU21 4HX
) 01483 756362

Kettlewell House offers care for 40 residents, some with dementia, physical disability or sensory impairment. It is in a semi-rural location, a short drive from Woking town centre. The home's gardens are open plan and many residents need the help of a carer to access them. There is an accessible courtyard area in which to sit during fine weather. The home has also planted a sensory garden. The home uses the local authority transport to take residents on outings to, for example, Guildford Cathedral, garden centres and on a boat trip.

Registered places: 40
Guide weekly rate: £450–£550
Specialist care: Dementia, physical disability
Medical services: Podiatry, hygienist, optician, physiotherapy
Qualified staff: Exceeds standard: 96% at NVQ Level 2

Home details
Location: Village location, 1 mile from Woking centre
Communal areas: 3 lounges, 2 dining rooms, garden
Accessibility: *Floors:* 3 • *Access:* Lift • *Wheelchair access:* Good
Smoking: ✗
Pets: At manager's discretion
Routines: Flexible

Room details
Single: 34
Shared: 3
En suite: Undisclosed
Facilities: TV point, telephone point

Door lock: ✓
Lockable place: ✓

Services provided
Beauty services: Hairdressing, aromatherapy, manicures
Mobile library: ✗
Religious services: ✗
Transport: ✗
Activities: *Coordinator:* ✗ • *Examples:* Flower arranging, musical entertainment, Pets As Therapy • *Outings:* ✓
Meetings: ✓

Registered places: 43
Guide weekly rate: £550–£1,800
Specialist care: Nursing, physical disability, respite
Medical services: Podiatry, hygienist, optician, physiotherapy
Qualified staff: Meets standard

Home details

Location: Village location, 4 miles from Redhill
Communal areas: 2 lounges, dining room, conservatory, activities
room, physiotherapy room, patio and garden
Accessibility: *Floors:* 2 • *Access:* Lift • *Wheelchair access:* Good
Smoking: In designated area
Pets: ✗
Routines: Flexible

Room details

Single: 33
Shared: 5
En suite: 38
Facilities: TV point, telephone point

Door lock: ✓
Lockable place: ✓

Services provided

Beauty services: Hairdressing, aromatherapy, manicures
Mobile library: ✗
Religious services: Monthly church service
Transport: ✗
Activities: *Coordinator:* ✓ • *Examples:* Computer lessons, flower
arranging, music sessions • *Outings:* ✓
Meetings: ✓

Kings Lodge

Manager: Vacant
Owner: Alum Care Ltd
Contact: Kings Cross Lane,
South Nutfield, Surrey RH1 5PA
☎ 01737 822221
@ crabhill@bmlhealthcare.co.uk
🖰 www.bmlhealthcare.co.uk

Kings Lodge is a large detached Edwardian building close to South Nutfield's railway station. The home's communal rooms mostly look over an attractive safe garden with patio area. Residents go on various outings, to for example Boxhill National Trust, Lingfield Race Course, pubs and garden centres. The home has a volunteer computer teacher who teaches basic IT skills to anyone who is interested. Residents are encouraged to participate in a full list of weekly activities, examples of which include gentle keep fit exercises, speech and music sessions and flower arranging.

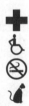

Registered places: 72
Guide weekly rate: £650–£800
Specialist care: Nursing, dementia, learning disability, physical
disability, sensory impairment
Medical services: Physiotherapy, Podiatry, optician
Qualified staff: Undisclosed

Home details

Location: Residential area. 0.5 miles from Camberley centre
Communal areas: 6 lounges, dining room, conservatory,
hairdressing salon/therapy room, patio and garden
Accessibility: *Floors:* 2 • *Access:* 2 lifts • *Wheelchair access:* Good
Smoking: ✗
Pets: At manager's discretion
Routines: Structured

Room details

Single: 70
Shared: 1
En suite: 10
Facilities: TV point

Door lock: ✓
Lockable place: ✗

Services provided

Beauty services: Hairdressing, massages, aromatherapy
Mobile library: ✓
Religious services: Monthly Catholic visits
Transport: ✗
Activities: *Coordinator:* ✓ • *Examples:* Cooking, gardening, quizzes
Outings:
Meetings: ✓

Kingsclear Nursing and Residential Home

Manager: Susan Allen
Owner: Caring Homes Group
Contact: Park Road, Camberley, Surrey
GU15 2LN
☎ 01276 21211
@ kingsclear@caringhomes.org
🖰 www.caringhomes.org

Kingsclear Nursing and Residential Home is set in four acres of landscape grounds in a quiet residential area. The house is a detached Edwardian building where original architectural features combine with the modern, purpose-built facilities. The home was converted from a hotel in the 1950s. The home is a few minutes' walk from Camberley town centre, down a slight slope. The home is split into four units, each with a lounge area. Three part-time activities coordinators ensure there are activities Monday to Friday. There is a monthly 'meet the chef', where residents can advise the chef on dishes they liked, or request alternatives.

Kingsleigh Resource Centre

Manager: Karen Seabrook
Owner: Care UK Community Partnerships Ltd
Contact: Kingfield Road, Woking, Surrey GU22 9EQ
☏ 01483 740750
🖰 www.careuk.com

Kingsleigh Resource Centre is built on one level and is therefore fully wheelchair accessible. Bedrooms are arranged in five suites, all of which have their own lounge, diner, kitchenette and access to a pleasant courtyard and gardens. Doors to the garden have sensors on to let the staff know when a resident has left the building. The care home is set in attractive and secure grounds, ideally located close to shops and local amenities. Residents in this home are encouraged to lead a fulfilling life and to maintain their independence though day-to-day choices.

Registered places: 50
Guide weekly rate: £689–£725
Specialist care: Dementia, sensory impairment
Medical services: Podiatry, hygienist, optician, physiotherapy
Qualified staff: Meets standard

Home details
Location: Residential area, 2 miles from Woking centre
Communal areas: 5 lounge/dining rooms, hairdressing salon, garden
Accessibility: *Floors:* 1 • *Wheelchair access:* Good
Smoking: ✗
Pets: At manager's discretion
Routines: Flexible

Room details
Single: 50
Shared: 0
En suite: 20
Facilities: TV point, telephone point
Door lock: ✗
Lockable place: ✓

Services provided
Beauty services: Hairdressing, massages
Mobile library: ✓
Religious services: ✓
Transport: ✗
Activities: *Coordinator:* ✓ • *Examples:* Bingo, crafts, seasonal activities • *Outings:* ✗
Meetings: ✓

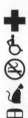

Kingswood Court

Manager: Ann Sayers
Owner: Balcombe Care Homes Ltd
Contact: Warren Lodge Drive, Kingswood, Surrey KT20 6QN
☏ 01737 830480
@ kingswood@balcombe carehomes.co.uk
🖰 www.balcombecarehomes.co.uk

Kingswood Court is a Georgian mansion adapted to its present use as a care home. It has large, landscaped gardens and is situated in a secluded village location. The home offers a variety of activities including film shows and a gardening club. The home is affiliated with Age Concern who take residents out to concerts and on other trips. As well as a residents association the home has residents' meetings every three months. There are also two resident cats. The home aims to create a relaxing retirement amid elegant surroundings.

Registered places: 59
Guide weekly rate: £600–£900
Specialist care: Nursing, day care, dementia, physical disability, respite
Medical services: Podiatry, dentist, optician, physiotherapy
Qualified staff: Meets standard

Home details
Location: Village location, 3 miles from Tadworth
Communal areas: 3 lounges, 3 dining room, patio and garden
Accessibility: *Floors:* 3 • *Access:* Lift • *Wheelchair access:* Good
Smoking: ✗
Pets: At manager's discretion
Routines: Flexible

Room details
Single: 43
Shared: 8
En suite: 18
Facilities: TV, telephone
Door lock: ✓
Lockable place: ✓

Services provided
Beauty services: Hairdressing
Mobile library: ✓
Religious services: Monthly Anglican, Baptist, Catholic and Greek Orthodox services
Transport: Minibus
Activities: *Coordinator:* ✓ • *Examples:* Film shows, gardening club, movement to music • *Outings:* ✓
Meetings: ✓

Registered places: 26
Guide weekly rate: £600–£750
Specialist care: Nursing, dementia, mental disorder, respite
Medical services: Podiatry, dentist, optician, physiotherapy
Qualified staff: Meets standard

Home details
Location: Residential area, 1 mile from Epsom centre
Communal areas: 2 lounges, dining room, activities room,
    patio and garden
Accessibility: *Floors:* 2 • *Access:* Lift • *Wheelchair access:* Good
Smoking: In designated area
Pets: ✗
Routines: Flexible

Room details
Single: 23
Shared: 3
En suite: 18
Facilities: TV point, telephone point

Door lock: ✓
Lockable place: ✓

Services provided
Beauty services: Hairdressing
Mobile library: ✓
Religious services: Weekly Communion service,
    monthly Anglican service
Transport: ✗
Activities: *Coordinator:* ✓ • *Examples:* Films, skittles, target
    throwing • *Outings:* ✓
Meetings: ✓

Leighton House

Manager: Eileen Spacey
Owner: Azher Hashmi
Contact: 59 Burgh Heath Road,
Epsom, Surrey KT17 4NB
☎ 01372 720908
🖰 www.leightonhouse-carehomes.co.uk

Leighton House is a large, detached property in a residential area of Epsom on top of a hill. It is within the M25 and close to public transport links. The home has an activities coordinator who is keen to create links with Age Concern to take residents out on trips. There is no residents association as most of the residents suffer from dementia. The home holds reviews with family members instead, to keep them up to date and involved in the care of their relatives.

Registered places: 32
Guide weekly rate: £395–£570
Specialist care: Dementia
Medical services: Podiatry, optician physiotherapy
Qualified staff: Meets standard

Home details
Location: Residential area, 1 mile from Epsom centre
Communal areas: 3 lounges, 2 dining rooms, garden
Accessibility: *Floors:* 2 • *Access:* Lift • *Wheelchair access:* None
Smoking: In designated area
Pets: At manager's discretion
Routines: Flexible

Room details
Single: 32
Shared: 0
En suite: 32
Facilities: Telephone point

Door lock: ✗
Lockable place: ✓

Services provided
Beauty services: Hairdressing
Mobile library: ✓
Religious service: ✓
Transport: ✗
Activities: *Coordinator:* ✓ • *Examples:* Debate lunches, skittles,
    walks • *Outings:* ✗
Meetings: ✓

Linden House

Manager: Mr Harvey
Owner: Mr Harvey
Contact: 9 College Road,
Epsom, Surrey KT17 4HF
☎ 01372 721447
@ ukcarehomes@supanet.co.uk

Linden House is a privately owned care home which used to be a hotel. It is situated on a quiet residential road in Epsom about one mile from the nearest local shops. It is near a few recreational grounds, and often, mobile residents go for walks around either Alexandra or Elizabeth Welschman gardens. There are also other activities planned on a weekly basis such as debate lunches, bingo night and cards. The home has a large garden which is well kept which those who are keen on gardening are welcome to help maintain it.

Linwood

Manager: Lorraine Hills-Avery
Owner: Anchor Trust
Contact: 9 Mercer Close, Thames Ditton, Surrey KT7 0BS

- ☏ 020 8335 6800
- @ valerie.snow@anchor.org.uk
- 🖱 www.anchor.org.uk

Linwood is located in a residential area within walking distance of Thames Ditton with its shops and other amenities. There is a GP surgery close by at which all residents are registered. There is car parking to the front of the building with additional more parking and an enclosed, well-maintained garden to the rear. Regular activities are planned for the residents including day trips to Hampton Court Palace. Activities coordinators also organise daily activities such as bingo, knitting and flower arranging to keep the residents stimulated.

Registered places: 66
Guide weekly rate: Undisclosed
Specialist care: Dementia, physically disabled
Medical services: Podiatry, optician, physiotherapy
Qualified staff: Exceeds standard: 60% at NVQ Level 2

Home details
Location: Residential area, 0.5 miles from Thames Ditton centre
Communal areas: 4 lounges, dining room, garden
Accessibility: *Floors:* 3 • *Access:* Lift • *Wheelchair access:* Good
Smoking: In designated area
Pets: ✓
Routines: Flexible

Room details
Single: 66
Shared: 0
En suite: 66
Facilities: TV point, telephone point

Door lock: ✗
Lockable place: ✓

Services provided
Beauty services: Hairdressing
Mobile library: ✗
Religious services: ✓
Transport: ✗
Activities: *Coordinator:* ✓ • *Examples:* Cooking, flower arranging, knitting, bingo • *Outings:* ✓
Meetings: ✓

Lodore Nursing Home

Manager: Stephen Pittman
Owner: Stephen Pittman
Contact: 9 Mayfield Road, Sutton, Surrey SM2 5DU

- ☏ 020 8642 3088

Lodore Nursing Home is set in an Edwardian building, on a pleasant tree-lined road in Sutton. The staff endeavour to maintain a friendly and homely atmosphere for the residents. They have many activities including musical entertainers and reading for the deaf. Special days are always marked, such as pancakes on Shrove Tuesday and birthdays.

Registered places: 36
Guide weekly rate: £675–£815
Specialist care: Nursing, dementia, physical disability, terminal care
Medical services: Podiatry, hygienist, optician, physiotherapy
Qualified staff: Exceeds standard: 100% at NVQ Level 2

Home details
Location: Residential area, 0.75 miles from Sutton centre
Communal areas: Lounge, dining room, garden
Accessibility: *Floors:* 3 • *Access:* Lift and stair lift *Wheelchair access:* Good
Smoking: ✗
Pets: ✗
Routines: Structured

Room details
Single: 18
Shared: 9
En suite: 0
Facilities: TV point

Door lock: ✓
Lockable place: ✓

Services provided
Beauty services: Hairdressing
Mobile library: ✓
Religious services: ✗
Transport: ✗
Activities: *Coordinator:* ✓ • *Examples:* Exercise classes, musical entertainment, singing • *Outings*
Meetings: ✗

Registered places: 23
Guide weekly rate: £550
Specialist care: Dementia
Medical services: Podiatry, dentist, optician, occupational therapy
Qualified staff: Meets standard

Home details

Location: Residential area, 1 mile from Caterham centre
Communal areas: Lounge, dining room, conservatory,
library, garden
Accessibility: *Floors:* 3 • *Access:* Lift • *Wheelchair access:* Good
Smoking: ✗
Pets: At manager's discretion
Routines: Flexible

Room details

Single: 15
Shared: 4
En suite: 6
Facilities: TV point, telephone point

Door lock: ✓
Lockable place: ✓

Services provided

Beauty services: Hairdressing
Mobile library: ✓
Religious services: Catholic, Anglican and Baptist church visit
Transport: Car
Activities: *Coordinator:* ✗ • *Examples:* Exercises, reminiscence
therapy, poetry readings, music evenings • *Outings:* ✓
Meetings: ✓

Longmead House

Manager: Bridget McAleese
Owner: Bridget McAleese
Contact: 1 Buxton Lane, Caterham,
Surrey CR3 5HG
☎ 01883 340686

Longmead House is a Victorian property situated in Caterham. The home has a garden with conservatory to enjoy the good weather outside and inside. Regular outings are organised with trips to garden centres and afternoon teas. Garden parties are arranged for residents to enjoy during the summer. Activities are varied with poetry readings and musical evenings. There is a resident cat and the owner's dogs are around frequently. Meetings with residents take place every week so any issues or concerns can be voiced.

Registered places: 19
Guide weekly rate: Undisclosed
Specialist care: Dementia, mental disorder, physical disability,
sensory impairment
Medical services: Podiatry, dentist, optician, physiotherapy
Qualified staff: Exceeds standard: 100% at NVQ Level 2

Home details

Location: Residential area, 0.5 miles from East Molesey centre
Communal areas: Lounge, dining room, conservatory,
patio and garden
Accessibility: *Floors:* 3 • *Access:* Lift • *Wheelchair access:* Good
Smoking: ✗
Pets: ✓
Routines: Structured

Room details

Single: 19
Shared: 0
En suite: 19
Facilities: TV, telephone point

Door lock: ✓
Lockable place: ✓

Services provided

Beauty services: Hairdressing, manicures
Mobile library: ✓
Religious services: ✓
Transport: ✗
Activities: *Coordinator:* ✓ • *Examples:* Bingo, organ music,
visiting entertainers • *Outings:* ✗
Meetings: ✓

Malmesbury House

Manager: Mary Gajraj
Owner: Dr and Mrs Gajraj
Contact: 18 Beauchamp Road,
East Molesey, Surrey KT8 0PA
☎ 020 8783 0444

Malmesbury House is a large, detached property situated in a residential area close to the local shops of West Molesey. The home has good travel links by bus and a large garden with a seating area and conservatory. Several bedrooms are located on the ground floor and have access to the rear garden. There are three floors serviced by a lift and good wheelchair access throughout. The residents have a structured daily routine and set meal times and the home has its own activities coordinator. There are a range of activities on offer such as games and occupational therapy exercises and musical entertainment.

Manor House

Manager: Helene Sessford
Owner: Mr and Mrs Sessford
Contact: London Road, Morden,
Surrey SM4 5QT

☎ 020 8648 3571

Manor House is a detached property situated in a residential area of Morden. There are parking spaces at the side of the home and public transport bus links within a short distance. The home offers a varied menu with many options and residents are involved in menu choices. Special diets are catered for including diabetes and low fat. Activities are offered for residents to get involved and socialise with their fellow residents, such as painting, drawing and indoor games. Outings are also organised with trips to the shops and afternoon teas.

Registered places: 23
Guide weekly rate: £485–£500
Specialist care: Dementia, respite
Medical services: Podiatry, dentist, optician, physiotherapy
Qualified staff: Meets standard

Home details
Location: Residential area, in Morden
Communal areas: Lounge, dining room, library, conservatory, garden
Accessibility: *Floors:* 2 • *Access:* Lift • *Wheelchair access:* Good
Smoking: In designated area
Pets: At manager's discretion
Routines: Flexible

Room details
Single: 19
Shared: 2
En suite: 21
Facilities: TV, telephone point

Door lock: ✓
Lockable place: ✓

Services provided
Beauty services: Hairdressing
Mobile library: ✗
Religious services: Anglican and Catholic ministers visit
Transport: ✗
Activities: *Coordinator:* ✓ • *Examples:* Bingo, drawing, painting *Outings:* ✓
Meetings: ✓

Marlyna Lodge

Manager: Desline Davis
Owner: Redstone Care Ltd
Contact: 37 Mitcham Park, Mitcham,
Surrey CR4 4ER

☎ 020 8687 2199

Marlyna Lodge is situated in a residential area, approximately one mile from Mitcham town centre. The home has a garden and there are regular outings organised to the local garden centre. The home also provides a daily activities programme for residents to participate in. There are also regular residents meetings to discuss any issues residents may have.

Registered places: 10
Guide weekly rate: Undisclosed
Specialist care: Respite
Medical services: Podiatry, dentist, optician
Qualified staff: Undisclosed

Home details
Location: Residential area, 0.7 miles from Mitcham
Communal areas: Lounge, garden
Accessibility: *Floors:* 2 • *Access:* Lift • *Wheelchair access:* Good
Smoking: In designated area
Pets: ✗
Routines: Flexible

Room details
Single: 6
Shared: 2
En suite: 2
Facilities: TV point, telephone point

Door lock: ✓
Lockable place: ✓

Services provided
Beauty services: Hairdressing
Mobile library: ✓
Religious services: ✓
Transport: ✗
Activities: *Coordinator:* ✗ • *Examples:* Bingo, games • *Outings:* ✓
Meetings: ✓

Registered places: 11
Guide weekly rate: £425–£500
Specialist care: None
Medical services: None
Qualified staff: Meets standard

Home details

Location: Residential area, 0.5 miles from Cheam centre
Communal areas: Lounge, dining room, garden
Accessibility: *Floors:* 2 • *Access:* Lift • *Wheelchair access:* Good
Smoking: ✗
Pets: ✗
Routines: Flexible

Room details

Single: 9
Shared: 1
En suite: 2
Facilities: TV point, telephone point

Door lock: ✓
Lockable place: ✗

Services provided

Beauty services: Hairdressing
Mobile library: ✗
Religious services: ✓
Transport: ✗
Activities: *Coordinator:* ✗• *Examples:* Painting, tea afternoons,
    walks • *Outings:* ✗
Meetings: ✓

Mayfield Lodge

Manager: Maleenee Cooppen
Owner: Mr and Mrs Cooppen
Contact: 19 Burdon Lane, Cheam,
Surrey SM2 7PP
  ☎ 020 8770 0935
  @ cooppencare@yahoo.co.uk

Mayfield Lodge is located in a quite residential road in Cheam. The home is on a bus route which takes passengers into Cheam Village. The village provides an abundance of amenities including shops, restaurants, beauty salons and a leisure centre. The well being of the residents is the main concern in this small home, and as a result the staff plan different activities for the residents such as walks for the mobile, and games such as bingo and skittles on a daily basis. There are also themed nights such as painting evenings.

Registered places: 53
Guide weekly rate: £800–£1,100
Specialist care: Nursing
Medical services: Podiatry, dentist, optician, physiotherapy
Qualified staff: Exceeds standard: 65% at NVQ Level 2

Home details

Location: Village location, 1.5 miles to Virginia Water
Communal areas: Lounge, 2 dining rooms, library,
    hairdressing salon, chapel, garden
Accessibility: *Floors:* 1 • *Wheelchair access:* Good
Smoking: ✗
Pets: ✗
Routines: Flexible

Room details

Single: 53
Shared: 0
En suite: 53
Facilities: TV point, telephone point

Door lock: ✓
Lockable place: ✓

Services provided

Beauty services: Hairdressing
Mobile library: Library facilities
Religious services: Weekly church service
Transport: Minibus
Activities: *Coordinator:* ✓ • *Examples:* Craft, exercise, films,
    visiting entertainers • *Outings:* ✓
Meetings: ✓

Merlewood Nursing and Residential Home

Manager: Michael Maher
Owner: Elizabeth Finn Homes Ltd
Contact: Hollow Lane, Callow Hill,
Virginia Water, Surrey GU25 4LR
  ☎ 01344 845 314
  @ merlewood@efhl.co.uk
  ⌂ www.efhl.co.uk

Merlewood is a Victorian building, set in 23 acres of ground with a summerhouse. The home has extensive communal areas, with a lounge, two dining rooms, a library periodically updated by the local library, a chapel and a hairdressing salon. The home has its own minibus in which it makes regular trips to local sites such as to Windsor or out for lunch. There are also in-house activities including musical entertainers that come and perform to residents.

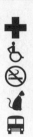

Moorhouse

Manager: Sharon Egan
Owner: Timothy Shepherd
Contact: Tilford Road, Hindhead,
Surrey GU26 6RA
☎ 01428 604381

Moorhouse is situated in the village of Hindhead, around nine miles from Farnham town. The home has four close care units and offers nursing care. There are regular entertainers and musicians who come in for residents to enjoy. The home also goes on outings such as theatre trips. In the home's garden, there is a terrace and patio area as well as two fishponds.

Registered places: 36
Guide weekly rate: £650–£950
Specialist care: Nursing, respite
Medical services: Podiatry, dentist, optician, physiotherapy
Qualified staff: Exceeds standard: 97% at NVQ Level 2

Home details
Location: Village location, 0.5 miles from Hindhead centre
Communal areas: Lounge, dining room, day room, patio and garden
Accessibility: *Floors:* 3 • *Access:* Lift • *Wheelchair access:* Good
Smoking: ✗
Pets: At manager's discretion
Routines: Flexible

Room details
Single: 36
Shared: 0
En suite: 0
Facilities: TV point, telephone point

Door lock: ✗
Lockable place: ✓

Services provided
Beauty services: Hairdressing
Mobile library: ✓
Religious services: Weekly Anglican and Catholic services
Transport: Cars
Activities: *Coordinator:* ✗ • *Examples:* Music and movement, speakers, word games • *Outings:* ✓
Meetings: ✗

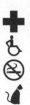

Moorlands Nursing Home

Manager: Kathleen Buckley
Owner: Moorlands Ltd
Contact: Macdonald Road, Lightwater,
Surrey GU18 5US
☎ 01276 473140

Built in the early 1900s, Moorlands is set in its own grounds, one mile from Lightwater village centre and two miles from Camberley town centre. The home is tastefully decorated and furnished, with lounges and quiet areas overlooking well-kept gardens. Pets As Therapy visits alongside other activities, which include dominoes, quizzes and occasionally visiting entertainers.

Registered places: 41
Guide weekly rate: £675–£775
Specialist care: Nursing, dementia, physical disability, respite
Medical services: Podiatry, optician, physiotherapy
Qualified staff: Fails standard: at NVQ Level 2

Home details
Location: Village location, 2 miles from Camberley
Communal areas: 2 lounges, coffee lounge, dining room, garden
Accessibility: *Floors:* 2 • *Access:* Lift • *Wheelchair access:* Good
Smoking: ✗
Pets: At manager's discretion
Routines: Flexible

Room details
Single: 33
Shared: 4
En suite: 25
Facilities: TV point, telephone point

Door lock: ✓
Lockable place: ✓

Services provided
Beauty services: Hairdressing
Mobile library: ✓
Religious services: ✓
Transport: ✗
Activities: *Coordinator:* ✓ • *Examples:* Entertainers, games, quizzes • *Outings:* ✗
Meetings: ✓

Registered places: 38
Guide weekly rate: Undisclosed
Specialist care: Nursing, physical disability, palliative care, respite, terminal care
Medical services: Podiatry, occupational therapy, physiotherapy
Qualified staff: Undisclosed

Home details

Location: Village location, 3 miles from Woking
Communal areas: Lounge, activities room, library, conservatory, hairdressing salon, garden
Accessibility: *Floors:* 2 • *Access:* Lift • *Wheelchair access:* Good
Smoking: In designated area
Pets: ✓
Routines: Flexible

Room details

Single: 36
Shared: 2
En suite: 38
Facilities: TV, telephone point

Door lock: ✓
Lockable place: ✗

Services provided

Beauty services: Hairdressing, aromatherapy, hydrotherapy
Mobile library: ✗
Religious services: ✓
Transport: ✓
Activities: *Coordinator:* ✓ • *Examples:* Crosswords, knitting, painting • *Outings:* ✓
Meetings: ✗

Oakcroft House

Manager: Vivien Grieve
Owner: BUPA Care Homes Ltd
Contact: Oakcroft Road, West Byfleet, Surrey KT14 6JG
) 0113 3816100
@ OakcroftHouseALL@BUPA.com
🖰 www.bupacarehomes.co.uk

Originally an imposing private residence, Oakcroft House is situated in a residential area within walking distance of the village of West Byfleet. A conservatory overlooks the mature landscaped gardens and leads on to a sun terrace, as does the lounge. There is a dedicated activities room and daily activities are offered with painting, gardening, crosswords and trips to the theatre particularly popular. A pianist comes in fortnightly to play in the lounge. The home has two resident cats and pets are welcome. Oakcroft House also offers care to a number of younger physically disabled residents.

Registered places: 61
Guide weekly rate: £528–£850
Specialist care: Nursing, day care, dementia, respite
Medical services: Podiatry, dentist, optician
Qualified staff: Undisclosed

Home details

Location: Residential area, 0.5 miles from Croydon centre
Communal areas: 3 lounges, 3 dining rooms, garden
Accessibility: *Floors:* 3 • *Access:* Lift • *Wheelchair access:* Good
Smoking: In designated area
Pets: ✗
Routines: Flexible

Room details

Single: 41
Shared: 10
En suite: 51
Facilities: TV point, telephone point

Door lock: ✓
Lockable place: ✓

Services provided

Beauty services: Hairdressing
Mobile library: ✗
Religious services: Anglican and Catholic services
Transport: Minibus
Activities: *Coordinator:* ✓ • *Examples:* Arts and crafts, entertainment, games • *Outings:* ✓
Meetings: ✓

Oban House

Manager: Zelina Ramdhan
Owner: Southern Cross Healthcare Ltd
Contact: 42–46 Bramley Hill, South Croydon, Surrey CR2 6NS
) 020 8649 8866
@ Oban.house@ashbourne.co.uk
🖰 www.ashbourne.co.uk

Oban House is a purpose-built care home. There are three floors, each with its own facilities including a dining room and lounge for each floor. There is a large landscaped garden for residents to enjoy during fine weather. The home organises a range of activities including arts and crafts. There are also outings including trips to Brighton and the theatre in Croydon, made possible by the home's minibus. The home is situated near a train station and on a main bus route.

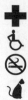

Orchard House Nursing Home

Manager: Emma Langbridge
Owner: Stephen Pittman
Contact: 35 Hallmead Road, Sutton, Surrey SM1 1RD
☎ 020 8644 5095

Orchard House Nursing Home is involved in the Gold standards programme, and specialises in palliative care. There is a patio and garden area with fruit trees that are picked and their fruits enjoyed by residents. Music is very important at Orchard House and the matron plays both the guitar and organ to residents. The home also offers outings to pantomimes.

Registered places: 44
Guide weekly rate: £600–£1,050
Specialist care: Nursing, day care, respite, terminal care
Medical services: Podiatry, hygienist, optician, physiotherapy
Qualified staff: Exceeds standard: 80% at NVQ Level 2

Home details

Location: Residential area, in Sutton
Communal areas: 4 lounges, 3 dining rooms, quiet lounge, chapel, patio and garden
Accessibility: *Floors:* 2 • *Access:* Lift • *Wheelchair access:* Good
Smoking: ✗
Pets: At manager's discretion
Routines: Flexible

Room details

Single: 22
Shared: 11
En suite: 5
Facilities: TV point, telephone point

Door lock: ✓
Lockable place: ✓

Services provided

Beauty services: Hairdressing, aromatherapy
Mobile library: ✓
Religious services: ✓
Transport: ✗
Activities: *Coordinator:* ✗ • *Examples:* Bingo, quizzes, music, themed events • *Outings:* ✓
Meetings: ✓

Pickering House

Manager: Helen Tomlinson
Owner: Journalists' Charity
Contact: Ridgeway Road, Dorking, Surrey RH4 3AY
☎ 01306 888077
@ Helen.tomlinson@pickeringhouse.org.uk

Pickering House is owned by the Journalists' Charity and all the residents have worked in or been connected to journalism. The home is located in a rural area, approximately one mile from Dorking. There is a computer with internet access and a wide range of books and DVDs for residents to enjoy as well as a daily activities program. There is an Anglican and Catholic service held every two weeks and the home arranges regular outings for the residents.

Registered places: 20
Guide weekly rate: £500–£650
Specialist care: Nursing, dementia, respite
Medical services: Physiotherapy
Qualified staff: Meets standard

Home details

Location: Rural area, 1 mile from Dorking
Communal areas: 5 lounges, dining room, library, bar, chapel, garden
Accessibility: *Floors:* 3 • *Access:* Lift • *Wheelchair access:* Good
Smoking: In designated area
Pets: At manager's discretion
Routines: Flexible

Room details

Single: 20
Shared: 0
En suite: 20
Facilities: TV, telephone

Door lock: ✓
Lockable place: ✓

Services provided

Beauty services: Hairdressing salon
Mobile library: Library facilities
Religious services: Fortnightly Anglican and Catholic services
Transport: ✗
Activities: *Coordinator:* ✗ • *Examples:* Games • *Outings:* ✓
Meetings: ✓

Registered places: 35
Guide weekly rate: £495–£675
Specialist care: Dementia
Medical services: Podiatry, dentist, optician, physiotherapy
Qualified staff: Exceeds standard: 98% at NVQ Level 2

Home details
Location: Village location, 2 miles from Guilford
Communal areas: Lounge, dining room,
   hairdressing salon, garden
Accessibility: *Floors:* 4 • *Access:* Lift and stair lift
   Wheelchair access: Good
Smoking: ✗
Pets: At manager's discretion
Routines: Flexible

Room details
Single: 29
Shared: 3
En suite: 32
Facilities: TV point

Door lock: ✓
Lockable place: ✓

Services provided
Beauty services: Hairdressing, aromatherapy
Mobile library: ✗
Religious services: ✗
Transport: ✗
Activities: *Coordinator:* ✓ • *Examples:* Flower arranging, musical
   events, talks • *Outings:* ✓
Meetings: ✓

Pilgrim Wood

Manager: Emily Hayward
Owner: Jean Walker and John Flexer
Contact: Sandy Lane, Guildford,
Surrey GU3 1HF
☏ 01483 573111

Pilgrim Wood is set in three acres of ground and overlooks the North Downs, a few miles from Guildford town centre. The home has one large lounge, which can be split into three areas, including a quiet room, a large dining room and gardens which are safe and accessible for residents. A recent extension has added a hairdressing salon to the home's facilities. Residents regular go on shopping trips and visit places of interest.

Registered places: 19
Guide weekly rate: £695–£795
Specialist care: Dementia, mental disorder, respite
Medical services: Podiatry, dentist, optician, physiotherapy
Qualified staff: Exceeds standard: 100% at NVQ Level 2

Home details
Location: Village location, 2 miles from Dorking
Communal areas: Lounge, dining room, patio and garden
Accessibility: *Floors:* 2 • *Access:* Lift • *Wheelchair access:* Good
Smoking: In designated area
Pets: ✓
Routines: Flexible

Room details
Single: 14
Shared: 2
En suite: 10
Facilities: TV point, telephone point

Door lock: ✓
Lockable place: ✓

Services provided
Beauty services: Hairdressing
Mobile library: ✓
Religious services: Weekly Anglican service
Transport: 2 cars
Activities: *Coordinator:* ✓ • *Examples:* Art, exercises, music for
   therapy • *Outings:* ✓
Meetings: ✓

Pinehurst

Manager: Theresa Schneider
Owner: Theresa Schneider
Contact: National Trust Road, Boxhill,
Mickleham, Surrey RH5 6BY
☏ 01306 889942

Pinehurst has a secure private garden which overlooks beautiful National Trust-owned land. The home has a wealth of activities and outings for residents to get involved in. These include classical and modern concerts, film afternoons, poetry, and visiting students who come in to chat to the residents once a week. Outings are also arranged once a week to markets, shopping in Dorking and coffee mornings, to name a few. The home arranges parties weekly and acoustic concerts twice a week. Two drivers are available to take residents out shopping or out for tea at their request. The home also has two resident cats.

Priors Mead Retirement Home

Manager: Lynette Pearman
Owner: Nightingale Retirement Care Ltd
Contact: 26 Blanford Road, Reigate, Surrey RH2 7DR
☎ 01737 224334
@ admin@nightingales.co.uk
🖱 www.nightingales.co.uk

Priors Mead Retirement Home is a redbrick Victorian property set in a tranquil, residential avenue. Reigate centre is a 15-minute level walk away with shops, pubs, churches; other local amenities are available closer to hand. The home has a conservatory which leads out onto a large decked patio area. There are two resident cats but no other pets are allowed in the home. The home can cater for specific dietary requirements and visitors are always welcome.

Registered places: 21
Guide weekly rate: £418–£600
Specialist care: Dementia, physical disability, respite
Medical services: Podiatry, dentist, optician, physiotherapy
Qualified staff: Meets standard

Home details
Location: Residential area, 1 mile from Reigate centre
Communal areas: Lounge, dining room, conservatory, patio and garden
Accessibility: *Floors:* 3 • *Access:* Lift • *Wheelchair access:* Good
Smoking: In designated area
Pets: ✗
Routines: Flexible

Room details
Single: 21	**Door lock:** ✓
Shared: 0	**Lockable place:** ✓
En suite: 21	
Facilities: TV point, telephone point	

Services provided
Beauty services: Hairdressing
Mobile library: ✓
Religious services: ✗
Transport: ✗
Activities: *Coordinator:* ✗ • *Examples:* Bingo, music, skittles
  Outings: ✗
Meetings: ✗

Purley View Nursing Home

Manager: Anna Cunningham
Owner: Glancestyle Care Homes Ltd
Contact: 30 Addiscombe Grove, Croydon, Surrey CR9 5AY
☎ 020 8645 0174
@ purleyanna@aol.com

Purley View Nursing Home is a purpose-built nursing home situated close to Croydon centre, within walking distance from Purley train station. The home offers recreational movement to music designed especially for the elderly, run by a qualified therapist. Activities such as art classes, bingo and aromatherapy constitute part of the events programme. There is a large open plan lounge and dining area, with a quiet corner. Outside, a small decking area is provided. At Purley View, emphasis is put on residents' independence and this is encouraged where possible.

Registered places: 39
Guide weekly rate: £525–£740
Specialist care: Nursing, respite, palliative care
Medical services: Podiatry
Qualified staff: Exceeds standard: 100% at NVQ Level 2

Home details
Location: Residential area, in Croydon
Communal areas: Lounge/dining room, patio
Accessibility: *Floors:* 3 • *Access:* Lift • *Wheelchair access:* Good
Smoking: ✗
Pets: At manager's discretion
Routines: Flexible

Room details
Single: 24	**Door lock:** ✓
Shared: 5	**Lockable place:** ✓
En suite: 29	
Facilities: TV, telephone point	

Services provided
Beauty services: Hairdressing, aromatherapy
Mobile library: ✗
Religious services: ✗
Transport: ✗
Activities: *Coordinator:* ✓ • *Examples:* Art classes, bingo, exercise • *Outings:* ✗
Meetings: ✓

Registered places: 77
Guide weekly rate: £650–£900
Specialist care: Nursing, dementia, respite
Medical services: Podiatry, dentist, optician
Qualified staff: Meets standard

Home details

Location: Residential area, 2.5 miles from Guildford
Communal areas: 5 lounges, 1 quiet lounge,
    3 dining rooms, garden
Accessibility: *Floors:* 3 • *Access:* Lift • *Wheelchair access:* Good
Smoking: ✗
Pets: ✓
Routines: Flexible

Room details

Single: 77
Shared: 0
En suite: 77
Facilities: TV, telephone point

Door lock: ✗
Lockable place: ✗

Services provided

Beauty services: Hairdressing, manicure
Mobile library: ✓
Religious services: Monthly Communion service
Transport: ✗
Activities: *Coordinator:* ✓ • *Examples:* Arts and crafts, bridge,
    concerts, discussion • *Outings:* ✓
Meetings: ✓

Queen Elizabeth Park

Manager: Katarina Parr
Owner: CareBase Ltd
Contact: 1–72 Hallowes Close,
Guildford, Surrey GU2 9LL
☏ 01483 531133
@ Katarina.parr@carebase.org.uk
🖥 www.qepprivatecarehome.co.uk

Queen Elizabeth Park home is set at the edge of 57 acres of wooded parkland. Purpose-built, the home believes residents should treat it exactly like their own home but without added worry. Therefore, there are no timetables or visiting hours. Music and theatrical groups visit the home and activities organised by the activities coordinator include an adaptation of *The Times* quiz and bridge games. Residents are also encouraged to participate in gardening. The home celebrates Burns' night, St George's day and individual birthdays. There is a comprehensive website with the option of increased font size.

Registered places: 32
Guide weekly rate: Undisclosed
Specialist care: Nursing, palliative care, respite, terminal care
Medical services: Podiatry, physiotherapy
Qualified staff: Exceeds standard: 85% at NVQ Level 2

Home details

Location: Residential area, 1 mile from Croydon centre
Communal areas: 3 lounges, 2 dining rooms, activities room,
    hairdressing salon, garden
Accessibility: *Floors:* 3 • *Access:* Lift • *Wheelchair access:* Good
Smoking: In designated area
Pets: ✗
Routines: Flexible

Room details

Single: 32
Shared: 0
En suite: 14
Facilities: TV, telephone point

Door lock: ✓
Lockable place: ✗

Services provided

Beauty services: Hairdressing, aromatherapy
Mobile library: ✓
Religious services: ✓
Transport: ✓
Activities: *Coordinator:* ✓ • *Examples:* Art sessions, visiting
    entertainers • *Outings:* ✓
Meetings: ✓

Red Court Nursing Home

Manager: Palace Chivero
Owner: BUPA Care Homes Ltd
Contact: 27 Stanhope Road,
Croydon, Surrey CR0 5NS
☏ 020 8681 2359
@ RedCourtALL@BUPA.com
🖥 www.bupacarehomes.co.uk

Red Court is conveniently situated a short distance from the centre of Croydon, and stands in several acres of landscaped gardens with seating areas. This grade II listed Edwardian house has been refurbished and extended, and offers a choice of lounges and a cottage-style dining room overlooking the gardens. Entertainers and guest speakers regularly visit the home, and local attractions such as the Whitgift Centre and Fairfield Halls can be visited on organised trips or with friends and family. Red Court also offers care to people with Parkinson's disease, have suffered a stroke or require terminal care.

Redwood Care Centre

Manager: Rosalyn Hampson
Owner: Care UK Community Partnerships Ltd
Contact: 179 Epsom Road, Merrow, Guildford, Surrey GU1 2QY
☎ 01483 532562
@ Admin.redwood@careuk.com
🖰 www.careuk.com

The Redwood care centre is a ground-level building comprising of five units, three of which are for permanent residents. The home is located in a village, a 20-minute walk from Guildford. There are 30 places for permanent residents and all the rooms are single occupancy. There is a lounge/dining room in each unit as well as a large communal lounge. There are some quiet areas and the home is surrounded by a large garden. There are no pets allowed but there are visits from Pets As Therapy.

Registered places: 50
Guide weekly rate: Undisclosed
Specialist care: Nursing, respite
Medical services: Podiatry, dentist, optician
Qualified staff: Exceeds standard: 75% at NVQ Level 2

Home details

Location: Village location, 2 miles from Guildford
Communal areas: 5 lounges, 5 lounge/dining rooms, garden
Accessibility: *Floors:* 1 • *Wheelchair access:* Good
Smoking: ✗
Pets: ✗
Routines: Structured

Room details

Single: 50	**Door lock:** ✓
Shared: 0	**Lockable place:** ✗
En suite: 50	
Facilities: TV	

Services provided

Beauty services: Hairdressing, manicures
Mobile library: ✓
Religious services: ✓
Transport: ✗
Activities: *Coordinator:* ✓ • *Examples:* Arts and crafts, music, visiting entertainers • *Outings:* ✗
Meetings: ✗

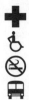

Reigate Beaumont

Manager: John Levan
Owner: Barchester Healthcare Ltd
Contact: Colley Lane, Reigate, Surrey RH2 9JB
☎ 01737 225544
@ reigate@barchester.com
🖰 www.barchester.com

Reigate Beaumont is a relaxed care home situated in its own private woodlands, conveniently placed just one mile from Reigate town centre. It has well-kept gardens with pathways ensuring wheelchair access and shaded outside seating areas. The home's full-time activities coordinator organises an activities schedule each month that is discussed beforehand with residents. Services offered include a hairdresser who visits three times a week, aromatherapy sessions and local sightseeing trips to the local vineyard and visiting musicians such as harpists and organists.

Registered places: 60
Guide weekly rate: From £850
Specialist care: Nursing, day care, emergency admissions, respite
Medical services: Podiatry, dentist, hygienist, optician, physiotherapy
Qualified staff: Exceeds standard: 80% at NVQ level 2

Home details

Location: Rural area, 1 mile from Reigate centre
Communal areas: 3 lounges, 3 dining rooms, bar, library, 2 patios and garden
Accessibility: *Floors:* 2 • *Access:* Lift • *Wheelchair access:* Good
Smoking: ✗
Pets: ✗
Routines: Flexible

Room details

Single: 60	**Door lock:** ✗
Shared: 0	**Lockable place:** ✗
En suite: 60	
Facilities: TV, telephone	

Services provided

Beauty services: Hairdressing, aromatherapy
Mobile library: ✗
Religious services: Monthly church services
Transport: Minibus
Activities: *Coordinator:* ✓ • *Examples:* Exercises, flower arranging, visiting musicians • *Outings:* ✓
Meetings: ✗

Registered places: 16
Guide weekly rate: £540–£580
Specialist care: Dementia
Medical services: Podiatry, optician
Qualified staff: Meets standard

Home details

Location: Residential area, 1 mile from Farnham
Communal areas: 2 lounges, dining room, conservatory, garden
Accessibility: *Floors:* 2 • *Access:* Lift • *Wheelchair access:* Good
Smoking: ✗
Pets: ✗
Routines: Flexible

Room details

Single: 16
Shared: 0
En suite: 16
Facilities: Telephone

Door lock: ✓
Lockable place: ✓

Services provided

Beauty services: Hairdressing, manicures
Mobile library: ✓
Religious services: Monthly Communion service
Transport: ✗
Activities: *Coordinator:* ✓ • *Examples:* Bingo, games, music
        Outings: ✓
Meetings: ✓

Ridgway Court

Manager: Julie Hynd
Owner: Abbeyfield Wey Valley Society Ltd
Contact: 48 Ridgway Road, Farnham,
Surrey GU9 8NW
✆ 01252 715921
@ Julie.hynd@btconnect.com

Ridgway Court is located in a residential area, one mile from Farnham. The home has two lounges, a dining room and a conservatory. There is also a garden. The home arranges for a mobile library to visit and there is a Communion service held on a monthly basis. There are regular residents meetings and there are also outings on offer.

Registered places: 46
Guide weekly rate: £550–£951
Specialist care: Nursing, day care, dementia, mental disorder,
        physically disabled
Medical services: Podiatry, dentist, optician
Qualified staff: Exceeds standard: 75% at NVQ level 2

Home details

Location: Rural area, 1.5 miles from Addlestone
Communal areas: Lounge, dining room, conservatory, patio and
        garden
Accessibility: *Floors:* 2 • *Access:* Lift • *Wheelchair access:* Good
Smoking: ✗
Pets: At manager's discretion
Routines: Flexible

Room details

Single: 30
Shared: 8
En suite: 38
Facilities: TV point, telephone point

Door lock: ✓
Lockable place: ✓

Services provided

Beauty services: Hairdressing
Mobile library: ✓
Religious services: Weekly Anglican service
Transport: ✗
Activities: *Coordinator:* ✓ • *Examples:* Art group, films,
        one-to-one sessions • *Outings:* ✓

Meetings: ✓

Rodwell Farm

Manager: Karen Raggett
Owner: Rodwell Farm Nursing Home Ltd
Contact: Row Town, Addlestone,
Surrey KT15 1HH
✆ 01932 853371
@ grahamcare@msn.com
🖳 www.rodwellfarmnursinghome.co.uk

Rodwell Farm is located in a rural area, one and a half miles from Addlestone. The home is set in four acres of land and arranges an Anglican service to take place on a weekly basis and there are also regular outings. There is an activities coordinator in the home who arranges group activities such as an art group and film showing as well as one-to-one sessions. There are regular residents meetings held to discuss any issues that may arise.

Rosina Lodge

Manager: Ginige Balachandran
Owner: Balasubramaniam and Ginige Balachandran
Contact: 76 St Augustine's Avenue, South Croydon, Surrey CR2 6JH
) 020 8760 0735
@ rosina@blueyonder.co.uk

Rosina Lodge is a converted, detached family home located in South Croydon. The home is an eight-minute walk from the town centre. The home has two lounges, a dining room, a garden and a patio. A mobile library does not visit, but the home has its own books. The home offers religious services to a variety of denominations. The home arranges activities such as bingo, painting, an exercise session three times a week and arts and crafts. There are outings to the seaside and local concerts. There is a payphone in the hallway.

Registered places: 19
Guide weekly rate: From £374
Specialist care: None
Medical services: Podiatry, dentist, optician
Qualified staff: Exceeds standard: 86% at NVQ Level 2

Home details
Location: Residential area, 1.5 miles from Croydon.
Communal areas: 2 lounges, dining room, patio and garden
Accessibility: *Floors:* 3 • *Access:* Lift
Wheelchair access: Limited
Smoking: ✗
Pets: ✗
Routines: Flexible

Room details
Single: 15
Shared: 2
En suite: 0
Facilities: TV point

Door lock: ✓
Lockable place: ✓

Services provided
Beauty services: Hairdressing, manicures
Mobile library: Library facilities
Religious services: ✓
Transport: ✗
Activities: *Coordinator:* ✗ • *Examples:* Bingo, movement to music, painting • *Outings:* ✓
Meetings: ✓

Rutland Care Home

Manager: Joan Mullooly-Coomb
Owner: Joan Mullooly-Coomb
Contact: 46 West Street, Reigate, Surrey RH2 9DB
) 01737 242188
@ Mulloolycoomb@aol.com

Rutland Care Home is a large Edwardian detached house set on a main road between Reigate and Dorking. The home is about four minutes from the town centre; a bus service is available. The home is set back from the road with a sweeping driveway leading up to it. There is a large, terraced garden at the back of the house and many of the rooms have views onto this. The home prides itself on offering compassion and humour in equal measure and the staff, who live onsite, strive to achieve this balance. The home has its own dog.

Registered places: 18
Guide weekly rate: From £550
Specialist care: Dementia, physical disability, mental disorder
Medical services: Podiatry, dentist, optician
Qualified staff: Falls standard: 20% at NVQ level 2

Home details
Location: Residential area, 0.5 miles from Reigate centre
Communal areas: 2 lounges, 2 dining rooms, library, patio and garden
Accessibility: *Floors:* 2 • *Access:* Stair lift
Wheelchair access: Limited
Smoking: ✓
Pets: At manager's discretion
Routines: Flexible

Room details
Single: 13
Shared: 2
En suite: 2
Facilities: TV point, telephone point

Door lock: ✓
Lockable place: ✓

Services provided
Beauty services: Hairdressing, aromatherapy
Mobile library: Library facilities
Religious services: ✓
Transport: ✗
Activities: *Coordinator:* ✓ • *Examples:* arts and crafts, gentle exercise, singalongs • *Outings:* ✗
Meetings: ✓

Sheerwater House

Manager: Teresa Denton
Owner: Mr and Mrs Oozeerally
Contact: Sheerwater Road, Woodham, Woking, Surrey GU21 5TT
☎ 01932 349959

Sheerwater House is a modestly sized property located in Addlestone, close to Woking. The home is very accessible as West Byfleet station is only half a mile away, and Woking town centre is two and a half miles away where there is an abundance of shops and facilities. The home has a large garden with decking areas boasting awning for the residents to sit outside and enjoy. There are also weekly activities organised including walks along the local canal to watch local wildlife, as well as singalongs, bingo and games. Pets are welcome at the vicinity making it a lively yet homely residency.

Registered places: 20
Guide weekly rate: £350–£550
Specialist care: Dementia, respite
Medical services: None
Qualified staff: Exceeds standard: 60% at NVQ level 2

Home details

Location: Village location, 2.5 miles from Woking centre
Communal areas: Lounge, dining room, patio and garden
Accessibility: *Floors:* 3 • *Access:* Lift • *Wheelchair access:* Good
Smoking: ✗
Pets: ✓
Routines: Flexible

Room details

Single: 14
Shared: 3
En suite: 0
Facilities: TV point

Door lock: ✓
Lockable place: ✓

Services provided

Beauty services: Hairdressing
Mobile library: ✗
Religious services: ✓
Transport: ✗
Activities: *Coordinator:* ✗ • *Examples:* Bingo, gentle exercise, singalongs, walks • *Outings:* ✗
Meetings: ✓

Southborough Nursing Home

Manager: Mrs Litster
Owner: London Residential Healthcare Ltd
Contact: 12–14 Langley Avenue, Surbiton, Surrey KT6 6QL
☎ 020 8390 3366
@ info@lrh-homes.com
🖥 www.lrh-homes.com

Situated at the heart of Southborough conservation area of the Royal Borough of Kingston-upon-Thames, Southborough Nursing Home provides care and support close to an accommodating town centre. Offering a warm environment, visitors are welcome at all times and residents are kept entertained and active by the full-time activities coordinator. The home has two large lounges and a smaller sitting room for communing with friends or finding a quiet place to sit. The landscaped garden is easily accessed from the house and a conservatory provides a pleasant place to sit in colder weather. Their latest newsletter is available online.

Registered places: 56
Guide weekly rate: £500–£825
Specialist care: Nursing, physical disability, respite
Medical services: Podiatry, dentist, occupational therapy, optician, physiotherapy, speech therapy
Qualified staff: Meets standard

Home details

Location: Residential area, in Surbiton
Communal areas: 2 lounges, quite lounge, dining room, conservatory, garden
Accessibility: *Floors:* 2 • *Access:* 2 lifts *Wheelchair access:* Good
Smoking: ✗
Pets: ✗
Routines: Structured

Room details

Single: 34
Shared: 11
En suite: 7
Facilities: TV

Door lock: ✗
Lockable place: ✓

Services provided

Beauty services: Hairdressing
Mobile library: ✗
Religious services: Monthly Anglican service
Transport: ✗
Activities: *Coordinator:* ✓ • *Examples:* Bingo, crafts, visiting entertainers • *Outings:* ✓
Meetings: ✓

Southlands Rest Home

Manager: Angela Sohun
Owner: Mr and Mrs Sohun
Contact: 7 Linkfield Lane, Redhill,
Surrey RH1 1JF
☏ 01737 769146
@ southlandsresthome@hotmail.com
🖰 www.southlandsresthome.co.uk

Southlands is a large, detached property set in its own grounds. The home is situated in a residential street close to Redhill town centre and all amenities including shops, post office, theatre, cinema and good transport links to London and the south-east. The home provides a taxi service for residents who would like to go to church. The home has an activities coordinator who carries out exercise sessions, arts and craft, and outings.

Registered places: 19
Guide weekly rate: £380–£450
Specialist care: Dementia, mental disorder, respite
Medical services: Podiatry, dentist, optician, physiotherapy
Qualified staff: Exceeds standard: 70% at NVQ Level 2

Home details
Location: Residential area, 0.5 miles from Redhill centre
Communal areas: 2 lounges, dining room, patio and garden
Accessibility: *Floors:* 3 • *Access:* Lift • *Wheelchair access:* Good
Smoking: In designated area
Pets: ✓
Routines: Flexible

Room details
Single: 11
Shared: 2
En suite: 4
Facilities: TV point, telephone point

Door lock: ✓
Lockable place: ✓

Services provided
Beauty services: Hairdressing
Mobile library: ✗
Religious services: ✓
Transport: ✗
Activities: *Coordinator:* ✓ • *Examples:* Arts and crafts, exercises
   Outings: ✓
Meetings: ✓

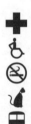

Springfield House

Manager: Ann Higgins
Owner: The Springfield Partnership
Contact: 6 Stoke Road, Cobham,
Surrey KT11 3AS
☏ 01932 862580
@ fothergills@aol.com

Springfield House is a detached property situated on a busy road in Cobham. The staff organise for musical groups and plays to visit as well as going on outings monthly. Outings occur on a monthly basis, in the home's own minibus. There is a substantial garden with two patio areas and a water fountain.

Registered places: 27
Guide weekly rate: From £880
Specialist care: Nursing, day care, dementia, respite
Medical services: Podiatry, hygienist, optician, physiotherapy
Qualified staff: Exceeds standard: 90% at NVQ level 2

Home details
Location: Residential area, 0.5 miles from Cobham centre
Communal areas: 2 lounges, 2 dining rooms, conservatory,
   hairdressing salon, 2 patios and garden
Accessibility: *Floors:* 3 • *Access:* Lift • *Wheelchair access:* Good
Smoking: ✗
Pets: At manager's discretion
Routines: Flexible

Room details
Single: 27
Shared: 0
En suite: 22
Facilities: TV point, telephone point

Door lock: ✗
Lockable place: ✓

Services provided
Beauty services: Hairdressing, aromatherapy
Mobile library: ✗
Religious services: Monthly Anglican service
Transport: Minibus
Activities: *Coordinator:* ✓ • *Examples:* Crosswords, quizzes and
   poetry • *Outings:* ✓
Meetings: ✓

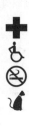

Registered places: 30
Guide weekly rate: £550–£750
Specialist care: Nursing, respite
Medical services: Podiatry, dentist, optician
Qualified staff: Meets standard

Home details

Location: Rural area, 5 miles from Guildford
Communal areas: patio and garden
Accessibility: *Floors:* 2 • *Access:* Lift • *Wheelchair access:* Good
Smoking: ✗
Pets: At manager's discretion
Routines: Flexible

Room details

Single: 24
Shared: 3
En suite: 12
Facilities: TV, telephone

Door lock: ✓
Lockable place: ✓

Services provided

Beauty services: Hairdressing
Mobile library: ✓
Religious services: Clergy visits
Transport: ✗
Activities: *Coordinator:* ✗ • *Examples:* Exercises, quizzes
    Outings: ✗
Meetings: ✗

Springfield Manor

Manager: Vacant
Owner: Springfield Manor UK Ltd
Contact: Hogs Back, Puttenham, Guildford, Surrey GU3 1AQ
☎ 01483 810177
@ Springfield.manoruk@virgin.net

Springfield Manor is located in a rural area, five miles from Guildford. Overlooking the Surrey countryside the home has a garden with a patio area. The home arranges for clergy of various denominations to visit at the residents' request. There is a range of activities on offer including performances by visiting entertainers.

Registered places: 31
Guide weekly rate: £400–£525
Specialist care: Dementia, physical disability, respite
Medical services: Podiatry, optician, physiotherapy
Qualified staff: Exceeds standard: 65% at NVQ Level 2

Home details

Location: Village location, in Hindhead
Communal areas: 2 lounges, dining room, garden
Accessibility: *Floors:* 3 • *Access:* 2 lifts
    Wheelchair access: Good
Smoking: ✗
Pets: ✗
Routines: Structured

Room details

Single: 31
Shared: 0
En suite: 15
Facilities: None

Door lock: ✗
Lockable place: ✓

Services provided

Beauty services: Hairdressing, manicures
Mobile library: ✗
Religious services: Weekly Communion service
Transport: ✗
Activities: *Coordinator:* ✗ • *Examples:* Arts and crafts, cooking,
    exercises, quizzes, gardening • *Outings:* ✗
Meetings: ✗

Springkell House

Manager: Karen Goddard
Owner: Madeprice Ltd
Contact: Wood Road, Hindhead, Surrey GU26 6PW
☎ 01428 605509
@ Springkel.care@btclick.com
 www.springkellcare.co.uk

Springkell House is a large detached Victorian property set in its own grounds in a residential part of Hindhead. A newly refurbished sitting and dining room has contributed to the homes features and environment. Pets As Therapy visits residents on a regular basis and staff organise various activities for residents, in the absence of an activities coordinator. A weekly Communion service takes place at the home.

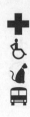

St Catherine's Manor

Manager: Susan Haslam

Owner: Mr Hasham

Contact: Portsmouth Road, Artington, Guildford, Surrey GU3 1LJ

☏ 01483 531181

St Catherine's Manor is a large detached house on the outskirts of Guildford. It is set in extensive gardens which are landscaped and very well maintained with shrubs, hedges and flowers. Those residents that enjoy gardening as a hobby are welcome to do gardening if they wish. An activities coordinator organises games, sing a longs and gentle exercise for the residents. The policy at this home is to keep residents as active and independent as possible, and by organising a variety of activities they achieve this.

Registered places: 34

Guide weekly rate: £525–£800

Specialist care: Nursing, dementia

Medical services: None

Qualified staff: Exceeds standard: 75% at NVQ Level 2

Home details

Location: Village location, 1.5 miles from Guildford

Communal areas: Lounge, dining room, patio and garden

Accessibility: *Floors:* 2 • *Access:* Lift • *Wheelchair access:* Good

Smoking: In designated area

Pets: ✓

Routines: Flexible

Room details

Single: 28	**Door lock:** ✗
Shared: 3	**Lockable place:** ✓
En suite: 20	

Facilities: TV point, telephone point

Services provided

Beauty services: Hairdressing, aromatherapy

Mobile library: ✓

Religious services: ✓

Transport: Minibus

Activities: *Coordinator:* ✓ • *Examples:* Arts and crafts, games, music • *Outings:* ✗

Meetings: ✓

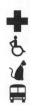

St George's Nursing Home

Manager: Carol Purdy

Owner: BUPA Care Homes Ltd

Contact: 5 Byfleet Road, Cobham, Surrey KT11 1DS

☏ 01932 868 111

@ StGeorge'sALL@BUPA.com

🖰 www.bupacarehomes.co.uk

St George's is designed to provide a safe environment for residents with all levels of dementia and related illnesses including Alzheimer's disease. The single-storey layout enables residents to walk around freely with each room opening onto the courtyard garden. An activities centre, reminiscence therapy and trips to local attractions all offer stimulation and enjoyment to residents. The staff are specially trained, and a consultant Psycho-Geriatrician is available for support and advice. Support is also provided to family and friends through a regular carers' group. The home provides a flexible pop-in service where people with dementia can use the home, giving carers access to help on an hour-by-hour basis.

Registered places: 60

Guide weekly rate: Undisclosed

Specialist care: Nursing, day care, dementia, mental disorder, respite

Medical services: Podiatry, dentist, occupational therapy, opticians, physiotherapy

Qualified staff: Undisclosed

Home details

Location: Rural area, on the outskirts of Cobham

Communal areas: 3 lounges, 2 dining rooms, hairdressing salon, patio and garden

Accessibility: *Floors:* 1 • *Wheelchair access:* Good

Smoking: In designated area

Pets: ✓

Routines: Flexible

Room details

Single: 50	**Door lock:** ✓
Shared: 4	**Lockable place:** ✗
En suite: 53	

Facilities: TV, telephone point

Services provided

Beauty services: Hairdressing, aromatherapy

Mobile library: ✓

Religious services: ✓

Transport: ✓

Activities: *Coordinator:* ✓ • *Examples:* Arts and crafts, games, reminiscence • *Outings:* ✓

Meetings: ✓

Registered places: 41
Guide weekly rate: £552–£700
Specialist care: Nursing, dementia
Medical services: Podiatry, dentist, optician, physiotherapy
Qualified staff: Meets standard

Home details

Location: Residential area, 0.5 miles from Sutton centre
Communal areas: 4 lounges, 2 dining rooms, hairdressing salon, library, garden
Accessibility: *Floors: 3 • Access:* 2 lifts and 2 stair lifts
Wheelchair access: Good
Smoking: ✗
Pets: ✗
Routines: Flexible

Room details

Single: 23
Shared: 9
En suite: 19
Facilities: TV point

Door lock: ✗
Lockable place: ✓

Services provided

Beauty services: Hairdressing
Mobile library: ✓
Religious services: ✓
Transport: ✗
Activities: *Coordinator:* ✗ • *Examples:* Karaoke, knitting, scrabble
Outings: ✓
Meetings: ✓

St Jude's Nursing Home

Manager: Sister Catherine Akhtar
Owner: Churchill Residential Care and Nursing Homes Ltd
Contact: 29–31 Mayfield Road, Sutton, Surrey SM2 5DU
☏ 020 8643 1335

St Jude's is situated in a residential area and is less than half a mile away from the town centre. There are two shopping centres in Sutton along with restaurants, hairdressers, and other amenities. Sutton has extensive public transport links with a mainline railway station and numerous bus routes passing through. The home was previously two large family houses that have been joined to form one large home. It has a garden with seating for residents to socialise as well as a hairdressing salon and library. These in-house facilities make it easier for residents to go about their daily activities.

Registered places: 40
Guide weekly rate: £400–£450
Specialist care: Dementia
Medical services: Podiatry, dentist, optician
Qualified staff: Meets standard

Home details

Location: Residential area, 0.5 miles from Sutton centre
Communal areas: 5 lounges, dining room, conservatory, garden
Accessibility: *Floors: 3 • Access:* Lift
Wheelchair access: Limited
Routines: Flexible
Pets: At manager's discretion
Smoking: In designated area

Room details

Single: 35
Shared: 5
En suite: 6
Facilities: TV point, telephone point

Door lock: ✓
Lockable place: ✓

Services provided

Beauty services: Hairdressing
Mobile library: ✗
Religious services: ✓
Transport: ✓
Activities: *Coordinator:* ✓ • *Examples:* Bingo, musical entertainment • *Outings:* ✓
Meetings: ✓

St Mary's Lodge

Manager: Jugdutt Dudhee
Owner: Jugdutt and Marietta Dudhee
Contact: 81–83 Cheam Road, Sutton, Surrey SM1 2BD
☏ 020 8661 6215

Comprised of two large Edwardian houses, St Mary's Lodge is situated within easy reach from Sutton town centre, on a main road. There is a secure garden which is accessible to residents. An activities coordinator provides residents with a range of activities, which include bingo and musical entertainment. With the home's own transport, outings are made possible.

Stanecroft

Manager: Jennifer Sharman
Owner: Care UK Community Partnerships Ltd
Contact: Spook Hill, North Holmwood, Dorking, Surrey RH5 4EG
) 01306 876567
@ Manager.burroughs@careuk.com
⌂ www.careuk.com

Stanecroft is a large care home situated in North Holmwood in Dorking. The home is on one level, divided into five units designed to maintain a sense of group living. An activities coordinator provides a range of activities for residents, such as dancing, dominoes, quizzes and visiting entertainers. Visits are made to the local garden centre, and often meals in the local pubs are arranged.

Registered places: 50
Guide weekly rate: £654
Specialist care: Day care, dementia, physical disability, respite
Medical services: Podiatry, hygienist, optician, physiotherapy
Qualified staff: Exceeds standard: 70% at NVQ Level 2

Home details
Location: Village location, 2 miles from Dorking centre
Communal areas: 5 lounges, 5 dining rooms, 2 conservatories, patio and garden
Accessibility: *Floors:* 1 • *Wheelchair access:* Good
Smoking: ✗
Pets: ✓
Routines: Flexible

Room details
Single: 50
Shared: 0
En suite: Undisclosed
Facilities: TV point, telephone point

Door lock: ✓
Lockable place: ✓

Services provided
Beauty services: Hairdressing, aromatherapy, manicures
Mobile library: ✓
Religious services: ✓
Transport: ✗
Activities: *Coordinator:* ✓ • *Examples:* Dancing, singing, quizzes
Outings: ✓
Meetings: ✓

Stokefield Care Home

Manager: Elizabeth Duddridge
Owner: Hanover Friends
Contact: St John's Hill Road, Woking, Surrey GU21 1RG
) 01483 761779
@ ann.duddridge@hanover.org.uk
⌂ www.hanover.org.uk

Stokefield Care Home is run by Hanover Friends and is situated close to Woking town centre. The garden contains seating areas for residents and the home's weekly activities are displayed on a notice board in the hall, for residents to choose what they attend. There are also frequent outings with shopping trips into town and day trips to the National Park's Clandon Park for afternoon teas and enjoying nature.

Registered places: 24
Guide weekly rate: From £497
Specialist care: Respite
Medical services: Podiatry, dentist, optician
Qualified staff: Undisclosed

Home details
Location: Residential area, 2 miles from Woking centre
Communal areas: 2 lounges, dining room, library, garden
Accessibility: *Floors:* 2 • *Access:* Lift • *Wheelchair access:* Good
Smoking: In designated area
Pets: ✗
Routines: Flexible

Room details
Single: 24
Shared: 0
En suite: 24
Facilities: TV point, telephone point

Door lock: ✓
Lockable place: ✓

Services provided
Beauty services: Hairdressing
Mobile library: ✗
Religious services: Monthly Anglican visits
Transport: Minibus
Activities: *Coordinator:* ✓ • *Examples:* Cards, scrabble, quizzes
Outings: ✓
Meetings: ✓

Registered places: 39
Guide weekly rate: £495–£679
Specialist care: Dementia, physical disability, respite
Medical services: Podiatry, hygienist, optician, physiotherapy
Qualified staff: Exceeds standard: 90% at NVQ Level 3

Home details
Location: Village location, 4 miles from Godalming
Communal areas: Lounge, dining room, conservatory, library, garden
Accessibility: *Floors:* 3 • *Access:* Lift • *Wheelchair access:* Good
Smoking: ✗
Pets: ✗
Routines: Flexible

Room details
Single: 24 Door lock: ✓
Shared: 4 Lockable place: ✓
En suite: Undisclosed
Facilities: None

Services provided
Beauty services: Hairdressing, aromatherapy, manicures
Mobile library: ✗
Religious services: Monthly church service
Transport: ✗
Activities: *Coordinator:* ✓ • *Examples:* Exercise, knitting, puzzles, quizzes • *Outings:* ✓
Meetings: ✓

Surrey Heights

Manager: Michele Woodger
Owner: Mr and Mrs Hasham
Contact: Brook Road, Wormley, Surrey GU8 5UA
☎ 01428 682734
@ g.john@carehomesofdistinction.co.uk
🖥 www.carehomesofdistinction.co.uk

Surrey Heights is a large detached building set in acres of mature south facing grounds on the crest of the Surrey Hills. There is an accessible garden and decking area. The activities coordinator works three days a week, and a programme of activities is drawn up with the help of residents. The activities coordinators consult residents over a programme of activity to be established, thus the residents preferences are prioritised. A pianist visits every other week.

Registered places: 28
Guide weekly rate: Undisclosed
Specialist care: physical disability, palliative care, respite, terminal care
Medical services: Podiatry, physiotherapy
Qualified staff: Undisclosed

Home details
Location: Residential area, 1 miles from Weybridge
Communal areas: 3 lounges, dining room, conservatory, hairdressing salon, garden
Accessibility: *Floors:* 3 • *Access:* Lift • *Wheelchair access:* Good
Smoking: ✗
Pets: ✗
Routines: Flexible

Room details
Single: 20 Door lock: ✓
Shared: 5 Lockable place: ✗
En suite: 23
Facilities: TV, telephone point

Services provided
Beauty services: Hairdressing, aromatherapy, massage
Mobile library: ✓
Religious services: Anglican vicar and Catholic priest visit once a month
Transport: ✓
Activities: *Coordinator:* ✓ • *Examples:* Barbecues, flower arranging, jazz evenings • *Outings:* ✓
Meetings: ✓

Sutton Lodge

Manager: Jackie Tout
Owner: BUPA Care Homes Ltd
Contact: 87 Oatlands Drive, Weybridge, Surrey KT13 9LN
☎ 01932 222184
@ SuttonLodgeALL@BUPA.com
🖥 www.bupacarehomes.co.uk

This Edwardian residence is situated in a residential area of Weybridge, a short distance from the town centre with its village atmosphere and traditional shops. The garden offers mature trees and flowerbeds and a pergola with climbing plants. Daily activities are offered, often in the activities room. Residents enjoy visiting speakers, and trips to local attractions such as the Savill Garden and Virginia Water in Windsor Great Park. Sutton Lodge also provides care to a number of people with physical disabilities, those who have had a stroke or require palliative or terminal care.

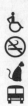

Sydenhurst

Manager: David White
Owner: Association of Ukrainians in Great Britain
Contact: Mill Lane, Chiddingfold, Surrey GU8 4SJ
☎ 01428 683124

Sydenhurst is a large detached property in its own enclosed grounds in the village of Chiddingfold. The village has a variety of local amenities, including shops, restaurants, pubs and a village green. As the Association of Ukrainians in Britain owns the home, the food reflects the Ukrainian culture. The home's extensive grounds measure 33 acres, all of which is accessible to the residents. The home also offers a separate day centre equipped with staff who provide assisted living.

Registered places: 32
Guide weekly rate: £400–£550
Specialist care: Dementia, mental disorder
Medical services: Podiatry, dentist, optician
Qualified staff: Exceeds standard: 63% at NVQ Level 2

Home details
Location: Village location, 7 miles from Godalming
Communal areas: 2 lounges, dining room, conservatory, garden
Accessibility: *Floors:* 3 • *Access:* Lift • *Wheelchair access:* Good
Smoking: ✗
Pets: ✓
Routines: Flexible

Room details
Single: 23
Shared: 4
En suite: 12
Facilities: None

Door lock: ✓
Lockable place: ✓

Services provided
Beauty services: Hairdressing, aromatherapy
Mobile library: ✗
Religious services: Monthly visits from ministers
Transport: Minibus
Activities: *Coordinator:* ✗ • *Examples:* Ball games, darts, exercise • *Outings:* ✓
Meetings: ✓

Tandridge Heights, Memorial Care Home

Manager: Joy Seymour
Owner: Barchester Healthcare Ltd
Contact: Memorial Close, off Barnett's Shaw, Oxted, Surrey RH8 0NH
☎ 01883 715595
@ tandridge@barchester.com
🖳 www.barchester.com

Tandridge Heights is situated in the town of Oxted, close to local shops and amenities. There are lounge and dining facilities on each of the three floors as well as smaller sitting areas at the end of each wing. There are pleasant garden areas with garden furniture. Activities include a variety of outings to golf ranges and pub lunches.

Registered places: 75
Guide weekly rate: Up to £1,050
Specialist care: Nursing, dementia, respite
Medical services: Podiatry, dentist, optician, physiotherapy
Qualified staff: Meets standard

Home details
Location: Village location, in Oxted
Communal areas: 3 lounges, 3 dining rooms, patio and garden
Accessibility: *Floors:* 3 • *Access:* Lift • *Wheelchair access:* Good
Smoking: In designated area
Pets: ✓
Routines: Flexible

Room details
Single: 75
Shared: 0
En suite: 75
Facilities: TV point, telephone point

Door lock: ✓
Lockable place: ✓

Services provided
Beauty services: Hairdressing, aromatherapy, manicures
Mobile library: ✓
Religious services: Weekly church service
Transport: ✗
Activities: *Coordinator:* ✓ • *Examples:* Carpet bowls, golf, pub lunches • *Outings:* ✓
Meetings: ✓

Registered places: 39
Guide weekly rate: £528–£915
Specialist care: Respite
Medical services: Podiatry, dentist, optician
Qualified staff: Exceeds standard: 75% at NVQ level 2

Home details
Location: Urban area, 1 mile from Croydon
Communal areas: Lounge, dining room, conservatory, garden
Accessibility: *Floors:* 3 • *Access:* Lift • *Wheelchair access:* Good
Smoking: x
Pets: x
Routines: Flexible

Room details
Single: 39
Shared: 0
En suite: 39
Facilities: None

Door lock: x
Lockable place: x

Services provided
Beauty services: Hairdressing

Mobile library: x

Religious services: Monthly Communion

Transport: x
Activities: *Coordinator:* ✓ • *Examples:* Bingo, games, wine tasting
Outings: x
Meetings: ✓

Thackeray House

Manager: Thomas Ndebele
Owner: Barchester Healthcare Ltd
Contact: Thackeray House,
58 Addiscombe Road, Croydon,
Surrey CR0 5PH
) 020 8649 8800
@ thackerayhouse@barchester.net
www.barchester.com

Thackeray House is situated in an urban area, one mile from Croydon and its amenities. The home arranges a Communion service once a month and there are regular residents and relatives meetings. The home also has a quiet room for residents to relax in, in addition to a conservatory and a garden. The home employs an activities coordinator who arranges a variety of activities for the residents including bingo and wine tastings.

Registered places: 17
Guide weekly rate: £400–£500
Specialist care: Dementia
Medical services: Podiatry, optician
Qualified staff: Fails standard: 40% at NVQ Level 2

Home details
Location: Residential area. 0.5 miles from New Malden centre
Communal areas: Lounge, garden
Accessibility: *Floors:* 2 • *Access:* Stair lift
Wheelchair access: Limited
Smoking: In designated area
Pets: x
Routines: Flexible

Room details
Single: 13
Shared: 2
En suite: 2
Facilities: Telephone point

Door lock: ✓
Lockable place: ✓

Services provided
Beauty services: Hairdressing
Mobile library: x
Religious services: ✓
Transport: ✓
Activities: *Coordinator:* x • *Examples:* Light exercise,
board games • *Outings:* ✓
Meetings: ✓

Thetford Lodge

Manager: Sue Martin
Owner: CHD Ltd
Contact: 16 Thetford Road, New Malden,
Surrey KT3 5DT
) 020 8942 6049

Thetford Lodge is situated in a residential street in New Malden, a short walk from the high street. The home is a converted building, with a small garden to the side of the property with seating areas. In the summer months, outings are organised to places of interest such as Worthing, Farnham and Little Hampton. The home also caters for the residents' needs as much as possible and organises activities on a weekly basis, for example board games, quizzes and light exercises.

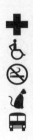

Tupwood Gate Nursing Home

Manager: Jennifer Roach
Owner: Cygnet Health Care Ltd
Contact: 74 Tupwood Lane, Caterham, Surrey CR3 6YE

✆ 01883 342275
@ tupwood@cygnethealth.co.uk
🖰 www.cygnethealth.co.uk

Tupwood House is an historic building overlooking Caterham town. As the home is on a steep hill, access is preferable by car and the home benefits from its own minibus. The home organises regular outings to restaurants and places of historic interest and entertainment from visitors at the home itself. A heated conservatory overlooks the landscaped garden and is a pleasant place to sit even in the winter months. The home also offers this as a venue for private parties with relatives. There is a quiet lounge in the drawing room and there is also a library which contains a TV.

Registered places: 34
Guide weekly rate: £850
Specialist care: Nursing, day care, dementia, palliative, respite
Medical services: Podiatry, dentist, occupational therapy, physiotherapy
Qualified staff: Exceeds standard: 75% at NVQ level 2

Home details

Location: Residential area, 0.5 miles from Caterham centre
Communal areas: Lounge, 2 dining rooms, library, conservatory, garden
Accessibility: *Floors:* 3 • *Access:* Lift • *Wheelchair access:* Good
Smoking: ✗
Pets: ✓
Routines: Structured

Room details

Single: 27
Shared: 4
En suite: 31
Facilities: Telephone point

Door lock: ✓
Lockable place: ✓

Services provided

Beauty services: Hairdressing
Mobile library: Library facilities
Religious services: Monthly Anglican service
Transport: Minibus
Activities: *Coordinator:* ✓ • *Examples:* Exercises, gardening, music sessions • *Outings:* ✓
Meetings: ✓

Upalong

Manager: Mrs McTeggart
Owner: Mrs McTeggart
Contact: 16 Castle Road, Camberley, Surrey GU15 2DS

✆ 01276 682132

Upalong is one mile from the centre of Canterbury in a quiet residential location on a bus route. The activities coordinator is trained to do physiotherapy with the residents as well as arranging games and entertainment. The home also arranges visits to the countryside for picnics, facilitated by the home's minibus. There is a religious service once a month and the home supplies books for the residents. The residents have a flexible daily routine with set meal times. Each resident has a three-course meal everyday with wine or sherry. There is also access to a medi-bath with a jacuzzi and a relaxing heated chair.

Registered places: 9
Guide weekly rate: From £500
Specialist care: None
Medical services: Podiatry, dentist, optician, physiotherapy
Qualified staff: Exceeds standard: 100% at NVQ Level 2

Home details

Location: Residential area, 1 mile from Camberley
Communal areas: Lounge, dining room, patio and garden
Accessibility: *Floors:* 2 • *Access:* Stair lift
Wheelchair access: Good
Smoking: ✗
Pets: ✓
Routines: Flexible

Room details

Single: 9
Shared: 0
En suite: 9
Facilities: TV point, telephone point

Door lock: ✓
Lockable place: ✓

Services provided

Beauty services: Hairdressing
Mobile library: Library facilities
Religious service: ✓
Transport: Minibus
Activities: *Coordinator:* ✓ • *Examples:* Exercises, games, entertainment • *Outings:* ✓
Meetings: ✓

Registered places: 26
Guide weekly rate: £525–£800
Specialist care: Nursing, emergency admissions, terminal care
Medical services: Podiatry, dentist, optician
Qualified staff: Exceeds standard: 100% at NVQ level 2

Home details

Location: Residential area, 1 mile from Croydon centre
Communal areas: Lounge, quiet lounge, activities room, dining room, conservatory, hairdressing salon, garden
Accessibility: *Floors:* 2 • *Access:* Lift • *Wheelchair access:* Good
Smoking: ✗
Pets: ✓
Routines: Structured

Room details

Single: 14
Shared: 6
En suite: 4
Facilities: TV, telephone

Door lock: ✓
Lockable place: ✓

Services provided

Beauty services: Hairdressing, aromatherapy
Mobile library: ✓
Religious services: Weekly Anglican and Catholic services
Transport: 9-seater ambulance
Activities: *Coordinator:* ✗ • *Examples:* Barbecues, floor games, reminiscence quizzes, shows, visiting artists • *Outings:* ✓
Meetings: ✗

Villa Maria Nursing Home

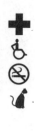

Manager: Maureen Donnelly
Owner: Jean Hedgeland and Linda Thompson
Contact: 62–68 Croham Road, South Croydon, Surrey CR2 7BB
☏ 020 8680 1777
@ villa@villamaria.co.uk
🖱 www.villamaria.co.uk

Villa Maria provides for 26 residents, aiming to create a caring family atmosphere. The home is situated in south Croydon and is near a main train station. All communal rooms overlook the large and attractive garden, which is well used in summer months. Animals are welcome in the home as it already has a dog and a cat to keep residents company. For residents that are able, outings are organised on a regular basis. These include trip to the pub for lunch, to the seaside and Bluewater shopping centre.

Registered places: 36
Guide weekly rate: £575 – £850
Specialist care: Nursing, dementia, respite
Medical services: Podiatry, dentist, optician
Qualified staff: Fails standard: 30% at NVQ Level 2

Home details

Location: Residential area, 8 miles from Leatherhead
Communal areas: Lounge, dining room, patio and garden
Accessibility: *Floors:* 2 • *Access:* Lift • *Wheelchair access:* Good
Smoking: ✗
Pets: At manager's discretion
Routines: Flexible

Room details

Single: 22
Shared: 7
En suite: 19
Facilities: TV point, telephone point

Door lock: ✓
Lockable place: ✓

Services provided

Beauty services: Hairdressing
Mobile library: ✓
Religious services: Monthly Anglican visit
Transport: Minibus
Activities: *Coordinator:* ✓ • *Examples:* Bingo, painting, pottery • *Outings:* ✓
Meetings: ✗

Warrengate Nursing Home

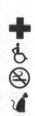

Manager: Catherine Blatcher
Owner: Claremont Care Services Ltd
Contact: De Vere House, 63 Woodland Way, Kingswood, Surrey KT20 6NN
☏ 01737 833359

Warrengate Nursing home is a large, detached building standing in its own grounds on the edge of a private estate. It benefits from large gardens and is about eight miles from Leatherhead town. The home arranges a lot of activities and outings as well as external shows once a month. The home aims to create a welcoming and caring atmosphere for residents to enjoy.

Westcott House

Manager: Eduardo Dela Cruz
Owner: Mr and Mrs Charalambous
Contact: Guildford Road, Westcott, Dorking, Surrey RH4 3QD
) 01306 881421
@ info@westcotthouse.co.uk
⌂ www.westcotthouse.co.uk

Westcott House is a large property situated in its own grounds, one and a half miles from the town centre. The home consists of a large house and an adjoining annexe plus spacious gardens. All parts of the property are accessible to wheelchairs. The home has a purpose-built day centre and a day centre manager who organises activities for residents including cookery classes, wine tasting and quizzes. There are also organised outings. The home has several lounges, a few dining rooms and a garden with a patio area. The home offers religious services and there are visits from a mobile library.

Registered places: 54
Guide weekly rate: Undisclosed
Specialist care: Nursing, day care, dementia, mental disorder, respite
Medical services: Podiatry, dentist, optician
Qualified staff: Meets standard

Home details
Location: Village location, 1.5 miles from Dorking
Communal areas: Lounges, dining rooms, conservatory/activities room, day centre, patio and garden
Accessibility: *Floors:* 3 • *Access:* Lift • *Wheelchair access:* Good
Smoking: In designated area
Pets: At manager's discretion
Routines: Flexible

Room details
Single: 39
Shared: 7
En suite: 39
Facilities: TV and telephone

Door lock: ✓
Lockable place: ✓

Services provided
Beauty services: Hairdressing, aromatherapy
Mobile library: ✓
Religious services: ✓
Transport: ✗
Activities: *Coordinator:* ✓ • *Examples:* Arts and crafts, cooking, films, wine tasting • *Outings:* ✓
Meetings: ✓

Westside Care Home

Manager: Mary Sogeler
Owner: Hill House Nursing Home Ltd
Contact: 106 Foxley Lane, Purley, Surrey CR8 3NB
) 020 8660 6453
@ hillho@freenetname.co.uk
⌂ www.hillhousecare.co.uk

Westside Care Home is situated in residential Purley, just south of Croydon, and is close to Purley crossroads. There are two lounges both with TV and video facilities, a hairdressing salon and garden with a pond at the rear. The home's motto is 'comfort with care', aiming to provide a home from home for its residents. There are two activities coordinators who organise in-house activities such as twice weekly exercise classes to music and board games. Opportunity is given for residents to be involved in activities outside the home, to ensure independence and social links are maintained.

Registered places: 31
Guide weekly rate: £620–£875
Specialist care: Nursing, respite
Medical services: Podiatry, hygienist, optician, physiotherapy
Qualified staff: Meets standard

Home details
Location: Residential area, 1 mile from Purley
Communal areas: 2 lounges, dining room, hairdressing salon, garden
Accessibility: *Floors:* 3 • *Access:* Lift • *Wheelchair access:* Good
Smoking: ✗
Pets: At manager's discretion
Routines: Flexible

Room details
Single: 20
Shared: 5
En suite: 12
Facilities: TV, telephone point

Door lock: ✓
Lockable place: ✓

Services provided
Beauty services: Hairdressing, aromatherapy, beauticians
Mobile library: ✓
Religious services: ✓
Transport: ✗
Activities: *Coordinator:* ✓ • *Examples:* Arts and crafts, pampering days, visiting entertainers • *Outings:* ✓
Meetings: ✓

Registered places: 27
Guide weekly rate: From £480
Specialist care: Respite, dementia, physical disability
Medical services: Podiatry, hygienist, optician, physiotherapy
Qualified staff: Exceeds standard: 80% at NVQ level 2

Home details

Location: Residential area, in Farnham
Communal areas: Lounge, dining room, patio and garden
Accessibility: *Floors:* 2 • *Access:* Lift • *Wheelchair access:* Good
Smoking: ×
Pets: ×
Routines: Flexible

Room details

Single: 27   Offer Door lock: ✓
Shared: 0   Lockable place: ✓
En suite: 3
Facilities: TV point, telephone point

Services provided

Beauty services: Hairdressing
Mobile library: ✓
Religious services: Fortnightly Anglican Communion service
Transport: ×
Activities: *Coordinator:* × • *Examples:* Basketball, walks, yoga
      Outings: ✓
Meetings: ✓

Wey Valley House

Manager: Shelley Hartley
Owner: Abbeyfield Society Ltd
Contact: Mike Hawthorn Drive, Farnham, Surrey GU9 7UQ
☎ 01252 712021
@ weyvalleyhouse@ukonline.co.uk

Wey Valley Home is situated in the centre of Farnham and is close to local amenities. This long-standing home is part of a charitable organisation that runs two residences and one support-living home. The residents are encouraged to be independent and active with walks along the nearby River Wey. The home also has strong links with the local community, such as the Friends of River Wey Society who take the residents on outings. Outings for residences are also organised by the home along with many other activities.

Registered places: 25
Guide weekly rate: £503–£675
Specialist care: Nursing
Medical services: Podiatry, optician
Qualified staff: Meets standard

Home details

Location: Residential area, 0.5 miles from New Malden centre
Communal areas: Lounge, dining room, garden
Accessibility: *Floors:* 2 • *Access:* Lift • *Wheelchair access:* Good
Smoking: ×
Pets: ✓
Routines: Flexible

Room details

Single: 25   Door lock: ✓
Shared: 0   Lockable place: ×
En suite: 0
Facilities: TV point

Services provided

Beauty services: Hairdressing
Mobile library: ✓
Religious services: Monthly church visits
Transport: ×
Activities: *Coordinator:* ✓ • *Examples:* Bingo, crosswords, quizzes
      • *Outings:* ✓
Meetings: ✓

The White House Nursing Home

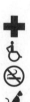

Manager: Lesley Carnegie
Owner: Badru and Sater Manji
Contact: 274 Malden Road, New Malden, Surrey KT3 6AR
☎ 020 8949 0747
@ thewhitehousenursinghome@
      btopenworld.com

The White House Nursing Home is situated on a main road close to the centre of New Malden. Public transport, shops and other amenities are within close distance of the home. There is an activities coordinator who organises daily activities for the residents such as giant crosswords, bingo and quizzes. There are also regular outings around the area for pub lunches or river walks. There is a garden with seating at the rear which residents can use to socialise or take visitors; this is used in finer weather for barbecues and outside afternoon tea.

Whitebourne

Manager: Rosaline Stevenson
Owner: Care UK Ltd
Contact: Burleigh Road, Frimley, Surrey GU16 2EP

☏ 01276 20723
@ Manager.whitebourne@careuk.com
🖰 www.careuk.com

Whitebourne is situated in a residential area, within walking distance to the local shops. The home consists of five units, each with their own lounges and communal areas. There is a pleasant grass area enclosed by fencing. Residents can participate in various days out, such as trips to the park to feed the ducks, or to the pub or a museum, which occur around twice a week. The Friends of Whitebourne, a group of family and friends of residents are regularly involved with the home's activities.

Registered places: 63
Guide weekly rate: £750–£850
Specialist care: Day care, dementia, sensory impairment
Medical services: Podiatry, optician
Qualified staff: Exceeds standard: 70% at NVQ Level 2

Home details
Location: Residential area, 2 miles from Farnborough
Communal areas: 5 lounges, 3 dining rooms, garden
Accessibility: *Floors:* 2 • *Access:* Lift • *Wheelchair access:* Good
Smoking: In designated area
Pets: ✗
Routines: Flexible

Room details
Single: 63
Shared: 0
En suite: 63
Facilities: TV point, telephone point

Door lock: ✓
Lockable place: ✓

Services provided
Beauty services: Hairdressing
Mobile library: ✗
Religious services: Weekly Anglican and Catholic Communion services
Transport: ✗
Activities: *Coordinator:* ✓ • *Examples:* Arts and crafts, cooking, orientation memory games • *Outings:* ✓
Meetings: ✓

Whitgift House

Manager: Philomena Kavanagh
Owner: The Whitgift Foundation
Contact: 76 Brighton Road, South Croydon, Surrey CR2 6AB

☏ 020 8760 0472
🖰 www.whitgiftfoundation.co.uk

Owned and managed by the charitable trust, The Whitgift Foundation, Whitgift House shares its grounds with a secondary school and the home is active within the wider community. With well-maintained grounds that include a chapel as well as lawns and a cricket ground, residents and staff play croquet on the lawn. Many of the residents take part in social activities such as the lunch club, aerobics and the arts and crafts summer fair. There is a bus stop just outside the house which provides residents with easy access to nearby facilities.

Registered places: 20
Guide weekly rate: £524–£695
Specialist care: Nursing
Medical services: Podiatry, dentist, optician, physiotherapy
Qualified staff: Exceeds standard: 65% at NVQ level 2

Home details
Location: Residential area, 1 mile from Croydon
Communal areas: Lounge, dining room, chapel, garden
Accessibility: *Floors:* 3 • *Access:* Lift • *Wheelchair access:* Good
Smoking: ✗
Pets: At manager's discretion
Routines: Flexible

Room details
Single: 20
Shared: 0
En suite: 0
Facilities: TV point, telephone point

Door lock: ✗
Lockable place: ✓

Services provided
Beauty services: Hairdressing
Mobile library: ✗
Religious services: ✓
Transport: Minibus
Activities: *Coordinator:* ✓ • *Examples:* Crafts, exercise, musical entertainment, reminiscence sessions • *Outings:* ✗
Meetings: ✓

Registered places: 12
Guide weekly rate: From £700
Specialist care: Nursing, respite
Medical services: Podiatry, dentist, optician, physiotherapy
Qualified staff: Exceeds standard: 70% at NVQ Level 2

Home details

Location: Residential area, in East Molsey
Communal areas: 4 lounges, dining room, patio and garden
Accessibility: *Floors:* 2 • *Access:* Stair lift
    Wheelchair access: Good
Smoking: In designated area
Pets: ✓
Routines: Flexible

Room details

Single: 12
Shared: 0
En suite: 12
Facilities: TV, telephone

Offer of Door lock: ✓
Lockable place: ✓

Services provided

Beauty services: Hairdressing, manicure, personal trainer
Mobile library: ✗
Religious services: ✗
Transport: Minibus
Activities: *Coordinator:* ✓ • *Examples:* Crossword, music
    performances, quizzes • *Outings:* ✓
Meetings: ✓

Willowmead Residential Home

Manager: Marion Davies
Owner: Marion Davies
Contact: Summer Road, East Molesey, Surrey KT8 9LR
☏ 020 8398 8664
@ willowmead@mariondavies.fsnet.co.uk

Willowmead Residential Home is located in the village of East Molsey and is within walking distance from shops and facilities on East Molsey high street. The home has a garden to the rear with a patio area that leads down to a summerhouse overlooking the River Thames. In the summer months, the home aims to provide a weekly outing for its residents in the home's minibus and is conveniently only half a mile from Hampton Court Palace.

Registered places: 73
Guide weekly rate: Undisclosed
Specialist care: Nursing, learning disability, palliative care,
    physical disability, respite, terminal care
Medical services: Podiatry, physiotherapy
Qualified staff: Undisclosed

Home details

Location. Village location, 1 mile from Esher centre
Communal areas: 5 lounges, 3 dining room, kitchenette,
    hairdressing salon, café/bar, computer room, garden
Accessibility: *Floors:* 2 • *Access:* Lift • *Wheelchair access:* Good
Smoking: In designated area
Pets: ✓
Routines: Flexible

Room details

Single: 73
Shared: 0
En suite: 73
Facilities: TV

Door lock: ✓
Lockable place: ✗

Services provided

Beauty services: Hairdressing, aromatherapy
Mobile library: ✓
Religious services: ✓
Transport: ✓
Activities: *Coordinator:* ✓ • *Examples:* Crafts, quizzes,
    visiting entertainers • *Outings:* ✓
Meetings: ✓

Wingham Court

Manager: Jacky Sylvester
Owner: BUPA Care Homes Ltd
Contact: Oaken Lane, Claygate, Surrey KT10 0RQ
☏ 01372 464612
@ WinghamCourtALL@BUPA.com
🖳 www.bupacarehomes.co.uk

Wingham Court is situated in Claygate, near local shops and public transport; the home is on a main bus route and close to Claygate BR Station. The home is a purpose-built building set in four acres of grounds and is designed specifically to meet the needs of elderly residents who require nursing care and also provides care for younger physically disabled people. The home also has a bowling green and tennis courts. Regular activities are arranged such as crafts, quizzes and general entertainment. Trips are also taken to local places of interest such as Hampton Court and boat trips taken along the River Thames.

Woking Homes

Manager: Mavis Phair
Owner: Woking Homes
Contact: Oriental Road, Woking,
Surrey GU22 7BE
☎ 01483 763558
@ administrator@woking-homes.co.uk
🖱 www.woking-homes.co.uk

Woking Homes is a care home run by a registered charity of the same name, providing accommodation mostly for ex-employees of the rail network and their spouses. Residents have access to the home's indoor swimming pool, sauna and gym. The home also boasts a small bowling alley, and residents regularly use the garden to play bowls or croquet during the warmer months. The home offers outings to theatres and other places of interest for residents to enjoy. There is also a book club.

Registered places: 50
Guide weekly rate: Undisclosed
Specialist care: Dementia, respite
Medical services: Podiatry
Qualified staff: Meets standard

Home details
Location: Residential area, 1 mile from Woking centre
Communal areas: 5 lounges, quiet lounge, swimming pool, sauna and gym, bowling alley, conservatory, garden
Accessibility: *Floors:* 1 • *Wheelchair access:* Good
Smoking: ✗
Pets: At manager's discretion
Routines: Flexible

Room details
Single: 48	**Door lock:** ✓
Shared: 2	**Lockable place:** ✓
En suite: 50	
Facilities: TV point, telephone point	

Services provided
Beauty services: Hairdressing
Mobile library: ✓
Religious services: Monthly Communion service
Transport: ✓
Activities: *Coordinator:* ✗ • *Examples:* Arts and crafts, croquet
Outings: ✓
Meetings: ✓

Wolf House

Manager: Yvonne Gomes
Owner: Yvonne Gomes
Contact: Wolf's Row, Oxted,
Surrey RH8 0EB
☎ 01883 716627

Wolf House is situated in a quiet residential area and is an adapted, detached house set in its own grounds. To the front of the building, there is a small car park with a seating area overlooking a cottage garden. The home has a secluded rear garden with small a patio area. Though set in a rural location Wolf House is only a short distance from Oxted town centre. Here there is a wide range of shops and community amenities. Pub lunches are also offered to residents as part of their programme of outings.

Registered places: 13
Guide weekly rate: £330–£650
Specialist care: Dementia, mental disorder, respite
Medical services: Podiatry, hygienist, optician, physiotherapy
Qualified staff: Exceeds standard: 60% at NVQ Level 2

Home details
Location: Village location, 1 mile from Oxted centre
Communal areas: Lounge, dining room, conservatory, garden
Accessibility: *Floors:* 3 • *Access:* Stair lift
Wheelchair access: Limited
Smoking: ✓
Pets: ✓
Routines: Flexible

Room details
Single: 11	**Door lock:** ✓
Shared: 1	**Lockable place:** ✓
En suite: 2	
Facilities: TV point, telephone point	

Services provided
Beauty services: Hairdressing, aromatherapy, manicures
Mobile library: ✗
Religious services: ✓
Transport: ✗
Activities: *Coordinator:* ✓ • *Examples:* Arts and crafts, cookery, occupational therapy • *Outings:* ✓
Meetings: ✓

Registered places: 51
Guide weekly rate: £526–£854
Specialist care: Day care, dementia, respite, terminal care
Medical services: Podiatry, dentist, optician, physiotherapy
Qualified staff: Fails standards

Home details

Location: Residential area, 1 mile from Redhill
Communal areas: 3 lounges, dining room, garden
Accessibility: *Floors:* 2 • *Access:* Lift • *Wheelchair access:* Good
Smoking: ✗
Pets: At manager's discretion
Routines: Structured

Room details

Single: 41
Shared: 5
En suite: 14
Facilities: TV point, telephone point

Door lock: ✗
Lockable place: ✓

Services provided

Beauty services: Hairdressing
Mobile library: ✓
Religious services: ✓
Transport: ✗
Activities: *Coordinator:* ✓ • *Examples:* Discussion, quizzes,
   music • *Outings:* ✗
Meetings: ✗

Wray Common Nursing Home

Manager: Karin Edgren
Owner: Dovestone Estates Ltd
Contact: Wray Common Road,
Reigate, Surrey RH2 0ND
☎ 01737 242647

Wray Common Nursing Home is a family-run home, and staff pride themselves on being able to offer a service with a personal touch. The home offers a range of activities and focuses on the care of the resident. They offer a wide range of care and aim for a friendly and caring environment. Various ministers visit the home at the request of residents.

Registered places: 24
Guide weekly rate: From £525
Specialist care: Dementia, physical disability, mental disorder,
   sensory impairment
Medical services: Podiatry, dentist, optician
Qualified staff: Exceeds standard: 68% at NVQ Level 2

Home details

Location: Residential area, 1.5 miles from Reigate centre
Communal areas: 2 lounges, dining room, garden
Accessibility: *Floors:* 3 • *Access:* Lift and stair lift
   Wheelchair access: Good
Smoking: In designated area
Pets: At manager's discretion
Routines: Flexible

Room details

Single: 16
Shared: 4
En suite: 14
Facilities: TV point, telephone point

Door lock: ✗
Lockable place: ✓

Services provided

Beauty services: Hairdressing, aromatherapy
Mobile library: ✗
Religious services: Monthly Anglican visits
Transport: Minibus
Activities: *Coordinator:* ✓ • *Examples:* Arts and craft, music,
   reminiscence • *Outings:* ✓
Meetings: ✓

Wray Park Care Home

Manager: Antony Coomb
Owner: Care Homes Of Distinction Ltd
Contact: 55 Alma Road, Reigate,
Surrey RH2 0DN
☎ 01737 242778
@ wraypark@btconnect.com

Wray Park Care Home is a detached, Georgian property in Reigate. The home is set in substantial grounds with a well-maintained garden including various features such as a birdbath donated by a previous resident. Reigate town centre and its amenities is a 15-minute walk from the home and Reigate railway station is a 10-minute walk. The home has its own minibus in which to take residents on outings. There is also an activities coordinator at the home who organises activities such as reminiscence sessions and musical entertainment.

Wychwood

Manager: Mumtaz Lalani
Owner: Mumtaz Lalani
Contact: Headley Road, Hindhead,
Surrey GU26 6TN
☎ 01428 607014

Comprising of two properties that are set in the home's grounds, Wychwood is situated in the village of Hindhead, 10 minutes from local shops and amenities. The home is set in an acre of grounds that are maintained by a gardener who comes weekly. Residents are free to walk around the well-kept grounds, which has level access in most parts. On a weekly basis activities are planned such as country walks, gardening and games.

Registered places: 24
Guide weekly rate: £450–£799
Specialist care: Dementia, mental disorder, physical disability
Medical services: Podiatry, dental, optician, physiotherapy
Qualified staff: Meets standard

Home details

Location: Village location, in Hindhead
Communal areas: 2 lounges, dining room, garden
Accessibility: *Floors:* 2 • *Access:* Lift
   Wheelchair access: Limited
Smoking: In designated area
Pets: At manager's discretion
Routines: Flexible

Room details

Single: 18	**Door lock:** ✗
Shared: 3	**Lockable place:** ✓
En suite: 6	
Facilities: TV point, telephone point	

Services provided

Beauty services: Hairdressing
Mobile library: ✓
Religious services: ✗
Transport: ✗
Activities: *Coordinator:* ✗ • *Examples:* Gardening, quizzes, walks • *Outings:* ✗
Meetings: ✗

Wykeham House

Manager: Naresh Mapara
Owner: Barchester Healthcare Ltd
Contact: 21 Russells Crescent, Horley, Surrey RH6 7DJ
☎ 01293 823835
@ naresh.mapara@barchester.com
🖰 www.barchester.com

Wykeham House is located in a residential area approximately one mile from the town centre of Horley. The home has four lounges, two dining rooms and large gardens for the residents to enjoy. The home has its own minibus for outings and there are two activities coordinators employed at the home. There are regular residents meetings held and daily activities include performances by visiting entertainers and visits from PAT dogs.

Registered places: 76
Guide weekly rate: £750–£775
Specialist care: Nursing, dementia, mental disorder, physically disabled, respite
Medical services: Podiatry, dentist, optician
Qualified staff: Fails standard

Home details

Location: Residential area, 0.7 miles from Horley
Communal areas: 4 lounges, 2 dining rooms, garden
Accessibility: *Floors:* 2 • *Access:* 2 lifts
   Wheelchair access: Good
Smoking: ✗
Pets: ✗
Routines: Flexible

Room details

Single: 76	**Door lock:** Undisclosed
Shared: 0	**Lockable place:** ✓
En suite: 76	
Facilities: TV point, telephone	

Services provided

Beauty services: Hairdressing room
Mobile library: Undisclosed
Religious services: Undisclosed
Transport: Minibus
Activities: *Coordinator:* ✓ • *Examples:* Pets as Therapy, visiting entertainers • *Outings:* ✓
Meetings: ✓

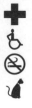

Abbas Combe Nursing Home

Manager: Victoria Barkaway
Owner: Lotus Care Group
Contact: 94 Whyke Road, Chichester, West Sussex PO19 8JF
☎ 01243 789826

Abbas Combe is a care home offering nursing, situated near the ring road south of Chichester. The home was originally a detached house, which has now been extended and renovated. The home is approximately 20 minutes walk from Chichester town centre. They have regular visits from visiting entertainers and also a clothes show. Any religious services can be arranged on request. The home aims to have a happy atmosphere for residents and their families to feel at home.

Registered places: 25
Guide weekly rate: £550–£700
Specialist care: Nursing, respite
Medical services: Podiatry, optician
Qualified staff: Fails standard: 45% at NVQ Level 2

Home details
Location: Residential area, 1.5 miles from Chichester centre
Communal areas: Lounge, dining room, conservatory, patio and garden
Accessibility: *Floors:* 2 • *Access:* Lift • *Wheelchair access:* Good
Smoking: ✗
Pets: At manager's discretion
Routines: Flexible

Room details
Single: 21
Shared: 2
En suite: 8
Facilities: TV point

Door lock: ✓
Lockable place: ✓

Services provided
Beauty services: Hairdressing
Mobile library: ✗
Religious services: ✓
Transport: ✗
Activities: *Coordinator:* ✗ • *Examples:* Clothes show, entertainers, quizzes • *Outings:* ✗
Meetings: ✗

Abbey Dean

Manager: Laramie Dean
Owner: Mr and Mrs Dean
Contact: 102 Barnham Road, Barnham, Chichester, West Sussex PO22 0EW
☎ 01243 554535

Abbey Dean is a semi-detached property with well-kept gardens with lawns and walkways. The home is situated in the village of Barnham, nine miles from Chichester and five miles from Bognor Regis. The home has a wealth of activities to choose form including flower arranging and arts and crafts. There are also outings for shopping trips and local points of interest. The home aims for a caring environment for both the residents and relatives to enjoy.

Registered places: 14
Guide weekly rate: From £475
Specialist care: None
Medical services: Podiatry, dentist, optician
Qualified staff: Meets standard

Home details
Location: Village location, 5 miles from Bognor Regis
Communal areas: Lounge, dining room, garden
Accessibility: *Floors:* 2 • *Access:* Lift • *Wheelchair access:* Good
Smoking: ✗
Pets: Pets welcome
Routines: Flexible

Room details
Single: 14
Shared: 0
En suite: 14
Facilities: TV point, telephone point

Door lock: ✓
Lockable place: ✓

Services provided
Beauty services: Hairdressing
Mobile library: ✓
Religious services: Monthly Anglican service
Transport: Minibus
Activities: *Coordinator:* ✓ • *Examples:* Crafts, flower arranging, beetle drive • *Outings:* ✓
Meetings: ✗

Adelaide House

Manager: Mr Philip
Owner: Adelaide Health Care Ltd
Contact: 13 Oathall Road, Haywards Heath, West Sussex RH16 3EG

☎ 01444 441244
@ ashtongrpade@aol.com

Adelaide House is a large, detached Victorian building situated half a mile from the local shops. There is a lounge, dining room, sun lounge and garden with a paved area. The home has an activities coordinator who devises a one-to-one programme for those who do not wish to participate in group activities in addition to the group programme. These activities include quizzes, singing, visiting entertainers and exercise sessions. There are special events such as fêtes and barbecues and birthdays and anniversary celebrations. Pets are allowed at the manager's discretion, if the resident can care for the animal.

Registered places: 40
Guide weekly rate: £519–£750
Specialist care: Physical disability
Medical services: Podiatry, dentist, optician, physiotherapy
Qualified staff: Exceeds standard: 75% at NVQ Level 2

Home details
Location: Residential area, 0.5 miles from Haywards Heath centre
Communal areas: Lounge, dining room, conservatory, garden
Accessibility: *Floors:* 3 • *Access:* Lift • *Wheelchair access:* Good
Smoking: In designated area
Pets: At manager's discretion
Routines: Flexible

Room details
Single: 26
Shared: 7
En suite: 23
Facilities: TV, telephone point

Door lock: ✓
Lockable place: ✓

Services provided
Beauty services: Hairdressing, aromatherapy, manicures
Mobile library: ✓
Religious services: ✓
Transport: ✗
Activities: *Coordinator:* ✓ • *Examples:* Exercise, quizzes, visiting entertainers • *Outings:* ✓
Resident meetings: ✗

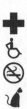

Aldersmead Residential and Nursing Home

Manager: Mrs Pauline Borland
Owner: Balcombe Care Homes Ltd
Contact: 17–19 Upper Bognor Road, Bognor Regis, West Sussex PO21 1AJ

☎ 01243 827619
@ Aldermead@
    balcombecarehomes.co.uk
🖰 www.balcombecarehomes.co.uk

Aldersmead is situated on the outskirts of Bognor Regis, close to the railway station and all local amenities. The home is undergoing an extension and improvements to the facilities are being made. Families are welcomed into the home and are able to join residents for lunch. Residents have the option to partake in organised activities, or to leisurely carry out their day as they please. Parties are held to celebrate residents' birthdays.

Registered places: 35
Guide weekly rate: £600–£750
Specialist care: Nursing, respite
Medical services: Podiatry, optician
Qualified staff: Meets standard

Home details
Location: Residential area, 0.5 miles from Bognor Regis centre
Communal areas: Lounge, dining room, patio and garden
Accessibility: *Floors:* 3 • *Access:* Lift • *Wheelchair access:* Good
Smoking: ✗
Pets: At manager's discretion
Routines: Flexible

Room details
Single: 35
Shared: 0
En suite: 35
Facilities: TV point

Door lock: ✓
Lockable place: ✓

Services provided
Beauty services: Hairdressing
Mobile library: ✗
Religious services: ✗
Transport: ✗
Activities: *Coordinator:* ✓ • *Examples:* Bingo, exercise, quizzes
Meetings: ✓

Registered places: 32
Guide weekly rate: Undisclosed
Specialist care: Nursing, dementia, mental disorder
Medical services: Podiatry
Qualified staff: Meets standard

Home details
Location: Residential area, 0.5 miles from Bognor Regis centre
Communal areas: Lounge, dining room, conservatory, garden
Accessibility: *Floors:* 2 • *Access:* Lift • *Wheelchair access:* Good
Smoking: In designated area
Pets: ✗
Routines: Structured

Room details
Single: 30
Shared: 1
En suite: Undisclosed
Facilities: TV, telephone

Door lock: ✓
Lockable place: ✓

Services provided
Beauty services: Hairdressing, aromatherapy, massage
Mobile library: ✗
Religious services: ✗
Transport: ✗
Activities: *Coordinator:* ✗ *Examples:* • Gardening, painting, visiting entertainers • *Outings:* ✗
Meetings: ✗

Aldwick House

Manager: Simon Hollis
Owner: New Century Care Ltd
Contact: Nyewood Lane, Bognor Regis, West Sussex PO21 2SJ
☏ 01243 842244
@ aldwickhouse@new-meridan.co.uk
🖰 www.newcenturycare.co.uk

Aldwick House is situated in a residential area a quarter of a mile from local amenities, theatres and the seafront. The staff arrange daily activities and visits from entertainers such as magicians. The home is in the process of building a conservatory which will be used as a sensory room. There is a TV in each room and a telephone can be arranged. There are good train and bus services near the home with easy access to the local towns of Bognor, Brighton and Chichester. A monthly newsletter is handed out to relatives to ensure they are kept up-to-date with events in the home.

Registered places: 12
Guide weekly rate: £400–£453
Specialist care: Respite, mental disorder
Medical services: Podiatry, hygienist, optician, physiotherapy
Qualified staff: Exceeds standard: 75% at NVQ Level 2

Home details
Location: Residential area, 0.5 miles from Bognor Regis centre
Communal areas: 2 lounge/dining rooms, garden
Accessibility: *Floors:* 2 • *Access:* Lift
   Wheelchair access: Good
Smoking: ✗
Pets: ✓
Routines: Flexible

Room details
Single: 12
Shared: 0
En suite: 3
Facilities: TV point

Door lock: ✗
Lockable place: ✓

Services provided
Beauty services: Hairdressing
Mobile library: ✓
Religious services: ✓
Transport: Minibus
Activities: *Coordinator:* ✓ • *Examples:* Music and exercise, visiting entertainers twice weekly, musicians • *Outings:* ✓
Meetings: ✓

Amber Lodge

Manager: Patricia Simmonds
Owner: Patricia Simmonds
Contact: 12 Annandale Avenue, Bognor Regis, West Sussex PO21 2EU
☏ 01243 821550
@ p.simmonds@btconnect.com

Amber Lodge is located half a mile from Bognor Regis town centre, in a quiet residential area. It has well-kept gardens. The home has its own minibus which is used to take the residents out on regular day trips to Bognor centre. In the home there is also a video library and two resident cats and a dog. Residents' pets are always welcome. Coffee mornings are held daily, where residents discuss what they would like to do that day, and the home also organises visiting entertainment to come in twice a week, this includes a live musician and talks about the local area.

The Anchorage Rest Home

Manager: Sheila Wyatt
Owner: Rhymecare Ltd
Contact: Coombelands Lane, Pulborough, West Sussex RH20 1AG
☎ 01798 872779
@ theanchorage@rhymecare.co.uk
🖰 www.rhymecare.co.uk

The Anchorage is a detached property, situated near Pulborough. The home is set in its own grounds with views of the South Downs from many bedroom windows. There is a variety of activities on offer including a book club and garden parties. The full-time chefs use fresh, local produce, and regularly organise themed lunches for residents. The home is in a rural location, and without its own transport, residents could feel isolated.

Registered places: 30
Guide weekly rate: Undisclosed
Specialist care: Respite
Medical services: Podiatry, dentist, optician, physiotherapy
Qualified staff: Meets standard

Home details

Location: Rural area, 1 mile from Pulborough
Communal areas: Lounge, dining room, garden
Accessibility: *Floors:* 2 • *Access:* Lift
  Wheelchair access: Good
Smoking: In designated area
Pets: At manager's discretion
Routines: Flexible

Room details

Single: 30
Shared: 0
En suite: 22
Facilities: TV, telephone

Door lock: ✓
Lockable place: ✓

Services provided

Beauty services: Hairdressing
Mobile library: ✓
Religious services: Fortnightly Anglican and Catholic services
Transport: ✗
Activities: *Coordinator:* ✓ • *Examples:* Book club, garden parties • *Outings:* ✓
Meetings: ✗

Appletree House Care Home

Manager: Angelo Dalpadado
Owner: Mr and Mrs Dalpadado
Contact: 9 Pratton Avenue, Lancing, West Sussex BN159NU
☎ 01903 762102

Appletree House is a detached property located in a residential area of Lancing, three and a half miles from Worthing. The home is close to local amenities, and offers a large rear garden for residents to enjoy. An activities coordinator provides residents with activities such as quizzes, bingo and card making. Weekly visits are made by boys from a local independent school who either take residents for walks, talk or read to residents or play table games.

Registered places: 15
Guide weekly rate: £310–£400
Specialist care: Respite
Medical services: Podiatry, dentist, optician
Qualified staff: Meets standard

Home details

Location: Residential area, 3.5 miles from Worthing
Communal areas: 2 lounge/dining rooms, conservatory, garden
Accessibility: *Floors:* 2 • *Access:* Lift • *Wheelchair access:* Limited
Smoking: ✗
Pets: At manager's discretion
Routines: Structured

Room details

Single: 13
Shared: 1
En suite: 4
Facilities: TV point, telephone point

Door lock: ✓
Lockable place: ✓

Services provided

Beauty services: Hairdressing
Mobile library: ✗
Religious services: Communion service
Transport: ✗
Activities: *Coordinator:* ✓ • *Examples:* Quizzes, bingo, card making • *Outings:* ✓
Meetings: ✓

Registered places: 20
Guide weekly rate: £400–£480
Specialist care: Day care, respite
Medical services: Podiatry, dentist, optician
Qualified staff: Fails standard: 30% at NVQ Level 2

Home details

Location: Village location, 9 miles from Chichester
Communal areas: Lounge, dining room, garden
Accessibility: *Floors:* 2 • *Access:* Lift and stair lift
    Wheelchair access: Limited
Smoking: In designated area
Pets: At manager's discretion
Routines: Flexible

Room details

Single: 20   Door lock: ✓
Shared: 0   Lockable place: ✓
En suite: 7
Facilities: TV, telephone point

Services provided

Beauty services: Hairdressing
Mobile library: ✗
Religious services: Monthly visit from vicar
Transport: ✗
Activities: *Coordinator:* ✓ • *Examples:* Concerts, music for health,
    walks • *Outings:* ✗
Meetings: ✗

April Cottage

Manager: Elaine Davitt
Owner: Dr Hugh and
Dr Catherine Condon
Contact: 1 Park Road, Selsey,
Chichester, West Sussex PO20 0PR
☎ 01243 602450

April Cottage is a detached property with a spacious garden close to the seafront in Selsey. There are activities in the home available for residents to get involved in and residents are also encouraged to join activities in the local community such as art clubs and church. The activities organiser also takes residents for walks by the sea. The home has strong ties with the community for example local school children come in to help at supper times. The home is a quarter mile from shops, a post office and bus stop.

Registered places: 38
Guide weekly rate: From £480
Specialist care: Nursing
Medical services: Podiatry, dentist, optician, physiotherapy
Qualified staff: Exceeds standard: 80% at NVQ level 2

Home details

Location: Residential area, 0.5 miles from Bognor Regis centre
Communal areas: Lounge, dining room, patio and garden
Accessibility: *Floors:* 2 • *Access:* Lift • *Wheelchair access:* Good
Smoking: ✗
Pets: ✗
Routines: Flexible

Room details

Single: 34   Door lock: ✓
Shared: 2   Lockable place: ✓
En suite: 18
Facilities: TV point, telephone point

Services provided

Beauty services: Hairdressing
Mobile library: ✓
Religious services: ✓
Transport: Minibus
Activities: *Coordinator:* ✓ • *Examples:* Gardening club, pilates,
    reminiscence • *Outings:* ✓
Meetings: ✓

Aronel Cottage

Manager: Julian Hitchcock
Owner: Aronel Cottage Care Home Ltd
Contact: 5–11 Highfield Road,
Bognor Regis, West Sussex PO22 8BQ
☎ 01243 842000
@ enquiries@aronelcottage.co.uk
🖳 www.aronelcottage.co.uk

A family-run care home that has been established for 32 years, Aronel Cottage is situated in a quiet residential area and was once a private school. The home is situated half a mile from Bognor Regis and is located on a bus route. The residents have a flexible routine with set meal times. The home offers a comprehensive activities programme that includes a gardening club, pilates and musical therapy. There are also monthly outings in the summer to places of local interest and the home has its own trolley shop and produces a newsletter every month in conjunction with the residents' meetings.

Arun Lodge Rest Home

Manager: Vacant
Owner: Annette Rawlins
Contact: 6–8 Stocker Road, Bognor Regis, West Sussex PO21 2QF
☎ 01243 866056

Arun Lodge is situated close to the seafront in Bognor Regis. There is good wheelchair access with the exception of four rooms that are reached only by stairs and therefore inaccessible for wheelchairs. In the garden decking and a gazebo for shade make pleasant seating areas. Outings are organised such as a day trip to Spinnaker Tower. There is a Pets For Therapy scheme.

Registered places: 21
Guide weekly rate: £331–£440
Specialist care: Respite
Medical services: Podiatry, dentist, optician, physiotherapy
Qualified staff: Meets standard

Home details
Location: Residential area, 1 mile from Bognor Regis centre
Communal areas: 2 lounges, dining room, garden
Accessibility: *Floors:* 2 • *Access:* Lift • *Wheelchair access:* Good
Smoking: In designated area
Pets: At manager's discretion
Routines: Flexible

Room details
Single: 21
Shared: 0
En suite: 19
Facilities: TV point, telephone point
Door lock: ✓
Lockable place: ✓

Services provided
Beauty services: Hairdressing
Mobile library: ✓
Religious services: Fortnightly Anglican Communion service
Transport: Car
Activities: *Coordinator:* ✗ • *Examples:* Exercise, fêtes, quizzes • *Outings:* ✓
Meetings: ✓

Ashbourne

Manager: Natasha Gould
Owner: Mr and Mrs Wilford
Contact: Byways, Selsey, West Sussex PO20 0HY
☎ 01243 604612

Ashbourne is detached house in a quiet area of Selsey a few yards from the seafront and half a mile from the town centre. The home is close to local amenities. The home has its own cat and organises a variety of activities. There is also musical entertainment brought in for residents to enjoy.

Registered places: 18
Guide weekly rate: £400–£445
Specialist care: Day care, Respite
Medical services: Podiatry, optician, physiotherapy
Qualified staff: Meets standard

Home details
Location: Village location, 9 miles from Chichester
Communal areas: Lounge, dining room, patio and garden
Accessibility: *Floors:* 2 • *Access:* Lift • *Wheelchair access:* Good
Smoking: In designated area
Pets: At manager's discretion
Routines: Flexible

Room details
Single: 18
Shared: 0
En suite: 18
Facilities: TV point, telephone point
Door lock: ✓
Lockable place: ✓

Services provided
Beauty services: Hairdressing
Mobile library: ✗
Religious services: ✗
Transport: ✗
Activities: *Coordinator:* ✗ • *Examples:* Bingo, music and movement, skittles • *Outings:* ✓
Meetings: ✗

Registered places: 13
Guide weekly rate: £317–£489
Specialist care: Respite
Medical services: Podiatry, hygienist, optician, physiotherapy
Qualified staff: Meets standard

Home details
Location: Residential area, 1.5 miles from Littlehampton
Communal areas: Lounge, dining room, patio and garden
Accessibility: *Floors:* 2 • *Access:* Lift • *Wheelchair access:* Good
Smoking: ✗
Pets: ✓
Routines: Flexible

Room details
Single: 13
Shared: 0
En suite: 4
Facilities: TV point, telephone point

Door lock: ✓
Lockable place: ✓

Services provided
Beauty services: Hairdressing, manicures
Mobile library: Library facilities
Religious services: Monthly Anglican and Catholic services
Transport: ✗
Activities: *Coordinator:* ✗ • *Examples:* Bingo, quizzes, walks • *Outings:*
Meetings: ✓

Ashdown Lodge

Manager: Julie Clear
Owner: Janet Tucker
Contact: 2 Wendy Ridge, North Lane, Rustington, Littlehampton, West Sussex BN16 3PJ
☏ 01903 785251

Ashdown Lodge is a semi-detached two-storey home in the village of Rustingdon, close to local shops. There is no mobile library but the home gets their books from the local library. There is also a resident dog and other pets are welcome. There are a lot of different activities for residents to get involved in, board games and going for walks to keep active or even some fresh air.

Registered places: 50
Guide weekly rate: £259–£601
Specialist care: Nursing, respite
Medical services: Podiatry, hygienist, optician, physiotherapy
Qualified staff: Meets standard

Home details
Location: Residential area, 0.5 miles from Worthing centre
Communal areas: 4 lounges, dining room, conservatory, patio and garden
Accessibility: *Floors:* 4 • *Access:* Lift • *Wheelchair access:* Good
Smoking: ✗
Pets: ✗
Routines: Flexible

Room details
Single: 50
Shared: 0
En suite: 2
Facilities: TV point, telephone point

Door lock: ✓
Lockable place: ✓

Services provided
Beauty services: Hairdressing
Mobile library: ✗
Religious services: Monthly Communion service
Transport: ✗
Activities: *Coordinator:* ✓ • *Examples:* Bingo, quizzes • *Outings:* ✓
Meetings: ✓

Ashmount Residetial and Nursing Home

Manager: Alison Wiles
Owner: Guild Care
Contact: 10 Southey Road, Worthing, West Sussex BN11 3HT
☏ 01903 528500
@ ashmount@guildcare.org
🖰 www.guildcare.org.uk

Backing directly onto a main road in a residential area of Worthing, Ashmount is a Victorian building that is located 300 yards from the seafront and shopping areas. Activities coordinators supply a programme of activities, ranging from bingo, quizzes, and shopping and theatre trips. A recently founded 'gourmet dining club' activity has also been set up to allow residents to dress and dine in smart attire.

Ashtonleigh

Manager: Nicola Ambler
Owner: Ashtonleigh Residential Care Home Ltd
Contact: 4 Wimblehurst Road, Horsham, West Sussex RH12 2ED
☏ 01403 259217

Purpose-built in 1996, Ashtonleigh is situated on the outskirts of Horsham in a small village. It is close to local shops and has ample transport links into Horsham town centre. The home also has its own minibus to transport residents into town or on outings. The house comprises of a large, well-kept garden leading from the lounge. It is also a short walk from Warnham Mill Pond, which is a picturesque spot for residents to enjoy. It is also close to the bustling city centre of Brighton, which is a 15-minute drive away.

Registered places: 30
Guide weekly rate: £335–£550
Specialist care: Respite
Medical services: Podiatry, dentist, optician, hygienist
Qualified staff: Meets standard

Home details

Location: Residential area, 1 mile from Horsham centre
Communal areas: Lounge, dining room, garden
Accessibility: *Floors:* 2 • *Access:* Lift • *Wheelchair access:* Good
Smoking: In designated area
Pets: At manager's discretion
Routines: Flexible

Room details

Single: 22	Door lock: ✗
Shared: 4	Lockable place: ✓
En suite: 18	
Facilities: TV point, telephone point	

Services provided

Beauty services: Hairdressing
Mobile library: ✗
Religious services: Monthly church visits
Transport: Minibus
Activities: *Coordinator:* ✓ • *Examples:* Bingo, musical exercises, quizzes • *Outings:* ✗
Meetings: ✓

Balcombe Place

Manager: Jill De Le Vingne
Owner: Balcombe Care Homes Ltd
Contact: Haywards Heath Road, Balcombe, West Sussex RH17 6QJ
☏ 01444 811066
@ balcombe@balcombecarehomes.co.uk
🖥 www.balcombecarehomes.co.uk

Balcombe Place is situated in a private estate, 1.5 miles south of the village of Balcombe where there are local shops and amenities. The property is a listed country house set within 12 acres of ground. The home has been modified but all the original features remain intact. To the rear of the home is a secure garden with seating area, which provides residents with views across the grounds. There are regular activities planned such as arts and crafts, bingo, film night and quizzes.

Registered places: 40
Guide weekly rate: £600–£900
Specialist care: Nursing, respite
Medical services: Podiatry, dentist, optician, physiotherapy
Qualified staff: Exceeds standard: 60% at NVQ Level 2

Home details

Location: Rural area, 4 miles from Haywards Heath
Communal areas: Lounge, dining room, library, music room, patio and garden
Accessibility: *Floors:* 3 • *Access:* Lift • *Wheelchair access:* Good
Smoking: In designated area
Pets: ✓
Routines: Flexible

Room details

Single: 33	Door lock: ✗
Shared: 5	Lockable place: ✓
En suite: 24	
Facilities: TV point, telephone point	

Services provided

Beauty services: Hairdressing
Mobile library: Library facilities
Religious services: ✓
Transport: ✓
Activities: *Coordinator:* ✗ • *Examples:* Arts and crafts, exercise, films • *Outings:* ✗
Meetings: ✓

Registered places: 64
Guide weekly rate: From £575
Specialist care: Dementia, mental disorder, respite
Medical services: Podiatry, dentist, optician, physiotherapy
Qualified staff: Meets standard

Home details

Location: Rural area, 2.5 miles from Petworth
Communal areas: Lounge, dining room, den, garden
Accessibility: *Floors:* 2 • *Access:* Lift • *Wheelchair access:* Good
Smoking: In designated area
Pets: At manager's discretion
Routines: Flexible

Room details

Single: 60
Shared: 2
En suite: 51
Facilities: TV point, telephone point

Door lock: ✓
Lockable place: ✓

Services provided

Beauty services: Hairdressing, manicures
Mobile library: ✓
Religious services: Weekly Catholic Communion service
Transport: People carrier
Activities: *Coordinator:* ✓ • *Examples:* Arts and crafts, music,
   quizzes • *Outings:* ✗
Meetings: ✗

Barlavington Manor

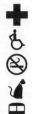

Manager: Lisa Ryan
Owner: Realmpark Health Care Ltd
Contact: Burton Park Road, Heath End,
Petworth, West Sussex GU28 0JS
) 01798 343309
@ info@barlavingtonmanor.co.uk
🖰 www.barlavingtonmanor.co.uk

Barlavington Manor is in a rural location,
south of Petworth village. It stands in four
acres of grounds, with views of the South
Downs enjoyed from most bedrooms. The
main part of the home is for 43 elderly
residents and there is separate, newly
built accommodation for residents with
dementia. The home offers a selection
of activities and musical entertainment
in the summer months. Specific dietary
requirement can be catered to with a
choice of menu for all.

Registered places: 23
Guide weekly rate: £375–£500
Specialist care: Nursing
Medical services: Podiatry
Qualified staff: Meets standard

Home details

Location: Village location, 5 miles from Bognor Regis
Communal areas: Lounge, dining room, garden
Accessibility: *Floors:* 2 • *Access:* Lift • *Wheelchair access:* Good
Smoking: ✗
Pets: At manager's discretion
Routines: Flexible

Room details

Single: 17
Shared: 3
En suite: All
Facilities: TV point, telephone point

Door lock: ✓
Lockable place: ✗

Services provided

Beauty services: Hairdressing
Mobile library: ✓
Religious services: Monthly Communion service
Transport: Car
Activities: *Coordinator:* ✗ • *Examples:* Bingo,
   visiting entertainers • *Outings:* ✗
Meetings: ✗

Barnham Manor

Manager: Sivagamee Curpen
Owner: Barnham Manor Ltd
Contact: 150 Barnham Road,
Barnham, Bognor Regis, West Sussex
PO22 0EH
) 01243 551190
@ barnhammanorLtd@aol.com

Barnham Manor is set in a rural location
on the outskirts of Barnham village, less
than a mile from local facilities which
include a pub, shops and a railway
station. There is a lounge and a garden
and the residents are offered the option
to have a lock on their door. The home
arranges activities such as bingo and
visiting entertainers and pets are allowed
at the manager's discretion. The home
has its own transport and has a monthly
Communion service as well as monthly
visits from a mobile library.

Beech Hurst Nursing Home

Manager: Jacqueline Cox
Owner: Care UK Ltd
Contact: Butlers Green Road, Haywards Heath, West Sussex RH16 4DA
) 01444 412208
⊕ www.careuk.com

Beech Hurst is located on the outskirts of Haywards Heath a short drive away from shops and other amenities. The home has a lounge, a dining room and a garden, accessible for the residents to enjoy. The home has its own activities coordinator and services such as hairdressing and visits from a mobile library are offered. There is the option to attend a church service once a month and the residents benefit from a flexible routine as well as flexible meal times.

Registered places: 60
Guide weekly rate: £535–£770
Specialist care: Nursing, dementia, mental disorder, physical disability
Medical services: Podiatry, dentist, hygienist, optician, physiotherapy
Qualified staff: Fails standard: 48% at NVQ Level 2

Home details
Location: Residential area, 0.5 miles from Haywards Heath centre
Communal areas: Lounge, dining room, garden
Accessibility: *Floors:* 2 • *Access:* Undisclosed
  Wheelchair access: Undisclosed
Smoking: ×
Pets: ×
Routines: Flexible

Room details
Single: 52
Shared: 4
En suite: 60
Facilities: TV, telephone point

Door lock: ×
Lockable place: ×

Services provided
Beauty services: Hairdressing
Mobile library: ✓
Religious services: Monthly church service
Transport: ×
Activities: *Coordinator:* ✓ • *Examples:* Exercises • *Outings:* ×
Meetings: ×

The Beeches

Manager: Christine Heffron
Owner: Diana Wyatt
Contact: 45 Wordsworth Road, Worthing, West Sussex BN11 3JB
) 01903 239875
@ info@thebeechesnursinghome.co.uk
⊕ www.thebeechesnursinghome.co.uk

The Beeches is a three-storey, converted and extended building, on a characteristic road. Entertainment comes in monthly for the residents to enjoy. The home focuses on the individual and aims to make the residents remain active with exercises twice a week. Outings are also arranged at the home, as well as film showings and arts and crafts. A monthly Communion service takes place at the home, as well as weekly prayer meetings.

Registered places: 43
Guide weekly rate: £500–£750
Specialist care: Nursing, respite, physical disability
Medical services: Podiatry, optician
Qualified staff: Meets standard

Home details
Location: Residential area, 0.5 miles from Worthing centre
Communal areas: Lounge, dining room, patio and garden
Accessibility: *Floors:* 3 • *Access:* Lift • *Wheelchair access:* Good
Smoking: ×
Pets: ×
Routines: Flexible

Room details
Single: 34
Shared: 4
En suite: 38
Facilities: TV point, telephone point

Door lock: ✓
Lockable place: ✓

Services provided
Beauty services: Hairdressing
Mobile library: ✓
Religious services: Monthly Communion service, weekly prayer service
Transport: ×
Activities: *Coordinator:* × • *Examples:* Arts and crafts, music and movement, film shows • *Outings:* ✓
Meetings: ✓

Registered places: 34
Guide weekly rate: £448
Specialist care: Physical disability, respite
Medical services: Podiatry, dentist, optician
Qualified staff: Exceeds standard: 70% at NVQ level 2

Home details

Location: Residential area, 0.5 miles from Horsham
Communal areas: 7 lounges, dining room, patio and garden
Accessibility: *Floors:* 2 • *Access:* Lift
    Wheelchair access: Limited
Smoking: In designated area
Pets: ✓
Routines: Flexible

Room details

Single: 34
Shared: 0
En suite: 0
Facilities: TV point, telephone point

Offer Door lock: ✓
Lockable place: ✓

Services provided

Beauty services: Hairdressing, manicures
Mobile Library: ✓
Religious services: Monthly Communion service
Transport: ✗
Activities: *Coordinator:* ✗ • *Examples:* Arts and crafts, bingo,
    storytelling • *Outings:* ✗
Meetings: ✓

Bryce Lodge

Manager: Rosemary Howard
Owner: Shaw Healthcare Ltd
Contact: New Street, Horsham, West Sussex RH13 5EL
☏ 01403 254251
@ Bryce.lodge@shaw.co.uk
🖰 www.shaw.co.uk

A purpose-built home that has stood for more than 40 years, Bryce Lodge offers a friendly and homely environment on the outskirts of Horsham. The home offers residents with a range of activity programmes coordinated by an activities coordinator, all of which are optional for residents to partake. These include storytelling and singalongs. Themed meals, such as Chinese, are often enjoyed by residents and are a popular treat.

Registered places: 16
Guide weekly rate: £285–£450
Specialist care: Day care, respite
Medical services: Podiatry, dentist, optician
Qualified staff: Meets standard

Home details

Location: Village location, 3 miles from Bognor Regis
Communal areas: Lounge, dining room, garden
Accessibility: *Floors:* 2 • *Access:* Lift • *Wheelchair access:* Good
Smoking: ✗
Pets: ✗
Routines: Flexible

Room details

Single: 12
Shared: 2
En suite: 13
Facilities: TV point, telephone point

Door lock: ✓
Lockable place: ✓

Services provided

Beauty services: Hairdressing
Mobile library: ✗
Religious services: Weekly Catholic and Anglican service
Transport: 7-seater vehicle
Activities: *Coordinator:* ✓ • *Examples:* Bingo, games, music,
    quizzes • *Outings:* ✓
Meetings: ✗

Byway House

Manager: Christine Tidmarsh
Owner: Mary Ross
Contact: Middleton Road, Middleton-on-Sea, Bognor Regis, West Sussex PO22 6DR
☏ 01243 583346

Byway House is a two-storey, detached house in the village of Middleton-on-Sea, on a main bus route to Bognor Regis. The home offers a wealth of activities including board games, music and quizzes, organised by an activities coordinator. Meals can be flexible depending on when or where residents want to eat. The home caters to residents' desires at all times, organising outings and activities as requested.

Caer Gwent Care Home with Nursing

Manager: Alison Williams
Owner: Guild Care
Contact: Downview Road, Worthing, West Sussex BN11 4TA
) 01903 536649
www.guildcare.org

Caer Gwent Care Home comprises a purpose-built premises and a converted smaller building. It is situated on the outskirts on Worthing, a couple of miles from the town centre. The home is on a main bus route into town and less than half a mile from Worthing seafront. There is an enclosed garden with handrails in some parts, which has been newly reconstructed to provide level access for residents. The home also has its own African grey parrot and a few budgies. Activities are planned on a daily basis, and often outings are taken down to Worthing seafront.

Registered places: 61
Guide weekly rate: £450–£850
Specialist care: Nursing, respite
Medical services: Podiatry, dentist, optician, physiotherapy
Qualified staff: Exceeds standard: 60% at NVQ Level 2

Home details

Location: Residential area, 1 mile from Worthing centre
Communal areas: 4 lounges, 3 dining rooms, hairdressing salon, kitchenette, computer room/library, garden
Accessibility: *Floors:* 3 • *Access:* 2 lifts • *Wheelchair access:* Good
Smoking: ✗
Pets: ✗
Routines: Flexible

Room details

Single: 61
Shared: 0
En suite: 61
Facilities: TV point, telephone point

Door lock: ✗
Lockable place: ✓

Services provided

Beauty services: Hairdressing
Mobile library: Library facilities
Religious services: Monthly church service
Transport: ✗
Activities: *Coordinator:* ✓ • *Examples:* Charades, coffee mornings, jigsaws • *Outings:* ✗
Meetings: ✓

Challcraft Hall Care Home

Manager: Angela Barton
Owner: Anra Care Home Ltd
Contact: 76 Chalcraft Lane, North Bersted, Bognor Regis, West Sussex PO21 5TS
) 01243 821368

Challcraft Hall is situated in a quiet, residential area on the outskirts of Bognor Regis close to a local shopping parade. The town centre is a 10-minute drive away with its train station, shops and other amenities. The detached building is set in attractive gardens consisting of paved and lawned areas, most with level access for wheelchair users. There is a seating area for residents to sit outside. Outings to the seaside are frequent where residents have fish and chips and observe the sea views. There are also regular daily activities in the home such as exercise, gardening and games.

Registered places: 20
Guide weekly rate: £350–£500
Specialist care: Dementia
Medical services: Podiatry, optician
Qualified staff: Exceeds standard: 75% at NVQ Level 2

Home details

Location: Residential area, 1.5 miles from Bognor Regis
Communal areas: 2 lounges, dining room, garden
Accessibility: *Floors:* 2 • *Access:* Lift • *Wheelchair access:* Good
Smoking: In designated area
Pets: ✓
Routines: Flexible

Room details

Single: 20
Shared: 0
En suite: 17
Facilities: TV point, telephone point

Door lock: ✗
Lockable place: ✓

Services provided

Beauty services: Hairdressing
Mobile library: ✓
Religious services: Monthly church service
Transport: ✓
Activities: *Coordinator:* ✗ • *Examples:* Bingo, exercises, games, gardening • *Outings:* ✗
Meetings: ✓

Registered places: 18
Guide weekly rate: £375–£400
Specialist care: Residential
Medical services: Podiatry, hygienist, optician, physiotherapy
Qualified staff: Fails standard: 30% at NVQ Level 2

Home details
Location: 0.5 miles from Worthing centre
Communal areas: 2 lounges, dining room, garden
Accessibility: *Floors:* 2 • *Access:* Lift • *Wheelchair access:* Good
Smoking: ✗
Pets: ✗
Routines: Structured

Room details
Single: 16
Shared: 1
En suite: 17
Facilities: TV point, telephone point

Door lock: ✓
Lockable place: ✓

Services provided
Beauty services: Hairdressing, manicures
Mobile library: ✗
Religious services: ✓
Transport: ✗
Activities: *Coordinator:* ✓ • *Examples:* Games, bingo,
movement to music • *Outings:* ✓
Meetings: ✓

Chiltingtons
Manager: Sherifan Saheid
Owner: Mr and Mrs Saheid
Contact: 127–131 Lyndhurst Road,
Worthing, West Sussex BN11 2DE
☎ 01903 234409

Chiltingtons is a detached property located half a mile from the town centre of Worthing. The home provides a range of activities and outings, such as bingo, movement to music and shopping trips. The home provides individual care to residents and will provide personal trips if required. Chiltingtons is family run and puts strong emphasis on its home cooked meals.

Registered places: 7
Guide weekly rate: £331–£401
Specialist care: Respite
Medical services: Podiatry, optician, physiotherapy
Qualified staff: Exceeds standard: 80% at NVQ Level 2

Home details
Location: Residential area, in Littlehampton
Communal areas: Lounge, dining room, library, patio and garden
Accessibility: *Floors:* 2 • *Access:* Stair lift
Wheelchair access: Good
Smoking: In designated area
Pets: ✓
Routines: Flexible

Room details
Single: 5
Shared: 1
En suite: 0
Facilities: TV, telephone point

Door lock: ✓
Lockable place: ✓

Services provided
Beauty services: Hairdressing
Mobile library: ✗
Religious services: Monthly Anglican service
Transport: People carrier
Activities: *Coordinator:* ✗ • *Examples:* Bingo, music,
reminiscence games • *Outings:* ✓
Meetings: ✗

Chippers
Manager: Pauline Shanahan
Owner: Pauline Shanahan
Contact: 68 Arundel Road,
Littlehampton, West Sussex BN17 7DF
☎ 01903 725097

Chippers is an extended terraced house with good local shops and all amenities within half a mile. It is also half a mile away from the seafront in Littlehampton. The staff aim to provide the atmosphere of a family home and though there are no formal meetings for residents there are informal discussions. The home focuses on maintaining a homely and friendly atmosphere. There is a resident dog and many outings including trips to the theatre.

Church Farm Residential Home

Manager: Phyllis Jeffery
Owner: BUPA Care Homes Ltd
Contact: Church Farm Lane,
East Wittering, Chichester,
West Sussex PO20 8PT
☎ 01243 672999
@ ChruchFarmResALL@BUPA.com
🖰 www.bupacarehomes.co.uk

Purpose-built in a traditional style, Church Farm is located in pleasant countryside and is a short distance from Chichester and the coast. The home offers modern convenience combined with traditional style. There are several lounges in which residents can meet to chat or enjoy a game of cards. A garden and patio are enjoyed by residents and guests on a sunny afternoon. Many bedrooms enjoy garden views, and all have en suite facilities. Personal interests are encouraged and activities offered include gardening, keep fit, reminiscence therapy, theatre trips and mystery tours.

Registered places: 60
Guide weekly rate: Undisclosed
Specialist care: Day care, respite, palliative care
Medical services: Podiatry, physiotherapy
Qualified staff: Undisclosed

Home details
Location: Rural area, 1 mile from East Wittering
Communal areas: 4 lounges, dining room, conservatory,
hairdressing salon, patio and garden
Accessibility: *Floors:* 2 • *Access:* Lift • *Wheelchair access:* Good
Smoking: In designated area
Pets: ✓
Routines: Flexible

Room details
Single: 50
Shared: 2
En suite: 52
Facilities: TV, telephone point

Door lock: ✓
Lockable place: ✓

Services provided
Beauty services: Hairdressing, aromatherapy
Mobile library: ✓
Religious services: Monthly Communion service
Transport: Minibus
Activities: *Coordinator:* ✓ • *Examples:* Entertainers, quizzes
Outings: ✓
Meetings: ✓

Clapham Lodge Residential Home

Manager: Christine Woods
Owner: Clapham Lodge Ltd
Contact: Woodland Close, Clapham
Village, Worthing, West Sussex BN13 3XR
☎ 01903 871326
@ paulren@lineone.net
🖰 www.claphamlodge.co.uk

Set in a bright, spacious Edwardian redbrick building, Clapham Lodge Residential Home is located in the Downland village of Clapham. Set in one and a half acres of gardens, Clapham Lodge offers panoramic views over the South Downs and across to Worthing and the English Channel. The home has been modernised and extended, still retaining the individual character and charm of a country house. A large, heated, conservatory overlooks the gardens with ramped access to both the adjoining terrace and flower gardens. All bedrooms have their own remote-controlled colour television.

Registered places: 26
Guide weekly rate: £270–£720
Specialist care: Nursing
Medical services: Podiatry, hygienist, optician, physiotherapy
Qualified staff: Meets standard

Home details
Location: Village location, 6 miles from Worthing
Communal areas: Lounge, dining room, garden
Accessibility: *Floors:* 2 • *Access:* Lift • *Wheelchair access:* Good
Smoking: ✗
Pets: At manager's discretion
Routines: Flexible

Room details
Single: 26
Shared: 0
En suite: 0
Facilities: TV

Door lock: ✗
Lockable place: ✓

Services provided
Beauty services: Hairdressing, massages
Mobile library: ✓
Religious services: ✓
Transport: ✗
Activities: *Coordinator:* ✓ • *Examples:* Bowling, quizzes, walks
Outings: ✗
Meetings: ✓

Registered places: 35
Guide weekly rate: £600–£650
Specialist care: Nursing, physically disabled, respite
Medical services: Podiatry, dentist, optician
Qualified staff: Meets standard

Home details

Location: Residential area, 1 mile from Selsey
Communal areas: Lounge, dining room, garden
Accessibility: *Floors:* 2 • *Access:* Lift • *Wheelchair access:* Good
Smoking: ×
Pets: ×
Routines: Flexible

Room details

Single: 27
Shared: 4
En suite: 31
Facilities: TV

Door lock: ✓
Lockable place: ✓

Services provided

Beauty services: Hairdressing, massage
Mobile library: Library facilities
Religious services: ✓
Transport: ×
Activities: *Coordinator:* ✓ • *Examples:* Music, fête • *Outings:* ✓
Meetings: ✓

Cornelia Gardens

Manager: Felicity Hillary-Warnett
Owner: Stephen Geach
Contact: Ursula Square, Seal Road, Selsey, West Sussex PO20 0HS
) 01243 606060
@ gardens@corneliacarehomes.co.uk
🖰 www.corneliacarehomes.co.uk

Cornelia Gardens is situated in a residential area, one mile from Selsey. The garden leads down to the nearby seafront and inside the home there is ample communal space with a lounge and dining room. There is a monthly newsletter produced and there are also regular residents meetings. The home employs an activities coordinator and arranges music sessions and special sessions such as a summer fête and birthday parties.

Registered places: 20
Guide weekly rate: £520–£620
Specialist care: Respite
Medical services: Podiatry, dentist, optician, physiotherapy
Qualified staff: Meets standard

Home details

Location: Residential area, 1 mile from Chichester centre
Communal areas: 2 lounges, dining room, garden
Accessibility: *Floors:* 3 • *Access:* Lift • *Wheelchair access:* Good
Smoking: ×
Pets: ×
Routines: Flexible

Room details

Single: 20
Shared: 0
En suite: 20
Facilities: TV point, telephone point

Door lock: ✓
Lockable place: ✓

Services provided

Beauty services: Hairdressing
Mobile library: ✓
Religious services: Fortnightly Catholic Communion service
Transport: Van
Activities: *Coordinator:* × • *Examples:* Crafts, keep fit, music and movement • *Outings:* ×
Meetings: ×

Cornelius House

Manager: Pamela Venus
Owner: Cornelius House Ltd
Contact: 114 Fishbourne Road West, Chichester, West Sussex PO19 3JR
) 01243 779372
@ Cornelius.house@btconnect.com

Cornelius House is a spacious three-storey establishment in Fishbourne, with a large garden at the front with a summerhouse and lawn. The home offers breakfast in bed, coffee and treats mid-morning as well as afternoon teas and cakes. Visiting entertainers are frequently engaged to entertain the residents. Though no pets are allowed to stay at the home, they can visit with friends and family.

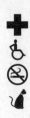

Country Lodge Nursing Home

Manager: Deborah Spokes

Owner: Mr and Mrs Wright

Contact: Cote Street,
Worthing, West Sussex BN13 3EX

☎ 01903 830600

@ enquiries@countrylodgenursing.co.uk

🖰 www.countrylodgenursing.co.uk

Country Lodge is a detached, two-storey property found on the outskirts of Worthing. Residents go on regular trips to pubs, beach and Worthing town. There are weekly visit's from an occupational therapist in addition to the activities in house. There is a pick up of books on tape for residents from the local library. The home has it's own summer garden party and organises larger parties for residents and relatives to get involved.

Registered places: 25

Guide weekly rate: £615–£850

Specialist care: Nursing, respite

Medical services: Podiatry, hygienist, optician, physiotherapy

Qualified staff: Meets standard

Home details

Location: Village location, 3 miles from Worthing

Communal areas: Lounge, dining room, garden

Accessibility: *Floors:* 2 • *Access:* Lift • *Wheelchair access:* Good

Smoking: ✗

Pets: At manager's discretion

Routines: Flexible

Room details

Single: 21

Shared: 1

En suite: 12

Facilities: TV, telephone

Door lock: ✗

Lockable place: ✓

Services provided

Beauty services: Hairdressing

Mobile library: Library facilities

Religious services: Monthly Anglican service

Transport: ✗

Activities: *Coordinator:* ✓ • *Examples:* Arts and crafts, exercise, games • *Outings:* ✓

Meetings: ✗

Courtlea

Manager: Anna Seago

Owner: Shaw Healthcare Ltd

Contact: Wyndham Road, Petworth, West Sussex GU28 0BZ

☎ 01798 342717

Courtlea is a purpose-built care home constructed in the 1960s found in the centre of Petworth. The home centres on personal care so all residents have their own carers and therefore receive focused individual care. Religious services are offered at residents' request and all denominations can be catered for. The home aims to create a homely and friendly atmosphere and while pets are not allowed there is a resident cat.

Registered places: 35

Guide weekly rate: £415–£483

Specialist care: Respite

Medical services: Podiatry, hygienist, optician

Qualified staff: Fails standards

Home details

Location: Village location, in Petworth

Communal areas: Lounge, dining room, garden

Accessibility: *Floors:* 3 • *Access:* Lift • *Wheelchair access:* Good

Smoking: ✗

Pets: ✗

Routines: Flexible

Room details

Single: 35

Shared: 0

En suite: 0

Facilities: TV point

Door lock: ✗

Lockable place: ✓

Services provided

Beauty services: Hairdressing

Mobile library: ✓

Religious services: ✗

Transport: ✗

Activities: *Coordinator:* ✓ • *Examples:* Exercise, group discussions, musical entertainment • *Outings:* ✗

Meetings: ✓

Registered places: 27
Guide weekly rate: Undisclosed
Specialist care: Dementia, respite
Medical services: Podiatry, dentist, optician, physiotherapy
Qualified staff: Meets standard

Home details

Location: Village location, in Steyning
Communal areas: Lounges, dining room, smoking room, garden
Accessibility: *Floors:* 2 • *Access:* Lift • *Wheelchair access:* Good
Smoking: In designated area
Pets: At manager's discretion
Routines: Flexible

Room details

Single: 27
Shared: 0
En suite: 0
Facilities: TV point

Door lock: ✓
Lockable place: ✓

Services provided

Beauty services: Hairdressing, aromatherapy
Mobile library: ✗
Religious services: Monthly Anglican service
Transport: ✗
Activities: *Coordinator:* ✗ • *Examples:* Armchair exercise, bowles, reminiscence • *Outings:* ✓
Meetings: ✗

Croft Meadow

Manager: Vacant
Owner: Shaw Healthcare Ltd
Contact: Tanyard Lane, Steyning, West Sussex BN44 3RJ
☏ 01903 814956

Croft Meadow is situated in the centre of Steyning, close to local shops, a health centre, the library and pubs. There is a two-weekly activities programme which includes games and exercises. The home focuses on the well being of the individual providing active options and those for the more restful resident. Attached to the home are secluded gardens accessible to residents.

Registered places: 25
Guide weekly rate: £345–£700
Specialist care: None
Medical services: Podiatry
Qualified staff: Fails standards

Home details

Location: Village location, 1.5 miles from Haywards Heath
Communal areas: Lounge, dining room, quiet room, garden
Accessibility: *Floors:* 2 • *Access:* Lift and stair lift
 Wheelchair access: Good
Smoking: ✗
Pets: At manager's discretion
Routines: Flexible

Room details

Single: 19
Shared: 3
En suite: 18
Facilities: TV point, telephone point

Door lock: ✗
Lockable place: ✓

Services provided

Beauty services: Hairdressing
Mobile library: ✗
Religious services: ✗
Transport: ✗
Activities: *Coordinator:* ✗ • *Examples:* Art classes, board games • *Outings:* ✓
Meetings: ✓

Crossways Care Home

Manager: Deepwantee Mannick
Owner: Crossways Healthcare Ltd
Contact: 2 Sunte Avenue, Lindfield, Haywards Heath, West Sussex RH16 2AA
☏ 01444 416841

Crossways is a large detached property in Lindfield village, 15 minutes drive from Haywards Heath. The home is close to local shops and the main public transport links into Haywards Heath. It is very close to Haywards Heath Golf Club, which has picturesque grounds and can be visited at any time by non-members. There is a large garden for residents to enjoy, and activities and outings are organised on a regular basis to keep the residents active and stimulated.

Darlington Court Care Home

Manager: Sandra Daniels
Owner: Care UK Ltd
Contact: The Leas, off Station Road, Rustington, West Sussex BN16 3SE

☎ 01903 850232
@ manager.darlington@careuk.com
🖰 www.careuk.com

A purpose-built building situated in a residential area just off a main road, Darlington Court is a home whose two floors denote dementia care and care for those experiencing physical frailty. The home caters mainly towards respite and rehab care after hospital stays but provides Gold Standard terminal care with doctors on hand every day. The home has an internal library and provides activities such as arts and crafts, cooking classes and visiting entertainers.

Registered places: 61
Guide weekly rate: £675
Specialist care: Nursing, dementia, physical disability, respite, terminal care
Medical services: Podiatry, dentist, occupational therapy, optician, physiotherapy
Qualified staff: Fails standard: 35% at NVQ level 2

Home details
Location: Residential area, 3 miles from Littlehampton
Communal areas: 2 lounges, 2 dining rooms, kitchenette, 2 conservatories, library, garden
Accessibility: *Floors:* 2 • *Access:* Lift • *Wheelchair access:* Good
Smoking: In designated area
Pets: ✗
Routines: Flexible

Room details
Single: 57	**Door lock:** ✓
Shared: 4	**Lockable place:** ✓
En suite: 61	
Facilities: TV, telephone	

Services provided
Beauty services: Hairdressing, aromatherapy
Mobile library: Library facilities
Religious services: ✗
Transport: ✗
Activities: *Coordinator:* ✗ • *Examples:* Arts and crafts, cooking classes, visiting entertainers • *Outings:* ✗
Meetings: ✓

Dean House

Manager: Allan Rollason
Owner: Maria Eagland and Dean Williams
Contact: 67 Sea Lane, Angmering-on-Sea, Littlehampton, West Sussex BN16 1ND

☎ 01903 784217
@ Deanhouse1@aol.co.uk

Dean House is a detached property set only yards from the sea in the village of East Preston. Local amenities are close to the home if residents choose to visit. Monthly religious services are provided, and residents are frequently reminded of activities taking place and are asked whether they wish to participate, examples of which include bingo, gentle exercise and flower arranging. Relatives are welcome to visit at any time. Residents are able to personalise their rooms to suit their tastes and preferences which helps to form a relaxed and homely feel.

Registered places: 27
Guide weekly rate: Up to £450
Specialist care: Respite
Medical services: Podiatry, hygienist, optician, physiotherapy
Qualified staff: Exceeds standard: 100% at NVQ Level 2

Home details
Location: Village location, 4 miles from Littlehampton
Communal areas: 3 lounges, dining room, conservatory, garden
Accessibility: *Floors:* 2 • *Access:* Lift • *Wheelchair access:* Good
Smoking: In designated area
Pets: ✓
Routines: Flexible

Room details
Single: 22	**Door lock:** ✓
Shared: 3	**Lockable place:** ✓
En suite: 25	
Facilities: TV, telephone	

Services provided
Beauty services: Hairdressing
Mobile library: ✗
Religious services: ✓
Transport: ✗
Activities: *Coordinator:* ✗ • *Examples:* Baking, flower arranging, quizzes • *Outings:* ✗
Meetings: ✓

Registered places: 28
Guide weekly rate: £445–£575
Specialist care: Nursing, respite
Medical services: Podiatry, optician
Qualified staff: Exceeds standard: 60% at NVQ Level 2

Home details

Location: Village location, 1.5 miles from Chichester centre
Communal areas: 2 lounges, dining room, conservatory, garden
Accessibility: *Floors:* 2 • *Access:* Lift • *Wheelchair access:* Good
Smoking: ✗
Pets: At manager's discretion
Routines: Flexible

Room details

Single: 28
Shared: 0
En suite: 5
Facilities: TV point, telephone point

Door lock: ✓
Lockable place: ✓

Services provided

Beauty services: Hairdressing
Mobile library: ✓
Religious services: Monthly Anglican Communion service
Transport: ✗
Activities: *Coordinator:* ✗ • *Examples:* Reminiscence,
visiting entertainers • *Outings:* ✓
Meetings: ✓

Donnington House

Manager: Anne Bareham
Owner: Donnington House Care
Home Ltd
Contact: 12 Birdham Road, Chichester,
West Sussex PO19 8TE
☏ 01243 783883
@ matron@donningtonhouse.co.uk
⌂ www.donningtonhouse.co.uk

Donnington House has large landscaped gardens at the rear of the building. It is also a registered charity. The home is closely linked with the local hospice. Chosen for the Gold Standards Framework. There are frequent entertainers coming into the home to perform, such as SG Productions, who put on productions in the home four times a year and a voluntary keyboard player. Regular activities including games and bingo, also there are rare outings to the theatre. The home has budgerigars. There are also monthly residents meetings.

Registered places: 26
Guide weekly rate: £425–£520
Specialist care: Respite
Medical services: Podiatry, optician
Qualified staff: Exceeds standard: 80% at NVQ Level 2

Home details

Location: Near Chichester
Communal areas: Lounge, dining room, patio and garden
Accessibility: *Floors:* 2 • *Access:* Lift • *Wheelchair access:* Good
Smoking: ✗
Pets: ✓
Routines: Flexible

Room details

Single: 26
Shared: 0
En suite: 19
Facilities: TV point, telephone point

Door lock: ✓
Lockable place: ✓

Services provided

Beauty services: Hairdressing
Mobile library: ✗
Religious services: ✗
Transport: ✗
Activities: *Coordinator:* ✓ • *Examples:* Arts and crafts,
music, quizzes • *Outings:* ✓
Meetings: ✓

Dovecote View

Manager: Julie Buck
Owner: Dovecote View Ltd
Contact: Claypit Lane, Westhampnett,
Chichester, West Sussex PO18 0NT
☏ 01243 779080

Dovecote View is a purpose-built detached property with a large garden. The home provides organised activities daily, in the mornings and afternoons, and has a designated activities coordinator. Great emphasis is placed on physical well-being and all residents are encouraged to go for a daily walk in the landscaped gardens, with a member of staff if they wish.

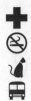

Downlands Park Nursing Home

Manager: Nicola Palladino
Owner: BUPA Care Homes Ltd
Contact: Isaacs Lane, Haywards Heath, West Sussex RH16 4BQ

☏ 01444 457871
@ DownlandsParkALL@BUPA.com
🖰 www.bupacarehomes.co.uk

Downlands Park is a converted large private house and former school. It is set in its own landscaped grounds with extensive lawns, mature trees, a patio and gazebo. Daily activities are offered, and personal interests are encouraged, including flower arranging, music, gardening and scrabble. Local attractions such as the West Sussex coast and Ditchling Beacon may be enjoyed on organised trips. Links with the local community are maintained by offering day care to local older people. Downlands Park is able to offer post-operative care rehabilitation, care to people with Parkinson's disease, motor neurone disease and those who have had strokes.

Registered places: 46
Guide weekly rate: Undisclosed
Specialist care: Nursing, respite
Medical services: Podiatry, physiotherapy
Qualified staff: Undisclosed

Home details
Location: Rural area, 1 mile from Haywards Heath centre
Communal areas: 2 lounges, dining room, hairdressing salon, kitchenette, garden
Accessibility: *Floors:* 2 • *Access:* Lift and stair lift
   Wheelchair access: Good
Smoking: ✗
Pets: ✓
Routines: Flexible

Room details
Single: 29
Shared: 6
En suite: 31
Facilities: TV, telephone point

Door lock: ✓
Lockable place: ✗

Services provided
Beauty services: Hairdressing
Mobile library: ✗
Religious services: ✓
Transport: ✓
Activities: *Coordinator:* ✓ • *Examples:* Flower arranging, music, gardening and scrabble • *Outings:* ✓
Meetings: ✗

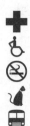

Drumconner

Manager: Roger Kinsman
Owner: Drumconner Ltd
Contact: 13–21 Brighton Road, Lancing, West Sussex BN15 8RJ

☏ 01903 753516

Drumconner is a large detached building which stands in its own, well-maintained gardens. It is situated in a residential area on the main coast road from Worthing to Brighton in the village of Lancing. Local shops and other community facilities are close by. Some of the bedrooms in the home have sea views, and the beach is literally across the main road. Seafront walks and fish and chips occur regularly, as staff like to take advantage of the location of the home. The gardens are well maintained and have shrubbery and flower beds making it a pleasant environment to relax in.

Registered places: 48
Guide weekly rate: £500–£800
Specialist care: Nursing, physical disability
Medical services: Podiatry, dentist, optician, physiotherapy
Qualified staff: Meets standard

Home details
Location: Village location, 1 mile from Worthing centre
Communal areas: 4 lounges, dining room, hairdressing salon, garden
Accessibility: *Floors:* 2 • *Access:* Lift • *Wheelchair access:* Good
Smoking: ✗
Pets: ✓
Routines: Flexible

Room details
Single: 42
Shared: 2
En suite: 21
Facilities: TV point, telephone point

Door lock: ✗
Lockable place: ✓

Services provided
Beauty services: Hairdressing
Mobile library: ✓
Religious services: Monthly church visits
Transport: ✓
Activities: *Coordinator:* ✗ • *Examples:* Keep fit, gardening, singalongs • *Outings:* ✓
Meetings: ✓

Registered places: 22
Guide weekly rate: £363–£550
Specialist care: Dementia
Medical services: Podiatry, dentist, optician
Qualified staff: Exceeds standards

Home details

Location: Residential area, in Burgess Hill
Communal areas: Lounge, garden
Accessibility: *Floors:* 2 • *Access:* Lift • *Wheelchair access:* Good
Smoking: ×
Pets: At manager's discretion
Routines: Flexible

Room details

Single: 20
Shared: 1
En suite: 7
Facilities: TV point

Door lock: ✓
Lockable place: ✓

Services provided

Beauty services: Hairdressing
Mobile library: ×
Religious services: ×
Transport: ×
Activities: *Coordinator:* ✓ • *Examples:* Musical entertainers
   Outings: ×
Meetings: ×

Edward House

Manager: Christine Gamlin
Owner: Nicholas James Care Homes Ltd
Contact: 86 Mill Road, Burgess Hill,
West Sussex RH15 8DZ
☎ 01444 248080

Edward House is situated in a residential area in the centre of Burgess Hill. The staff work on developing a close rapport with the residents. Routines are flexible, which allows for a laid back environment. Residents choose when to get up and go to bed, where they eat their meals and when to have a bath. Residents, if they wish, are also taken on outings, for example, to the garden centre.

Registered places: 60
Guide weekly rate: Undisclosed
Specialist care: Dementia, respite
Medical services: Podiatry
Qualified staff: Meets standard

Home details

Location: Urban area, 0.5 miles from Bognor Regis
Communal areas: Lounge, garden
Accessibility: *Floors:* 3 • *Access:* 2 lifts • *Wheelchair access:* Good
Smoking: In designated area
Pets: ×
Routines: Flexible

Room details

Single: 60
Shared: 0
En suite: 60
Facilities: TV point, telephone point

Door lock: ✓
Lockable place: ✓

Services provided

Beauty services: Hairdressing
Mobile library: ×
Religious services: Catholic Communion service
Transport: Minibus
Activities: *Coordinator:* ✓ • *Examples:* Exercise, singing
   Outings: ✓
Meetings: ✓

Elizabeth House

Manager: Marion Drake
Owner: Shaw Healthcare Ltd
Contact: Victoria Drive, Bognor Regis,
West Sussex PO21 2TB
☎ 02920 364411
@ Elizabeth.house@shaw.co.uk
🖰 www.shaw.co.uk

Elizabeth House is a purpose-built home located in an urban area, approximately half a mile from the town centre of Bognor Regis. The home has an activities coordinator who arranges outings for the residents as well as internal activities such as exercise sessions and singing and dancing. The home has its own minibus to use for outings. The home arranges a Catholic Communion service and there are also residents meetings held on a monthly basis.

Elton Lodge

Manager: Susan Lamb
Owner: Elton Lodge Ltd
Contact: 22–24 Selden Road, Worthing, West Sussex BN11 2LN
☎ 01903 230798

Elton Lodge is an Edwardian property that comprises of two large converted houses joined together and is close to the seafront. The home offers a variety of activities with an exercise club and arts and crafts. Outings are offered frequently, and include trips to the seafront, Beach House Park, the bowling green and cafés that are along the seafront. The residents also enjoy trips to garden centres where they can see the changing of the seasons. The home has informal monthly meetings with the residents.

Registered places: 21
Guide weekly rate: £490–£665
Specialist care: Nursing, physical disability, respite
Medical services: Podiatry, dentist, optician
Qualified staff: Exceeds standard: 75% at NVQ Level 2

Home details
Location: Residential area, 0.5 miles from Worthing centre
Communal areas: Lounge, lounge/dining room, library, patio and garden
Accessibility: *Floors:* 2 • *Access:* Lift • *Wheelchair access:* Good
Smoking: ✗
Pets: ✗
Routines: Flexible

Room details
Single: 21	**Door lock:** ✓
Shared: 0	**Lockable place:** ✓
En suite: 9	
Facilities: TV point, telephone point	

Services provided
Beauty services: Hairdressing
Mobile library: ✗
Religious services: ✗
Transport: ✗
Activities: *Coordinator:* ✓ • *Examples:* Bingo, crafts, exercise club • *Outings:* ✓
Meetings: ✓

Fairlight Nursing Home

Manager: Paula Hamat
Owner: Forever Care Ltd
Contact: 121 Worthing Road, Rustington, West Sussex BN16 3LX
☎ 01903 772444
🖱 www.fairlightnursinghome.co.uk

Fairlight is located in the seaside resort of Rustington, near Littlehampton. It has recently been re-registered following the extension and refurbishment of the original building. There is a large garden to the rear with a patio area. Each resident is encouraged to determine their own schedule. Activities offered include arts and crafts, voice therapy and entertainers come in. Residents are taken on outings and have formerly been to theatre shows, such as *The King and I*.

Registered places: 44
Guide weekly rate: £500–£750
Specialist care: Nursing, respite, physical disability
Medical services: Podiatry, dentist, optician, physiotherapy
Qualified staff: Meets standard

Home details
Location: Residential area, 2 miles from Littlehampton centre
Communal areas: Lounge, dining room, patio and garden
Accessibility: *Floors:* 2 • *Access:* 2 lifts • *Wheelchair access:* Good
Smoking: ✗
Pets: At manager's discretion
Routines: Flexible

Room details
Single: 38	**Door lock:** ✓
Shared: 3	**Lockable place:** ✓
En suite: 35	
Facilities: TV point, telephone point	

Services provided
Beauty services: Hairdressing
Mobile library: ✓
Religious services: Weekly Anglican and Catholic services
Transport: ✗
Activities: *Coordinator:* ✓ • *Examples:* Arts and crafts, exercise, music • *Outings:* ✓
Meetings: ✗

Registered places: 14
Guide weekly rate: £495–£510
Specialist care: Respite
Medical services: Podiatry, dentist, optician, physiotherapy
Qualified staff: Meets standard

Home details

Location: Village location, 1.5 miles from Goring-by-Sea
Communal areas: Lounge, dining room, library, garden
Accessibility: *Floors:* 2 • *Access:* Lift • *Wheelchair access:* Good
Smoking: ×
Pets: ×
Routines: Flexible

Room details

Single: 12
Shared: 1
En suite: 13
Facilities: TV point, telephone point

Door lock: ✓
Lockable place: ✓

Services provided

Beauty services: Hairdressing
Mobile library: ×
Religious services: Monthly visit from local minister
Transport: ×
Activities: *Coordinator:* × • *Examples:* Bingo, films,
    scrabble • *Outings:* ✓
Meetings: ×

Ferringham House

Manager: Susan Leaney
Owner: Ferringham House Ltd
Contact: 58 Ferringham Lane, Ferring,
Worthing, West Sussex BN12 5LU
☎ 01903 242334

Ferringham House is in the village of
Ferring, on the south coast. Many of the
home's residents have lived in the village
where the home is situated. They belong
to a five-day retirement club in the village
where they can maintain their social
contacts. Though no pets are allowed to
stay at the home they are allowed to visit.
There are no large group outings; instead
they are arranged on a one-to-one basis,
with individuals going for shopping trips
or the theatre.

Registered places: 24
Guide weekly rate: £325–£400
Specialist care: None
Medical services: Podiatry, optician
Qualified staff: Undisclosed

Home details

Location: Residential area, 0.5 miles from Worthing centre
Communal areas: 2 lounges, dining room, garden
Accessibility: *Floors:* 2 • *Access:* Lift • *Wheelchair access:* Good
Smoking: ×
Pets: ×
Routines: Flexible

Room details

Single: 24
Shared: 0
En suite: 2
Facilities: None

Door lock: ✓
Lockable place: ×

Services provided

Beauty services: Hairdressing
Mobile library: ×
Religious services: ×
Transport: ×
Activities: *Coordinator:* × • *Examples:* Exercise, musical
    entertainment, dancing classes • *Outings:* ×
Meetings: ×

Fitzroy Lodge

Manager: Vacant
Owner: Ramprakash Beeharry
Contact: 4 Windsor Road,
Worthing, West Sussex BN11 2LX
☎ 01903 233798

Fitzroy Lodge is a detached property
located in a residential area of Worthing,
close to the seafront and approximately
half a mile from the town centre.
Residents have a good choice at meal
times and are offered dessert. The home
offers residents a key for their door if they
are deemed capable of possessing one.
There are photographs in the hallway
showing residents enjoying a dancing
class.

Forest View

Manager: Paula Devonport
Owner: Shaw Healthcare Ltd
Contact: Southway, Burgess Hill,
West Sussex RH15 9SU
☎ 01444 245749
@ Nicola.kelly@shaw.co.uk
🖥 www.shaw.co.uk

Forest View is situated on the outskirts of Burgess Hill and is a purpose-built home that stands in its own grounds. It is divided into six units each with its own lounge, dining room and kitchen area. The majority of residents of Forest View need care appropriate to their dementia. An activities coordinator arranges several appropriate activities for residents, including ball games and reminiscence sessions.

Registered places: 60
Guide weekly rate: £669
Specialist care: Day care, dementia, respite
Medical services: Podiatry, hygienist, optician, psychiatry, physiotherapy
Qualified staff: Meets standard

Home details
Location: Residential area, 0.5 miles from Burgess Hill centre
Communal areas: 6 lounges, 6 dining rooms, garden room, garden
Accessibility: *Floors:* 2 • *Access:* Lift • *Wheelchair access:* Good
Smoking: In designated area
Pets: At manager's discretion
Routines: Flexible

Room details
Single: 60
Shared: 0
En suite: 60
Facilities: TV point, telephone point

Door lock: ✓
Lockable place: ✓

Services provided
Beauty services: Hairdressing, aromatherapy
Mobile library: ✗
Religious services: ✗
Transport: ✗
Activities: *Coordinator:* ✓ • *Examples:* Ball games, reminiscence, singalongs • *Outings:* ✗
Meetings: ✓

Foxmead

Manager: Silvia Curry
Owner: Shaw Healthcare Ltd
Contact: Meadowside, Storrington, West Sussex RH20 4EG
☎ 01903 743867
🖥 www.shaw.co.uk

Foxmead is based in a residential area of Storrington. The accommodation is on a ground floor and a lower ground floor. There is a garden but because it is on a steep incline it is considered unsuitable for the elderly and frail. The home is being replaced by a new building in Pulborough, which will be ready for 2009. Carers run activities when they get some free time, as there is not a designated coordinator. This includes monthly exercise classes and a monthly visit from an entertainer.

Registered places: 34
Guide weekly rate: £428–£528
Specialist care: Physical disability, respite
Medical services: Podiatry, hygienist, optician, physiotherapy
Qualified staff: Undisclosed

Home details
Location: Residential area. 0.5 miles from Storrington centre
Communal areas: Lounge, dining room, garden
Accessibility: *Floors:* 2 • *Access:* Lift • *Wheelchair access:* Good
Smoking: In designated area
Pets: ✓
Routines: Flexible

Room details
Single: 34
Shared: 0
En suite: 0
Facilities: TV point, telephone point

Door lock: ✓
Lockable place: ✓

Services provided
Beauty services: Hairdressing
Mobile library: ✓
Religious services: Weekly nondenominational service
Transport: ✗
Activities: *Coordinator:* ✗ • *Examples:* Exercise classes, games, visiting entertainers • *Outings:* ✓
Meetings: ✓

Registered places: 56
Guide weekly rate: From £619
Specialist care: Nursing, dementia
Medical services: Podiatry, optician
Qualified staff: Meets standard

Home details

Location: Village location, 2.5 miles from Crawley centre
Communal areas: Lounge, dining room, garden
Accessibility: *Floors:* 2 • *Access:* Lift • *Wheelchair access:* Good
Smoking: ✗
Pets: ✓
Routines: Flexible

Room details

Single: 52
Shared: 2
En suite: 26
Facilities: TV point, telephone point

Door lock: ✗
Lockable place: ✓

Services provided

Beauty services: Hairdressing
Mobile library: ✓
Religious services: Monthly Communion service
Transport: ✗
Activities: *Coordinator:* ✓ • *Examples:* Arts and crafts, bingo, music and movement • *Outings:* ✗
Meetings: ✓

The Gables Nursing Home

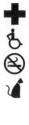

Manager: Sara-Jane Barrington
Owner: Excel Care Homes Ltd
Contact: 56 Ifield Green, Crawley, West Sussex RH11 0NU
☎ 01293 552022
@ info@gableshome.com
🖰 www.gableshome.com

The Grey Gables Nursing Home is located on Ifield Green. Local shops and a pleasant local pub are within walking distance from the home. Bus services are available to and from the home. Crawley town centre and amenities are approximately 10 minutes drive away. The home has two gardens available to the residents: one is an enclosed garden in the centre of the premises and the second is to the front of the home and has shrubbery and flowerbeds. There are organised outings to local sites of interest such as museums, and regular activities in the home.

Registered places: 40
Guide weekly rate: £428–£528
Specialist care: Respite
Medical services: Podiatry, hygienist, optician
Qualified staff: Undisclosed

Home details

Location: Village location, 4 miles from Havant
Communal areas: Lounge/dining room, 3 dining rooms, garden
Accessibility: *Floors:* 2 • *Access:* Lift • *Wheelchair access:* Good
Smoking: In designated area
Pets: At manager's discretion
Routines: Flexible

Room details

Single: 40
Shared: 0
En suite: 40
Facilities: TV point, telephone point

Door lock: ✓
Lockable place: ✓

Services provided

Beauty services: Hairdressing
Mobile library: ✓
Religious services: Weekly Anglican service
Transport: ✗
Activities: *Coordinator:* ✓ • *Examples:* Bingo, bowles, quizzes • *Outings:* ✓
Meetings: ✗

Glebe House

Manager: Mrs Parsons
Owner: Shaw Healthcare Ltd
Contact: Stein Road, Southborne, West Sussex PO10 8LB
☎ 01243 379179
🖰 www.shaw.co.uk

Glebe House is situated near the seafront in Southboune, which is between Havant and Chichester towns. The home is purpose-built on two floors and is divided into four units comprising 10 bedrooms per unit and each unit has its own dining room. There is a single, secure front entrance and secluded garden areas. It has a variety of activities for residents to enjoy including classic board games and quizzes. There are also many outings that residents are taken on to local points of interest and for afternoon teas. The home's aim is to meet the individual needs of every resident.

Gracelands

Manager: Margaret Kerbey
Owner: Macleod Pinsent Care Ltd
Contact: 42–48 Richmond Avenue,
Bognor Regis, West Sussex
PO21 2YE
📞 01243 867707

Gracelands is situated in a residential street in Bognor Regis within half a mile of local shops and the seafront. The home has a medium-sized garden at the rear of the property which offers seating and decking areas for residents to sit outside. There is an activities coordinator who organises activities such as bingo, music afternoon and movement to music to keep residents active and agile. There are also monthly outings to various places, but a favorite is to the beach for fish and chips.

Registered places: 31
Guide weekly rate: Dementia
Specialist care: £400–£600
Medical services: Podiatry, optician, physiotherapy
Qualified staff: Meets standard

Home details
Location: Residential area, 1 mile from Bognor Regis centre
Communal areas: 4 lounges, dining room, garden
Accessibility: *Floors:* 2 • *Access:* Lift • *Wheelchair access:* Good
Smoking: In designated area
Pets: ✗
Routines: Flexible

Room details
Single: 25	**Door lock:** ✗
Shared: 3	**Lockable place:** ✓
En suite: 8	
Facilities: TV point, telephone point	

Services provided
Beauty services: Hairdressing
Mobile library: ✗
Religious services: ✓
Transport: ✗
Activities: *Coordinator:* ✓ • *Examples:* Bingo, movement to music, music afternoon • *Outings:* ✓
Meetings: ✗

Grasmere Nursing Home

Manager: Yvonne Evans
Owner: Kargini Care Services Ltd
Contact: 51 Manor Road, Worthing,
West Sussex BN11 4SH
📞 01903 201281

Grasmere Nursing Home is situated in a residential area one mile from the town centre of Worthing, which offers a variety amenities and good transport links. The home is a two-story detached property, that offers nursing care to the elderly. It has a garden at the rear which is accessible to wheelchair users. There are regular outings and trips planned for the residents such as visits to the seafront for fish and chips, trips to local garden centres and visits to history points in the local area. There are also visiting entertainers who come into the home on a regular basis.

Registered places: 21
Guide weekly rate: £550–£700
Specialist care: Nursing
Medical services: Podiatry, optician
Qualified staff: Meets standard

Home details
Location: Residential area, 1 mile from Worthing centre
Communal areas: 2 lounges, dining room, patio
Accessibility: *Floors:* 2 • *Access:* Lift and stair lift
Wheelchair access: Good
Smoking: ✗
Pets: ✓
Routines: Flexible

Room details
Single: 21	**Door lock:** ✗
Shared: 0	**Lockable place:** ✓
En suite: 8	
Facilities: TV point	

Services provided
Beauty services: Hairdressing
Mobile library: ✓
Religious services: ✓
Transport: ✗
Activities: *Coordinator:* ✓ • *Examples:* Film afternoon, knitting, walks • *Outings:* ✗
Meetings: ✗

Registered places: 22
Guide weekly rate: £389–£600
Specialist care: Respite
Medical services: Podiatry, dentist, optician, physiotherapy
Qualified staff: Exceeds standard: 90% at NVQ Level 2

Home details

Location: Residential area, 0.5 miles from Littlehampton centre
Communal areas: Lounge, dining room, library, garden
Accessibility: *Floors:* 2 • *Access:* Lift • *Wheelchair access:* Good
Smoking: In designated area
Pets: At manager's discretion
Routines: Flexible

Room details

Single: 16
Shared: 3
En suite: 6
Facilities: TV point, telephone point

Door lock: ✓
Lockable place: ✓

Services provided

Beauty services: Hairdressing
Mobile library: Library facilities
Religious services: ✓
Transport: ✗
Activities: *Coordinator:* ✓ • *Examples:* Music and exercise, reminiscence, quizzes • *Outings:* ✓
Meetings: ✓

Gratwick House

Manager: Lorraine Barclay
Owner: Mr and Mrs Hitchens
Contact: 55 Norfolk Road,
Littlehampton, West Sussex BN17 5HE
☏ 01903 716022

Gratwick House is a large, converted house with a paved front yard and a large secluded garden at the rear. It is half a mile from the seafront and town centre. The home arranges for religious services depending on personal choice: there are Catholic and Anglican services on offer. The home goes on local outings to the town centre for afternoon teas and also the seaside. The home has monthly meetings and there is a meetings coordinator.

Registered places: 18
Guide weekly rate: £595–£700
Specialist care: Respite
Medical services: Podiatry, dentist, optician, physiotherapy
Qualified staff: Exceeds standard: 70% at NVQ Level 2

Home details

Location: Village location, 5 miles from Littlehampton
Communal areas: Lounge, dining room, conservatory, library, patio and garden
Accessibility: *Floors:* 1 • *Wheelchair access:* Good
Smoking: ✗
Pets: ✗
Routines: Flexible

Room details

Single: 14
Shared: 2
En suite: 16
Facilities: TV point, telephone point

Door lock: ✓
Lockable place: ✓

Services provided

Beauty services: Hairdressing, aromatherapy
Mobile library: Library facilities
Religious services: Monthly Anglican service
Transport: People carrier
Activities: *Coordinator:* ✓ • *Examples:* Exercises, games, story time • *Outings:* ✓
Meetings: ✓

Green Willow Residential Home

Manager: Julie Howard
Owner: Green Willow Care Ltd
Contact: 21–23 Vicarage Lane,
East Preston, Littlehampton,
West Sussex BN16 2SP
☏ 01903 775009

Green Willow is a two-storey building with all residents living on the ground floor only. The home is situated in East Preston village and most of the residents lived locally before moving into the home. Though no pets are allowed to stay at the home they can visit. The home organises an array of activities for residents of all abilities to enjoy and owns a people carrier in which residents are taken on trips.

Hambrook Meadows

Manager: Brigid Cullen
Owner: Mr and Mrs Cullen
Contact: Broad Road, Hambrook, Chichester, West Sussex PO18 8RF
☎ 01243 572922

Hambrook Meadows is a large, detached house in Hambrook village a few miles from Chichester and close to local transport. The staff aim for a friendly atmosphere and to create a home from home for the residents. The daily routine is focused around the residents' interests and activities are organised accordingly. The home has its own cat and religious services can be arranged at residents request.

Registered places: 15
Guide weekly rate: £330–£385
Specialist care: Respite
Medical services: Podiatry, optician
Qualified staff: Meets standard

Home details

Location: Village location, 7 miles from Chichester
Communal areas: Lounge, dining room, conservatory, patio and garden
Accessibility: *Floors:* 2 • *Access:* Lift • *Wheelchair access:* Good
Smoking: In designated area
Pets: ✓
Routines: Flexible

Room details

Single: 11	**Door lock:** ✓
Shared: 2	**Lockable place:** ✓
En suite: 4	
Facilities: TV, telephone point	

Services provided

Beauty services: Hairdressing
Mobile library: ✗
Religious services: ✗
Transport: Car
Activities: *Coordinator:* ✗ • *Examples:* Exercise, games, reminiscence • *Outings:* ✓
Meetings: ✗

Hampton House

Manager: April Mitchell
Owner: Shaw Healthcare Ltd
Contact: West Way, Wick, Littlehampton, West Sussex BN17 7NB
☎ 01903 715348

Hampton House is a care home providing care for up to 35 residents and is in Wick, on the outskirts of Littlehampton. The building was built in 1967 and is typical of this period. Forthcoming events and activities are displayed on a notice board, so that residents can plan when their visitors come and visit. The large gardens are accessible to residents and there is seating for them to sit and enjoy the grounds. There are local shops a five-minute drive away in Wick, however the more extensive facilities are in Littlehampton which is around a mile away.

Registered places: 45
Guide weekly rate: £427–£527
Specialist care: Learning disability, physical disability
Medical services: Podiatry, optician
Qualified staff: Fails standard: 35% at NVQ Level 2

Home details

Location: Residential area, 1 mile from Littlehampton centre
Communal areas: Lounge, dining room, garden
Accessibility: *Floors:* 2 • *Access:* Lift • *Wheelchair access:* Good
Smoking: In designated area
Pets: ✗
Routines: Structured

Room details

Single: 45	**Door lock:** ✗
Shared: 0	**Lockable place:** ✓
En suite: 0	
Facilities: TV point	

Services provided

Beauty services: Hairdressing
Mobile library: ✗
Religious services: ✗
Transport: ✗
Activities: *Coordinator:* ✗ • *Examples:* Bingo, cards, scrabble • *Outings:* ✗
Meetings: ✓

Registered places: 21
Guide weekly rate: £430–£500
Specialist care: Physical disability, respite
Medical services: Podiatry, optician
Qualified staff: Exceeds standard: 70% at NVQ Level 2

Home details
Location: Village location, 6 miles from Chichester
Communal areas: Dining room, lounge, patio and garden
Accessibility: *Floors:* 2 • *Access:* Lift • *Wheelchair access:* Good
Smoking: In designated area
Pets: ✗
Routines: Flexible

Room details
Single: 21
Shared: 0
En suite: 10
Facilities: TV point, telephone point

Door lock: ✓
Lockable place: ✓

Services provided
Beauty services: Hairdressing, aromatherapy
Mobile library: ✓
Religious services: Monthly visits from vicar
Transport: ✗
Activities: *Coordinator:* ✗ • *Examples:* Bingo, exercises,
    floor games • *Outings:* ✓
Meetings: ✓

Heathfield Care Home

Manager: Jacqueline Ovington
Owner: Intercare Orthopaedic Services Ltd
Contact: Main Road, West Wittering, Nr Chichester, West Sussex PO20 8QA
) 01243 511040
@ Heathfield@tesco.net

Heathfield is a detached property in its own attractive grounds, six miles from Chichester and two miles from West Wittering village. Though pets are not allowed in the home they are allowed to visit. The home aims to create a homely atmosphere with friendly service. There is no activities coordinator at the home but outings and in-house activities are organised by staff. These include various games such as skittles and bingo.

Registered places: 20
Guide weekly rate: £455–£630
Specialist care: Respite
Medical services: Podiatry, optician
Qualified staff: Exceeds standard: 60% at NVQ Level 2

Home details
Location: Residential area, 2 miles from Worthing centre
Communal areas: 2 lounges, dining room, conservatory, garden
Accessibility: *Floors:* 2 • *Access:* Lift • *Wheelchair access:* Good
Smoking: In designated area
Pets: At manager's discretion
Routines: Flexible

Room details
Single: 16
Shared: 2
En suite: All
Facilities: TV point, telephone point

Door lock: ✗
Lockable place: ✓

Services provided
Beauty services: Hairdressing
Mobile library: ✓
Religious services: Monthly nondenominational service
Transport: ✗
Activities: *Coordinator:* ✓ • *Examples:* Exercises, t'ai chi,
    visiting musicians • *Outings:* ✗
Meetings: ✓

Highgrove House

Manager: Clive Neil-Smith
Owner: Clive and Sally Neil-Smith
Contact: 32–34 Winchester Road, Worthing, West Sussex BN11 4DH
) 01903 230487
@ care@highgrove-house.net
🖰 www.heaton-house.net

Highgrove House is owned by Sally and Clive Neil-Smith who established their first care home in March 1974 in Worthing. The home is situated near the centre of Worthing, the seafront and local amenities. The home provides a variety of activities, including t'ai chi once a week and visiting musicians. There is a piano in one of the lounges for residents to play. There is ample communal space in the home, with lounges, the dining room and conservatory as well as landscaped gardens, where residents can take their visitors for tea and a slice of cake.

Hilgay

Manager: Judi Shearn
Owner: Dr and Mrs Shearn
Contact: Keymer Road, Burgess Hill, West Sussex RH15 0AL
- ☏ 01444 244756
- @ judi@hilgaycare.co.uk
- 🖥 www.hilgaycare.co.uk

Hilgay offers long-term, short-term and holiday stays and is situated in the centre of Burgess Hill. The manager is a qualified District Nurse and Health Visitor, and her husband, the other owner is a local GP. Activities are arranged by staff such as quiz and bingo afternoons, music and movement and local walks are arranged. The home is also visited by local theatrical and vocal groups. There is a shop that is open weekly, selling toiletries, sweets and stationery.

Registered places: 36
Guide weekly rate: Undisclosed
Specialist care: Respite
Medical services: Podiatry, physiotherapy, dentist, optician
Qualified staff: Undisclosed

Home details
Location: Residential area, in Burgess Hill
Communal areas: 2 lounges, 2 dining rooms, conservatory, garden
Accessibility: *Floors:* 3 • *Access:* Lift • *Wheelchair access:* Good
Smoking: ✗
Pets: ✗
Routines: Flexible

Room details
Single: 28	Door lock: ✓
Shared: 4	Lockable place: ✓
En suite: 15	
Facilities: TV	

Services provided
Beauty services: Hairdressing
Mobile library: ✗
Religious services: ✗
Transport: ✗
Activities: *Coordinator:* ✗ • *Examples:* Bingo, music and movement, quizzes • *Outings:* ✗
Meetings: ✗

Hollymead House

Manager: Michael Martin
Owner: Hugh, Michael and June Martin
Contact: 3 Downview Road, Felpham, Bognor Regis, West Sussex PO22 8HG
- ☏ 01243 868826
- @ hollymeadhouse@aol.com

Hollymead House is a purpose-built care home and therefore has good wheelchair access throughout. The front garden has been designed to encourage residents to walk independently and also provides good access. It is a community and family-run home that focuses on individual care and promotes independence. There is an activities coordinator who organises in-house activities and entertainment as well as outings for residents, facilitated by the home's people carrier.

Registered places: 35
Guide weekly rate: £400–£440
Specialist care: Day care, respite
Medical services: Podiatry, hygienist, optician, physiotherapy
Qualified staff: Exceeds standard: 80% at NVQ Level 2

Home details
Location: Village location, 2 miles from Bognor Regis
Communal areas: Lounge, dining room, 2 conservatories, garden
Accessibility: *Floors:* 2 • *Access:* Lift • *Wheelchair access:* Good
Smoking: ✗
Pets: At manager's discretion
Routines: Flexible

Room details
Single: 33	Door lock: ✓
Shared: 1	Lockable place: ✓
En suite: 30	
Facilities: TV point, telephone point	

Services provided
Beauty services: Hairdressing, aromatherapy
Mobile library: ✓
Religious services: Weekly Anglican service
Transport: People carrier
Activities: *Coordinator:* ✓ • *Examples:* Music for health, visiting guitarist • *Outings:* ✓
Meetings: ✓

Registered places: 40
Guide weekly rate: £400–£650
Specialist care: Learning disability, respite
Medical services: Podiatry, dentist, optician, physiotherapy
Qualified staff: Meets standard

Home details

Location: Residential area, 1 mile from Worthing centre
Communal areas: Lounge, dining room, conservatory,
    patio and garden
Accessibility: *Floors:* 2 • *Access:* Lift • *Wheelchair access:* Good
Smoking: ✗
Pets: At manager's discretion
Routines: Flexible

Room details

Single: 35
Shared: 3
En suite: 21
Facilities: TV, telephone point

Door lock: ✓
Lockable place: ✓

Services provided

Beauty services: Hairdressing, aromatherapy, massage, manicures
Mobile library: ✓
Religious services: ✓
Transport: Minibus
Activities: *Coordinator:* ✓ • *Examples:* Games, keep fit,
    visiting entertainers • *Outings:* ✓
Meetings: ✗

Hollywynd Rest Home

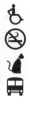

Manager: Barbara Giles
Owner: Techcrown Ltd
Contact: 5–9 St Botolph's Road,
Worthing, West Sussex BN11 4JN
❫ 01903 210681

Hollywynd is a detached home, located on the outskirts of Worthing and is close to the shops and other local amenities. The home is a 15-minute walk to the town centre and there is a bus service. The home has a large lounge and a dining room, as well as a hairdressing salon. There is also a garden with a conservatory. The home has an activities coordinator who arranges a varied programme for the residents including exercise sessions, visiting entertainers and fêtes. The home has its own minibus and takes residents on outings once a week. These outings include trips to the seafront and local garden centres.

Registered places: 66
Guide weekly rate: £350–£700
Specialist care: Nursing, physical disability
Medical services: Podiatry, dentist, optician, physiotherapy
Qualified staff: Meets standard

Home details

Location: Residential area, 0.5 miles from Bognor Regis
Communal areas: 3 lounges, conservatory, dining room, garden
Accessibility: *Floors:* 2 • *Access:* Lift • *Wheelchair access:* Good
Smoking: ✗
Pets: ✗
Routines: Structured

Room details

Single: 47
Shared: 3
En suite: 0
Facilities: TV point, telephone point

Door lock: ✗
Lockable place: ✓

Services provided

Beauty services: Hairdressing
Mobile library: ✗
Religious services: Monthly church service
Transport: ✗
Activities: *Coordinator:* ✗ • *Examples:* Bingo, games, music
    Outings: ✗
Meetings: ✓

Homebeech

Manager: Marie-Claire Vallerich
Owner: Safronland Homes
Contact: 19–21 Stocker Road, Bognor
Regis, West Sussex PO21 2QH
❫ 01243 823389
🖥 www.homebeechltd.co.uk

Homebeech is a large extended building that was originally four separate houses. It is based a few minutes walk from Aldwych town centre and only a 10-minute drive from Bognor Regis. A two-minute stroll away there is the beach and public garden. Homebeech offers full nursing care for residents, within attractive and comfortable surroundings. The Daffodil Suite, which is a separate unit, located in the grounds of Homebeech, offers dedicated specialist nursing care for younger residents aged 18–65 years. There is a roof garden and several different patio areas with flowers for the residents to sit outside and enjoy.

Homelands Nursing Home

Manager: Frances Price
Owner: Medicrest Ltd
Contact: Horsham Road, Cowfold,
West Sussex RH13 8AJ

) 01403 864581

Homelands Nursing Home is located in a pleasant village, which contains two pubs and some shops. The home is also surrounded by beautiful countryside which is full of local wildlife. The home is split between two houses each of which has two floors and a lift. The residents are encouraged to undertake activities, such as playing cards, feeding the wild birds, walking in the garden and in the grounds. Residents are able to keep contact with family and friends as and when they wish. They are also aided in exercising choice and control over their lives.

Registered places: 43
Guide weekly rate: £575–£650
Specialist care: Nursing, dementia
Medical services: Podiatry, dentist, optician, physiotherapy
Qualified staff: Exceeds standards

Home details
Location: Village location, 7 miles from Horsham
Communal areas: Lounge, dining room, conservatory, patio and garden
Accessibility: *Floors:* 2 • *Access:* Lift • *Wheelchair access:* Good
Smoking: In designated room
Pets: ✗
Routines: Flexible

Room details
Single: 17	**Door lock:** ✓
Shared: 13	**Lockable place:** ✓
En suite: Undisclosed	
Facilities: TV, telephone point	

Services provided
Beauty services: Hairdressing
Mobile library: ✗
Religious services: Weekly church visits
Transport: ✗
Activities: *Coordinator:* ✗ • *Examples:* Arts and crafts, movement to music, singalongs • *Outings:* ✗
Meetings: ✗

Homeleigh

Manager: Roma Wood
Owner: Homebeech Ltd
Contact: 24–28 Stocker Road,
Bognor Regis, West Sussex PO21 2QF

) 01243 863373
✆ www.homebeechltd.co.uk

Homeleigh is situated very near the seafront in a residential area of Bognor Regis. The home can hold 40 residents and has one double room. There are qualified nurses on duty 24 hours per day. Though there are no formal association meeting there are regular relatives meetings. The home will offer religious services if requested. There are also a range of activities from watching films to weekly keep fit classes and gardening.

Registered places: 40
Guide weekly rate: £450–£650
Specialist care: Nursing, respite
Medical services: Podiatry, optician
Qualified staff: Fails standard: 45% at NVQ Level 2

Home details
Location: Residential area, 1 mile from Bognor Regis centre
Communal areas: 2 lounges, dining room, conservatory, garden
Accessibility: *Floors:* 3 • *Access:* Lift
  Wheelchair access: Limited
Smoking: ✗
Pets: ✓
Routines: Flexible

Room details
Single: 38	**Door lock:** ✓
Shared: 1	**Lockable place:** ✓
En suite: 39	
Facilities: TV point	

Services provided
Beauty services: Hairdressing
Mobile library: ✓
Religious services: ✗
Transport: ✗
Activities: *Coordinator:* ✗ • *Examples:* Crafts, keep fit, movie shows • *Outings:* ✓
Meetings: ✓

Registered places: 22
Guide weekly rate: £511–£575
Specialist care: Nursing
Medical services: Podiatry, optician
Qualified staff: Exceeds standard: 64% at NVQ level 2

Home details

Location: Residential area, 1 mile from Worthing
Communal areas: Lounge, dining room, garden
Accessibility: *Floors:* Undisclosed • *Access:* Lift
  Wheelchair access: Undisclosed
Smoking: In designated area
Pets: ✗
Routines: Flexible

Room details

Single: 20
Shared: 2
En suite: 4
Facilities: TV point, telephone point

Door lock: ✗
Lockable place: ✓

Services provided

Beauty services: Hairdressing
Mobile library: ✓
Religious services: Monthly church services
Transport: ✗
Activities: *Coordinator:* ✓ • *Examples:* Cards, charades,
  singalongs • *Outings:* ✓
Meetings: ✓

The Hurst Nursing Home

Manager: Sheila Sheriff
Owner: Sheila Sheriff
Contact: 1 Mill Road, Worthing,
West Sussex BN11 4JR
☎ 01903 236935

The Hurst Nursing Home is located in Worthing, close to shops and other local amenities. The home has a small, secluded garden, which is well kept and has shrubbery and flowers for residents to sit outside and enjoy. Activities are arranged on a daily basis and include singalongs, charades, karaoke and cards. The daily routine at the home is flexible, meaning residents can choose when they get up and their bed times according to what suits them, although there is some structure around meal times.

Registered places: 12
Guide weekly rate: £360–£380
Specialist care: Respite
Medical services: Podiatry, dentist, optician, physiotherapy
Qualified staff: Exceeds standard: 90% at NVQ level 2

Home details

Location: Residential area, 0.7 miles from Worthing
Communal areas: Lounge, dining room, conservatory, garden
Accessibility: *Floors:* 2 • *Access:* None
  Wheelchair access: Limited
Smoking: In designated area
Pets: At manager's discretion
Routines: Flexible

Room details

Single: 12
Shared: 0
En suite: 6
Facilities: TV point, telephone point

Door lock: ✓
Lockable place: ✓

Services provided

Beauty services: Hairdressing
Mobile library: ✓
Religious services: Catholic and Anglican visit
Transport: People carrier
Activities: *Coordinator:* ✓ • *Examples:* Bingo,
  monthly rotary club, quizzes • *Outings:* ✓
Meetings: ✓

Jacaranda

Manager: Rachel Winter
Owner: Mr and Mrs Winter
Contact: 98 Broadwater Road, Worthing,
West Sussex BN14 8AW
☎ 01903 235371

Jacaranda is a detached property with a small garden. Nearby are local churches for residents to attend and the home is also close to local amenities and train stations. Activities take place regularly with a monthly rotary club and board games. Outings are also frequent with trips to garden centres and the beach, good weather permitting. Jacaranda publishes its own quarterly newsletter for residents, staff and relatives.

Knowle House Nursing Home

Manager: Bernadine Dias-Jayasinghe
Owner: Yourcare Ltd
Contact: Lingfield Road, East Grinstead, West Sussex RH19 2EJ
) 01342 317740

Knowle House is a large detached building situated on a residential road near the town centre of East Grinstead. It is a 10-minute drive from local amenities. There is a large well-kept garden for residents to enjoy, and when the weather is colder there are regular activities such as skittles, cards, giant crossword and topical debates around the daily newspaper articles. There is wheelchair access throughout, and 24 hour nursing care. The home arranges a monthly religious service and there are also regular residents meetings.

Registered places: 35
Guide weekly rate: £518–£610
Specialist care: Nursing
Medical services: Podiatry, dentist, optician, physiotherapy
Qualified staff: Meets standard

Home details
Location: Residential area, 0.5 miles from East Grinstead
Communal areas: 2 lounges, dining room/conservatory, garden
Accessibility: *Floors:* 2 • *Access:* Lift • *Wheelchair access:* Good
Smoking: ✗
Pets: ✗
Routines: Flexible

Room details
Single: 19
Shared: 8
En suite: 14
Facilities: TV point

Door lock: ✗
Lockable place: ✓

Services provided
Beauty services: Hairdressing
Mobile library: ✓
Religious services: Monthly
Transport: ✗
Activities: *Coordinator:* ✓ • *Examples:* Arts, skittles, cards
   Outings: ✗
Meetings: ✓

Ladymead Nursing Home

Manager: Motilall Jagannath
Owner: Warren Ball and Philip Hale
Contact: Albourne Road, Hurstpierpoint, Haywards Heath, West Sussex BN6 9ES
) 01273 834873

Ladymead is a large detached house set in the village of Hurstpierpoint. The home's large gardens overlook the South Downs. There are two home cats in residence. There is no smoking area at present as there are no smokers in residence, but smokers are accepted so one can be arranged. The home accommodates all faiths and arranges visits on requested. There are residents meetings monthly to twice monthly. The home also arranges outings for the residents and has its own car for this purpose.

Registered places: 27
Guide weekly rate: From £550
Specialist care: Nursing
Medical services: Podiatry, dentist, optician, physiotherapy
Qualified staff: Fails standard: 47% at NVQ level 2

Home details
Location: Village location, 9 miles from Haywards Heath
Communal areas: Lounge, dining room, conservatory, patio and garden
Accessibility: *Floors:* 2 • *Access:* Lift • *Wheelchair access:* Good
Smoking: ✓
Pets: ✗
Routines: Flexible

Room details
Single: 17
Shared: 5
En suite: 2
Facilities: TV point

Door lock: ✗
Lockable place: ✓

Services provided
Beauty services: Hairdressing
Mobile library: ✓
Religious services: ✓
Transport: Car
Activities: *Coordinator:* ✓ • *Examples:* Singing, music and
   movement, quizzes • *Outings:* ✓
Meetings: ✓

Registered places: 18
Guide weekly rate: £331–£395
Specialist care: Respite
Medical services: Podiatry, dentist, optician
Qualified staff: Exceeds standard: 60% at NVQ level 2

Home details
Location: Residential area, 1 mile from Worthing
Communal areas: Lounge/dining room, private lounge, garden
Accessibility: *Floors:* 2 • *Access:* Lift • *Wheelchair access:* Good
Smoking: In designated area
Pets: ✗
Routines: Flexible

Room details
Single: 18
Shared: 0
En suite: 12
Facilities: TV point, telephone point

Door lock: ✓
Lockable place: ✓

Services provided
Beauty services: Hairdressing
Mobile library: ✓
Religious services: Fortnightly Catholic Communion, monthly
   Anglican service
Transport: ✗
Activities: *Coordinator:* ✓ • *Examples:* Accordionist visits,
   board games, puzzles • *Outings:* ✗
Meetings: ✓

Larkswood

Manager: Marilyn Jones
Owner: Sound Homes Ltd
Contact: 3 St Botolph's Road, Worthing,
West Sussex BN11 4JN
☏ 01903 202650

Larkswood is a large detached property situated close to parks and gardens. The home aims to create a friendly atmosphere and a home from home for residents. There is a small staff turnover so there is a sense of continuity for residents. In the home there is a resident cat and occasional dog, every two weeks there is a Pets As Therapy scheme. The home arranges a residents meeting once a month and there are both Anglican and Catholic services on offer.

Registered places: 54
Guide weekly rate: £558–£711
Specialist care: Nursing, dementia, physical disability
Medical services: Podiatry, hygienist, optician
Qualified staff: Exceeds standard: over 60% at NVQ level 2

Home details
Location: Residential area, 0.5 miles from Worthing
Communal areas: 5 lounges, 2 dining rooms, activities room,
   hairdressing salon, patio and garden
Accessibility: *Floors:* 3 • *Access:* lift • *Wheelchair access:* Good
Smoking: In designated area
Pets: At manager's discretion
Routines: Flexible

Room details
Single: 54
Shared: 0
En suite: 54
Facilities: TV point, telephone point

Door lock: ✗
Access to Lockable place: ✓

Services provided
Beauty services: Hairdressing
Mobile library: ✓
Religious services: Fortnightly Catholic visits
Transport: ✓
Activities: *Coordinator:* ✗ • *Examples:* Bingo, bowls night
   Outings: ✓
Meetings: ✓

Linfield Care Home

Manager: Patricia Hall
Owner: Guild Care
Contact: 18–22 Wykeham Road,
Worthing, West Sussex BN11 4JD
☏ 01903 529629
@ linfield@guildcare.org
⌨ www.guildcare.org

Linfield Care Home is a large, purpose-designed facility with a secure garden and an additional roof garden. There are four cluster areas each with a lounge and kitchen in addition to the communal spaces provided for the whole home. There are pleasant views of Victoria Park and Sussex Downs and the home is close to local shops, a library and the seafront. The home also has a dedicated room for painting, pottery and craftwork. Broadband and computer access points are available. The home also has a communal pet dog in the dementia unit, a parrot, budgies and a fish tank.

Littlefair

Manager: Susan Dorman

Owner: Mr and Mrs Kennedy

Contact: Warburton Close, East Grinstead, West Sussex RH19 3TX

) 01342 318008

@ Sue.dorman@littlefair.net

www.littlefair.net

Littlefair is a purpose-built care home located in a residential area of East Grinstead. There are gardens to the front and rear of the building and a central, secluded garden with seating. There is a range of activities for residents to choose from including carpet Bowles and flower arranging. The home focuses on keeping the independence and dignity of the residents intact while also keeping them active. The home takes the residents on outings to this end and arranges a nondenominational service once a month.

Registered places: 41

Guide weekly rate: £345–£525

Specialist care: Physical disability, respite

Medical services: Podiatry, dentist, optician, physiotherapy

Qualified staff: Exceeds standard: 57% at NVQ level 2

Home details

Location: Residential area, 1 mile from East Grinstead

Communal areas: 2 lounges, dining room, garden

Accessibility: *Floors:* 3 • *Access:* 2 lifts
Wheelchair access: Good

Smoking: ✗

Pets: At manager's discretion

Routines: Flexible

Room details

Single: 41

Shared: 0

En suite: Undisclosed

Facilities: TV point, telephone point

Door lock: ✓

Lockable place: ✓

Services provided

Beauty services: Hairdressing

Mobile library: ✓

Religious services: Monthly nondenominational service

Transport: ✗

Activities: *Coordinator:* ✓ • *Examples:* Flower arranging, carpet Bowles, quizzes • *Outings:* ✓

Meetings: ✗

Longacre Nursing Home

Manager: Diane Thorpe

Owner: John Mayer

Contact: 12–14 Chute Way, High Salvington, Worthing, West Sussex BN13 3EA

) 01903 261648

Longacre is a converted, detached, two-storey building in a quiet, residential area, three miles from the sea. The home has well-maintained gardens with a seating area. Activities are organised regularly including crafts and music and movement. Outings are also frequent with trips to garden centres, the beach and the theatre. The home has meetings as and when the residents request them or when the manager feels they are needed. Religious services are offered and the home also arranges for a mobile library to visit.

Registered places: 30

Guide weekly rate: £550–£800

Specialist care: Nursing

Medical services: Podiatry, dentist, optician, physiotherapy

Qualified staff: Meets standard

Home details

Location: Residential area, 3 miles from Worthing

Communal areas: Lounge, dining room, 2 conservatories, garden

Accessibility: *Floors:* 2 • *Access:* Lift • *Wheelchair access:* Good

Smoking: ✗

Pets: At manager's discretion

Routines: Flexible

Room details

Single: 24

Shared: 3

En suite: 9

Facilities: TV point, telephone point

Door lock: ✓

Lockable place: ✓

Services provided

Beauty services: Hairdressing

Mobile library: ✓

Religious services: ✓

Transport: ✗

Activities: *Coordinator:* ✓ • *Examples:* Crafts, games, movement and music • *Outings:* ✓

Meetings: ✓

Registered places: 54
Guide weekly rate: £500–£700
Specialist care: Nursing, day care, dementia, respite
Medical services: Podiatry, dentist, optician, physiotherapy
Qualified staff: Meets standard

Home details

Location: Residential area, 0.5 miles from Billinghurst
Communal areas: Dining room, garden
Accessibility: *Floors:* 2 • *Access:* Lift • *Wheelchair access:* Good
Smoking: ✓
Pets: ✓
Routines: Flexible

Room details

Single: 46
Shared: 4
En suite: 50
Facilities: TV point, telephone point

Door lock: ✗
Lockable place: ✓

Services provided

Beauty services: Hairdressing
Mobile library: ✓
Religious services: Monthly
Transport: ✓
Activities: *Coordinator:* ✓ • *Examples:* Bowls, quizzes, singing
    Outings: ✓
Meetings: ✓

Longfield Manor

Manager: Shafik Sachedina and Shiraz Boghani
Owner: Jessica Dabalus-Pinson
Contact: West Street, Billingshurst, West Sussex RH14 9LX
✆ 01403 786832
🖰 www.longfield@sussexhealthcare.org

Longfield Manor is a two-storey building standing in its own grounds. It has an attached day care centre. The home is led by an experienced Home Manager and is staffed with a qualified nurse 24 hours a day. The home is located in a residential area, half a mile from Billingshurst. There is a dedicated activities coordinator who arranges outings for the residents as well as daily events such as bowls and quizzes. The bedrooms are situated around a quiet courtyard garden giving a peaceful setting. There are plenty of communal areas with four lounges, a quiet room and a spacious dining room overlooking the gardens.

Registered places: 18
Guide weekly rate: £600–£800
Specialist care: Respite
Medical services: Podiatry, dentist, optician, physiotherapy
Qualified staff: Fails standards

Home details

Location: Rural area, 8 miles from Chichester.
Communal areas: Lounge, dining room, patio and garden
Accessibility: *Floors:* 2 • *Access:* Lift • *Wheelchair access:* Good
Smoking: ✗
Pets: ✗
Routines: Flexible

Room details

Single: 18
Shared: 0
En suite: 18
Facilities: TV point, telephone point

Door lock: ✗
Lockable place: ✓

Services provided

Beauty services: Hairdressing
Mobile library: ✓
Religious services: Monthly Anglican Communion service
Transport: Car
Activities: *Coordinator:* ✗ • *Examples:* Art classes, barbecues,
    piano recitals • *Outings:* ✗
Meetings: ✗

Lordington Park

Manager: Mrs Smith
Owner: Mr and Mrs Rutland
Contact: Lordington, Chichester, West Sussex PO18 9DX
✆ 01243 371536

Lordington Park is a large, detached property set in 30 acres of grounds and eight miles from Chichester. The home allows the residents to organise their own activities and outings, focusing on a very independent atmosphere. Within the grounds there is a heated swimming pool and a crocket lawn for the residents to enjoy. The home can arrange for a Catholic priest to visit if requested and there is a monthly Anglican Communion service.

Manorfield

Manager: Christina Buckley
Owner: Mr, Mrs and Miss Buckley and Mrs Leach
Contact: Clappers Lane, Earnley, Chichester, West Sussex PO20 7JJ
) 01243 673023

Manorfield is a modern building with a purpose-built extension and is situated in a small village seven miles from Chichester. The garden has recently been landscaped so provides a relaxing area for use in warmer months. The home provides its own transport for residents. The home has many resident animals: a cat, parrot, some fish and a dog. There are also regular visits from visiting entertainers for residents to enjoy.

Registered places: 22
Guide weekly rate: £425–£675
Specialist care: Physical disability, respite
Medical services: Podiatry, optician, physiotherapy
Qualified staff: Meets standard

Home details
Location: Village location, 7 miles from Chichester
Communal areas: 2 lounges, dining room, patio and garden
Accessibility: *Floors:* 1 • *Wheelchair access:* Good
Smoking: In designated area
Pets: At manager's discretion
Routines: Flexible

Room details
Single: 20
Shared: 1
En suite: 21
Facilities: TV point, telephone point

Door lock: ✓
Lockable place: ✓

Services provided
Beauty services: Hairdressing
Mobile library: ✓
Religious services: Monthly Anglican Communion service
Transport: Minibus
Activities: *Coordinator:* ✓ • *Examples:* Crafts, music, bridge club
  Outings: ✓
Meetings: ✗

Marriott House and Lodge

Manager: Sandra Owens
Owner: Barchester Healthcare Ltd
Contact: Tollhouse Close, Chichester, West Sussex PO19 1SG
) 01243 536652
@ sandy.owens@barchester.com
www.barchester.com

Marriott House and Lodge is a large property that has been divided into two separate units. Marriott Lodge is a residential unit providing care for 47 residents and Marriott House provides nursing and residential care for 72 residents. The home is located in an urban area, half a mile from Chichester town centre. The home has a varied activities programme, which includes one-to-one sessions and seasonal events such as a cruise night. There is a vicar who visits the home and there is a Communion service held on a monthly basis.

Registered places: 119
Guide weekly rate: £331–£1,000
Specialist care: Nursing, physically disabled, respite
Medical services: Podiatry, optician
Qualified staff: Meets standard

Home details
Location: Urban area, 0.5 miles from Chichester
Communal areas: Lounges, dining room, hairdressing salon, garden
Accessibility: *Floors:* 3 • *Access:* Lift • *Wheelchair access:* Good
Smoking: In designated area
Pets: ✗
Routines: Flexible

Room details
Single: 119
Shared: 0
En suite: 118
Facilities: TV, telephone point

Door lock: ✓
Lockable place: ✓

Services provided
Beauty services: Hairdressing, manicures
Mobile library: ✓
Religious services: Monthly Communion service
Transport: Minibus
Activities: *Coordinator:* ✓ • *Examples:* Monthly tea dance, seasonal events • *Outings:* ✓
Meetings: ✓

Registered places: 20
Guide weekly rate: £375–£450
Specialist care: Day care, respite
Medical services: Podiatry, dentist, optician
Qualified staff: Meets standard

Home details

Location: Residential area, 0.5 miles from Shoreham-By-Sea
Communal areas: 2 lounges, dining room, patio and garden
Accessibility: *Floors:* 3 • *Access:* Lift • *Wheelchair access:* Good
Smoking: ✗
Pets: At manager's discretion
Routines: Flexible

Room details

Single: 20
Shared: 0
En suite: 10
Facilities: TV point, telephone point

Door lock: ✓
Lockable place: ✓

Services provided

Beauty services: Hairdressing
Mobile library: ✗
Religious services: Monthly Anglican, weekly Catholic service
Transport: ✗
Activities: *Coordinator:* ✓ • *Examples:* Bingo, scrabble, quizzes
    Outings: ✓
Meetings: ✓

Meadowcroft

Manager: Nada Mitrovic-Wakeford
Owner: Marlene Sanders
Contact: 30 Buckingham Road,
Shoreham-by-Sea, West Sussex
BN43 5UB
☎ 01273 452582

Meadowcroft is located in a residential area, half a mile from Shoreham-by-Sea. The home has a large garden for residents to enjoy. They have a wealth of activities for both frail and more active residents. There are trips to the theatre and pantomimes as well as afternoon teas. Visiting entertainment also comes in frequently. The home arranges regular meetings to allow residents to voice their opinions on any issues or concerns they may have.

Registered places: 20
Guide weekly rate: £615–£700
Specialist care: Nursing, respite
Medical services: Podiatry, dentist, optician, physiotherapy
Qualified staff: Exceeds standard: 75% at NVQ level 2

Home details

Location: Residential area, 0.5 miles from Worthing
Communal areas: Lounge, dining room, patio and garden
Accessibility: *Floors:* 2 • *Access:* Lift • *Wheelchair access:* Good
Smoking: ✗
Pets: At manager's discretion
Routines: Flexible

Room details.

Single: 16
Shared: 2
En suite: 11
Facilities: TV point, telephone point

Door lock: ✓
Lockable place: ✓

Services provided

Beauty services: Hairdressing, manicure, foot massage
Mobile library: ✗
Religious services: Local ministers visit
Transport: Minibus
Activities: *Coordinator:* ✓ • *Examples:* Games, singalongs, bingo
    Outings: ✓
Meetings: ✗

Melrose Care Home

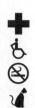

Manager: Elizabeth Seymour
Owner: Melrose Care Ltd
Contact: 9–11 Wykeham Road,
Worthing, West Sussex BN11 4JG
☎ 01903 230406
@ melrose.care@tiscali.co.uk
🖰 www.melrosecare.org.uk

Melrose is a large, detached Victorian property that has been converted into a care home. In each room there are large bay windows. The home arranges barbecues and parties for the residents to enjoy. The minibus is used to take residents to hospital and dentist while also for the more agile residents to go on outings and shopping trips. In the lounge there is a large television and video equipment for residents to watch films.

Millfield

Manager: Pauline Shanahan
Owner: Pauline Shanahan
Contact: 9 St Catherine's Road, Littlehampton, West Sussex BN17 5HS
✆ 01903 714992

Millfield is a semi-detached, spacious, Edwardian house, which overlooks a park. As it is a small home, members of staff are able to spend quality, individual time with residents. Home-cooked food prepared from fresh ingredients is also regarded as a high point by residents. The home also has its own GP. If requested by the residents the home can arrange visits from Anglican and Catholic clergy to give Communion. The home also has its own transport to take residents on outings.

Registered places: 11
Guide weekly rate: £331–£401
Specialist care: Respite
Medical services: Podiatry, optician, hygienist, physiotherapy
Qualified staff: Exceeds standard: 90% at NVQ level 2

Home details
Location: Residential area, 0.2 miles from Littlehampton
Communal areas: Lounge, dining room, patio and garden
Accessibility: *Floors:* 2 • *Access:* Lift • *Wheelchair access:* Good
Smoking: In designated area
Pets: ✗
Routines: Flexible

Room details
Single: 11
Shared: 0
En suite: 2
Facilities: TV point, telephone point
Door lock: ✓
Lockable place: ✓

Services provided
Beauty services: Hairdressing
Mobile library: ✗
Religious services: Anglican and Catholic visits
Transport: People carrier
Activities: *Coordinator:* ✗ • *Examples:* Arts and crafts, music and movement, bingo • *Outings:* ✓
Meetings: ✗

Nightingales Nursing Home

Manager: Cadogan Care Ltd
Owner: Tracey Elizabeth Searle
Contact: 43 Beach Road, Littlehampton, West Sussex BN17 5JG
✆ 01903 717376

Nightingales Nursing Home is a detached Edwardian house situated within Littlehampton, two minutes' walk from all shops and amenities. The home overlooks a park and is a few minutes' walk from the public transport, local amenities and the seafront. Residents are provided with the choice of participating in a number of activities and staff organise themed days on a monthly basis. This has included French and Hawaiian days, where dress, music and food are all themed. Resident's pets are welcome to visit the home.

Registered places: 35
Guide weekly rate: £600–£725
Specialist care: Nursing
Medical services: Podiatry, optician, physiotherapy
Qualified staff: Meets standard

Home details
Location: Residential area, 0.5 miles from Littlehampton
Communal areas: 2 lounges, 2 dining rooms, garden
Accessibility: *Floors:* 2 • *Access:* Lift • *Wheelchair access:* Good
Smoking: ✗
Pets: ✗
Routines: Flexible

Room details
Single: 31
Shared: 2
En suite: 3
Facilities: TV point, telephone point
Door lock: ✗
Lockable place: ✓

Services provided
Beauty services: Hairdressing
Mobile library: Library access
Religious services: Monthly
Transport: ✗
Activities: *Coordinator:* ✓ • *Examples:* Games, music, cooking *Outings:* ✓
Meetings: ✓

Registered places: 26
Guide weekly rate: £325–£475
Specialist care: Dementia, respite
Medical services: Podiatry, dentist, optician, physiotherapy
Qualified staff: Meets standard

Home details

Location: Residential area, 1 mile from Bognor Regis
Communal areas: Lounge, dining room, garden
Accessibility: *Floors:* 2 • *Access:* Lift • *Wheelchair access:* Good
Smoking: In designated area
Pets: x
Routines: Flexible

Room details

Single: 24
Shared: 1
En suite: 9
Facilities: TV point, telephone point

Door lock: ✓
Lockable place: ✓

Services provided

Beauty services: Hairdressing
Mobile library: ✓
Religious services: x
Transport: x
Activities: *Coordinator:* x • *Examples:* Bingo, keep fit, quizzes
  Outings: ✓
Meetings: x

Normanton Lodge

Manager: Susan English
Owner: Normanton Ltd
Contact: 14–16 Normanton Avenue,
Bognor Regis, West Sussex PO21 2TX
☎ 01243 821763

Local amenities such as shops are within walking distance of Normanton Lodge, and the seafront is a short drive away. Activities are organised frequently including painting, bingo and games. Visiting musical entertainers and mobile shops come often for residents to enjoy. Outings also take place, such as visits to the local shops, or attending shows and concerts. Relatives are allowed to visit at any time and are given privacy with their family. The home has two cats and two dogs.

Registered places: 47
Guide weekly rate: Undisclosed
Specialist care: Nursing, dementia, respite
Medical services: Podiatry, occupational therapy, physiotherapy
Qualified staff: Undisclosed

Home details

Location: Urban area, 1 mile from Horsham centre
Communal areas: 3 lounges, 2 dining rooms, activities room,
  kitchenette, garden
Accessibility: *Floors:* 2 • *Access:* Lift • *Wheelchair access:* Good
Smoking: In designated area
Pets: ✓
Routines: Flexible

Room details

Single: 45
Shared: 2
En suite: 34
Facilities: TV point, telephone point

Door lock: ✓
Lockable place: x

Services provided

Beauty services: Hairdressing, aromatherapy
Mobile library: ✓
Religious services: ✓
Transport: Minibus
Activities: *Coordinator:* ✓ • *Examples:* Reminiscence therapy
  Outings: ✓
Meetings: ✓

Oakhill House

Manager: Jane Marquis
Owner: BUPA Care Homes Ltd
Contact: Eady Close, Highlands Road,
Horsham, West Sussex RH13 5NA
☎ 01403 260801
@ OakHillHouseAll@BUPA.com
🖰 www.bupacarehomes.co.uk

Situated in a quiet cul-de-sac a short distance from Horsham, Oakhill House is purpose-designed to provide a safe environment and specialist care for residents with dementia. The carefully planned layout enables residents to walk around freely, and ground floor bedrooms have French doors onto the enclosed gardens. There are also two double rooms. There is a practically designed activities centre, and regular reminiscence therapy, trips to local places of interest and visiting entertainers. Support is also provided to family and friends, individually and through a regular carers' group.

Oakhurst Court Rest Home

Manager: Mrs Lawson and Mr Elliot
Owner: I, G and H Elliott
Contact: Carron Lane, Midhurst, West Sussex GU29 9LF
☎ 01730 816242

Oakhurst Court is a detached property, set in its own grounds in a rural area, one mile from Midhurst. The home focuses on a friendly atmosphere and organises many different activities for the residents to enjoy. They also go on outings such as to Bluebell Railway to ride the steam train. The home tries to keep them as active as possible going for walks or taking them out into the garden during the summer.

Registered places: 6
Guide weekly rate: From £420
Specialist care: Day care, respite
Medical services: Podiatry, dentist, optician, physiotherapy
Qualified staff: Undisclosed

Home details
Location: Residential area, 1 mile from Midhurst
Communal areas: Lounge, dining room, garden
Accessibility: *Floors:* 2 • *Access:* None
  Wheelchair access: Limited
Smoking: ✗
Pets: ✗
Routines: Flexible

Room details
Single: 6	**Door lock:** ✓
Shared: 0	**Lockable place:** ✓
En suite: 2	

Facilities: TV point, telephone point

Services provided
Beauty services: Hairdressing
Mobile library: ✗
Religious services: Monthly Communion service
Transport: ✗
Activities: *Coordinator:* ✗ • *Examples:* Musical entertainment, tea parties • *Outings:* ✓
Meetings: ✗

Oakhurst Grange

Manager: Frankie Deane
Owner: BUPA Care Homes Ltd
Contact: Goffs Park Road, Crawley, West Sussex RH11 8AY
☎ 01293 536481
@ OakhurstGrangeALL@BUPA.com
🖰 www.bupacarehomes.co.uk

Oakhurst Grange is situated in a residential area of Crawley. This modern, purpose-built single-storey home has been designed specifically to meet the needs of elderly residents. Oakhurst Grange comprises four separate houses, each with its own character. Two are registered for nursing care, one for dementia nursing care and one for dementia residential care. Each house has a comfortable, well-furnished lounge, dining area and conservatory which provide places for residents and guests to meet. All houses also have access to the large landscaped gardens and patio area. Daily activities are arranged, including board games, reminiscence sessions and gardening.

Registered places: 120
Guide weekly rate: Undisclosed
Specialist care: Nursing, dementia, palliative care, physical disability, respite, terminal care
Medical services: Podiatry
Qualified staff: Undisclosed

Home details
Location: Residential area, 1 mile from Crawley centre
Communal areas: 4 lounges, 4 dining rooms, hairdressing salon, garden
Accessibility: *Floors:* 1 • *Wheelchair access:* Good
Smoking: In designated area
Pets: ✗
Routines: Flexible

Room details
Single: 120	**Door lock:** ✓
Shared: 0	**Lockable place:** ✗
En suite: 0	

Facilities: TV point, telephone point

Services provided
Beauty services: Hairdressing, aromatherapy
Mobile library: ✓
Religious services: ✓
Transport: ✓
Activities: *Coordinator:* ✓ • *Examples:* Arts and crafts, ball games, musical entertainers • *Outings:* ✓
Meetings: ✓

Registered places: 37
Guide weekly rate: £450–£580
Specialist care: Respite
Medical services: Podiatry, dentist, optician, physiotherapy
Qualified staff: Exceeds standard: 55% at NVQ level 2

Home details

Location: Village location, 1.5 miles from Bognor Regis
Communal areas: 2 lounges, dining room, garden
Accessibility: *Floors:* 3 • *Access:* Lift • *Wheelchair access:* Good
Smoking: ✗
Pets: At manager's discretion
Routines: Flexible

Room details

Single: 37	Door lock: ✓
Shared: 0	Lockable place: ✓
En suite: 37	
Facilities: TV, telephone	

Services provided

Beauty services: Hairdressing
Mobile library: ✓
Religious services: Weekly Catholic and Anglican service
Transport: ✗
Activities: *Coordinator:* ✗ • *Examples:* Arts and crafts, exercises, weekly music • *Outings:* ✓
Meetings: ✓

Oakland Court

Manager: Julie VanBiene
Owner: Oakland Court Ltd
Contact: 26 Admiralty Road, Felpham, Bognor Regis, West Sussex PO22 7DW
☏ 01243 842400

Oakland Court is a converted building situated in a village one and a half mile outside Bognor Regis. The lounge and dining room open out onto attractive, secluded gardens. The home is only a short walk from the seafront for residents to enjoy a day with their family or for outings. The home offers a range of activities including arts and crafts and exercise classes to keep residents active.

Registered places: 42
Guide weekly rate: £420–£543
Specialist care: Day care, respite
Medical services: Podiatry, hygienist, optician, physiotherapy
Qualified staff: Fails standard: 29% at NVQ level 2

Home details

Location: Residential area, 1 mile from Littlehampton
Communal areas: 2 lounges, dining room, patio and garden
Accessibility: *Floors:* 3 • *Access:* 2 lifts • *Wheelchair access:* Good
Smoking: ✗
Pets: ✗
Routines: Flexible

Room details

Single: 40	Door lock: ✓
Shared: 2	Lockable place: ✓
En suite: 42	
Facilities: TV point, telephone point	

Services provided

Beauty services: Hairdressing
Mobile library: ✗
Religious services: Monthly Anglican service
Transport: ✗
Activities: *Coordinator:* ✓ • *Examples:* Bingo, quiz nights, music for health • *Outings:* ✓
Meetings: ✓

Oakland Grange

Manager: Philip Peart
Owner: Oakland Ltd
Contact: St Floras Road, Littlehampton, West Sussex BN17 6B
☏ 01903 715995
🖰 www.oaklandcare.co.uk

Oakland Grange was originally a large private home and is close to local amenities such as shops, churches and post offices. The home has its own chef who tailors menus to suit all dietary requirements. The garden is being re-designed with ponds and summerhouses for residents to enjoy during the warmer months. There are also many themed nights including French and cowboy nights and they have musical entertainment every weekend. Some rooms have views of the garden while others can see the Downs.

Oaklodge Nursing Home

Manager: Dhananjay Dalmond
Owner: Dhananjay Dalmond
Contact: 2 Silverdale Road, Burgess Hill, West Sussex RH15 0EF
) 01444 243788

Oaklodge Nursing Home is situated in Burgess Hill town. The home is close to local amenities and a train station. There are no pets allowed to stay in the home, but they can visit with family or friends. The home has a wealth of activities including visiting entertainers, summer barbecues and a Christmas party. There are also film nights when the residents all watch a film together. The home also arranges for Anglican and Catholic services to take place once a month.

Registered places: 25
Guide weekly rate: £525–£650
Specialist care: Nursing, respite
Medical services: Podiatry, dentist, optician
Qualified staff: Meets standard

Home details
Location: Residential area, 1 mile from Burgess Hill
Communal areas: 2 lounges, dining room, patio and garden
Accessibility: *Floors:* 3 • *Access:* Lift • *Wheelchair access:* Good
Smoking: ✗
Pets: ✗
Routines: Flexible

Room details
Single: 17
Shared: 4
En suite: 1
Facilities: TV point

Door lock: ✓
Lockable place: ✓

Services provided
Beauty services: Hairdressing
Mobile library: ✓
Religious services: Monthly Catholic and Anglican services
Transport: ✗
Activities: *Coordinator:* ✓ • *Examples:* Bingo, cards, exercise • *Outings:* ✓
Meetings: ✗

Oban House

Manager: Eve Kent
Owner: Eve Kent and Ronald Rook
Contact: 9–11 Victoria Drive, Bognor Regis, West Sussex PO21 2RH
) 01243 863564

Oban House is a large property, consisting of two detached houses, linked to form one establishment. The home is located in the costal town of Bognor Regis, close to the seafront and shops. The home organises outings, as the home has its own minibus which makes this easier. There are frequent summer outings to nearby Arundel and Chichester, or simply seafront walks at Bognor for fish and chips. Residents are encouraged to stay as active as possible, so there are frequent exercise lessons, movement to music and seafront walks.

Registered places: 30
Guide weekly rate: £256–£390
Specialist care: None
Medical services: Podiatry, optician, physiotherapy
Qualified staff: Meets standard

Home details
Location: Residential area, 1 mile from Bognor Regis
Communal areas: Lounge, dining room, garden
Accessibility: *Floors:* 2 • *Access:* Lift • *Wheelchair access:* Good
Smoking: In designated area
Pets: ✗
Routines: Flexible

Room details
Single: 24
Shared: 3
En suite: 17
Facilities: TV point, telephone point

Door lock: ✓
Lockable place: ✓

Services provided
Beauty services: Hairdressing
Mobile library: ✓
Religious services: Monthly
Transport: ✓
Activities: *Coordinator:* ✗ • *Examples:* Arts and crafts, exercise, music and movement • *Outings:* ✓
Meetings: ✓

Registered places: 23
Guide weekly rate: Undisclosed
Specialist care:
Medical services: Podiatry, dentist, optician, physiotherapy
Qualified staff: Undisclosed

Home details

Location: Residential area, 3 miles from Worthing
Communal areas: Lounge, conservatory, garden
Accessibility: *Floors:* 2 • *Access:* Lift • *Wheelchair access:* Good
Smoking: In designated area
Pets: ✗
Routines: Flexible

Room details

Single: 22
Shared: 1
En suite: 13
Facilities: TV point, telephone point

Door lock: ✗
Lockable place: ✓

Services provided

Beauty services: Hairdressing
Mobile library: ✓
Religious services: monthly
Transport: ✗
Activities: *Coordinator:* ✓ • *Examples:* Knitting, bingo, darts, visiting entertainers • *Outings:* ✓
Meetings: ✓

Offington Park Care Home

Manager: Jacqueline McCurd
Owner: Claremont Care Service Ltd
Contact: 145 Offington Drive, Worthing, West Sussex BN14 9PU
☎ 01903 260202

Offington Park Care Home is a detached building situated in a residential road on the outskirts of Worthing. Worthing is a seaside town, approximately three miles away, with shops, train stations and other amenities. The home has a lovely large garden at the rear which is well kept, and offers seating and decking for residents to socialise. In summer months barbecues and outside coffee mornings are frequent. There is a resident cat at the home, and pets are allowed to visit the home. Residents meetings take place once a month to discuss any issues they may have.

Registered places: 34
Guide weekly rate: £359.74–£798
Specialist care: Nursing, physical disability, respite
Medical services: Podiatry, dentist, optician, physiotherapy
Qualified staff: Exceeds standard: 70% at NVQ level 2

Home details

Location: Village location, 8.3 miles from Chichester
Communal areas: 2 lounges, dining room, garden
Accessibility: *Floors:* 2 • *Access:* Lift • *Wheelchair access:* Good
Smoking: In designated area
Pets: At manager's discretion
Routines: Flexible

Room details

Single: 30
Shared: 2
En suite: 31
Facilities: TV point, telephone point

Door lock: ✓
Lockable place: ✓

Services provided

Beauty services: Hairdressing, aromatherapy, massage
Mobile library: Local library facilities
Religious services: Varying clergy visit, Anglican service
Transport: ✗
Activities: *Coordinator:* ✓ • *Examples:* Bingo, card games, reminiscence sessions • *Outings:* ✓
Meetings: ✗

The Old Malthouse

Manager: Laura Bow
Owner: Timothy Whites Ltd
Contact: 33 High Street, Selsey, Chichester, West Sussex PO20 0RB
☎ 01243 605410

The Old Malthouse is a large detached property located in the village of Selsey, around eight and a half miles from Chichester. It is within easy walking distance of the seafront and village shops. A full-time activities coordinator is employed and a board in reception displays the weekly activities. These include bingo, card games, board games and reminiscence classes. Though the home doesn't have any transport local outings are organised for residents. The home also organises for local clergy to visit the home, in addition to a regular Anglican service.

Parkside Lodge

Manager: Ann Smith
Owner: Mr and Mrs Nanji
Contact: 28 Wykeham Road, Worthing, West Sussex BN11 4JF
☎ 01903 235393

Parkside Lodge is a large, detached house in the centre of town. The home is also close to Victoria Park. All religions are catered for with the home organising transport to local Catholic and Methodist churches. There are residents meetings orgainsed every two months. The home also has an activities coordinator who arranges outings as well as daily activities such as art classes.

Registered places: 20
Guide weekly rate: £350–£475
Specialist care: Respite
Medical services: Podiatry, physiotherapy
Qualified staff: Meets standard

Home details
Location: Residential area, 0.5 miles from Worthing
Communal areas: 2 lounges, dining room, patio and garden
Accessibility: *Floors:* 3 • *Access:* Lift • *Wheelchair access:* Good
Smoking: In designated area
Pets: ✗
Routines: Flexible

Room details
Single: 18
Shared: 2
En suite: 3
Facilities: TV point, telephone point
Door lock: ✓
Lockable place: ✓

Services provided
Beauty services: Hairdressing
Mobile library: ✓
Religious services: Anglican service
Transport: ✗
Activities: *Coordinator:* ✓ • *Examples:* Mosaics, art classes, card making • *Outings:* ✓
Meetings: ✓

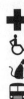

Pendean House

Manager: Jackie Travers
Owner: BUPA Care Homes Ltd
Contact: West Lavington, Midhurst, Chichester, West Sussex GU29 0ES
☎ 01730 812896
@ PendeanHouseALL@BUPA.com
🖰 www.bupacarehomes.co.uk

A beautifully situated country house of warm red brick and stone, with spectacular views across the South Downs, Pendean House has been sympathetically converted and extended. Just one mile from the market town of Midhurst, it boasts extensive, well-maintained mature gardens and a large pond. Daily activities offered include garden and cocktail parties and trips to the theatre, museums and local gardens. A car service takes residents to Midhurst for shopping and appointments. Pendean House also offers care to a number of younger residents with physical disabilities, and to those requiring palliative or terminal care.

Registered places: 44
Guide weekly rate: Undisclosed
Specialist care: Nursing, palliative care, respite, terminal care
Medical services: Podiatry, physiotherapy
Qualified staff: Undisclosed

Home details
Location: Rural area, 1 mile from Midhurst centre
Communal areas: 2 lounges, dining room, hairdressing salon, garden
Accessibility: *Floors:* 2 • *Access:* Lift • *Wheelchair access:* Good
Smoking: In designated area
Pets: ✓
Routines: Flexible

Room details
Single: 24
Shared: 10
En suite: 34
Facilities: TV, telephone point
Door lock: ✓
Lockable place: ✗

Services provided
Beauty services: Hairdressing, aromatherapy
Mobile library: ✓
Religious services: ✓
Transport: ✓
Activities: *Coordinator:* ✓ • *Examples:* Parties, quizzes *Outings:* ✓
Meetings: ✓

Registered places: 21
Guide weekly rate: £600–£700
Specialist care: Nursing, respite
Medical services: Podiatry, dentist, optician, physiotherapy
Qualified staff: Exceeds standard: 90% at NVQ level 2

Home details

Location: Rural area, 5.5 miles from Chichester
Communal areas: Lounge, dining room, patio and garden
Accessibility: *Floors:* 2 • *Access:* Lift • *Wheelchair access:* Good
Smoking: ✗
Pets: At manager's discretion
Routines: Flexible

Room details

Single: 17
Shared: 2
En suite: 16
Facilities: TV point, telephone point

Door lock: ✓
Lockable place: ✓

Services provided

Beauty services: Hairdressing
Mobile library: ✓
Religious services: Clergy visits
Transport: ✗
Activities: *Coordinator:* ✓ • *Examples:* Bingo, bowles, gardening shows • *Outings:* ✓
Meetings: ✗

Pinewood Nursing and Convalescent Nursing Home

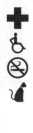

Manager: Deryl Marsh
Owner: Mr and Mrs Marsh
Contact: Conifers, Cot Lane, Chidham, Chichester, West Sussex PO18 8ST
☎ 01243 572480

Pinewood Nursing home is a detached house in beautiful grounds five and a half miles west of Chichester. It has stunning views of the sea and countryside. There are many activities for the residents to enjoy and outings are also arranged. Local clergy visit the home and there are also the facilities of a mobile library available.

Registered places: 50
Guide weekly rate: £650–£750
Specialist care: Nursing, physical disability
Medical services: Podiatry, dentist, optician, physiotherapy
Qualified staff: Undisclosed

Home details

Location: Residential area, 2 miles from Horsham
Communal areas: Lounge, quiet lounge, dining room, conservatory, garden
Accessibility: *Floors:* 2 • *Access:* 2 lifts • *Wheelchair access:* Good
Smoking: ✗
Pets: ✗
Routines: Flexible

Room details

Single: 50
Shared: 0
En suite: 5
Facilities: TV, telephone

Door lock: ✗
Lockable place: ✓

Services provided

Beauty services: Hairdressing, aromatherapy
Mobile library: ✓
Religious services: ✓
Transport: ✓
Activities: *Coordinator:* ✓ • *Examples:* Cooking, sewing, woodwork • *Outings:* ✓
Meetings: Undisclosed

Rapkyns

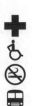

Manager: Michael Wooldridge
Owner: Shafik Sachedina
Contact: Guildford Road, Broadbridge Heath, Horsham, West Sussex RH12 3PQ
☎ 01403 265096
@ rapkyns@sussexhealthcare.org
🖰 www.sussexhealthcare.org

Rapkyns nursing home is a large detached property surrounded by countryside in the village of Broadbridge Heath, near Horsham. The home is two miles from the town centre and has large grounds for the residents to take walks in. The residents have a flexible daily routine which consists of the daily activities and outings the home offers. These activities include cooking, sewing and woodwork and there are outings to the theatre and the seaside. The home has a lounge, a dining room, a garden and a conservatory. The home also has its own transport.

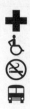

Rectory House Nursing Home

Manager: Patricia Hurst
Owner: Rectory House Ltd
Contact: West Street, Sompting, West Sussex BN15 0DA
📞 01206 828290

Rectory House is a detached property situated in Sompting village within easy distance of Lancing and Worthing. The home has a large conservatory which overlooks the garden, with seating areas outside if that is where residents wish to socialise. Daily activities include regular games, singalongs and gentle exercise to keep residents fit and agile. Residents pets are welcome to come and visit, which provides residents with entertainment. The home arranges a monthly religious service and for a mobile library to come to the home.

Registered places: 48
Guide weekly rate: £550–£650
Specialist care: Nursing
Medical services: Podiatry, dentist, optician, physiotherapy
Qualified staff: Meets standard

Home details
Location: Residential area, 3 miles from Worthing
Communal areas: 3 lounge/dining rooms, conservatory, garden
Accessibility: *Floors:* 3 • *Access:* Lift • *Wheelchair access:* Good
Smoking: ✗
Pets: ✗
Routines: Flexible

Room details
Single: 38
Shared: 5
En suite: 43
Facilities: TV point, telephone point

Door lock: ✗
Lockable place: ✓

Services provided
Beauty services: Hairdressing
Mobile library: ✓
Religious services: monthly
Transport: ✓
Activities: *Coordinator:* ✓ • *Examples:* Games, music, singalongs • *Outings:* ✗
Meetings: ✓

Red Oaks

Manager: Jacqueline Welch
Owner: Barchester Healthcare Ltd
Contact: The Hooks, Henfield, West Sussex BN5 9UY
📞 01273 493043
🖱 www.barchester.com

Red Oaks is situated on rising ground in a village just under a mile from Henfield. The home has both front and rear gardens and a patio area. Though pets are not allowed there is a resident cat at the home. The home also has a variety of activities with different options every day. There are two chefs employed by the home and every two months there is a food forum for residents to voice their opinions about the menus. The home arranges a wide variety of religious services for residents to partake in.

Registered places: 60
Guide weekly rate: £800–£1000
Specialist care: Nursing, physical disability, respite
Medical services: Podiatry, optician, physiotherapy
Qualified staff: Undisclosed

Home details
Location: Village location, 0.7 miles from Henfield
Communal areas: 4 lounges, dining room, patio and garden
Accessibility: *Floors:* 3 • *Access:* Lift • *Wheelchair access:* Good
Smoking: In designated area
Pets: ✗
Routines: Flexible

Room details
Single: 58
Shared: 1
En suite: 59
Facilities: TV point, telephone point

Door lock: ✓
Lockable place: ✓

Services provided
Beauty services: Hairdressing
Mobile library: ✓
Religious services: Weekly church service, weekly Catholic Communion service
Transport: Minibus and people carrier
Activities: *Coordinator:* ✓ • *Examples:* Arts and crafts, coffee mornings, talent contests • *Outings:* ✓
Meetings: ✓

Registered places: 18
Guide weekly rate: £400–£450
Specialist care: Day care, respite
Medical services: Podiatry, dentist, optician, physiotherapy
Qualified staff: Meets standard

Home details
Location: Residential area, 1 mile from Horsham
Communal areas: 3 lounges, dining room, hairdressing salon, garden
Accessibility: *Floors:* 2 • *Access:* Stair lift *Wheelchair access:* Good
Smoking: ✗
Pets: ✗
Routines: Flexible

Room details
Single: 11
Shared: 3
En suite: 4
Facilities: TV point, telephone point

Door lock: ✗
Lockable place: ✓

Services provided
Beauty services: Hairdressing
Mobile library: ✗
Religious services: Monthly Anglican and Catholic services
Transport: Car
Activities: *Coordinator:* ✗ • *Examples:* Arts and crafts, chair aerobics, quizzes • *Outings:* ✓
Meetings: ✓

Rosedale

Manager: Rosemary Pavoni
Owner: Mr and Mrs Pavoni
Contact: 25 Kings Road, Horsham, West Sussex RH13 5PP
☎ 01403 265236

Rosedale is a Victorian house with a large rear garden. The home is situated near Horsham rail station and approximately one mile from Horsham town centre. The home has many visiting entertainers and performers who lead singalong sessions. Over the Christmas period a theatre group perform a pantomime for the residents. The home also organises Anglican and Catholic services which take place once a month.

Registered places: 34
Guide weekly rate: £427–£527
Specialist care: Dementia
Medical services: Podiatry, optician
Qualified staff: Meets standard

Home details
Location: Residential area, 0.5 miles from Midhurst
Communal areas: 2 lounges, dining room, 2 gardens
Accessibility: *Floors:* 2 • *Access:* Lift • *Wheelchair access:* Good
Smoking: In designated area
Pets: At manager's discretion
Routines: Flexible

Room details
Single: 34
Shared: 0
En suite: 0
Facilities: TV point

Door lock: ✗
Lockable place: ✓

Services provided
Beauty services: Hairdressing
Mobile library: ✓
Religious services: Monthly
Transport: ✗
Activities: *Coordinator:* ✓ • *Examples:* Bingo, carpet bowls, exercises • *Outings:* ✗
Meetings: ✗

Rother House

Manager: Vacant
Owner: Shaw Healthcare Ltd
Contact: Lamberts Lane, Midhurst, West Sussex GU29 9DZ
☎ 01730 812759

Rother House is a care home for older people with a separate unit to care for residents with dementia. It is situated a few minutes' walk from the high street in Midhurst, a small country town with ample amenities. There are two gardens, to the side and the rear of the building. Most of it has level access for wheelchair users and seating areas for residents to socialise. An activities coordinator comes and organises activities for the residents, including reminiscence sessions, bingo and exercises sessions. There is a piano in the lounge for residents to play.

Royal Bay Nursing Home

Manager: Angela Ward
Owner: Royal Bay Care Homes Ltd
Contact: 86 Barrack Lane, Aldwick, Bognor Regis, West Sussex PO21 4DG
☎ 01243 267755
🖳 www.royalbay.co.uk

The Royal Bay Nursing Home is set in a quiet location in Aldwick, surrounded by mature gardens yet close to the sea. The home is two and a half miles from Bognor Regis. The home has a large conservatory that looks out over the gardens, which are well maintained and have a stonework fountain. The activities coordinator organises quiz and bingo nights to keep residents amused. There are monthly religious services in the home as well as regular residents meetings.

Registered places: 35
Guide weekly rate: £615–£695
Specialist care: Nursing, physical disability
Medical services: None
Qualified staff: Fails standard: 40% at NVQ level 2

Home details
Location: Residential area, 2.5 miles from Bognor Regis
Communal areas: Dining room, 2 conservatories, garden
Accessibility: *Floors:* 3 • *Access:* Lift • *Wheelchair access:* Good
Smoking: In designated area
Pets: At manager's discretion
Routines: Flexible

Room details
Single: 30
Shared: 3
En suite: 0
Facilities: TV point, telephone point

Door lock: ✗
Lockable place: ✓

Services provided
Beauty services: Hairdressing
Mobile library: ✓
Religious services: Monthly
Transport: ✗
Activities: *Coordinator:* ✓ • *Examples:* Bingo night, games, quiz night • *Outings:* ✗
Meetings: ✓

Royal Bay Residential Home

Manager: Beverley Treble
Owner: Royal Bay Care Homes Ltd
Contact: 83 Aldwick Road, Aldwick, Bognor Regis, West Sussex PO21 2PE
☎ 01243 864086
@ Beverley.treble@btconnect.com
🖳 www.royalbay.co.uk

Royal Bay is a detached, three-storey building situated close to local shops in Bognor Regis, a classic seaside town. The home employs a chef trained in nutrition for the elderly, so specified diets can be catered for. There is a range of activities for residents to get involved in, such as exercise sessions and music workshops. There are also outings offered for residents to take part in.

Registered places: 42
Guide weekly rate: £325–£475
Specialist care: Physical disability, respite
Medical services: Podiatry, dentist, optician, physiotherapy
Qualified staff: Exceeds standard: 55% at NVQ level 2

Home details
Location: Residential area, 1 mile from Bognor Regis
Communal areas: Lounge, dining room, garden
Accessibility: *Floors:* 2 • *Access:* Lift • *Wheelchair access:* Good
Smoking: In designated area
Pets: At manager's discretion
Routines: Flexible

Room details
Single: 28
Shared: 7
En suite: 35
Facilities: TV point, telephone point

Door lock: ✓
Lockable place: ✓

Services provided
Beauty services: Hairdressing
Mobile library: ✓
Religious services: Weekly Catholic and Anglican Communion services, monthly nondenominational service
Transport: ✗
Activities: *Coordinator:* ✓ • *Examples:* Bingo, exercises, music workshop • *Outings:* ✓
Meetings: ✓

Registered places: 36
Guide weekly rate: From £480
Specialist care: Respite
Medical services: Podiatry, physiotherapy
Qualified staff: Fails standard

Home details

Location: Residential area, 1 mile from Bognor Regis
Communal areas: Lounge, dining room, garden
Accessibility: *Floors:* 4 • *Access:* Lift • *Wheelchair access:* Good
Smoking: ✗
Pets: ✗
Routines: Flexible

Room details

Single: 20
Shared: 8
En suite: 28
Facilities: TV point, telephone point

Door lock: ✓
Lockable place: ✓

Services provided

Beauty services: Hairdressing
Mobile library: ✓
Religious services: Monthly nondenominational service
Transport: ✗
Activities: *Coordinator:* ✓ • *Examples:* Bingo, entertainment, quizzes • *Outings:* ✓
Meetings: ✓

Royal Garden Hotel

Manager: Martin Glass
Owner: Crescentworth Ltd
Contact: 1 Princess Avenue, Bognor Regis, West Sussex PO21 2QT
) 01243 841026
⌖ www.royalgarden.net

The Royal Garden Hotel is a purpose-built care home. The Beach Promenade and Marine Gardens are adjacent to the home and this location adds to the quality of residents' lives. The majority of rooms have a balcony and a sea view. The home's activities coordinator arranges daily activities for the residents such as quizzes and bingo and there are also outings around the local area. The home also organises a nondenominational religious service once a month.

Registered places: 45
Guide weekly rate: £550–£750
Specialist care: Nursing
Medical services: None
Qualified staff: Fails standard: 30% at NVQ level 2

Home details

Location: Village location, 5 miles from Haywards Heath
Communal areas: Lounge, dining room, garden
Accessibility: *Floors:* 2 • *Access:* Lift • *Wheelchair access:* Good
Smoking: ✗
Pets: ✓
Routines: Flexible

Room details

Single: 42
Shared: 2
En suite: 44
Facilities: TV point, telephone point

Door lock: ✗
Lockable place: ✓

Services provided

Beauty services: Hairdressing
Mobile library: ✓
Religious services: Monthly church service
Transport: ✓
Activities: *Coordinator:* ✓ • *Examples:* Bingo, flower arranging, music • *Outings:* ✓
Meetings: ✓

Russettings

Manager: Julie Jones
Owner: Alpha Health Care Ltd
Contact: Mill Lane, Balcombe, West Sussex RH17 6NP
) 01444 811630

Russettings is located in Balcombe village, within walking distance of local amenities. The village is situated between Haywards Heath and Crawley. The home has its own minibus which is very convenient for outings with the residents which means shopping trips can be as regular as twice a week. Often there are outings to other parts of West Sussex such as the seaside, Bluebell woods or other points of interest. Pets are welcome to visit residents, and can even be resident as long as the resident is capable of caring for it.

Sailaway

Manager: Rajendra Kumar
Owner: Rajendra and Nisha Kumar
Contact: Main Road, Bosham, Chichester, West Sussex PO18 8PH

) 01243 572556

Sailaway is a privately owned care home set back from a main road near the village of Bosham and approximately 20 minutes' walk from the nearest shop. It is a detached house which has been extended. Residents are able to participate in communal activities such as exercise and music sessions. Although the home has generally good wheelchair access, it does not have a lift so residents on the second floor must be able to manage the stairs. The home arranges religious services for the residents as well as the facilities of a mobile library.

Registered places: 18
Guide weekly rate: £425
Specialist care: Day care, respite
Medical services: Podiatry, optician
Qualified staff: Undisclosed

Home details
Location: Village location, 4 miles from Chichester
Communal areas: Lounge, dining room, patio and garden
Accessibility: *Floors:* 2 • *Access:* Lift • *Wheelchair access:* Limited
Smoking: x
Pets: At manager's discretion
Routines: Flexible

Room details
Single: 14
Shared: 2
En suite: 2
Facilities: TV point, telephone point

Door lock: ✓
Lockable place: ✓

Services provided
Beauty services: Hairdressing
Mobile library: ✓
Religious services: ✓
Transport: x
Activities: *Coordinator:* x • *Examples:* Exercise, music sessions, t'ai chi • *Outings:* x
Meetings: x

Sandmartins

Manager: Pauline Pink
Owner: Saffronland Homes
Contact: Kings Parade, Aldwick, Bognor Regis, West Sussex PO21 2QY

) 01243 864031
☝ www.homebeechltd.co.uk

Sandmartins is a large, detached building in a quiet area overlooking a park. The home lies one mile from Bognor Regis. The home organises a range of activities and outings for the residents. They hold residents' family meetings such as wine and cheese evenings and fêtes in the summer. There are also quiz nights and strawberry tea evenings for residents to enjoy. The home also has a monthly newsletter which is posted in the hall and in residents' bedrooms.

Registered places: 14
Guide weekly rate: £350–£500
Specialist care: Respite
Medical services: Podiatry, hygienist, optician, physiotherapy
Qualified staff: Meets standard

Home details
Location: Residential area, 1 mile from Bognor Regis
Communal areas: Lounge, dining room, garden
Accessibility: *Floors:* 2 • *Access:* Lift • *Wheelchair access:* Good
Smoking: x
Pets: At manager's discretion
Routines: Flexible

Room details
Single: 14
Shared: 0
En suite: 8
Facilities: TV point

Door lock: ✓
Lockable place: ✓

Services provided
Beauty services: Hairdressing
Mobile library: ✓
Religious services: Anglican visits
Transport: x
Activities: *Coordinator:* ✓ • *Examples:* Armchair exercise, bingo, music for health • *Outings:* ✓
Meetings: ✓

Registered places: 19
Guide weekly rate: £355–£425
Specialist care: None
Medical services: Podiatry, optician, physiotherapy
Qualified staff: Undisclosed

Home details

Location: Residential area, 0.5 miles from Bognor Regis
Communal areas: Lounge/dining room, lounge, conservatory, garden
Accessibility: *Floors:* 2 • *Access:* Stair lift
　Wheelchair access: Limited
Smoking: ✗
Pets: ✓
Routines: Flexible

Room details

Single: 19
Shared: 0
En suite: 4
Facilities: TV point, telephone point

Door lock: ✗
Lockable place: ✓

Services provided

Beauty services: Hairdressing, massage
Mobile library: ✗
Religious services: Weekly Catholic visits,
　Anglican visits every 3 months
Transport: ✗
Activities: *Coordinator:* ✗ • *Examples:* Bingo, movement
　to music, painting • *Outings:* ✗
Meetings: ✗

Saxby Lodge

Manager: Eileen McCarron
Owner: Eileen and Timothy McCarron
Contact: 124 Victoria Drive, Bognor
Regis, West Sussex PO21 2EJ
☏ 01243 828615
@ timgmaccarron@aol.com

Saxby Lodge is set in its own grounds, a mile from the seafront, and half a mile from local shops and services. There is a lounge and dining area on the ground floor and a conservatory and a lounge on the first floor looking out over the grounds. The home has no lift just a stair lift so wheelchair access is only on the first floor. Activities are organised for the residents, such as fortnightly music to movement sessions and a visiting entertainer each month.

Registered places: 25
Guide weekly rate: £575–£625
Specialist care: Respite
Medical services: Podiatry, dentist, optician, physiotherapy
Qualified staff: Exceeds standard: 60% at NVQ level 2

Home details

Location: Residential area, 4 miles from Worthing
Communal areas: Lounge, dining room, conservatory, garden
Accessibility: *Floors:* 2 • *Access:* Lift • *Wheelchair access:* Good
Smoking: ✗
Pets: At manager's discretion
Routines: Flexible

Room details

Single: 23
Shared: 1
En suite: 16
Facilities: TV point, telephone point

Door lock: ✓
Lockable place: ✓

Services provided

Beauty services: Hairdressing
Mobile library: ✓
Religious services: ✗
Transport: Car
Activities: *Coordinator:* ✗ • *Examples:* Bingo, exercises, shows
　Outings: ✓
Meetings: ✗

Scotch Dyke

Manager: Sharon Timmins
Owner: Westermain Ltd
Contact: 38 Beehive Lane, Ferring,
Worthing, West Sussex BN12 5NR
☏ 01903 242061

Scotch Dyke is a two-storey, detached house in Ferring, a village near Worthing It is situated half a mile from the seafront with a railway station less than a mile away. The home offers a range of activities including exercises and shows. There are also outings such as afternoon teas. The home has a conservatory for residents to relax in and a mobile library comes to the home.

The Shelley

Manager: Marlene Yvonne Sanders
Owner: The Shelley Ltd
Contact: 54 Shelley Road, Worthing,
West Sussex BN11 4BX
) 01903 237000
@ info@theshelley.com
✆ www.theshelley.com

The Shelley is situated in a residential area of Worthing close to the beachfront. There are good transport links into the town centre and shops within a few hundred yards. Each resident is allocated a carer who will offer as much or as little help as you need. The home offers a variety of activities including pottery, craft workshops and exercise classes. There are also outings such as shopping trips or recently trips to, a hotel for lunch and coffee mornings. The home has a library with an electric reader in it and there is a piano in the lounge.

Registered places: 32
Guide weekly rate: Undisclosed
Specialist care: Respite
Medical services: Podiatry, dentist, optician, physiotherapy
Qualified staff: Exceeds standard: 90% at NVQ level 2

Home details

Location: Residential area, 0.5 miles from Worthing
Communal areas: Lounge, dining room, library, IT room, hairdressing salon, garden
Accessibility: *Floors:* 2 • *Access:* Lift • *Wheelchair access:* Good
Smoking: In designated area
Pets: At manager's discretion
Routines: Flexible

Room details

Single: 32
Shared: 0
En suite: 32
Facilities: TV point, telephone point

Door lock: ✓
Lockable place: ✓

Services provided

Beauty services: Hairdressing, manicures
Mobile library: ✓
Religious services: Monthly nondenominational service
Transport: ✗
Activities: *Coordinator:* ✓ • *Examples:* Musical concerts, scrabble, t'ai chi • *Outings:* ✓
Meetings: ✓

St Clare

Manager: Christopher Thrower
Owner: Mr and Mrs Thrower
Contact: 14 Park Lane, Southwick, West Sussex BN42 4DL
) 01273 591695

St Clare is located five miles from Brighton town centre. The home has several communal areas and an easily accessible, well-maintained garden. Breakfast is normally served in residents' rooms while lunch and supper are more social occasions. The home has an activities coordinator who arranges regular activities such as arts and crafts, music to movement and classic board games. Outings are also frequently organised with shopping trips and visits to garden centres. Residents meetings take place as and when they are needed or residents request them.

Registered places: 18
Guide weekly rate: £390–£420
Specialist care: Day care, respite
Medical services: Podiatry, dentist, optician, physiotherapy
Qualified staff: Meets standard

Home details

Location: Residential area, 5 miles from Brighton
Communal areas: Lounge, dining room, library, garden
Accessibility: *Floors:* 3 • *Access:* Lift • *Wheelchair access:* Good
Smoking: ✗
Pets: ✗
Routines: Flexible

Room details

Single: 14
Shared: 2
En suite: 1
Facilities: TV, telephone point

Door lock: ✓
Lockable place: ✓

Services provided

Beauty services: Hairdressing
Mobile library: ✓
Religious services: Monthly Anglican service
Transport: ✗
Activities: *Coordinator:* ✓ • *Examples:* Arts and crafts, music and movement, quizzes • *Outings:* ✓
Meetings: ✓

Registered places: 26
Guide weekly rate: £380–£450
Specialist care: Respite
Medical services: Podiatry, hygienist, optician, physiotherapy
Qualified staff: Fails standard: 45% at NVQ level 2

Home details

Location: Residential area, 1 mile from Worthing
Communal areas: Lounge, dining room, garden
Accessibility: *Floors:* 2 • *Access:* Lift • *Wheelchair access:* Good
Smoking: ✗
Pets: ✓
Routines: Flexible

Room details

Single: 26
Shared: 0
En suite: 22
Facilities: TV, telephone point

Door lock: ✓
Lockable place: ✓

Services provided

Beauty services: Hairdressing
Mobile library: ✓
Religious services: Weekly Catholic Communion service
Transport: ✗
Activities: *Coordinator:* ✓ • *Examples:* Arts and crafts, music, skittles, exercise video • *Outings:* ✓
Meetings: ✓

St George's Lodge

Manager: Linda Young
Owner: Bushby Care Ltd
Contact: 46 Chesswood Road, Worthing, West Sussex BN11 2AG
) 01903 820633
⌂ www.stgeorgeslodge.com

St George's Lodge is a detached building in East Worthing and is relatively close to the sea and local parks. It has large gardens, which are being improved with the input of residents' suggestions. The home has a fish tank, a resident cat and two visiting dogs. The home goes on frequent outings, including shopping, trips to a local school for a music afternoon in the summer and a pre-Christmas music event. Entertainers also frequent the home. Residents meetings take place every four to six weeks.

Registered places: 24
Guide weekly rate: £525–£575
Specialist care: Nursing
Medical services: Podiatry, dentist, optician, physiotherapy
Qualified staff: Meets standard

Home details

Location: Residential area, 0.5 miles from Littlehampton
Communal areas: Lounge, dining room, garden
Accessibility: *Floors:* 2 • *Access:* Lift
Wheelchair access: Good
Smoking: ✗
Pets: ✗
Routines: Flexible

Room details

Single: 24
Shared: 0
En suite: 4
Facilities: TV point, telephone point

Door lock: ✓
Lockable place: ✓

Services provided

Beauty services: Hairdressing
Mobile library: ✓
Religious services: Daily Catholic service
Transport: Minibus and car
Activities: *Coordinator:* ✗ • *Examples:* Music and movement, quizzes • *Outings:* ✓
Meetings: ✗

St Joseph's Nursing Home

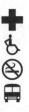

Manager: Angela Baughen
Owner: Franciscan Missionary Sisters of Littlehampton
Contact: East Street, Littlehampton, West Sussex BN17 6AU
) 01903 721053
⌂ www.franciscan.co.uk

St Joseph's Nursing Home is located in a residential area of Little hampton. The home has charitable status and therefore any extra services must be paid by the resident such as hairdressing. Pets are allowed to visit with family and friends but are not accepted to stay in the home. The home regularly goes on outings, for example, to see the Carpet of Flowers at Arundel. Residents are invited to join the sisters in prayer every day if desired.

Stanbridge House

Manager: Kim Sanders
Owner: Kim Sanders
Contact: 54–58 Kings Road, Lancing, West Sussex BN15 8DY

☎ 01903 753059
@ care@stanbridgehouse.com

Located in a quiet residential area, Stanbridge House is an extended property that is located approximately one mile from the sea and one mile from Lancing high street. The home has its own activities coordinator and the programme includes bingo, musical entertainment every fortnight and a quiz every afternoon. The home also takes residents on a drive through the local countryside for an hour and a half every week. On their return the residents are treated with fish and chips for lunch. The home allows pets and smoking is permitted outside. The residents have meetings once a month.

Registered places: 27
Guide weekly rate: Undisclosed
Specialist care: None
Medical services: Podiatry, dentist, optician
Qualified staff: Meets standard

Home details
Location: Residential area, 1 mile from Lancing
Communal areas: Lounge, 2 dining rooms, patio and 3 gardens
Accessibility: *Floors:* 2 • *Access:* Lift
 Wheelchair access: Limited
Smoking: ✗
Pets: ✗
Routines: Flexible

Room details
Single: 27
Shared: 0
En suite: 9
Facilities: TV point, telephone point

Door lock: ✗
Lockable place: ✓

Services provided
Beauty services: Hairdressing, manicures
Mobile library: ✓
Religious services: ✓
Transport: ✓
Activities: *Coordinator:* ✓ • *Examples:* Bingo, music, quizzes
 Outings: ✓
Meetings: ✓

Summerlands

Manager: Vacant
Owner: Paul and Annie Johnson
Contact: Summerhill Lane, Haywards Heath, West Sussex RH16 1RW

☎ 01444 459836
@ info@summerlandscarehome.co.uk
🖰 www.summerlandscarehome.co.uk

Sited in a residential area around one and a half miles from the centre of Haywards Heath, Summerlands is a large detached house within easy reach of local amenities and facilities. The home has sheltered gardens which consist of lawns, flowerbeds and a patio area that can be accessed from the main lounge. Residents are given the opportunity to take part in a weekly programme of activities arranged at the home, such as bingo, quizzes and art sessions. Religious services are also provided twice a month for residents.

Registered places: 31
Guide weekly rate: £585
Specialist care: Day care, respite
Medical services: Podiatry, optician, physiotherapy
Qualified staff: Fails standard: 30% at NVQ level 2

Home details
Location: Residential area, 1.3 miles from Hayward Seas
Communal areas: 2 lounges, dining room, patio and garden
Accessibility: *Floors:* 3 • *Access:* Lift • *Wheelchair access:* Limited
Smoking: ✗
Pets: ✓
Routines: Structured

Room details
Single: 29
Shared: 1
En suite: 30
Facilities: TV point, telephone point

Door lock: ✓
Lockable place: ✓

Services provided
Beauty services: Hairdressing
Mobile Library: ✓
Religious services: ✓
Transport: ✗
Activities: *Coordinator:* ✗ • *Examples:* Art sessions, bingo, quizzes • *Outings:* ✗
Meetings: ✓

Registered places: 40
Guide weekly rate: £400–£550
Specialist care: Nursing
Medical services: Podiatry, hygienist, optician
Qualified staff: Meets standard

Home details
Location: Residential area, 0.5 miles from Worthing
Communal areas: 2 lounges, dining room, garden
Accessibility: *Floors:* 2 • *Access:* Lift • *Wheelchair access:* Good
Smoking: In designated area
Pets: ✗
Routines: Flexible

Room details
Single: 22 | Door lock: ✓
Shared: 7 | Lockable place: ✓
En suite: 5
Facilities: TV point, telephone point

Services provided
Beauty services: Hairdressing
Mobile library: ✓
Religious services: Anglican visits
Transport: Minibus
Activities: *Coordinator:* ✗ • *Examples:* Music for health,
visiting musicians • *Outings:* ✗
Meetings: ✗

Sussex Clinic

Manager: E Baird
Owner: Sussex Clinic Ltd
Contact: 44–48 Shelley Road, Worthing,
West Sussex BN11 4BX
☎ 01903 239822

Sussex Clinic is a detached, two-storey building that was previously. Registered as a private hospital. The majority of the residents of the home are very frail and of a great age and require serious nursing care. Consequently, there are minimal organised activities. The staff aim to create a comfortable environment for the residents. There are visits from Anglican clergy and Communion is available. The home also has visits from a mobile library.

Registered places: 77
Guide weekly rate: £525–£750
Specialist care: Nursing, dementia, physically disabled, respite
Medical services: Podiatry, dentist, optician
Qualified staff: Meets standard

Home details
Location: Village location, 5 miles from Pulborough
Communal areas: Lounge, dining room, activities room, bar,
chapel, garden
Accessibility: *Floors:* 2 • *Access:* Lift • *Wheelchair access:* Good
Smoking: ✗
Pets: ✗
Routines: Flexible

Room details
Singlo: 75 | Door lock: ✓
Shared: 1 | Lockable place: ✓
En suite: 25
Facilities: TV

Services provided
Beauty services: Hairdressing
Mobile library: ✓
Religious services: Weekly Communion service
Transport: ✓
Activities: *Coordinator:* ✓ • *Examples:* Games, musical
entertainment • *Outings:* ✓
Meetings: ✓

Sussexdown

Manager: Laura Bale
Owner: Care South
Contact: Washington Road, Storrington,
Pulborough, West Sussex RH20 4DA
☎ 01903 744221
@ sussexdown@care-south.co.uk
🖱 www.care-south.co.uk

Sussexdown is situated in the village of Storrington, approximately five miles from Pulborough. The home has ample communal space with a lounge, a dining room, a bar and an activities room. There is also a chapel where a Communion service is held on a weekly basis. The home employs an activities coordinator who arranges games and musical entertainment for the residents. There are also regular outings arranged.

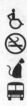

Sussex Grange

Manager: T Jameson
Owner: Sussex Grange
Contact: 14 Vincent Road, Selsey, Chichester, West Sussex PO20 9DH
☎ 01243 606262
🖰 www.sussexgrange.co.uk

Sussex Grange is a detached, two-storey building near Selsey village. As well as gardens, the outdoor area includes a paved area and a shaded area with a large pond. The home offers a range of activities including exercises and board games such as scrabble. Outings are arranged frequently, with trips to garden centres, the pub for lunches, the beach during fine weather and Arundel Wildlife Park. There is a resident budgie at the home and pets are allowed at manager's discretion. There are meetings four times a year for residents to voice any concerns. The home is also located near the seafront.

Registered places: 24
Guide weekly rate: £410–£500
Specialist care: Respite
Medical services: Podiatry, dentist, optician, physiotherapy
Qualified staff: Fails standard: 40% at NVQ level 2

Home details
Location: Residential area, 9 miles from Chichester
Communal areas: Lounge, dining room, garden
Accessibility: *Floors:* 2 • *Access:* Lift • *Wheelchair access:* Good
Smoking: ✗
Pets: At manager's discretion
Routines: Flexible

Room details
Single: 16
Shared: 4
En suite: 20
Facilities: TV point, telephone point

Door lock: ✓
Lockable place: ✓

Services provided
Beauty services: Hairdressing
Mobile library: Library facilities
Religious services: Monthly Anglican Communion service
Transport: Minibus
Activities: *Coordinator:* ✓ • *Examples:* Exercise class, games, music for health • *Outings:* ✓
Meetings: ✓

The Thatched House

Manager: Brigette Gosling
Owner: The Thatched House Residential Care Home Ltd
Contact: 32 Aldwick Avenue, Bognor Regis, West Sussex PO21 3AQ
☎ 01243 867921
@ info@thethatchedhouse.com
🖰 www.thethatchedhouse.com

The Thatched House is a detached, thatched, property with large gardens and is located on a private road close to the local beach. The staff aim to create a homely and exciting atmosphere for residents, this includes arranging a variety of activities. These include manicures, movie afternoons, dancing and frequent visiting musical entertainers. The home also arranges a Communion service every six weeks.

Registered places: 18
Guide weekly rate: £350–£600
Specialist care: Dementia, respite
Medical services: Podiatry, hygienist, optician, physiotherapy
Qualified staff: Meets standard

Home details
Location: Residential area, 1.5 miles from Bognor Regis
Communal areas: Lounge, dining room, garden
Accessibility: *Floors:* 2 • *Access:* Lift
Wheelchair access: Limited
Smoking: ✗
Pets: ✓
Routines: Flexible

Room details
Single: 12
Shared: 3
En suite: 5
Facilities: TV point, telephone point

Door lock: ✓
Lockable place: ✓

Services provided
Beauty services: Hairdressing, manicures
Mobile library: ✓
Religious services: Communion service every 6 weeks
Transport: ✗
Activities: *Coordinator:* ✗ • *Examples:* Armchair exercises, musical entertainers, reminiscence therapy • *Outings:* ✓
Meetings: ✗

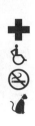

Registered places: 48
Guide weekly rate: £750–£800
Specialist care: Nursing, dementia, physical disability, respite
Medical services: Podiatry, dentist, optician, physiotherapy
Qualified staff: Fails standard: 33% at NVQ level 2

Home details

Location: Residential area, 0.5 miles from Henfield
Communal areas: 4 lounges, 2 dining rooms, library,
    quiet room, patio and garden
Accessibility: *Floors:* 2 • *Access:* Lift • *Wheelchair access:* Good
Smoking: ✗
Pets: ✓
Routines: Flexible

Room details

Single: 47
Shared: 1
En suite: 38
Facilities: TV point, telephone point

Door lock: ✓
Lockable place: ✓

Services provided

Beauty services: Hairdressing
Mobile library: Library facilities
Religious services: Weekly nondenominational service
Transport: ✗
Activities: *Coordinator:* ✓ • *Examples:* Quizzes, board games,
    parties for special occasions • *Outings:* ✓
Meetings: ✓

Upper Mead

Manager: Elizabeth Krandie
Owner: Shafik Sachedina and
Shiraz Boghani
Contact: Fabians Way, Henfield,
West Sussex BN5 9PX
☎ 01273 492870
@ uppermead@sussexhealthcare.org
🖱 www.sussexhealthcare.org

Upper Mead is a large detached property located in the West Sussex village of Henfield. It has pleasant accessible grounds and a patio. There are four lounges, two dining rooms, a library and quiet room. The home arranges for a hairdresser to visit and there are nondenominational religious services every week. Pets are allowed although smoking is not. There is a resident tenants association which meets every six months.

Registered places: 15
Guide weekly rate: £400–£420
Specialist care: None
Medical services: Podiatry, doctor optician, physiotherapy
Qualified staff: Meets standard

Home details

Location: Village location, 2 miles from Steyning
Communal areas: Lounge, dining room, study area,
    patio and garden
Accessibility: *Floors:* 1 • *Wheelchair access:* Good
Smoking: ✗
Pets: ✓
Routines: Flexible

Room details

Single: 13
Shared: 1
En suite: 13
Facilities: TV point, telephone point

Door lock: ✓
Lockable place: ✓

Services provided

Beauty services: Hairdressing, aromatherapy
Mobile library: ✗
Religious services: Anglican and Catholic visits
Transport: ✗
Activities: *Coordinator:* ✓ • *Examples:* Film shows,
    games, artwork • *Outings:* ✓
Meetings: ✓

Valerie Manor

Manager: Maureen Tiller
Owner: Mr and Mrs Tiller
Contact: Henfield Road, Upper Beeding,
West Sussex BN44 3TF
☎ 01903 812105

Valerie Manor is a 400-year-old manor house that has been skilfully converted for use as a care home. The history of the home is extensive, it was used by King Charles II, then as a hospital during the war and finally as a gentlemans' club. As well as a large garden, it is set in four acres of grounds. It is close to the village of Bramber which has shops and a bus service to Steyning, Shoreham and Worthing. There is also a bar on site. The home has its own dog and other pets are welcome.

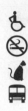

The Victoria Grand

Manager: Julie Courtnadge
Owner: Victoria Care Elite Ltd
Contact: 22 Mill Road, Worthing, West Sussex BN11 4LF
☏ 01903 248048

The Victoria Grand home is a detached Victorian building set in its own grounds and is one of several homes owned by Victoria Care Elite Ltd. The main lounge overlooks the gardens and a large fishpond. In the garden there is a special area for residents who enjoy gardening, including a greenhouse. Meals are freshly prepared using local produce, as well as creating specific meals for those with diabetes and any residents with specific dietary requirements. There are resident meetings every two months or when required. Religious services can be offered on request. The home is also located near the seafront.

Registered places: 26
Guide weekly rate: £450–£650
Specialist care: Day care, respite
Medical services: Podiatry, dentist, optician, physiotherapy
Qualified staff: Meets standard

Home details
Location: Residential area, 1mile from Worthing
Communal areas: 2 lounges, dining room, garden
Accessibility: *Floors:* 3 • *Access:* Lift • *Wheelchair access:* Good
Smoking: ✗
Pets: At manager's discretion
Routines: Flexible

Room details
Single: 20
Shared: 3
En suite: 11
Facilities: TV point, telephone point

Door lock: ✓
Lockable place: ✓

Services provided
Beauty services: Hairdressing
Mobile library: ✓
Religious services: ✓
Transport: Minibus
Activities: *Coordinator:* ✓ • *Examples:* Arts and crafts, bingo, quizzes • *Outings:* ✓
Meetings: ✓

The Victoria Lodge

Manager: Elaine Walker
Owner: Victoria Care Elite Ltd
Contact: 48–50 Shakespeare Road, Worthing, West Sussex BN11 4AS
☏ 01903 203049

The Victoria Lodge is one of several homes in the Worthing area owned by Victoria Care Elite Ltd. The home is not suitable for wheelchair users and is best suited to frail, but active clients. Organised outings occur very frequently. The garden of the home is small, but attractive. There is a residents meeting every three months. The home also arranges for a Catholic and Anglican Communion service to take place once a fortnight.

Registered places: 23
Guide weekly rate: £225–£450
Specialist care: Day care, respite
Medical services: Podiatry, dentist, optician
Qualified staff: Exceeds standard: 65% at NVQ level 2

Home details
Location: Residential area, 1 mile from Worthing
Communal areas: lounge, dining room, conservatory, library, patio and garden
Accessibility: *Floors:* 3 • *Access:* Lift • *Wheelchair access:* None
Smoking: In designated area
Pets: At manager's discretion
Routines: Flexible

Room details
Single: 23
Shared: 0
En suite: 12
Facilities: TV point, telephone point

Door lock: ✓
Lockable place: ✓

Services provided
Beauty services: Hairdressing
Mobile library: ✗
Religious services: Fortnightly Catholic and Anglican Communion service
Transport: Minibus
Activities: *Coordinator:* ✓ • *Examples:* Arts and crafts, music and movement, quizzes • *Outings:* ✓
Meetings: ✓

Registered places: 20
Guide weekly rate: £360–£650
Specialist care: Dementia, day care, respite
Medical services: Podiatry, dentist, optician, physiotherapy
Qualified staff: Meets standard

Home details

Location: Residential area, 1.2 miles from Worthing
Communal areas: Lounge, dining room, garden
Accessibility: *Floors:* 3 • *Access:* Lift • *Wheelchair access:* Good
Smoking: ✗
Pets: ✓
Routines: Flexible

Room details

Single: 17
Shared: 2
En suite: 19
Facilities: TV point, telephone point

Door lock: ✗
Lockable place: ✓

Services provided

Beauty services: Hairdressing
Mobile library: ✓
Religious services: ✓
Transport: ✓
Activities: *Coordinator:* ✗ • *Examples:* Bingo, tea parties, scrabble
　　• *Outings:* ✓
Meetings: ✓

The Victoria Mill

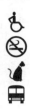

Manager: Denise Slaughter
Owner: Victoria Care Elite Ltd
Contact: 32 Mill Road, Worthing, West Sussex BN11 5DR
☏ 01903 249252

The Victoria Mill is situated just over a mile from Worthing. The home is set over three floors and access is provided via a lift to the first floor and up a flight of stairs to the second floor, therefore only those who are mobile stay on the top floor. Every fortnight, there is a minibus trip organised using the home's own transport to a number of places including the seafront and the garden centre. Along with this there are daily activities at the home such as bingo, tea parties and scrabble. The home can provide accommodation for relatives.

Registered places: 20
Guide weekly rate: £325–£650
Specialist care: Respite
Medical services: Podiatry, optician, physiotherapy
Qualified staff: Exceeds standard: 85% at NVQ level 2

Home details

Location: Residential area, 1.5 miles from Worthing
Communal areas: Lounge, dining room, quiet reading room, patio and garden
Accessibility: *Floors:* 3 • *Access:* Lift • *Wheelchair access:* Limited
Smoking: ✗
Pets: ✓
Routines: Flexible

Room details

Single: 20
Shared: 0
En suite: 13
Facilities: TV point, telephone point

Door lock: ✓
Lockable place: ✓

Services provided

Beauty services: Hairdressing
Mobile library: ✓
Religious services: ✗
Transport: Shared minibus
Activities: *Coordinator:* ✓ • *Examples:* cards, games, quizzes
　　Outings: ✓
Meetings: ✓

The Victoria Royal Beach

Manager: Coral Jackson
Owner: Victoria Care Elite Ltd
Contact: 12 Grand Avenue, Worthing, West Sussex BN11 5AW
☏ 01903 246499

The Victoria Royal Beach is one of several care homes owned by Victoria Care Elite Ltd. There is a company minibus for the home to use on its outings which take place every other week. There are many activities offered for residents including musical evenings. Pets are welcome at the home and there is already a resident cat. The home arranges regular meetings to allow residents to discuss any issues they may have.

The Victoria Parkview

Manager: Sheelagh Macey
Owner: Victoria Care Elite Ltd
Contact: 7 Madeira Avenue, Worthing, West Sussex BN11 2AT
☎ 01903 522022
@ victoriacare@freenet.co.uk
🖰 www.victoriacare.com

The Victoria Parkview is a detached two-storey property in the centre of Worthing, close to local shops, a park and the seafront. The home is a small property, with facilities for nine residents, giving the home a personalised service. There is a mobile library which visits and religious services are available. There is a company minibus which takes residents on an outing every fortnight. The home has an activities programme including activities such as arts and crafts and quizzes. There are regular residents meetings.

Registered places: 9
Guide weekly rate: Undisclosed
Specialist care: None
Medical services: Podiatry, dentist, optician
Qualified staff: Meets standard

Home details
Location: Urban area, 0.5 miles from Worthing
Communal areas: Lounge, dining room, patio and garden
Accessibility: *Floors:* 2 • *Access:* Lift • *Wheelchair access:* Good
Smoking: ✗
Pets: ✓
Routines: Flexible

Room details
Single: 9   **Door lock:** ✓
Shared: 0   **Lockable place:** ✓
En suite: 1
Facilities: TV, telephone

Services provided
Beauty services: Hairdressing, manicures
Mobile library: ✓
Religious services: ✓
Transport: Shared minibus
Activities: *Coordinator:* ✗ • *Examples:* quizzes, arts and crafts *Outings:* ✓
Meetings: ✓

Walstead Place

Manager: Jane Large
Owner: Caring Homes Ltd
Contact: Lewes Road, Walstead, Lindfield, West Sussex RH16 2QG
☎ 01444 483885
@ walstead@caringhomes.org
🖰 www.caringhomes.org

Walstead House dates back to 1852 and is in a pleasant rural setting, surrounded by its two and a half acres of land. The home employs a qualified chef and meals can be served with wine, and sherry is offered before a full Sunday Lunch. The home is within a mile of Lindfield village where there is a bank, shops and pubs. The home arranges religious services for the residents and shares a minibus with another home.

Registered places: 54
Guide weekly rate: £585–£650
Specialist care: Respite
Medical services: Podiatry, dentist, optician, physiotherapy
Qualified staff: Meets standard

Home details
Location: Rural area, 2.5 miles from Haywards Heath
Communal areas: Lounge, dining room, conservatory, patio and garden
Accessibility: *Floors:* 3 • *Access:* Lift • *Wheelchair access:* Good
Smoking: ✗
Pets: At manager's discretion
Routines: Flexible

Room details
Single: 40   **Door lock:** ✓
Shared: 7   **Lockable place:** ✓
En suite: 34
Facilities: TV point, telephone point

Services provided
Beauty services: Hairdressing
Mobile library: ✗
Religious services: Monthly Anglican Communion service
Transport: Shared minibus
Activities: *Coordinator:* ✓ • *Examples:* Crossword group, film night, poetry club • *Outings:* ✓
Meetings: ✓

Registered places: 13
Guide weekly rate: £480
Specialist care: Respite
Medical services: Podiatry, dentist, optician
Qualified staff: Fails standard: 45% at NVQ level 2

Home details
Location: Village location, 5 miles from Horsham
Communal areas: Lounge, dining room, patio and garden
Accessibility: *Floors:* 2 • *Access:* Lift • *Wheelchair access:* Good
Smoking: ✗
Pets: ✓
Routines: Structured

Room details
Single: 13
Shared: 0
En suite: 13
Facilities: TV point, telephone point

Door lock: ✗
Lockable place: ✗

Services provided
Beauty services: Hairdressing, aromatherapy
Mobile library: ✗
Religious services: Monthly
Transport: ✓
Activities: *Coordinator:* ✓ • *Examples:* Art classes, bingo, quizzes
   Outings: ✗
Meetings: ✓

Wayside
Manager: Carol Collins
Owner: Hope Keith Villagers Trust
Contact: High Street, Rusper, Horsham, West Sussex RH12 4PX
❯ 01293 871365
@ wayside@rusperwestsussex.freeserve.co.uk

Situated in the village of Rusper, five miles from Horsham, Wayside is located close to a local shop and church. Facing out onto the village high street, the home benefits from large grounds at the rear of the property. Promoting independence for its residents, individuals in the home are expected to make their own breakfast and have facilities in their room to enable them to do so. During the warmer months, residents enjoy undertaking small tasks in the garden. The home has two activities coordinators and there is a residents meeting twice a month.

Registered places: 42
Guide weekly rate: £600–£800
Specialist care: Nursing
Medical services: Podiatry
Qualified staff: Fails standard

Home details
Location: Village location, 2.5 miles from Horsham
Communal areas: 3 lounges, dining room, conservatory
Accessibility: *Floors:* 2 • *Access:* Lift • *Wheelchair access:* Good
Smoking: ✗
Pets: ✓
Routines: Flexible

Room details
Single: 30
Shared: 6
En suite: 32
Facilities: TV

Door lock: ✓
Lockable place: ✓

Services provided
Beauty services: Hairdressing
Mobile library: ✗
Religious services: ✗
Transport: ✗
Activities: *Coordinator:* ✓ • *Examples:* Flower arranging, quizzes
   Outings: ✗
Meetings: ✗

Wellcross Grange
Manager: Elizabeth Lawrence
Owner: Balcombe Care Homes Ltd
Contact: Lyons Corner, Five Oaks Road, Slinfold, Horsham, West Sussex RH13 0SY
❯ 01403 790388

Wellcross Grange is a detached house, originally built in the 1920s, set in its own extensive grounds and is located in the village of Slinfold, near Horsham. The home has three lounges and a conservatory for residents to relax in. There is an activities coordinator who arranges a variety of activities to stimulate residents including quizzes and flower arranging.

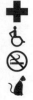

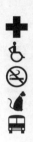

Westergate Care Home

Manager: Sharon McNamara
Owner: Barchester Healthcare Ltd
Contact: Denmans Lane, Fontwell, Arundel, West Sussex BN18 0SU
☎ 01243 544744
@ westergate@barchester.com
🖰 www.barchester.com

Westergate Care Home is a large Grade II listed building situated in a rural area, five miles from Arundel. The home has a garden with an area for residents to participate in gardening. There is an activities coordinator who arranges one-to-one sessions as well as group activities such as games and singing. There are regular religious visits to the home by local clergy and regular relatives meetings.

Registered places: 76
Guide weekly rate: £500–£1,100
Specialist care: Nursing, physically disabled, respite
Medical services: Podiatry, dentist, optician
Qualified staff: Meets standard

Home details
Location: Rural area, 5 miles from Arundel
Communal areas: 2 lounges, dining room, patio and garden
Accessibility: *Floors:* 2 • *Access:* Lift • *Wheelchair access:* Good
Smoking: ✗
Pets: At manager's discretion
Routines: Flexible

Room details
Single: 55
Shared: 19
En suite: 74
Facilities: TV point

Door lock: ✓
Lockable place: ✓

Services provided
Beauty services: Hairdressing
Mobile library: ✓
Religious services: ✓
Transport: Minibus and car
Activities: *Coordinator:* ✓ • *Examples:* Games, one-to-one sessions, singing • *Outings:* ✓
Meetings: ✓

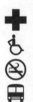

Westhampnett Nursing Home

Manager: Ignatius Gilarty
Owner: Philip and Mary Davis
Contact: Westhampnett Road, Chichester, West Sussex PO18 0NT
☎ 01243 782986

Westhampnett Nursing Home is a two storey listed Georgian building set in extensive gardens. The home has been sympathetically restored to provide nursing care. The gardens are well maintained and in some areas landscaped, making it a pleasant area for residents to enjoy, especially in good weather. The gardens are used regularly in good weather for barbecues and afternoon teas, and often the residents meeting are also held outside. The home has its own transport, and takes residents into the centre of town for shopping once a week.

Registered places: 32
Guide weekly rate: £625–£900
Specialist care: Nursing
Medical services: None
Qualified staff: Fails standard

Home details
Location: Village location, 2.5 miles from Chichester
Communal areas: 2 lounges, dining room, garden
Accessibility: *Floors:* 2 • *Access:* Lift • *Wheelchair access:* Good
Smoking: ✗
Pets: ✗
Routines: Flexible

Room details
Single: 24
Shared: 4
En suite: 18
Facilities: TV point, telephone point

Door lock: ✗
Lockable place: ✓

Services provided
Beauty services: Hairdressing
Mobile library: ✓
Religious services: Monthly
Transport: ✓
Activities: *Coordinator:* ✓ • *Examples:* Gardening, cooking, games • *Outings:* ✓
Meetings: ✓

Registered places: 56
Guide weekly rate: £820–£950
Specialist care: Nursing, respite
Medical services: Podiatry, dentist, optician, physiotherapy
Qualified staff: Meets standard

Home details

Location: Residential area, 2.5 miles from Horsham
Communal areas: Lounges, dining rooms
Accessibility: *Floors:* 2 • *Access:* Lift • *Wheelchair access:* Good
Smoking: ✗
Pets: Undisclosed
Routines: Flexible

Room details

Single: 52
Shared: 2
En suite: 52
Facilities: TV point, telephone

Door lock: Undisclosed
Lockable place: Undisclosed

Services provided

Beauty services: Hairdressing
Mobile library: Undisclosed
Religious services: Undisclosed
Transport: Minibus
Activities: *Coordinator:* ✓ • *Examples:* Games • *Outings:* ✓
Meetings: Undisclosed

Westlake

Manager: Christine van Klaveren
Owner: Barchester Healthcare Ltd
Contact: Pondtail Road, Horsham,
West Sussex RH12 5EZ
☎ 01403 270773
@ westlake@barchester.com
🖥 www.barchester.com

Westlake is located in a residential area, approximately two and a half miles from Horsham. The home has ample communal space for the residents including several lounges and a dining area. The home has its own minibus and often takes the residents on outings in the local area. The home has its own activities coordinator and the residents enjoy a flexible routine.

Registered places: 30
Guide weekly rate: £435–£600
Specialist care: None
Medical services: Dentist, optician
Qualified staff: Meets standard

Home details

Location: Residential area, 4.5 miles from Littlehampton
Communal areas: 2 lounges, dining room, conservatory,
   car park, patio and garden
Accessibility: *Floors:* 2 • *Access:* Lift • *Wheelchair access:* Good
Smoking: ✗
Pets: ✗
Routines: Flexible

Room details

Single: 27
Shared: 2
En suite: 29
Facilities: TV point, telephone point

Door lock: ✓
Lockable place: ✓

Services provided

Beauty services: Hairdressing
Mobile library: ✗
Religious services: ✓
Transport: ✗
Activities: *Coordinator:* ✓ • *Examples:* Bowls, darts,
   themed evenings • *Outings:* ✓
Meetings: ✓

White Lodge

Manager: Lesley Trudgett
Owner: South Coast Nursing Homes Ltd
Contact: South Strand, Angmering-
on-Sea, Littlehampton, West Sussex
BN16 1PN
☎ 01903 784415

White Lodge is a two storey extended, detached house, set in its own grounds approximately 200 yards from the sea and village centre. There is a communal area for television, as well as an area for reading. Residents are also welcome to go out on their own or with family and friends. The home also has a garden for residents to enjoy, and pets are welcome to come and visit. There is a residents meeting every six weeks.

White Waves

Manager: J M Satchell
Owner: Platinex Ltd
Contact: 17–19 Seal Road, Selsey,
Chichester, West Sussex PO20 0HW

) 01243 602379

@ whitewaves@fsmail.net

White Waves is a detached, two-storey building, one mile from Selsey. Residents make use of the Selsey Minibus to attend events in the village. Though no religious services are offered regularly a vicar or priest can visit by arrangement. The home is located near the seafront and there are regular activities arranged for the residents including games and music for health sessions.

Registered places: 19
Guide weekly rate: £460–£650
Specialist care: Day care, respite
Medical services: Podiatry, dentist, optician
Qualified staff: Fails standard: 18% at NVQ level 2

Home details

Location: Residential area, 1 mile from Selsey
Communal areas: Lounge, dining room, patio and garden
Accessibility: *Floors:* 2 • *Access:* Lift • *Wheelchair access:* Good
Smoking: ✗
Pets: At manager's discretion
Routines: Flexible

Room details

Single: 13
Shared: 3
En suite: 15
Facilities: TV point

Door lock: ✓
Lockable place: ✓

Services provided

Beauty services: Hairdressing
Mobile library: ✗
Religious services: ✓
Transport: ✗
Activities: *Coordinator:* ✗ • *Examples:* Music for health, games, music and movement • *Outings:* ✗
Meetings: ✗

Willett Lodge

Manager: Mary-Anne Lester
Owner: Mr and Mrs Simper
Contact: 4 Chaucer Road, Worthing,
West Sussex BN11 4PB

) 01903 235347

@ info@willettlodge.co.uk

🖰 www.willettlodge.co.uk

Willett Lodge is a family run, detached, two-storey house that has been extended. The home is within easy reach of local amenities and the promenade. Varied diets and specific dietary requirements can be catered for and in the summer the home has a barbecue. The home has its own budgerigar and a visiting dog. There are Methodist services once a month and the home arranges a residents meeting twice a month.

Registered places: 20
Guide weekly rate: £325–£550
Specialist care: Respite
Medical services: Podiatry, dentist, optician, physiotherapy
Qualified staff: Exceeds standard: 75% at NVQ level 2

Home details

Location: Residential area, 1 mile from Worthing
Communal areas: Lounge, dining room, conservatory, patio and garden
Accessibility: *Floors:* 2 • *Access:* Lift • *Wheelchair access:* Good
Smoking: ✗
Pets: At manager's discretion
Routines: Flexible

Room details

Single: 18
Shared: 1
En suite: 7
Facilities: TV point

Door lock: ✓
Lockable place: ✓

Services provided

Beauty services: Hairdressing
Mobile library: ✓
Religious services: Monthly Methodist service
Transport: ✗
Activities: *Coordinator:* ✓ • *Examples:* Bingo, quizzes, gentle exercise • *Outings:* ✓
Meetings: ✓

Registered places: 13
Guide weekly rate: £331–£400
Specialist care: Respite
Medical services: Podiatry, dentist, optician, physiotherapy
Qualified staff: Exceeds standard: 71% at NVQ level 2

Home details

Location: Residential area, 1 mile from Worthing
Communal areas: Lounge, dining room, garden
Accessibility: *Floors:* 2 • *Access:* Lift • *Wheelchair access:* Good
Smoking: In designated area
Pets: ✗
Routines: Flexible

Room details

Single: 11
Shared: 1
En suite: 4
Facilities: TV point, telephone point

Door lock: ✓
Lockable place: ✓

Services provided

Beauty services: Hairdressing
Mobile library: ✓
Religious services: Monthly Anglican service
Transport: 7-seater vehicle
Activities: *Coordinator:* ✓ • *Examples:* Musical entertainment, reminiscence • *Outings:* ✓
Meetings: ✗

Windsor Rest Home

Manager: Carol Pembrey
Owner: Mr and Mrs Pembrey
Contact: 52–54 Windsor Road, Worthing, West Sussex BN11 2LY
☏ 01903 235594

Windsor Rest Home is a large property converted from two terrace houses with a paved front area and a secluded rear garden with a summerhouse. The home has access to 250 books for residents to peruse. The home is pet-friendly, with a resident dog. Outings occur regularly to places such as the bluebell railway, Faulkner centre and to the beach for picnics. The home is also near the seafront. There is a monthly Anglican service and the home has its own transport.

Registered places: 29
Guide weekly rate: £325–£470
Specialist care: Respite
Medical services: Podiatry, dentist, optician, physiotherapy
Qualified staff: Meets standard

Home details

Location: Residential area, 1 mile from Bognor Regis
Communal areas: 2 lounges, dining room, conservatory, garden
Accessibility: *Floors:* 2 • *Access:* Lift • *Wheelchair access:* Good
Smoking: In designated area
Pets: At manager's discretion
Routines: Flexible

Room details

Single: 29
Shared: 0
En suite: 29
Facilities: TV point, telephone point

Door lock: ✓
Lockable place: ✓

Services provided

Beauty services: Hairdressing
Mobile library: ✓
Religious services: Catholic and Anglican service every 6 weeks
Transport: ✗
Activities: *Coordinator:* ✓ • *Examples:* Arts and crafts, bingo, music and movement • *Outings:* ✓
Meetings: ✓

Woodbine Manor

Manager: Peta Baldwinson
Owner: Peta Baldwinson
Contact: 25 Upper Bognor Road, Bognor Regis, West Sussex PO21 1JA
☏ 01243 841136

Woodbine Manor is a large, purpose-built, detached property in a quiet residential area on the outskirts of Bognor, approximately 10 minutes' walk from the town centre. The home arranges a lot of different activities for residents to take part in with therapists aiding such as music and movement therapy. The home also goes on outings to local places of interest. The home has residents meeting once every three months.

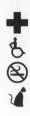

Woodlands Nursing Home

Manager: S Ratnasinkam

Owner: S Ratnasinkam

Contact: 23 Silverdale Road, Burgess Hill, West Sussex RH15 0ED

☏ 01444 243579

Woodlands is a large, Victorian property with extensive well-kept gardens and a patio area to the rear. There is a decking area with tables and chairs at the front of the home. The home has ties with the local community, using Bluebird buses to take residents on trips. The home visits the seafront in the summer and garden centres in the autumn and winter months. There is a summer fête for residents and relatives. Though there are no formal meetings there are occasionally informal ones, where families are welcome.

Registered places: 23

Guide weekly rate: £528–£560

Specialist care: Nursing, respite

Medical services: Podiatry, dentist, optician, physiotherapy

Qualified staff: Exceeds standard: 80% at NVQ level 2

Home details

Location: Residential area, 1 mile from Burgess Hill

Communal areas: Lounge, dining room, patio and garden

Accessibility: *Floors:* 3 • *Access:* Lift • *Wheelchair access:* Good

Smoking: ✗

Pets: At manager's discretion

Routines: Flexible

Room details

Single: 19	**Door lock:** ✗
Shared: 2	**Lockable place:** ✓
En suite: 8	
Facilities: TV point	

Services provided

Beauty services: Hairdressing, massage

Mobile library: ✗

Religious services: Monthly Catholic and Baptist service

Transport: ✗

Activities: *Coordinator:* ✓ • *Examples:* Bingo, music, quizzes
  Outings: ✓

Meetings: ✓

Yew Tree Nursing Home

Manager: Janette McCorquodale

Owner: Yew Tree Care Ltd

Contact: North End Road, Yapton, Arundel, West Sussex BN18 0DU

☏ 01243 552575

@ yewtree@sbdial.co.uk

The home is situated in the village of Yapton, around six miles from Bognor Regis. The home has a 'Friends of Yew Tree' association made up of relatives, ex-relatives and some residents. The home has two activities coordinators who organise activities such as games and weekly music sessions. The home has a basic structure to the day but the routine is open to change and caters to the residents needs. Pets are allowed to visit. The home arranges regular religious visits. The home has a sensory garden and portable telephone residents can use.

Registered places: 40

Guide weekly rate: From £550

Specialist care: Nursing, learning disability, physical disability

Medical services: Podiatry, dentist, optician, physiotherapy

Qualified staff: Exceeds standard

Home details

Location: Village location, 6 miles from Bognor Regis

Communal areas: 2 lounges, lounge/dining room, garden

Accessibility: *Floors:* 2 • *Access:* Lift • *Wheelchair access:* Good

Smoking: ✗

Pets: ✗

Routines: Structured

Room details

Single: 21	**Door lock:** ✗
Shared: 7	**Lockable place:** ✓
En suite: 12	
Facilities: TV	

Services provided

Beauty services: Hairdressing, aromatherapy, manicures

Mobile library: ✗

Religious services: ✓

Transport: ✗

Activities: *Coordinator:* ✓ • *Examples:* Exercise, games, weekly music sessions • *Outings:* ✗

Meetings: ✓

Useful contacts

Action on Elder Abuse (AEA)
- 0808 808 8141
- www.elderabuse.org.uk

Age Concern England
- 0808 808 6060
- www.ace.org.uk

British Red Cross Society
- 020 7235 5454
- www.redcross.org.uk

CareAware
- 0870 513 4925
- www.careaware.co.uk

Counsel and Care
- 0845 300 7585
- @ advice@counselandcare.org.uk
- www.counselandcare.org.uk

CSCI (Commission for Social Care Inspection)
- 0845015 0120/0191 233 3323
- @ enquiries@csci.gsi.gov.uk
- www.csci.org.uk

South-East regional contact team
- 01622 724950
- @ enquiries.southeast@csci.gsi.gov.uk

Elderly Accommodation Counsel (EAC)
- 020 7820 1343
- @ enquiries@e-a-c.demon.co.uk
- www.housingcare.org

Help The Aged
- 020 7278 1114
- www.helptheaged.org.uk

IFA Promotion
- 0800 085 3250
- @ contact@ifap.org.uk
- www.unbiased.co.uk

Local councils
- www.direct.gov.uk

Nursing Homes Fees Agency (NHFA)
- 0800 998 833
- @ enquiries@nhfa.co.uk
- www.hsbcpensions.co.uk

NHS Direct
- 0845 4647
- www.nhsdirect.nhs.uk

The Pension Service
- 0845 6060265
- www.thepensionservice.gov.uk

Relatives & Residents Association
- 020 7359 8136
- @ info@relres.org
- www.relres.org

Seniorline
- 0808 800 6565

University of the Third Age
- 020 8466 6139
- www.u3a.org.uk

Specific care information

Alzheimer's Society
- ☏ 0845 300 0336
- @ info@alzheimers.org.uk
- 🖰 www.alzheimers.org.uk

Provides support, information, advice and local services for those looking after someone with dementia.

Arthritis Care
- ☏ 0808 800 4050
- 🖰 www.arthritiscare.org.uk

Society for people with arthritis, helping to promote their health, well being and independence.

Dementia Information Service for Carers (DISC)
- ☏ 0845 120 4048

Advice and information for carers of older people with dementia.

Diabetes UK
- ☏ 020 7424 1000
- @ info@diabetes.org.uk
- 🖰 www.diabetes.org.uk

Works for people with diabetes, funding research, campaigning and helping people live with the condition.

Hearing Concern
- ☏ 020 7440 9871
- @ info@hearingconcern.org.uk
- 🖰 www.hearingconcern.org.uk

A national charity which provides support, advice and information for the deaf and hard of hearing.

Huntington's Disease Association
- ☏ 020 7223 7000
- 🖰 www.hda.org.uk

Local and regional advisers offer information, support and family visits to those with Huntington's Disease.

MIND (National Association for Mental Health)
- ☏ 0845 766 0163
- @ contact@mind.org.uk
- 🖰 www.mind.org.uk

A mental health charity working for everyone with experience of mental distress.

Parkinson's Disease Society
- ☏ 0845 608 445
- 🖰 www.parkinsons.org.uk

Provides help for people with Parkinson's Disease and their relatives.

The Stroke Association
- ☏ 0845 3033100
- 🖰 www.stroke.org.uk

Provides an advisory and information service for people who have had strokes, their families and carers.